ANNALS OF THE NEW YORK ACADEMY OF SCIENCES

VOLUME 156, ART. 1 PAGES 1–625

January 31, 1969

Editorial Director
PETER D. ALBERTSON

Editor-in-Chief
MARC KRAUSS

Associate Editor
HÉLÈNE RUTH BIELEFELD

EXPERIMENTAL "METABOLIC" CARDIOPATHIES AND THEIR RELATIONSHIP TO HUMAN HEART DISEASES*

Consulting Editor
EÖRS BAJUSZ

Conference Cochairmen
E. BAJUSZ AND F. HOMBURGER

CONTENTS

Foreword. *By* EÖRS BAJUSZ 5

Cardiomyopathy and Myocardial Degeneration: Problems of Terminology in Experimental and Clinical Pathology. *By* WILLIAM B. WARTMAN 7

Part I. Ultrastructure of Heart Muscle under Normal and Pathological Conditions

Microstructure of "Specialized" Tissues in the Mammalian Heart. *By* C. E. CHALLICE 14

Ultrastructure of Heart Muscle under Pathological Conditions. *By* R. POCHE 34

Electron Microscopical Studies on Experimental Ischemic Lesions of the Heart. *By* GERHARD KORB AND VLADIMIR TOTOVIĆ 48

Part II. Cardiopathies and Factors Influencing Myocardial Degeneration

Ischemic Injury of Myocardium. *By* ROBERT B. JENNINGS, HERBERT M. SOMMERS, PETER B. HERDSON, AND JOHN P. KALTENBACH 61

Mechanisms in the Development of Myocardial Lesions in Hemorrhagic Shock. *By* ARTHUR M. MARTIN, JR., DONALD B. HACKEL, MARK L. ENTMAN, M. PAUL CAPP, AND MADISON S. SPACH 79

* This series of papers is the result of a conference entitled Experimental "Metabolic" Cardiopathies and Their Relationship to Human Heart Diseases, held by The New York Academy of Sciences on January 9, 10, and 11, 1967.

Experimental Granulomatous Myocarditis: Genesis and Immunological Aspects. *By* Alexander Laufer and A. Michael Davies 91

Spontaneous, Hereditary Myocardial Degeneration and Congestive Heart Failure in a Strain of Syrian Hamsters. *By* E. Bajusz, J. R. Baker, C. W. Nixon, and F. Homburger 105

The Relationship of Nutrition to Fatty Degeneration of the Myocardium and Kidney. *By* Peter Rasmussen 130

Experimental Infection with *Trypanosoma cruzi* (Chagas' Disease): A Model of Acute and Chronic Myocardiopathy. *By* Walter H. Abelmann 137

Tryptophan Metabolism and Cardiac Disease. *By* Maria Spatz 152

Myofibrillar Degeneration: A Common Form of Cardiac Muscle Injury. *By* Dennis Reichenbach and Earl P. Benditt 164

Experimental Studies on the Healing of Cardiac Necrosis. *By* George Rona and David S. Kahn 177

Myocardial Toxicity of Cobalt in the Rat. *By* H. C. Grice, T. Goodman, I. C. Munro, G. S. Wiberg, and A. B. Morrison 189

Part III. Genesis and Prevention of Cardiopathies: Hormonal, Neural, Neuroendocrine, and Miscellaneous Mechanisms

The Pluricausal Cardiopathies. *By* Hans Selye 195

Studies on the "Nonspecific Mesenchymal Reaction" and the "Transit Zone" in Myocardial Lesions and Atherosclerosis. *By* W. H. Hauss, U. Gerlach, G. Junge-Hülsing, H. Themann, and W. Wirth 207

Regional Distribution of Catecholamines in the Hearts of Various Species. *By* E. T. Angelakos, M. P. King, and R. W. Millard 219

Central Nervous System Stimulation and Cardiac Ischemic Changes in Monkeys. *By* K. I. Melville, H. L. Garvey, H. E. Shister, and J. Knaack 241

Focal Myocytolysis and Fuchsinophilic Degeneration of the Myocardium of Patients Dying with Various Brain Lesions. *By* Richard C. R. Connor 261

Cardiotoxic Effects of Electrical Stimulation of the Stellate Ganglia. *By* Mary A. Klouda and G. Brynjolfsson 271

Pathophysiological Fundamentals of the Origin and Prevention of Degenerative Heart Disease. *By* W. Raab 281

Part IV. Cardiac Pathology Induced by Isoproterenol and Related Amines

Isoproterenol-Induced Cardiac Necrosis. *By* D. S. Kahn, G. Rona, and C. I. Chappel 285

Pharmacological Studies on Heart Muscle Lesions Induced by Isoproterenol. *By* Gerhard Zbinden and Robert A. Moe 294

Histochemical and Electron Microscopical Studies on the Cardiac Necroses Produced by Sympathomimetic Agents. *By* Victor J. Ferrans, Richard G. Hibbs, John J. Walsh, and George E. Burch 309

Factors Influencing the Production of Cardiomyopathies by Methoxamine and Metaraminol. *By* G. Jasmin 333

Tissue Electrolyte Alteration in Disseminated Myocardial Necrosis. *By* David Lehr 344

Part V. Progress in Studies on Cardiac Hypertrophy, Valvular Lesions, and Cardiac Failure

Effects of Heart Failure, Ventricular Hypertrophy, and Alterations in the Thyroid State on the Contractility of Isolated Cardiac Muscle. *By* EUGENE BRAUNWALD, EDMUND H. SONNENBLICK, JAMES F. SPANN, JR., AND ROBERT A. BUCCINO 379

The Interrelation between Myocardial Metabolism and Heart Failure. *By* HANS A. HOCHREIN AND KLAUS LOSSNITZER 387

Dissociation of Factors Influencing Myocardial Degeneration and Generalized Cardiocirculatory Failure. *By* E. BAJUSZ, F. HOMBURGER, J. R. BAKER, AND P. BOGDONOFF 396

Alterations in Water and Electrolyte Distribution in Congestive Heart Failure and Their Significance. By C. T. G. FLEAR 421

Experimental Cardiomegalies and "Cardiomegalies" in Free-Living Animals. *By* O. POUPA AND B. OŠŤÁDAL 445

A Quantitative Study of Myocardial Mitochondria in Experimental Cardiac Hypertrophy. *By* BEN D. MCCALLISTER AND ARNOLD L. BROWN, JR. 469

Interstitial Edema in Valvular Endocarditis. *By* A. ANGRIST, M. OKA, AND K. NAKAO 480

Part VI. Primary Cardiomyopathies and Congestive Heart Failure in Clinical Medicine

The African Cardiomyopathies. *By* J. N. P. DAVIES 498

Lack of Correlation between Coronary Thrombosis and Myocardial Infarction or Sudden "Coronary" Heart Death. *By* GIORGIO BAROLDI 504

A Distinctive Myocardiopathy Occurring in Omaha, Nebraska: Clinical Aspects. *By* JAMES F. SULLIVAN, JOHN D. EGAN, AND RALPH P. GEORGE 526

A Distinctive Myocardiopathy Occurring in Omaha, Nebraska: Pathological Aspects. *By* HENRY T. GRINVALSKY AND DONALD M. FITCH 544

Québec Beer-Drinkers' Cardiomyopathy: Clinical and Hemodynamic Aspects. *By* YVES MORIN, ANDRÉ TÊTU, AND GASTON MERCIER 566

Québec Beer-Drinkers' Myocardosis: Pathological Aspects. *By* JEAN-LOUIS BONENFANT, CARLTON AUGER, GEORGES MILLER, JACQUES CHENARD, AND PAUL-EMILE ROY 577

Molecular Changes in Myocardial Infarction in Heart Muscle. *By* RICHARD J. BING, SIGMUNDUR GUDBJARNASON, HANS TSCHOPP, AND WOLFGANG BRAASCH 583

Etiology of Congestive Heart Failure in Clinical Medicine. *By* RAYMOND T. BENACK 594

The Importance of Electrolyte Therapy in Heart Disease. *By* DEMETRIO SODI-PALLARES .. 603

Concluding Remarks. *By* EÖRS BAJUSZ 620

FOREWORD

Eörs Bajusz
Bio-Research Institute, Cambridge, Mass.

All branches of basic and clinical science require a periodic reassessment of previously reported work in relation to more modern investigative, diagnostic, and therapeutic methods, as well as an interdisciplinary search for a new research channels. The planning of such a reassessment for heart-muscle disease brought several difficulties to the fore. It was soon realized that the current literature contains a wide variety of opinions and some confusing viewpoints concerning the terminology, classification, interpretation, and significance of various types of heart-muscle disease. Virtually every author in the field has introduced his own variations in defining the terms, "cardiomyopathy," "primary myocardial disease," and "metabolic heart disease." Moreover, each author, either intentionally or unintentionally, is guilty of variations from paper to paper.

It may be true that among experts these variations in terminology appear to be trivial in many instances; however, when nonexperts, particularly students, attempt to study this complex subject, the terminological confusion becomes a significant barrier to understanding. Therefore, I am especially grateful to Dr. William B. Wartman who accepted the arduous task of dealing with such problems in his introductory lecture. We realize that many people regard the consideration of semantics as a waste of time, referring to it with prejorative overtones. We apologize to those who have this feeling, but would like to point out that, in the field of heart-muscle disease, progress is implemented by improved communication.

For the purpose of organizing this Conference program, I have accepted the following reasonings and views: *Cardiomyopathies* (heart-muscle diseases) comprise a large group of hereditary and acquired conditions, diseases of known and unknown etiology, degenerative and inflammatory processes affecting the myocardium, and a wide variety of aberrations characterized by idiopathic cardiac enlargement and heart failure. Cardiomyopathies are not necessarily "primary myocardial diseases," although the two terms are often used interchangeably in the literature. A cardiomyopathy may occur in the absence of any underlying disease elsewhere (primary cardiomyopathy, or primary myocardial disease) or in association with systemic diseases including endocrinopathies, viral infections, hemochromatosis, beriberi, and muscular dystrophy (secondary cardiomyopathy). All these diseases are essentially metabolic (nonocclusive) forms of heart-muscle disease, and experimental studies performed during the past decade have shown that such metabolic cardiomyopathies can be induced in laboratory animals by many techniques.

So far I have avoided the admission that the term cardiomyopathy was originally coined to designate disease processes that affect the myocardium, but spare or minimally involve other cardiovascular structures, and that this definition was intended to exclude such common etiological categories as coronary, hypertensive, pulmonary, and valvular heart diseases. It appears to me increasingly doubtful, in the light of recent developments, whether a clear distinction between coronary and noncoronary heart diseases is always really possible. There are no currently available methods for determining, in the absence of a recent occlusion, whether coronary atherosclerosis and myocardial degeneration in a particular patient are cause-and-effect related. Furthermore, an ischemic necrosis of the heart muscle (i.e., myocardial infarct) may develop not only as the secondary consequence of coronary artery occlusion (thrombosis, formation of atherosclerotic plaques, or stenosis), but also through a variety of other mechanisms (e.g. increased oxygen requirement of cardiac muscle cells, impairment of coronary compensatory dilatability, or peripheral circulatory collapse). I see no way out of this dilemma other than to accept that a discussion of ischemic heart-muscle lesions cannot be excluded from the program of a conference dealing with metabolic cardiomyopathies. While I do not intend to obscure the fact that a causal relationship often does exist between coronary atherosclerosis and the so-called "ischemic (or coronary) heart disease," including myocardial infarction, I would like to stress that from a theoretical point of view it is essential to distinguish between the atherogenesis itself and the factors that determine the resistance vs. susceptibility of the myocardium to pathogenic agents. The heart-muscle cell is the primary site of injury in most common cardiac diseases, and it appears to me that investigators are now wisely beginning to interpret the pathogenesis of all forms of cardiomyopathies as sequelae of metabolic derangements in the heart muscle influenced by electrolytes, hormones, hypoxia, and other sensitizing and desensitizing factors.

Of course, it would be unrealistic to expect that this Conference will solve all of our terminological difficulties or that it will result in the dramatic discovery of a simple answer to the entire metabolic cardiomyopathy problem. It is more reasonable to anticipate that the presentations will provide at least some insight into the sequence of events that participate in the pathogenesis of heart-muscle disease. The successful identification and delineation of one or another among the many steps leading to structural and functional alterations of heart muscle would constitute significant progress, since the modification, by appropriate measures, of even a single reaction may prevent the development of a given cardiomyopathy. I therefore look forward to hearing and sharing with the participants of this Conference their experiences with the various pertinent problems, and hope that the cumulative total will prove informative, interesting, and useful.

In opening the first session, I wish to express my cochairman's and my own personal thanks to Admiral Schanze for his meticulous attention to conference details, and to the editorial staff for the subsequent preparation of the monograph. I am sure that the published proceedings will prove to be a rather unique collection of papers on cardiomyopathies which should become valuable source material for all those wishing to study the problems of heart-muscle disease in man and animals.

CARDIOMYOPATHY AND MYOCARDIAL DEGENERATION: PROBLEMS OF TERMINOLOGY IN EXPERIMENTAL AND CLINICAL PATHOLOGY

William B. Wartman

Department of Pathology, Northwestern University Medical School, Chicago, Ill.

As can be seen from the contents of this monograph, the two chairmen, recognizing the importance of terminology, have scheduled this topic as the introductory lecture.

Although we are encountering increasing incidence of primary myocardial disease, little progress has been made toward effective treatment and prevention of this condition. The difficulty of research in this area has been compounded by two problems:

1. The tendency of each of us to focus complete attention on one aspect of the disease or on one way of approaching it rather than looking at the difficulties as part of a total picture.
2. The confusion that has been produced by the variety of terminology used in describing the cardiomyopathies.

Humpty Dumpty believed that when he used a word, it had the sense that he selected for it, neither more nor less, and there are those among us who share the same opinion. But if we are "to compare findings in different animal species or to integrate the results of workers from many disciplines, then the importance of the terms we use is inescapable. . . . If we are to advance our knowledge of myocardial disease then clinicians, pathologists, epidemiologists, biochemists and workers from many other disciplines must be able to understand each other; if the existing currency in terminology is debased, we must start afresh by looking, describing, classifying and comparing" (Mitchell & Schwartz, 1965).

The title of this monograph is "Experimental 'Metabolic' Cardiopathies and Their Relationship to Human Heart Diseases." Let us look first at the meaning of the word "cardiopathy." In the authoritative Shorter Oxford English Dictionary the word is defined as "disease of the heart." This is not very helpful. The British Medical Dictionary defines cardiopathy as "a collective term to include all diseases and disorders of the heart." Again, not a helpful definition. Under the heading "myocardiopathy," however, we get better results: "an abnormal condition of the heart muscle not due to a *known* infective agent. The term may be applied to disorders of the heart muscle due to abnormal infiltrations (glycogen, etc.) or to deficiency of Vitamin B or Fiedler's myocarditis (due to an *unknown* infective agent) and endomyocardial fibrosis. It excludes ischemic heart disease."

In Dorland's Medical Dictionary, we find confusion compounded: "Cardiopathy [is] any disorder or disease of the heart. In addition to heart disease of inflammatory origin there are," and the definition goes on to include almost everything.

Now let us look at that other word, "metabolic." The Shorter Oxford English Dictionary tells us that the word was first used in 1743, was derived from the Greek word meaning changeable, and is defined as "pertaining to or involving transition." The word "metabolism" is defined as "the processes in an organism or a single cell by which nutritive material is built up into living matter (constructive metabolism or anabolism), or by which protoplasm is broken down into simpler substances to perform special functions (destructive metabolism or catabolism)." This is a fine definition and acceptable to all of us. A moment's reflection will make clear, however, that when we speak of "metabolic cardiomyopathies" we are using the word "metabolic" in a special sense. What we mean is injury of the myocardium resulting from disturbance of its metabolism.

To summarize the foregoing and to give us a working definition for the purposes of this monograph I suggest that we define the term "metabolic cardiomyopathy" as a host reaction, either morphological, functional, or biochemical, to a congenital anomaly or to the ingestion or administration of injurious substances or procedures that interfere with the metabolism of the myocardial cells or of the heart as a whole.

Clinical and Experimental Disorders Considered To Be Cardiomyopathies

To clarify further our thoughts about the cardiomyopathies, it would be useful to survey the human and experimentally induced diseases and disorders that are usually called "cardiomyopathies."

The term "cardiomyopathy" in its current clinical sense was introduced in 1957 by Wallace Brigden of the National Heart Hospital and the London Hospital in London, England. He used the term cardiomyopathy "to indicate isolated non-coronary myocardial disease" (Brigden, 1957). By "isolated," he meant that disease of other systems of the body was either absent or of a minor degree and significant only as an aid to diagnosis.

Brigden gave an account of 50 patients with isolated heart-muscle disease (cardiomyopathy), none of whom "had evidence of coronary disease, hypertension, valve disease, rheumatism, syphilis, or diphtheria." These cases could be placed in broad etiological groups as follows: 7 cases with familial heart disease, 8 cases with myocarditis presumed to be caused by infection, 3 cases of puerperal myocarditis, 3 cases of collagen disease (not the well-known disseminated collagen disease), 1 case with acromegaly, 7 cases of primary cardiac amyloid disease, and 13 cases of alcoholic cardiomyopathy.

To Brigden this was, etiologically speaking, a heterogeneous group of cases, but he noted that they had a common factor—the presence of serious myocardial disease without significant disease elsewhere. Brigden, being a clinician, emphasized the clinical features: the insidious development of symptoms of biventricular failure; a high venous blood pressure and a characteristic wave of the venous pulse; triple rhythm in the absence of murmurs; diffuse electrocardiographic changes; and, on radiography, a relatively immobile heart with a clear silhouette. He also noted that the "cardiomyopathies may be caused by any of the known disease processes that affect other systems in man."

The findings at the necropsies on Brigden's cases were of two sorts: cardiac hypertrophy and myocardial lesions. The weight of the heart was increased in all cases and appeared to be due to muscle hypertrophy. Because the heart weights were less in patients with a relatively short history than in those who had survived a long time, Brigden regarded the length of survival as an important causal factor, and suggested that a nonspecific survival hypertrophy was the most probable explanation of the increased heart weight.

The myocardial lesions consisted of inflammation, necrosis, and repair, the subendocardial region being particularly affected. Fibrosis of the endomyocardium and thrombosis on the endocardium of the ventricles were common. Patchy endocardial fibrosis was believed to result from organization of the thrombi and possibly to be a recurring process leading to progressive deterioration through further interference with myocardial nutrition.

Thus the pathological observations, like the clinical features, were individually nonspecific, but collectively, formed a recognizable picture. It is perhaps worth noting here that such a situation is pregnant with possible diagnostic error, especially in the hands of the inexperienced and unwary.

After Brigden's paper appeared, other previously described clinical conditions were put in the category of the cardiomyopathies: conditions such as the cases of endomyocardial fibrosis observed in Africa and elsewhere, familial cardiomegaly, Friedreich's ataxia, acute and chronic isolated idiopathic myocarditis (often viral or protozoal), collagen disease, and nutritional heart disease.

Within a year of Brigden's work, another whole new group of clinical cardiomyopathies, characterized by hypertrophic muscular obstruction to outflow from the left ventricle, was described by R. D. Teare in England (Teare, 1958).

Results of Animal Studies and Experimentation

In addition to the natural occurrence of isolated cardiomegaly and cardiomyopathy in man, spontaneous myocardial degeneration with clinical congestive heart failure has been observed in other animals. As long ago as 1923, Herbert Fox reported his findings from 6,000 autopsies of captive wild animals that had died in the Philadelphia Zoo. He described myocardial degeneration (amyloid, hyaline, fatty metamorphosis, granular and cloudy degeneration) in 52 mammals and 46 birds of various orders. Myocarditis occurred in 52 mammals and 66 birds (Fox, 1923). Recently F. Homburger and his associates have observed spontaneous cardiomyopathy in a strain of Syrian hamsters (Homburger *et al.*, 1962). The cardiomyopathies have been studied from many different experimental approaches; some of the results of these studies are the subjects of papers in this monograph.

One of the important experimental approaches to the cardiomyopathies was provided by Hans Selye in his work on the so-called "pluricausal cardiopathies" (Selye, 1961). Cardiomyopathies also occur in uremia, following administration of certain proteolytic enzymes, particularly papain and bromelin, and after overdosage of various catecholamine derivatives, especially isoproterenol. Much of this work has been reviewed by Selye and by Bajusz (1965).

Two considerations should be borne in mind to avoid possible confusion in evaluating the results of animal experiments. The first point is that most of the so-called "cardiomyopathies" produced in experimental animals are actually examples of cardiac necrosis. To date there has been only slight morphological evidence to suggest that the lesions in animals bear a resemblance to many of the cardiomyopathies occurring naturally in humans.

The second point concerns the limitations imposed by the small number of possible morphological ways in which the heart can react to any sort of injury. Inflammation, hypertrophy, degeneration, necrosis and fibrosis just about cover the possibilities. Thus by necessity the heart muscle must show the same morphological response to a variety of injurious agents. For example, the finding of necrosis after administration of a toxic agent should not suggest that its pathogenesis is necessarily the same as the necrosis of an ischemic infarct. For this reason an experimental lesion is not necessarily a good model to use in studying the prevention and treatment of human disease. In fact, some experimental lesions may even provide misleading clues.

Suggested Classification of the Cardiomyopathies

Since the myocardium can develop either isolated injury, i.e., apparent primary idiopathic disease, or may be injured secondarily as part of a generalized disease, I have divided the cardiomyopathies int two large groups, the primary cardiomyopathies and the secondary cardiomyopathies. I have also qualified the word "cardiomyopathy" wherever possible so as to indicate its probable etiology (TABLE 1).

Even casual inspection of this classification of the cardiomyopathies makes it clear that we are dealing with a number of entities, many of which seem unrelated. Is it possible to discover among them some factor common to all? I believe that recent work in our own and other laboratories on the reversible and irreversible reactions of myocardial cells to injury may provide a clue to a general pattern of cellular reaction to a variety of injurious agents. However, before considering this question, it is necessary to mention briefly some of the special limitations inherent in a study of myocardial cells in living animals.

The heart muscle, because it is well differentiated and has complex physiological and biochemical functions, is easily injured by a large number of deleterious insults. Although we are beginning to understand the nature of some of the many injuries we know must occur, the study of cardiac muscle is difficult because the heart is necessary for maintaining life. Experimentally the heart of an animal may be injured acutely in a specific manner, but the animal may die before the injury can manifest itself. Another problem is our frequent inability to recognize the effects of an injury after it has occurred. This is especially true with respect to the very early stages of cellular injury. Thus we are dependent for our investigations upon the study of injuries that can be easily recognized in animals or upon isolated examples of disease in man. But in man there is the severe restriction that the inciting injury usually has occurred a long time prior to the investigation, and only the monuments of those ancient events remain for us to study.

TABLE 1

CLASSIFICATION OF CARDIOMYOPATHIES

A. Primary or isolated
   1. Congenital
      a. Familial cardiomegaly
      b. Friedreich's ataxia
      c. Gargoylism
      d. Hamster heart disease*
   2. Inflammatory
      a. Viral coxsackie, group B polio, encephalomyocarditis,* virus III*
      b. Bacterial
      c. Protozoal
   3. Collagen diseases: rheumatic, lupus, etc.
   4. Metabolic
      a. Amyloidosis, hemochromatosis, von Gierke's disease
      b. Experimental necrosis, "pluricausal cardiopathies," amines
   5. Nutritional: alcohol; K, Na, and Mg depletion
   6. Endocrine: acromegaly, thyroid disease
   7. Obstructive cardiomyopathy
      a. Subaortic hypertrophic type
      b. Secondary to ridges, etc.

B. Secondary
   1. Ischemia
   2. Hypertension
   3. Infection

* In experimental animals only.

TABLE 2

RESULTS OF EXPERIMENTAL ISCHEMIC INJURY TO THE MYOCARDIUM*

Ischemia	Endoplasmic Reticulum Changes	Mitochondrial Changes	Necrosis	ATP	Lactate	Pyruvate	Succinate	Na	K	H_2O	Fat Accumulation
Total, 15 minutes, no reflow	+	0	0	↓	↑	?	N	N	N	N	+
Total, 15 minutes, plus 5 minute reflow	+	0	0	N	N	N	N	N	N	N	N
Total, 60 minutes, no reflow	+	+	0	↓	↑	0	↓	N?	N?	N?	N
Total, 60 minutes, plus 5 minute reflow	+	++	+	0	0	0	↓	↑	↓	↑	+

Key: + = response; ++ = greater response: 0 = absent; N = normal; ↑ = increased level of compound tested; ↓ = decreased level of compound tested.

Bearing in mind these and other limitations of experiments on the living myocardium, we have devised, in our laboratory, ways of causing standardized ischemic injury to the myocardium under controlled conditions (Jennings & Wartman, 1957). Since 1957, the reactions of the myocardium have been studied by light and electron microscopy and by histochemical and biochemical methods, in a series of experiments, done chiefly by my colleagues (Jennings & Wartman, 1957; Wartman & Jennings, 1957; Herdson *et al.,* 1965; Jennings *et al.,* 1965). TABLE 2 briefly summarizes some of the results.

In all experiments the myocardium was examined after various intervals of total ischemia, both with and without subsequent release of the coronary ligature and restoration or reflow of the coronary circulation for a known period of time.

After 15 minutes of total ischemia we can see that slight endoplasmic reticulum changes occur and consist chiefly of swelling. The mitochondria, however, show no morphological changes, and there is no necrosis. After 60 minutes, however, marked alterations are seen electron microscopically in both the endoplasmic reticulum and mitochondria, and necrosis has developed; these changes persist or become even more intense when there is reflow of coronary blood.

Corresponding biochemical changes also occur. Adenosine triphosphate (ATP) and oxygen-consumption levels decrease drastically and lactate accumulates. Enzymatic activity in the mitochondria also drops, and there are serious ion shifts. At first these changes are reversible, but later they become irreversible. Thus the morphological and metabolic changes keep pace with each other. We can therefore draw up simple tables of correlations that give us hints of the emerging picture (TABLE 2).

We can indicate this emerging pattern in general terms, as in TABLE 3, which indicates the process by which a myocardial cell "changes from its normal steady state either to take up a new steady state or to be so disturbed that a new steady state is quite impossible. This can only mean total disorganization (or death)" (Judah *et al.,* 1965).

TABLE 3

FATE OF MYOCARDIAL CELL UNDER ATTACK*

Injurious agent

↓

Normal cell

⇆ ↘

Cell viable	Cell dying or dead
↓	↓
New steady state	Final events
a. Accumulation of normal cell components: fat, glycogen (reversible)	a. Calcification
b. Cloudy swelling; accumulation of water and salts from without (reversible)	b. Autolysis
c. Accumulation of foreign materials: amyloid (irreversible)	c. Replacement, regeneration, fibrosis

* Modified from Judah *et al.* (1965).

Summary

I have called attention to some of the misconceptions caused by drawing conclusions after insufficient evaluation of the many aspects of the cardiomyopathies. Other difficulties are based on our failure to standardize our usage of the word "cardiomyopathy." It is suggested that an acceptable definition of the term "metabolic cardiomyopathy" is a host reaction, either morphological, functional, or biochemical, to a congenital anomaly or to the ingestion or administration of injurious substances or procedures that interfere with the metabolism of the myocardial cells or of the heart as a whole.

The clinical and experimental features of the cardiomyopathies have been used as a basis for a clinical classification.

Brief consideration has been given to recent experimental work that suggests the pattern of reaction in a myocardial cell when it changes from its normal steady state either to a new steady state (reversible injury) or becomes so disturbed that a new steady state becomes impossible (irreversible injury).

References

BAJUSZ, E. 1965. Nutritional Aspects of Cardiovascular Disease. J. B. Lippincott Co. Philadelphia, Pa.

BRIGDEN, W. 1957. Uncommon myocardial diseases. The non-coronary cardiomyopathies. Lancet **ii**: 1179.

BRITISH MEDICAL DICTIONARY. 1961. 1st edit. The Caxton Publishing Co., Ltd. London.

DORLAND'S MEDICAL DICTIONARY. 1965. 24th edit. W. B. Saunders Co. Philadelphia, Pa.

FOX, H. 1923. Disease in Captive Wild Mammals and Birds. J. B. Lippincott Co. Philadelphia, Pa.

HERDSON, P. B., H. M. SOMMERS & R. B. JENNINGS. 1965. A comparative study of the fine structure of normal and ischemic dog myocardium with special reference to early changes following temporary occlusion of a coronary artery. Amer. J. Path. **46**: 367.

HOMBURGER, F., S. R. BAKER, C. W. NIXON & R. WHITNEY. 1962. Primary generalized polymyopathy and cardiac necrosis in an inbred line of Syrian hamsters. Med. Exp. (Basel) **6**: 339.

JENNINGS, R. B., J. P. KALTENBACH & H. M. SOMMERS. 1965. Cell death: electrolyte alterations in injured and dying myocardial cells. *In* Electrolytes and Cardiovascular Diseases. E. Bajusz, Ed.: 192–203. S. Karger. Basel, Switzerland.

JENNINGS, R. B. & W. B. WARTMAN. 1957. Production of an area of homogeneous myocardial infarction in the dog. Arch. Path. (Chicago) **63**: 580.

JUDAH, J. D., K. AHMED & A. E. M. MCLEAN. 1965. Pathogenesis of cell necrosis. Fed. Proc. **24**: 1217.

MITCHELL, J. R. A. & C. S. SCHWARTZ. 1965. Arterial Disease. Blackwell Sci. Publ. Oxford, England.

SELYE, H. 1961. The "Pluricausal" Cardiopathies. Charles C Thomas, Publ. Springfield, Ill.

SHORTER OXFORD ENGLISH DICTIONARY. 1959. 3rd edit. Oxford University Press. Oxford, England.

TEARE, R. D. 1958. Asymmetrical hypertrophy of the heart in young adults. Brit. Heart J. **20**: 1.

WARTMAN, W. B. & R. B. JENNINGS. 1957. Reactions of the myocardium to obstruction of the coronary arteries. Med. Clin. N. Amer. **41**: 3–15.

PART I. ULTRASTRUCTURE OF HEART MUSCLE UNDER NORMAL AND PATHOLOGICAL CONDITIONS

MICROSCTRUCTURE OF "SPECIALIZED" TISSUES IN THE MAMMALIAN HEART*

C. E. Challice

University of Calgary, Calgary, Alberta, Canada

INTRODUCTION

It seems scarcely necessary to emphasize the critical role of the heart's impulse initiation and conduction mechanism in the maintenance of life in higher animals. Various branches of science have contributed extensively to present-day knowledge of the structure and function of this system, and the work has been well summarized in recent reviews (Hoffman & Cranefield, 1960; Truex, 1961; Robb, 1965; Taccardi & Marchetti, 1965). Recently, electron microscopical studies have added to our knowledge about the structure of these tissues (Muir, 1957; Caesar *et al.*, 1958; Viragh & Porte, 1960, 1961a, b; Rhodin *et al.*, 1961; Torii, 1962; Trautwein & Uchizono, 1963; Ruska, 1965). In addition, some studies have attempted to correlate the electrophysiology and ultrastructure of these tissues with the techniques of the electrophysiologists to localize samples for electron microscopical study (Trautwein & Uchizono, 1963; Challice, 1965, 1966). The latter approach was pursued in the study described here, the aim being the correlation of cellular structure with electrophysiological properties, hopefully to provide some inferences as to the structural factors that give these cells their peculiar properties, and also, ultimately, some indications as to the subcellular changes, if any, which accompany failure of the system.

MATERIALS AND METHODS

Because of the extensive electrophysiological work done previously on the rabbit, this animal has formed the main source of material in our study. The electrophysiological technique has followed closely that used in the studies of Hoffman & Cranefield (1960), Paes de Carvalho & de Alameida (1960), and Paes de Carvalho (1961). Rabbits approximately one year of age were anesthetized with pentobarbital sodium (Nembutal®)†; the whole heart was removed and immersed in Tyrode solution at 37° C. While in Tyrode solution, the right atrium and most of the intraventricular septum were dissected from the heart; the areas thus exposed are illustrated in FIGURE 1. The tissue, with a small piece of foam plastic used as a mounting board, was immersed in oxygenated (95% oxygen, 5% carbon dioxide) Tyrode solution at 37° C (Paes de Carvalho, 1961). Electrical activity of the various regions was checked by means of microelectrode techniques, and the areas of particular interest were excised and cut into pieces of 1 mm^3 or less and immersed in fixative. Several larger blocks, in which special attention was paid to orientation, were also prepared. Some of these included and were at right angles to the sinoatrial (SA) ring bundle (Paes de Carvalho, 1961); others included the atrioventricular (AV) node, so that one end of the block was atrial tissue and the other end was part of

* This work was made possible by the support of the Alberta Heart Foundation and the National Research Council of Canada.

† Distributed by Abbott Laboratories, North Chicago, Ill.

the bundle of His (or in some cases, the ventricular myocardium). Details of the dissection of the AV nodal region are illustrated in FIGURES 2 and 3.

Tissue was fixed in glutaraldehyde (Sabatini *et al.*, 1963) or in a mixture of glutaraldehyde and acrolein (Sandborn, 1966). All specimens were post-fixed in a 2% solution of osmium tetroxide for two or three hours. The pieces of tissue were then dehydrated and embedded in epoxy resin. Sections were cut with glass or diamond knives, and some were stained with lead citrate (Reynolds, 1963) and uranyl acetate (Mercer, 1963).

Observations

An extensive survey of the evidence obtained is not possible here, and only a summary will be given. The results will be found in more complete form elsewhere (Challice, 1965; DeFelice & Challice, 1969).

Sinoatrial Node

Examination of tissue identified electrophysiologically as coming from the region of the primary pacemaker (SA node) shows that the fibers contain fibrils that are randomly oriented and pursue a tortuous course through the cell (FIGURE 4). The fibrils are poorly defined, with the characteristic cross-sectional closely packed hexagonal array of thick and thin filaments at best approximated (Huxley, 1956). The Z bands were poorly defined, and the other bands identi-

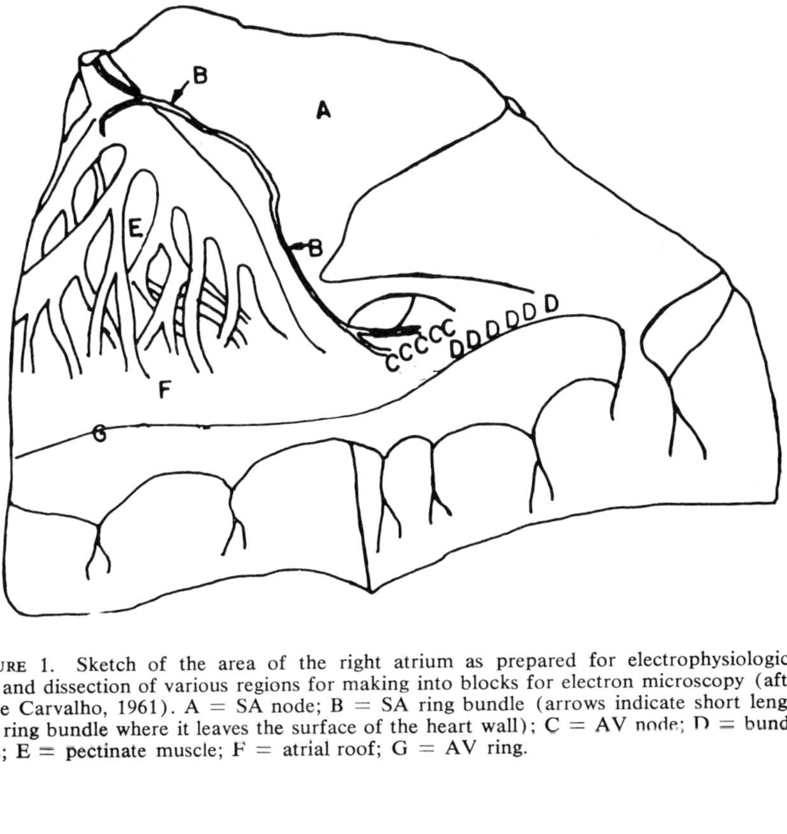

FIGURE 1. Sketch of the area of the right atrium as prepared for electrophysiological study, and dissection of various regions for making into blocks for electron microscopy (after Paes de Carvalho, 1961). A = SA node; B = SA ring bundle (arrows indicate short length of SA ring bundle where it leaves the surface of the heart wall); C = AV node; D = bundle of His; E = pectinate muscle; F = atrial roof; G = AV ring.

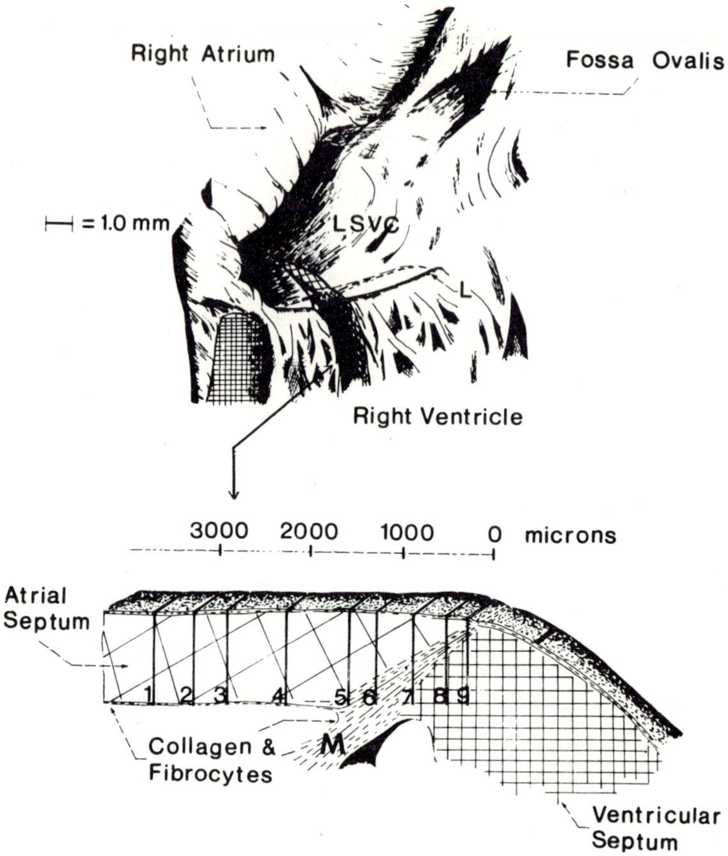

FIGURE 2. Dissection of the AV node. While the whole heart was in Tyrode solution, the tip of the ventricular chambers was removed so that an incision could be made along the outer walls of the right ventricle and atrium leading to the right superior vena cava.

(*Top*) The illustration shows the exposed orifice of the left superior vena cava (LSVC). The cut was made through the node, as identified by means of electrophysiological studies. The AV join is indicated by the dotted lines. The line of attachment (L) of the septal cusp of the tricuspid valve is not always contiguous with this join.

(*Bottom*) A block made by making a cut (solid arrow) as shown in the top illustration and a second cut parallel to it approximately 1 mm distant. The electrophysiological node forms part of the atrial septum. The AV ring is continuous with the aortic cusp of the mitral valve (M). Zones 1–9 are selected from 25 planes that were taken from this block and examined. The technique used allowed thick (1μ) sections to be cut and stained with toluidine blue for light microscopical examination, in addition to thin sections (~300 Å) for electron microscopy.

FIGURE 3. Zones 1–9 (FIGURE 2, bottom) schematically drawn from observations made by light microscopy on the toluidine blue-stained sections. Where cells were observed to be oriented, they have been drawn approximately to scale (i.e., overlay and transition muscle cells), but otherwise cross-hatching has been used (atrial myocardium and nodal cells). Blood vessels and nerves have not been drawn. It will be seen that nodal tissue begins on the atrial side at plane 3, extending into plane 9. The overlay cells become progressively more sparse and disappear around plane 6. In the particular series illustrated, planes 7–9 show nodal tissue insulated by connective tissue from ventricular myocardium. From a block made further to the right in FIGURE 2 (top) similar planes would show a transition to bundle of His cells (DeFelice & Challice, 1969).

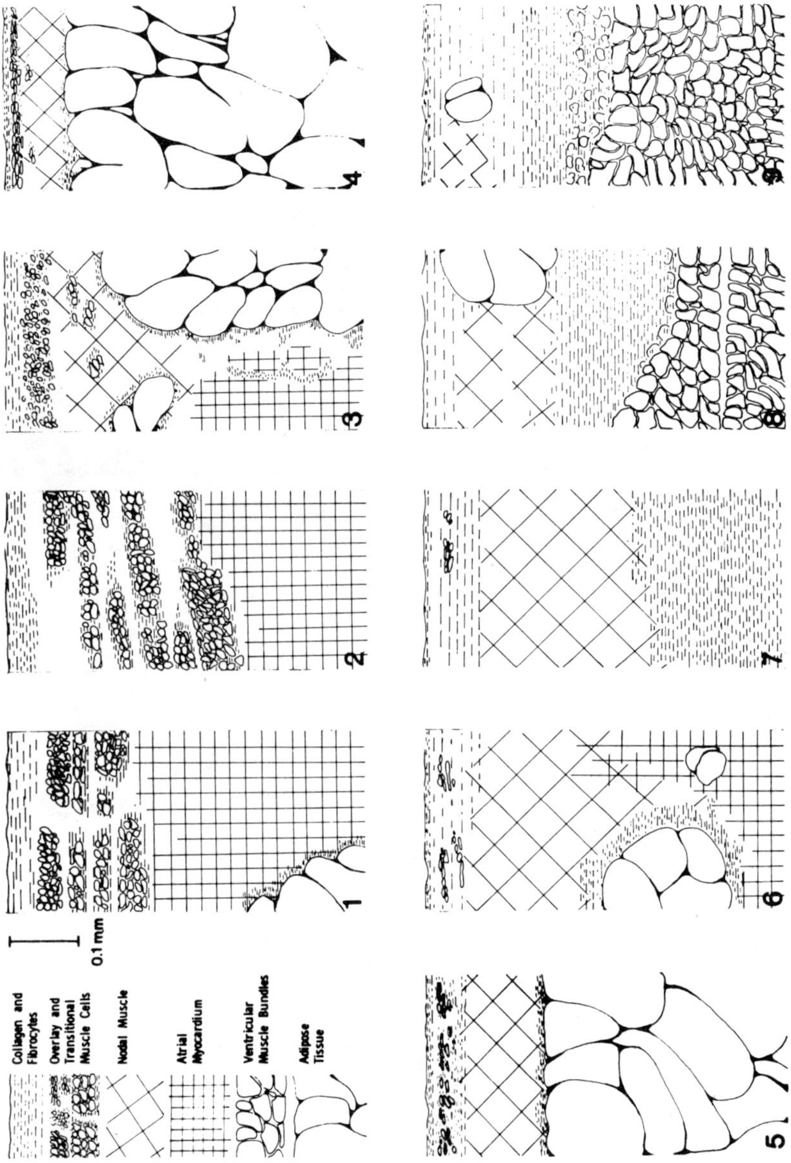
Collagen and Fibrocytes
Overlay and Transitional Muscle Cells
Nodal Muscle
Atrial Myocardium
Ventricular Muscle Bundles
Adipose Tissue
0.1 mm
1
2
3
4
5
6
7
8
9

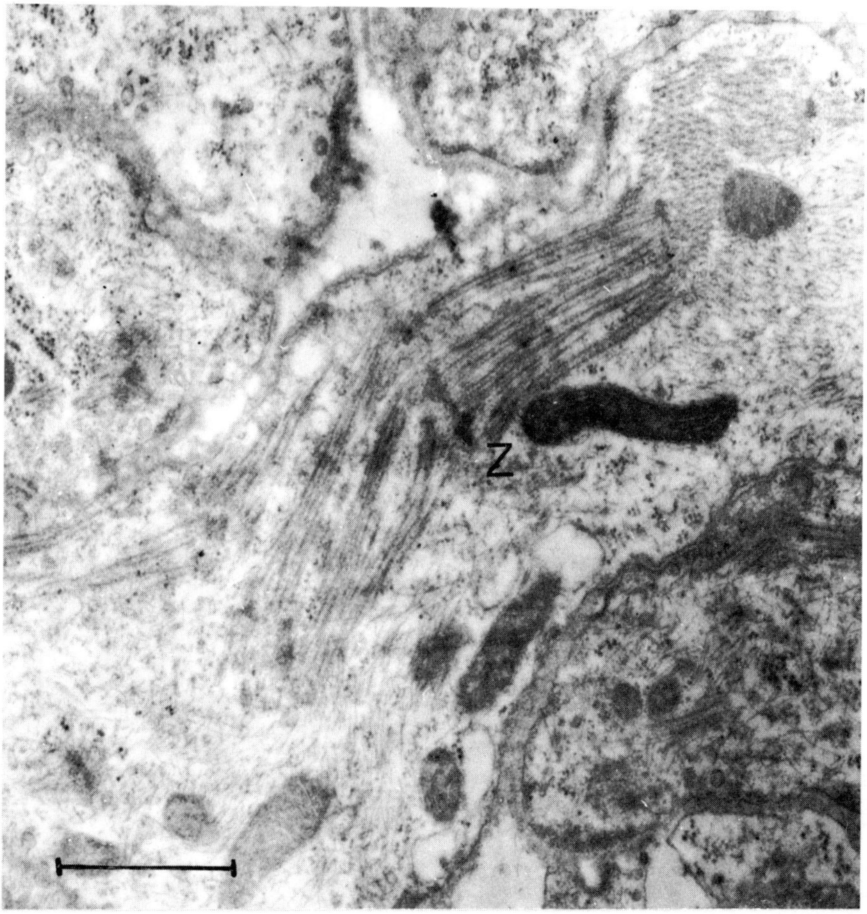

FIGURE 4. Sections of tissue from the SA node of the rabbit heart. Note the complete lack of orientation of the fibrils, and the unorganized filamentous material in the cytoplasm. The cells have a basement membrane surrounding them where they are not closely abutting on other cells. The Z bands (Z) are poorly defined, and, where the fibril is cut approximately in cross-section (top right), the closely packed hexagonal array of thin and thick filaments found in skeletal muscle is only approximated. Sarcoplasmic reticulum is very rare. Pinocytotic vesiculation can be seen at the plasma membrane. Scale = 1μ.

fied in skeletal muscle were scarcely detectable. Some membrane structures were observed in the sarcoplasm, but there was no evidence that the fibrils were surrounded by a sarcoplasmic reticulum (SR) sheath, such as that seen in mature skeletal and ventricular muscle (Porter, 1961). In those areas not occupied by definitive inclusions, there appeared a mass of apparently unorganized, thin filamentous material, of the same size as the thin filamentous component of the fibrils, along with granular material corresponding to that identified as glycogen (Fawcett & Selby, 1958). Cells appeared to be grouped together in twos and threes, with each group surrounded by a basement membrane and a larger interspace containing collagen. Where the cells were in close apposition, desmosomes were often observed, sometimes associated with a poorly defined Z band, but often with some of the thin filamentous component in the sarcoplasm associated with the intracellular component of the desmosome. Pinocytotic vesiculation was often observed at the plasma membrane. Where the cells were not closely abutting, a basement membrane approximately 50 mμ thick was apposed to the interstitial side of the plasma membrane. Nerve elements were frequently observed, but synaptic junctions between nerve and muscle have not been identified to date in this region.

Sinoatrial Ring Bundle

A survey has been conducted in which large areas taken from the region of the atrial wall containing the structure identified electrophysiologically as the SA ring bundle were examined by electron microscopy (Gray, 1966). It was established that there is a morphologically distinct bundle of cells in this region. Upon examination (Challice, 1966; Gray, 1966), a wide variation in morphology was observed between cells containing well-defined fibrils and ones in which characteristic fibrillar structures were scarcely detectable (FIGURE 5). The crude fibrils were oriented in the direction of the long axis of the fibers, and, although the fine filamentous component found in the cytoplasm of the SA nodal cells was present, it was not observed in such large quantity. Glycogen granules were observed within the crude fibrillar structures.

Again, some vestiges of sarcoplasmic membrane structures were seen, but there was no question of an SR sheath around the fibrils. Transverse membrane structures were comparatively well developed, especially in those cells in which

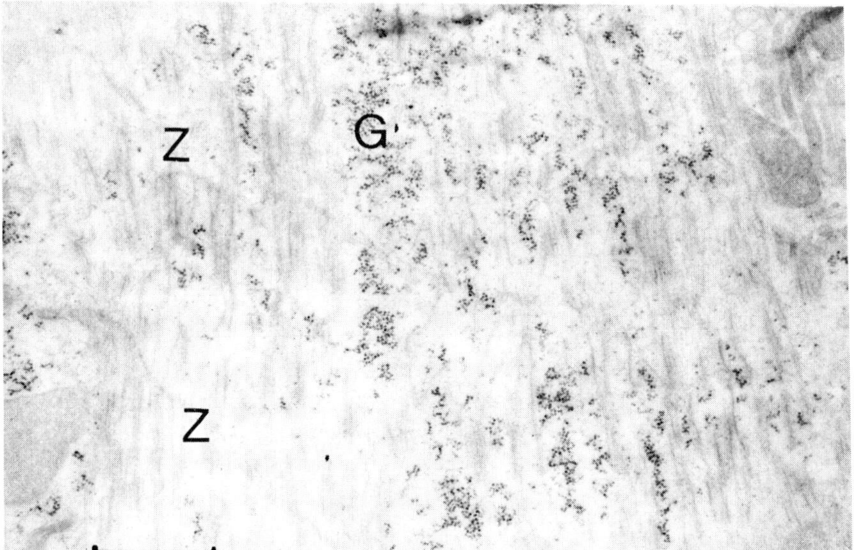

FIGURE 5. The SA ring bundle. Fibrillar orientation is from top to bottom of the micrograph, and suggestions of Z bands are seen running approximately across the micrograph. Fibrillar organization is very poorly developed. Glycogen (G) is seen in among the filaments. Sarcoplasmic reticulum is rare. Scale = 1μ.

the fibrillar structures were better differentiated. Also, the sarcolemma tended to invaginate at the Z line levels, as in Purkinje-type cells. Intercalated discs were observed where fibrillar continuity was interrupted by cellular abutments, but desmosome structures appeared to be less frequent than in SA nodal tissue.

Atrioventricular Node

A comprehensive study of this area is still in progress, and a picture of the cellular morphology and distribution is being assembled gradually. A detailed presentation of this material has yet to be given (DeFelice and Challice, 1969), and this paper briefly reports the progress on the material obtained to date.

The characteristic action potentials previously obtained by other workers have been confirmed, and serial sections at various levels were obtained from

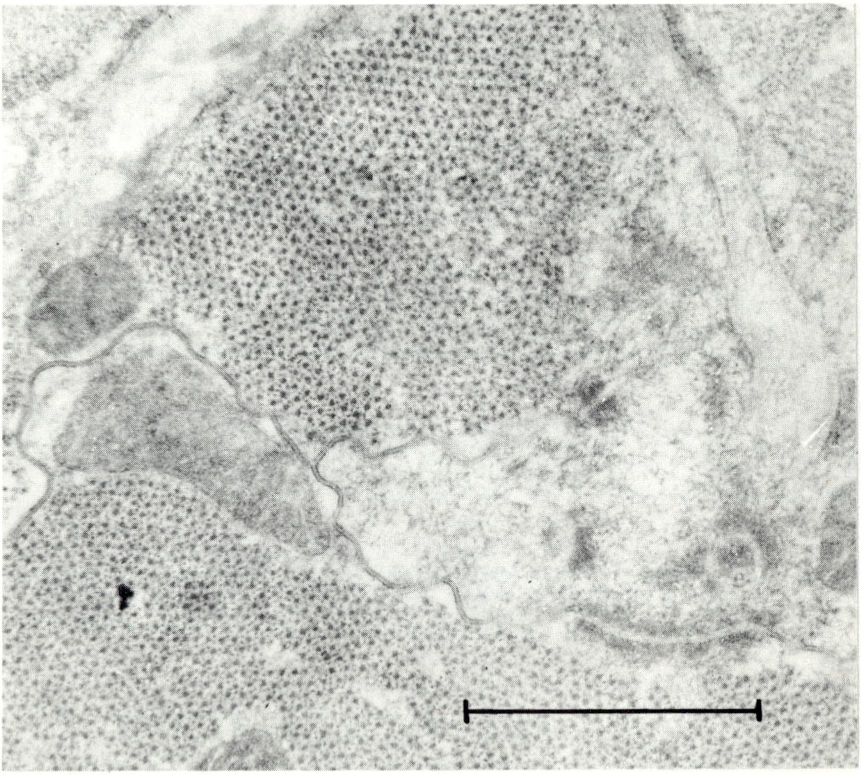

FIGURE 6. Section of a cell from zone 1 (FIGURES 2, bottom, and 3). This is in the atrial prenodal region. Fibrillar structure is readily recognizable in cross-section with the closely packed hexagonal array of thick and thin filaments not perfect but fairly well demonstrated. The area to the middle right is probably in the I region, showing thin filaments only, and where the array is not demonstrable as regular. The cellular abutment between the cells in the central part of the figure is close, corresponding in separation to that which has been designated a nexus (Dewey & Barr, 1962, 1964; Barr *et al.,* 1965). Sarcoplasmic reticulum is very sparse in this area and in all the nodal region until the bundle of His is reached. Scale = 1μ.

blocks which traversed the respective regions. FIGURE 2 illustrates the anatomy of the region, and FIGURE 3 schematically represents the changes in cellular morphology through the region at the light microscopical level. FIGURES 6–13 show some specimen electron micrographs of this area.

As shown in FIGURE 3, there are several distinguishable layers of cells, separated by spaces loosely filled with collagen. Although the surface layer of muscle, designated the overlay (which partly covers the area on the lumen side), may contribute in some manner to the characteristic action potentials, it is not these cells from which such potentials are recorded. This fact is known from the depth to which micropipettes must penetrate before the characteristic pulses are observed. The microscopical observations are from the second layer of cells, which appear to contain the specialized fibers.

The electrophysiological studies have established that the region (N region) in which the decremental conduction occurs (Hoffman & Cranefield, 1966) is a narrow band of at most 1-mm thickness running parallel to the join between the atrium and the ventricle. The techniques used to date in the present study do not permit identification of the cells in this region with as great a degree of accuracy as is felt desirable. Nevertheless, correlation between the regions identified electrophysiologically and those illustrated by electron micrographs has been made on a tentative basis. In fact, there does not seem to be a sharp line of demarcation between the regions from the standpoint of cellular micromorphology.

In cells located on the atrial side of the nodal region (FIGURE 6), the fibrils are comparatively well defined, showing the established band structure characteristic of skeletal and cardiac muscle. Intercalated discs are well developed, and there are desmosomes joining cells in other regions. There are also areas of close plasma membrane apposition between cells forming an intercellular junction described as a "nexus" (cf. Barr *et al.*, 1965).

There is normally only a negligible amount of randomly oriented fine filamentous components in the sarcoplasm (FIGURE 6), although in a few cells some may be seen (FIGURE 7). As one moves toward the nodal region, the cell fibrils become progressively less well oriented (FIGURES 8–10), and, in the area tentatively identified as the N region, there is a large amount of unorganized filamentous material in the cytoplasm (FIGURES 11–13), along with poorly defined fibrils arranged so haphazardly that they may be seen coursing in two directions at the same place in a given section (see FIGURE 11). Also, there is often a proliferation of the Z band or disc, which occasionally connects Z band with desmosome (FIGURES 10 and 11). There is sometimes a suggestion that this material, when not associated directly with a fibril, may be located preferentially at the plasma membrane, even though there is not necessarily a cellular abutment in these regions (FIGURE 9). Often this deposit displays a systematic distribution, sometimes connected by fine filaments oriented similarly to those described as leptofilaments (FIGURE 9). Disc and desmosome structures also sometimes display a broken and almost periodic structure (FIGURE 13).

In the central (N) region of the AV node, the cells themselves are poorly oriented, and have only intermittent contact with one another. Also, the close intercellular interdigitating abutments observed in other regions are infrequent in this region, although the haphazard angles at which the junctions occur make accurate and reliable measurements of separation difficult. Pinocytotic vesiculation is often apparent at the plasma membrane.

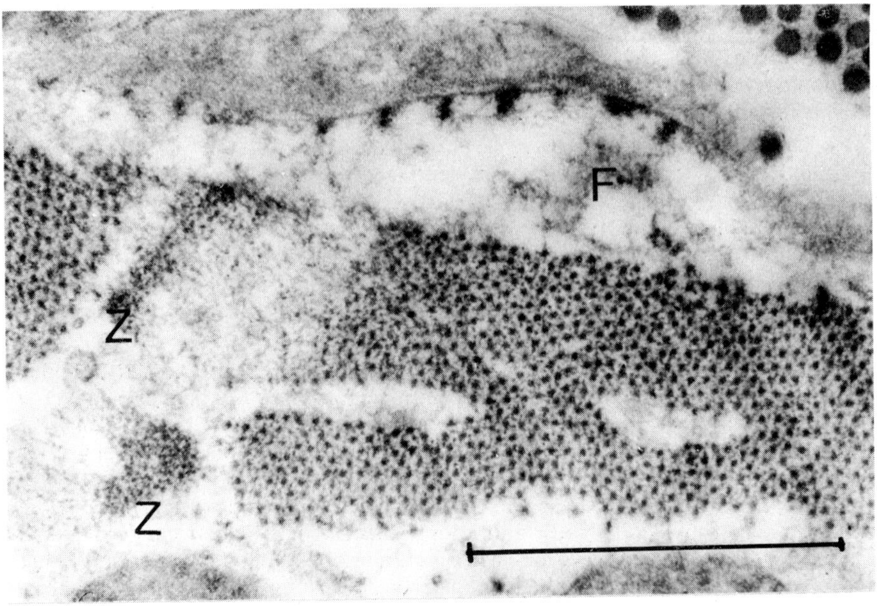

FIGURE 7. Cell from zone 3, showing a fairly well-differentiated fibril cut almost in cross-section, but sufficiently obliquely to traverse a Z band. In the A band the closely packed hexagonal array of thick and thin filaments, although not perfect, can be recognized, but large holes are seen. In the I band the hexagonal array is not readily recognizable. A more orderly array is seen in the Z band, but even this is broken into two parts. Some filamentous material (F) is seen in the cytoplasm, and against the cell membrane is an array resembling crude leptofibrils (Thoenes & Ruska, 1960). Scale = 1μ.

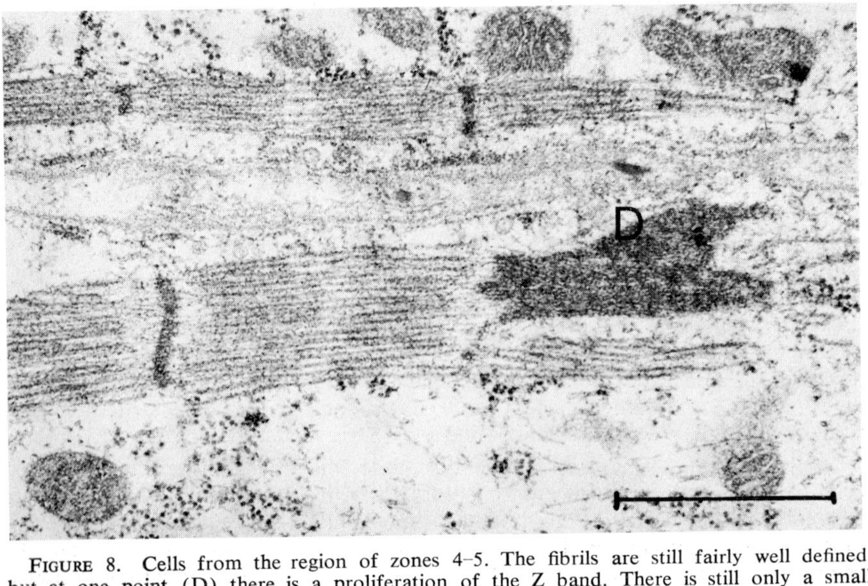

FIGURE 8. Cells from the region of zones 4–5. The fibrils are still fairly well defined, but at one point (D) there is a proliferation of the Z band. There is still only a small amount of unorganized filamentous material in the cytoplasm. Scale = 1μ.

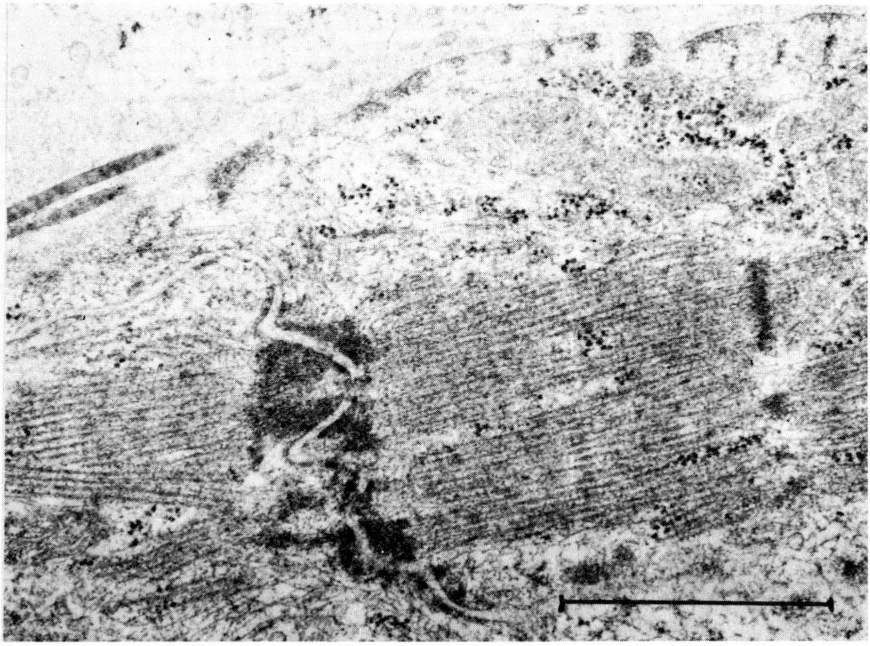

FIGURE 9. Cells from zones 5–6, the region surrounding an intercalated disc. Fibrillar orientation is not consistent (at left), disc structure is not regular, and the Z band is broken. Close apposition of cells (cf. FIGURE 6) is not apparent. There is now a greater density of unorganized filamentous material in the cytoplasm, and there is evidence of leptofibrils (top right). Glycogen granules are seen within the fibrillar structure. Scale = 1μ.

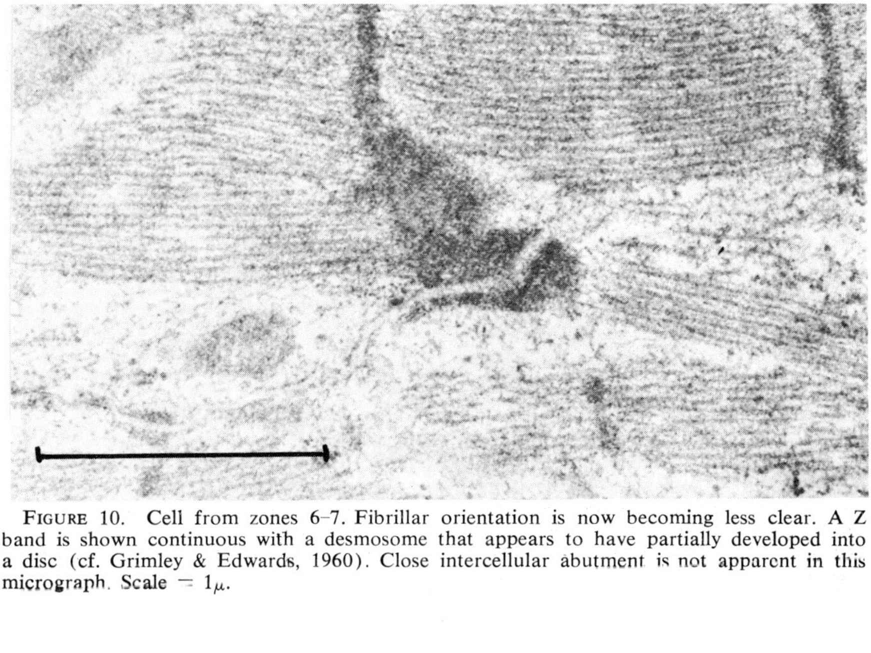

FIGURE 10. Cell from zones 6–7. Fibrillar orientation is now becoming less clear. A Z band is shown continuous with a desmosome that appears to have partially developed into a disc (cf. Grimley & Edwards, 1960). Close intercellular abutment is not apparent in this micrograph. Scale = 1μ.

Bundle of His

On the opposite side of the AV node there is also a transition in cellular morphology leading from the central region to the bundle of His. To date, this transition region has not been analyzed in as much detail as the atrial side of the node.

In the bundle of His the fibrils are well oriented but are not as closely packed as in the myocardium. They display the regular sarcomeric banding. Mitochondria are large, and the outer cell membrane invaginates deeply toward the Z

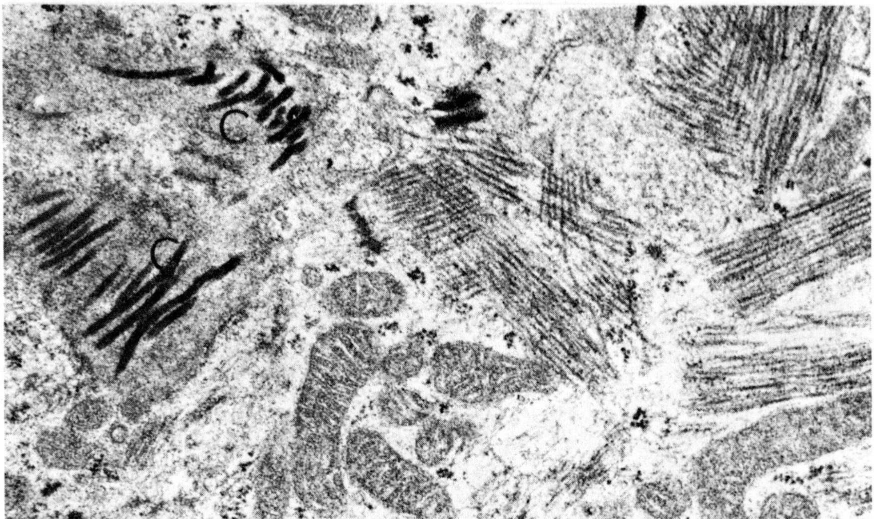

FIGURE 11. Cells from zone 7, believed to be in the middle of the physiological node. The almost complete random orientation of the fibrillar material can be seen, including fibrils coursing in more than one direction within the thickness of a single section (top right). Collagen (C) in the intercellular space is seen at the top left. Random filamentous material is seen in the cytoplasm. Scale = 1μ.

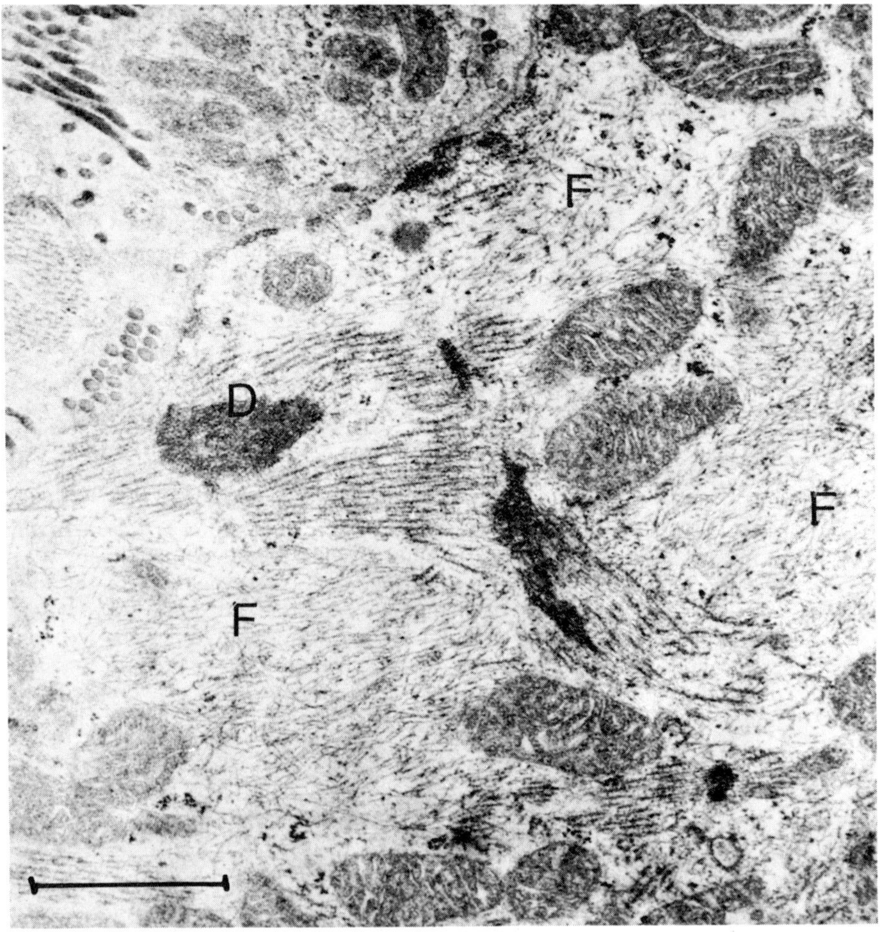

FIGURE 12. Zone 7, showing extremely poor organization of fibrils. Large dense areas associated with crude Z bands (D) and large amounts of unorganized filamentous material (F) are observed in the sarcoplasm. Scale = 1μ.

lines of the myofibrils, and also, although not quite so deeply, toward the M lines (FIGURE 14). The cells themselves are large, both long and large in cross-sectional area. There is a negligible amount of thin filamentous material in the ground cytoplasm, but there still seems to be a small amount associated with the plasma membrane. Intercalated discs are large, and desmosome structures between adjacent parallel interdigitating cells are common and extensive. Also, nexus-type intercellular abutments are common.

Sarcoplasmic reticulum is readily distinguishable, forming a network approximating a cylindrical sheath surrounding the sarcomeres (FIGURES 14 and 15). Transverse reticulum and triad structures are not usually well developed, but the SR shows intimate appositional contact with the outer plasma membrane itself at a number of points (FIGURE 14).

As yet the Purkinje fibers in the ventricle have not been examined in detail in the present study, but current information indicates that they appear to be essentially similar morphologically to the individual cells in the bundle of His. According to Truex (1961), light microscopical observations indicate that the rabbit heart is atypical in this respect.

Nerves

Nerve elements are frequently observed, particularly in the SA and AV nodal regions. However, synaptic junctions between nerve and muscle have not been observed. Occasionally, a myelinated axon can be seen.

Discussion

Neurogenic or Myogenic Conduction

Most investigators nowadays believe that the initiation and conduction of the electrical impulse in the heart is by means of specialized muscle cells rather than by nerves (cf. Hoffman & Cranefield, 1960). Recently, however, Wensing (1965) has claimed, primarily on the basis of morbid staining studies, that the heartbeat is neurogenic and not myogenic. A detailed criticism of this work will not be attempted here, but it must be observed that the present study does not support his views; therefore the myogenic theory will form the basis of the following discussion. Nerve elements were observed, but synaptic junctions of the type observed at skeletal muscle neuromuscular junctions were not seen. Also, studies performed in the author's laboratory have indicated that the distribution of neurons in the tissue is not nearly as extensive as claimed by Wensing (Gray, 1966).

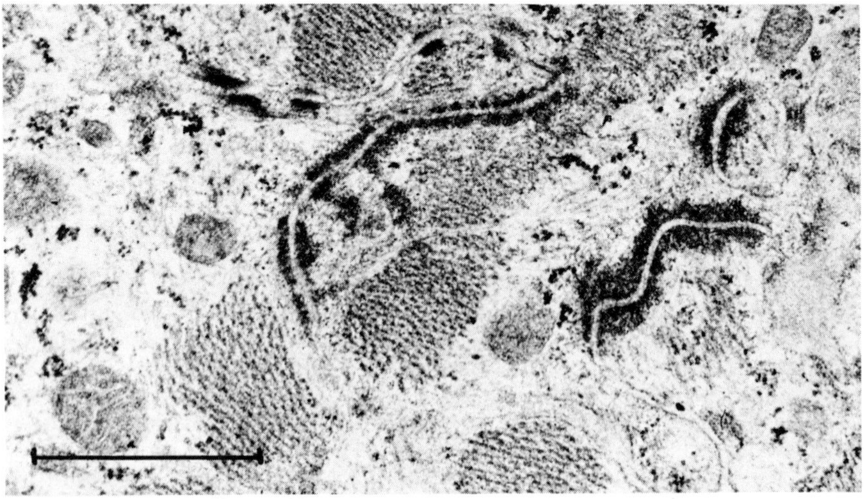

FIGURE 13. Intercellular connection showing randomness of orientation of both the poorly organized fibrils and also the cells. A poorly organized disc shows broken, almost periodic, structure. Unorganized filamentous material is seen in the background. Scale = 1μ.

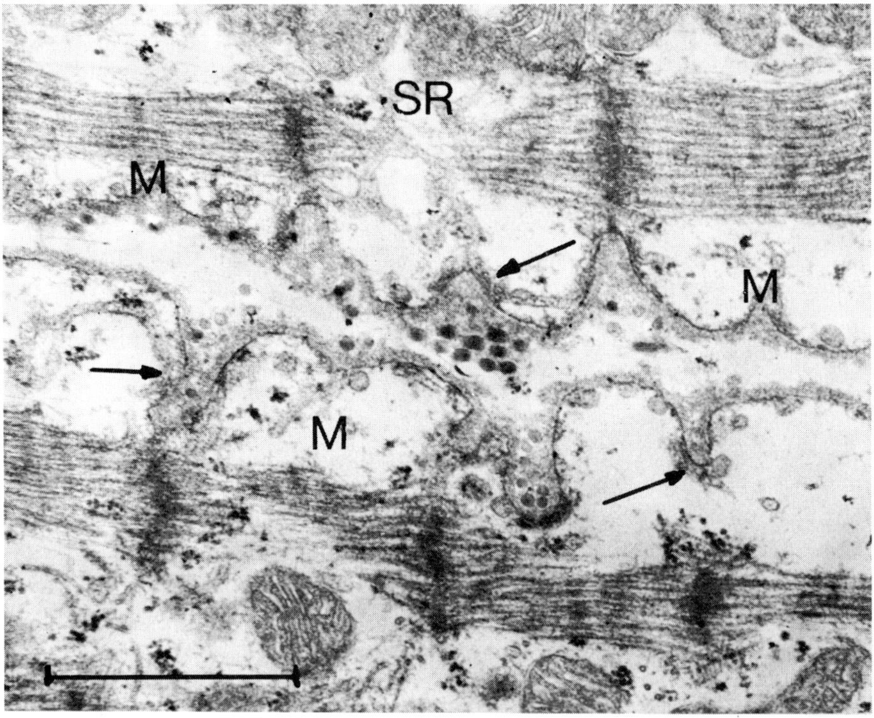

FIGURE 14. Section from the bundle of His. Fibrils are well defined and well oriented. There are invaginations of the sarcolemma at the Z band level and (to a lesser extent) at the M band level (M). Sarcoplasmic reticulum is readily seen, on occasion making direct appositional contact with the sarcolemma (arrows). Basement membrane is present, but unorganized filamentous material in the sarcoplasm is not readily seen. Scale = 1μ.

Relationship of Structure to Function

One problem in attempting to relate the morphology of cells with their physiological properties is that it is not immediately obvious which features lead to the observed electrophysiological properties and which occur as a result of these properties. In any case, different structures are in all likelihood intimately related by feedback mechanisms, making their separation a still more dubious matter. Tentatively, however, some inferences may be drawn at the present time.

Theories as to the fundamental processes involved in transmembrane potential phenomena, and particularly action potential phenomena, are by no means unanimous (Hodgkin & Huxley, 1952; Ling, 1962). However, no matter what may be the fundamental nature of the electrical events, an observation of transmembrane potential made by microelectrode techniques at any point in the tissue represents a combination of the effects of all the transmembrane phenomena of the entire system, since they affect the particular point of observation. Three factors appear to be of primary importance: (1) the electrical circuitry of the cell under examination, (2) the signal received from neighboring cells, and (3) the electrical junction between the cell and its neighbors.

Thus the system should be regarded as a complex electrical transmission line, the elements of the line being the individual cells linked together in parallel and in series with other cells, with the cells themselves consisting of a number of subelements.

Electrical Circuitry within a Cell

It is commonly assumed—albeit with reservations—that the active membrane phenomena of muscle are fundamentally similar to those in nerve (cf. Hoffman & Cranefield, 1960). Based on this assumption, the primary "active" phenomenon of the action potential would be associated with the outer plasma membrane. However, it would be reasonable to expect that the complex internal structure in a muscle cell (compared with the simple cylindrical structure of a nerve axon or dendrite) would give rise to a more complex action potential. The transverse tubular system (or T system), apparently regarded as essentially an invagination of the outer plasma membrane (Endo, 1964, Franzini-Arm-

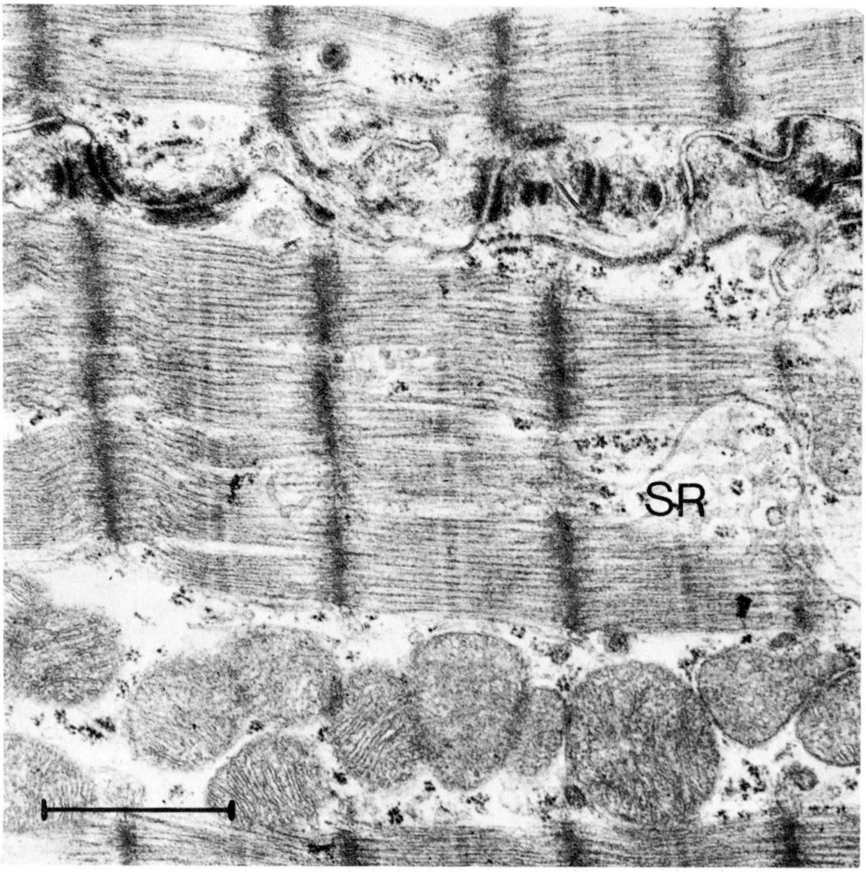

FIGURE 15. Bundle of His. Interdigitating cells with areas of close apposition and many desmosomes (region between top fibril and the wide fibril in the middle of the micrograph). Sarcoplasmic reticulum (SR) is evident. Scale = 1μ.

strong & Porter, 1964; Huxley, 1964), is believed to be part of the electrical link between the active plasma membrane and the contracting fibril. Furthermore, there is close association between the SR and T systems at the triad or dyad, and in the present study close association occasionally has been observed between the SR and the outer cell membrane (FIGURE 14). This observation has led to the inference that the action potential may be conveyed to the SR through these contacts (Peachey, 1966, Walker & Schrodt, 1966). There is evidence that membrane apposition as close as that observed at the triad represents a low resistance to ionic currents (Loewenstein & Kanno, 1964; Peachey, 1965; Loewenstein 1966). This electrical coupling could then be the mechanism that triggers the release of the Ca^{++} ions from the SR (Podolsky & Constantin, 1966), which in turn triggers the chemical reactions necessary for the contractile process in the myofibrils (Ebashi & Lipmann, 1962; Peachey, 1965). Evidence has also been produced that Ca^{++} ions are stored in the space enclosed by the SR membranes (Constantin *et al.,* 1965). If one takes this argument one step further, it is conceivable that the receipt of the action potential by the SR at the triad could trigger a Ca^{++}-selective membrane transport mechanism in the SR which might be comparable in some aspects with that responsible for the transport of Na^{+} ions in the case of the outer plasma membrane. Should this be the case, the presence of the SR could be expected to introduce an electrical effect that would modify the shape of the action potential produced by the cell, dependent in magnitude on the abundance of SR in the cell. The evidence of the present study is consistent with this idea. Electron-analogue studies also yield results that are consistent with this theory (Challice & Fry, 1966); it is also in agreement with the conclusion of Paes de Carvalho *et al.* (1966) that the cardiac action potential represents a summation of two distinct components.

The property of spontaneous depolarization, i.e., the condition in which the cell becomes self-oscillatory, appears to be governed by the ionic concentrations of the chemical environment on either side of the plasma membrane (Adelman *et al.,* 1965), and also by the properties of the membranes themselves. Little evidence along these lines can be inferred from the present study, although it is perhaps worth noting that in the nodal cells there is some evidence suggestive of a concentration of fine fibrillar components near the intracellular side of the cell membrane greater than in the other cells. It seems reasonable to suspect that this might alter the permeability properties of the membrane.

Effect of the Signal Transmitted by Neighboring Cells

In a system where a cell is a primary pacemaker (SA node) and has few contacts with other cells, the action potential is unlikely to be greatly affected by such contacts. It could be likened to an electronic oscillator coupled to a transmission line so that power is not drawn from the oscillator. Similarly, if the signal is accepted at one end of a long narrow cell (or bundle of cells) and conveyed along it and given to another cell (or cells) at the far end, when there is little or no contact along its length with other cells of different characteristics, the conduction cell (or cells) may be expected to behave like an active transmission line dissipating little energy (e.g. bundle of His and Purkinje fibers). However, where there is contact with different types of cells along the length of the path (as in the SA ring bundle), these cells cannot fail to have some effect, particularly on the velocity of propagation. Under these circumstances, it would be difficult for the impulse to travel much faster in the specialized tissue than in the surrounding tissue; hence, the suggestion that the role of the specialized fibers may be one of a *surer* pathway rather than a *faster* one (Paes de Carvalho, 1961).

The Atrioventricular Node

The AV nodal region provides a complex problem that has been analyzed in some detail in electrophysiological studies (Hoffman & Cranefield, 1960, Paes de Carvalho, 1961). The results demonstrate a slow conduction velocity of 0.05–0.02 meters per second over a distance of less than 1 mm, i.e., a very slow conduction velocity over a short distance. It has been suggested that this slow conduction "may be decremental," i.e., represent "a type of conduction in which the properties of the fiber change along its length in such a manner that the action potential becomes progressively less effective as a stimulus to the unexcited portion ahead of it" (Hoffman & Cranefield, 1960, p. 157). Evidence for this suggestion is inconclusive, but is not contradicted by any of the observations of transmembrane potentials. Hoffman and Cranefield further suggested that this decremental conduction takes place in a network of fibers of small diameter at the junction between the atrial and nodal fibers. They stated that studies of the type reported in this paper should provide a clear solution to the problem, but unfortunately, the present work shows that the solution is not as simple as it might have once appeared.

Electron microscopical observations have shown that, as Hoffman and Cranefield (1960) speculated, the cross-sectional diameter of the nodal cells is in fact smaller than that of myocardial cells, and they are not held together in bundles. This would, on the basis of nerve studies, imply a slower impulse conduction velocity, although it seems unlikely that this feature alone would produce the observed degree of slowing of the speed of pulse transmission. One is therefore led to seek other features that might be consistent with the electrophysiological observations.

Lowenstein (1966) reported extensive studies on the electrical resistance between the cytoplasm of adjacent tissue cells, and found that an abrupt resistance decrease was observed when a "tight" junction was made between two cells, in which the two plasma membranes of the opposing cells fused to form a single structural unit. These studies were made primarily on epithelial tissue, but Barr and co-workers (1965) have shown that a similar "tight" junction (or "nexus") occurs in heart-muscle cells. Lowenstein further found that the concentration of Ca^{++} ions was an important factor in the intercellular resistance. In addition, computer studies on the effect of variation of a number of parameters in the Hodgkin-Huxley equations (Hodgkin & Huxley, 1952) have indicated some conditions under which decremental conduction can occur in nerve; in terms of the ionic transport model of the action potential, this corresponds to a reduction in the sodium and potassium ionic transmembrane conductances (g_{Na} and g_K) to one-quarter or less of their normal values in these cells. Electron microscopical studies cannot provide direct evidence of these properties and can only point to observations that could be expected to be consistent with such properties.

1. There is an abundance of unorganized fine filamentous material in the cytoplasm of nodal cells, extending to the cell membrane, and possibly even preferentially greater there. This could be consistent with different transmembrane conductance properties.

2. Sarcoplasmic reticulum is scarce, and almost absent, in nodal cells. There is evidence that this structure is the site of Ca^{++} ion accumulation, and prob-

ably control. In the absence of this structure, which localizes Ca^{++} ions, it is conceivable that the Ca^{++} ion concentration could be greater in the cytoplasm, which, on the basis of Loewenstein's studies, would be consistent with a decrease in membrane permeability.

3. The nexus structure observable in most other parts of the heart is not frequent in the AV node, which would be consistent with the introduction of a time constant between the cells, and a slower rate of impulse conduction in the region.

From the standpoint of Cooley's and Dodge's (1966) computer studies, all three of these observations would be consistent with the occurrence of decremental conduction in the AV node.

It should be noted that some observations made on nodal tissue are similar to those made on embryonic heart and to others made on pathological muscle. The crude Z bands in the SA ring bundle are similar to those observed in developing myofibrils (Challice & Edwards, 1961), and the greatly enlarged Z bands seen in the AV node have been observed in muscle from patients with nemaline myopathy (Shy, 1966). Also, the unorganized fine filamentous material in the sarcoplasm has been found in dystrophic muscle (Milhorat *et al.*, 1966), where it has been identified as representing an early stage of regeneration. A comparison of these observations would seem to indicate that fibrillar development is incomplete in the nodal cells.

The morphological picture is at present incomplete. It is hoped that further studies in progress will clarify these points.

Bundle of His

It is noteworthy that the SR in the bundle of His is well developed and that it makes appositional contact with the plasma membrane. Cellular diameter is relatively large, and contact between cells in the bundle is close, with extensive desmosome attachments and nexus structures (cf. Rhodin *et al.*, 1961). The unorganized filamentous component in the cytoplasm is practically absent.

Summary

A progress report has been presented on electron microscopical studies of the structure of cells of the specialized fibers in the mammalian heart. Although this study is far from complete, an attempt has been made to correlate the structural variations observed to date with the variations in cellular electrophysiology. Particular attention has been paid to the structure and intracellular communications of the cells in the AV node in which decremental conduction is believed to occur. It is hoped that further studies will enable more precise correlations to be made.

Acknowledgments

The author is indebted to his graduate students for discussions and for some of the electron micrographs. He particularly would like to thank Dr. L. J. DeFelice for FIGURES 2 and 3, and for comments on the manuscript.

References

ADELMAN, JR., W. J., F. M. DYRO & J. P. SENFT. 1965. Spontaneous cardiac-like repetitive responses from internally perfused squid axons. Biophys. Soc. Abstr. : 14.

BARR, L., M. M. DEWEY & W. BERGER. 1965. Propagation of action potentials in the structure of the nexus in cardiac muscle. J. Gen. Physiol. **48:** 797–823.
CAESAR, R., G. A. EDWARDS & H. RUSKA. 1958. Electron microscopy of the impulse conducting system of the sheep heart. Z. Zellforsch **48:** 698–719.
CHALLICE, C. E. 1965. Some observations on the microstructure of the specialized tissue of the mammalian heart. *In* Muscle. : 71–83. Pergamon Press. Oxford, England.
CHALLICE, C. E. 1966. Studies on the microstructure of the heart. I. The sino-atrial node and the sino-atrial ring bundle. J. Roy. Micr. Soc. **85:** 1–21.
CHALLICE, C. E. & G. A. EDWARDS. 1961. The micromorphology of the developing ventricular muscle. *In* The Specialized Tissues of the Heart : 44–75. Elsevier Press, Inc. Amsterdam, The Netherlands.
CHALLICE, C. E. & D. J. I. FRY. 1966. Attempts to reproduce heart muscle action potentials by electronic circuits. Physics in Canada **22**(2): 55.
CONSTANTIN, L. L., C. FRANZINI-ARMSTRONG & R. J. PODOLSKY. 1965. Localization of calcium-accumulating structures in striated muscle fibers. Science **147:** 158–160.
COOLEY, J. W. & F. A. DODGE. 1966. Digital computer solutions for excitation and propagation of the nerve impulse. Biophys. J. **6:** 583–600.
DEFELICE, L. J. & C. E. CHALLICE. 1969. An anatomical and ultrastructural study of the electrophysiological A-V node. In preparation.
DEWEY, M. M. & L. BARR. 1962. Intercellular connection between smooth muscle cells: the nexus. Science **137:** 670-672.
DEWEY, M. M. & L. BARR. 1964. A study of the structure and distribution of the nexus. J. Cell Biol. **23:** 553–586.
EBASHI, S. & F. LIPMANN. 1962. Adenosine triphosphate-linked concentration of calcium ions in a particulate fraction of rabbit muscle. J. Cell Biol. **14:** 389–400.
ENDO, M. 1964. Entry of a dye into the sarcotubular system in muscle. Nature **202:** 1115–1116.
FAWCETT, D. W. & C. C. SELBY. 1958. Observations on the fine structure of the turtle atrium. J. Biophys. Biochem. Cytol. **4:** 63–72.
FRANZINI-ARMSTRONG, C. & K. R. PORTER. 1964. Sarcolemmal invaginations constituting the T system in fish muscle fibers. J. Cell Biol. **22:** 675–696.
GRAY, A. L. 1966. An investigation into the microstructure of an area of "specialized" atrial tissue present in the rabbit heart. M.Sc. Thesis. University of Calgary. Calgary, Alberta, Canada.
GRIMLEY, P. M. & G. A. EDWARDS. 1960. The ultrastructure of cardiac desmosomes in the toad and their relationship to the intercalated disc. J. Biophys. Biochem. Cytol. **8:** 305–318.
HODGKIN, A. L. & A. F. HUXLEY. 1952. A quantitative description of membrane current and its application to conduction and excitation in nerve. J. Physiol. (London) **117:** 500–544.
HOFFMAN, B. F. & P. F. CRANEFIELD. 1960 . *In* Electrophysiology of the Heart. McGraw-Hill Book Co. New York, N. Y.
HUXLEY, H. E. 1956. The ultra-structure of striated muscle. Brit. Med. Bull. **12:** 171–173.
HUXLEY, H. E. 1964. Evidence for continuity between the elements of the triad and extracellular space in frog sartorius muscle. Nature **202:** 1067–1071.
LING, G. N. 1962. A Physical Theory of the Living State. Blaisdell Publishing Co. New York, N. Y.
LOEWENSTEIN, W. R. 1966. Permeability of membrane junctions. Ann. N. Y. Acad. Sci. **137:** 441–472.
LOEWENSTEIN, W. R. & Y. KANNO. 1964. Studies on an epithelial (gland) cell junction. I. Modification of surface membrane permeability. J. Cell Biol. **22:** 565–586.
MERCER, E. H. 1963. A scheme for section staining in electron microscopy. J. Roy. Micr. Soc. **81:** 179–182.
MILHORAT, A. T., S. A. SHAFIQ & L. GOLDSTONE. 1966. Changes in muscle structure in dystrophic patients, carriers and normal sibling seen by electron microscopy; correlation with levels of serum creatinephosphokinase (CPK). Ann. N. Y. Acad. Sci. **138:** 246–292.
MUIR, A. R. 1957. Observations on the fine structure of the Purkinje fibres in the ventricles of the sheep's heart. J. Anat. **91:** 251–258.
PAES DE CARVALHO, A. 1961. Cellular electrophysiology of the atrial specialized tissues. *In* The Specialized Tissues of the Heart. : 115–133. Elsevier Press, Inc. Amsterdam, The Netherlands.
PAES DE CARVALHO, A. & D. F. DE ALAMEIDA. 1960. Spread of activity through the atrioventricular node. Circ. Res. **8:** 801–809.

PAES DE CARVALHO, A., B. F. HOFFMAN & W. B. LANGAN. 1966. Two components of the cardiac action potential. Nature **211**: 938–940.

PEACHEY, L. D. 1965. The transverse reticulum and transverse tubules of the frog's sartorius. J. Cell Biol. **25**: 209–232.

PEACHEY, L. D. 1966. The role of transverse tubules in excitation-contraction coupling in striated muscles. Ann. N. Y. Acad. Sci. **137**:1025–1037.

PODOLSKY, R. J. & L. L. CONSTANTIN. 1966. The internal membrane system and muscle activation. Ann. N. Y. Acad. Sci. **137**: 1038–1040

PORTER, K. R. 1961. The sarcoplasmic reticulum: Its recent history and present status. J. Biophys. Biochem. Cytol. **10**(4,II): 219–226.

REYNOLDS, E. S. 1963. The use of lead citrate at high pH as an electron opaque stain in electron microscopy. J. Cell Biol. **17**: 208–211.

RHODIN, J. A. G., P. DEL MISSIER & L. C. REID. 1961. The structure of the specialized impulse conducting system of the steer heart. Circulation **24**: 349–367.

ROBB, J. S. 1965. Comparative Basic Cardiology. Grune & Stratton. New York, N. Y.

RUSKA, H. 1965. Electron microscopy of the heart. *In* Electrophysiology of the heart. B. Taccardi & G. Marchetti, Eds. : 1–19. Pergamon Press. London, England.

SABATINI, D. D., D. BENSCH & R. J. BARRNETT. 1963. Cytochemistry and electron microscopy: The preservation of cellular ultrastructure and enzymatic activity by aldehyde fixation. J. Cell Biol. **17**: 19–58.

SANDBORN, E. B. 1966. Electron microscopy of neuron membrane systems and filaments. Canad. J. Physiol. Pharmacol. **44**: 329–338.

SHY, G. M. 1966. Chemical and morphological abnormalities in muscle disease. Ann. N. Y. Acad. Sci. **138**: 232–245.

TACCARDI, B. & G. MARCHETTI, Eds. 1965. Electrophysiology of the Heart. Pergamon Press. London, England.

TORII, H. 1962. Electron microscope observations of the S-A and A-V nodes and Purkinje fibers of the rabbit. Jap. Circ. J. **26**: 39–77.

TRAUTWEIN, W. & K. UCHIZONO. 1963. Electron microscopic and electrophysiologic study of the pacemaker in the sino-atrial node in the rabbit heart. Z. Zellforsch. **61**: 96–109.

THOENES, W. & H. RUSKA. 1960. Über leptomere Fibrillen in der Herzmuskelzelle. Z. Zellforsch. **51**: 560–570.

TRUEX, R. C. 1961. Comparative anatomy and functional considerations of the cardiac conduction system. *In* The Specialized Tissues of the Heart. : 22–43. Elsevier Press, Inc. Amsterdam, The Netherlands.

VIRAGH, S. & A. PORTE. 1960. Le Noued de Keith et Flack et les différentes fibres auriculaires de coeur du rat. Étude en microscopie optique et electronique. C. R. Acad. Sci. (Paris) **251**: 2086–2088.

VIRAGH, S. & A. PORTE. 1961a. Structure fine du tissu vecteur du rat. Z. Zellforsch. **55**: 263–281.

VIRAGH, S. & A. PORTE. 1961b. Elements nerveux intracardiaques et innervation du myocarde. Étude au microscope electronique du coeur du rat. Z. Zellforsch. **55**: 282–296.

WALKER, S. M. & G. R. SCHRODT. 1966. T system connections with the sarcolemma and sarcoplasmic reticulum. Nature **211**: 935–938.

WENSING, C. J. G. 1965. Evidence for neurogenic conduction in the mammalian heart. Nature **207**: 1375–1377.

ULTRASTRUCTURE OF HEART MUSCLE UNDER PATHOLOGICAL CONDITIONS*

R. Poche†

Pathologisches Institut der Universität Düsseldorf, Düsseldorf, Germany

The electron microscope has afforded insight into the ultrastructure of normal heart muscle, making possible a new understanding of the submicroscopical cellular pathology of the heart. This subject has recently been investigated by many research workers with great success. It would be quite impossible to give a comprehensive review of the submicroscopical pathology of the myocardium in this paper; therefore I shall confine myself to my own work, the results of which can be classified as: (1) changes in size and shape of the heart, (2) disorders of the myocardial electrolyte metabolism, and (3) disorders of myocardial energy exchange.

Changes in Heart Size and Shape

In classical pathology the anatomical basis of cardiac failure is dilatation of the heart. Two forms of dilatation are distinguishable: tonogenic and myogenic. "Tonogenic" dilatation can be produced experimentally by raising the extracellular potassium concentration. "Myogenic" dilatation usually develops gradually as a result of irreversible "plastic" displacements of muscle cells within the framework of the myocardium (*Gefügedilatation* of Linzbach).[1,2] Submicroscopically, myogenic dilatation is associated with changes of the intercalated discs *(Glanzstreifen)* which we call "dehiscences of the intercalated discs" *(Glanzstreifen-Dehiscenzen)*.[3]

The muscle cells of the heart are joined in line to form a myocardial fiber, and are firmly coupled together by interdigitation of neighboring cells at the level of the intercalated discs. If these junctions are loosened, the myocardial fiber will lengthen, and the heart dilates (FIGURE 1).[4,5] Dehiscences of the intercalated discs were found during electron microscopical studies of auricular appendages from patients with atrial septal defects or in cases of rheumatic mitral stenosis.[3] Overdosage with cortisol and aldosterone[6] also produced dehiscences of intercalated discs; orciprenaline sulfate or metaproterenol[7] (Alupent®)‡ had a similar effect, but to a lesser degree. Tonogenic dilatation can lead to myogenic dilatation, as confirmed by electron microscopical studies: Severe dehiscences of intercalated discs were seen after experimental cardioplegia induced by potassium citrate,[4,8,9] the method of induced cardiac arrest known to cause extreme degrees of cardiac dilatation.[10]

Atrophy, defined as diminution of the functioning mass of a previously normal myocardium, is usually an adaptation to reduced work. Localized atrophy is seen in certain valvular diseases, and diffuse atrophy in hypotension, senility, starvation, and cachexia. Rats fed on a diet that was insufficient in quantity, although qualitatively adequate, had their body weights reduced by about 50% in one group in 27 days (rapid emaciation) and in another group

* This work was supported in part by the Deutsche Forschungsgemeinschaft, Bad Godesberg, BRD.

† Present address: Pathologisches Institut der Städtischen Krankenanstalten Bielefeld, 48 Bielefeld, Oehlmühlenstrasse 26, BRD.

‡ Distributed by C. H. Boehringer Sohn, 6507 Ingelheim/Rhein, Germany.

in 52 days (slow emaciation).[3] The rats showed uniform atrophy of all organs, including the heart, without complicating edema. The myocardial fibers were 3–8 μ wide—only one-half their normal size—but the myofibrils were not significantly narrowed although less numerous. The mitochondria contained increased amounts of dark granules. The ratio of mitochondria to myofibrils was 0.85 in the control rats, but after rapid emaciation it fell to 0.65, and after slow emaciation to 0.50.[11]

In the shrunken myocardial fibers there were signs of myofibril breakdown, i.e., widening of the spaces between the myofilaments, and degenerative changes in the mitochondria with deposition of fine pigment granules. Lipofuscin, dense bodies, and osmiophilic bodies were increased, and the sarcoplasm contained strongly contrasting fine particles, up to 100 Å in diameter, which represented micelles of iron hydroxide liberated by the breakdown of myoglobin. The endoplasmic reticulum was somewhat increased, and the Golgi apparatus was usually very prominent, evidently unaffected by the atrophy. The nuclei of the myocardial cells were smaller than usual and had folded nuclear membranes with deep indentations.[3]

Hypertrophy, defined as an increase in the functioning mass of a previously normal myocardium, is usually an adaptation to increased work. The increase in mass is brought about by enlargement of each individual muscle cell. There is, however, a limit in size beyond which cells cannot grow, and this means that the heart has a critical weight; Linzbach gives this as about 500 g in man.[12] This limit in size is also referred to by Schoenmackers[13] as the upper myocardial limit weight, which he gives as 550 ± 50 g. Any enlargement of the heart beyond this limit can be achieved only by multiplication of cells, i.e., hyperplasia. As has been shown by light microscopical studies, the enlargement of myocardial cells takes place in small steps. Each step is preceded by a slight increase in the permeability of the cell membrane and an intake of water. Then the cell builds up an additional supply of various internal structures, such as myofibrils.[14] These findings have been confirmed by electron microscopy of

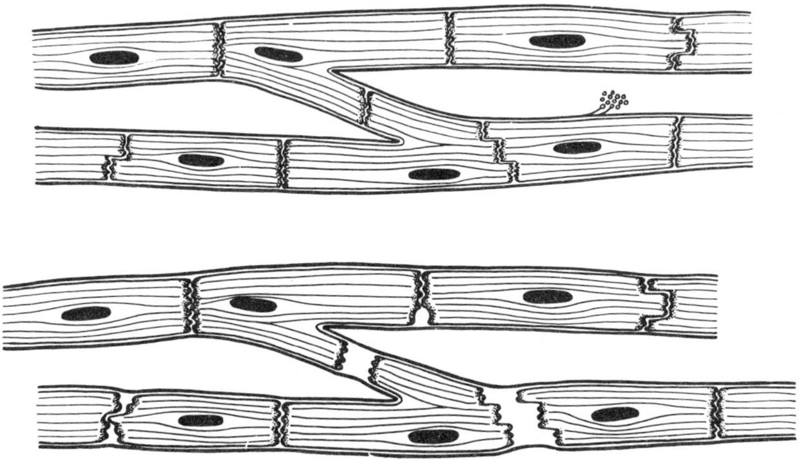

FIGURE 1. Scheme of the cellular architecture of the myocardial fibers. The upper figure shows the normal condition; the lower figure shows dehiscences of the intercalated discs, which cause dilatation of the heart (after Meessen and Poche[5]).

hypertrophied myocardial cells from the auricular appendages in cases of atrial septal defects and mitral stenosis,[3] from the walls of the right ventricle in cases of tetralogy of Fallot,[15] and from the wall of the left ventricle in rats with renal hypertension[16] or cardiac hypertrophy induced by intensive swimming exercise.[17] In myocardial cells that have enlarged up to twice their normal size, there was an increase in the subsarcolemmal sarcoplasm. The sarcoplasm was bent outward into arcades or protuded as diverticula. This was associated with an increase in the membrane vesiculation, which reflects augmented water transport or the increased permeability already referred to. The subsarcolemmal sarcoplasm contained increased numbers of ribosomes and ergastoplasmic membranes, which are, of course, not normally present in adult heart muscle. The transverse tubules were dilated or enlarged, and contained fine granular material. The myofibrils were not much thicker than those in normal myocardial cells, but they were more numerous. In such muscle cells, the ratio of mitochondria to myofibrils was smaller than normal. In rats with renal hypertension, the same ratio steadily diminished if the hypertension persisted, even though there was no further increase in hypertrophy. Hypertrophic myocardial cells usually contained numerous dense bodies and lipofuscin granules. Their nuclei were enlarged, and the nuclear membranes were often indented.

There are certain cases of idiopathic cardiac hypertrophy in which none of the known causes of hypertrophy can be found. A special subgroup has been split off from these cases[18] and is now referred to as "idiopathic hypertrophic subaortic stenosis"[19] or obstructive cardiomyopathy.[20] Five cases of this type were recently studied by light and electron microscopy.[21] In the hypertrophic area the muscle fibers branched more often than usual and showed an increase in the "intercalated sarcolemmas" *(Zwischensarkolemme)*. The myocardial cells were 25–50 μ wide. Electron microscopy revealed variable thickness of the myofibrils, and in some areas an increase in mitochondria, which were arranged in irregular clumps. The transverse tubules were enlarged and dilated, with the result that they sometimes fused and then appeared to run along the long axis of the muscle fibers. There were no sharp distinctions between the enlarged transverse tubules and the intercalated sarcolemmas. The subsarcolemmal sarcoplasm contained numerous glycogen granules and ergastoplasmic membranes. There were indications that new myofilaments were being formed. All these findings point to greatly enhanced growth activity, of a kind usually seen only in embryonic hearts (FIGURE 2).

Disorders of Myocardial Electrolyte Metabolism

The normal process of cardiac contraction depends on the maintenance of a constant ionic milieu. Disorders of myocardial electrolyte metabolism lead to functional impairment, and ultimately to heart failure. One of these disorders is potassium deficiency. By dietary deprivation of potassium it was possible to produce small areas of myocardial necrosis in animals.[22-27] Rats fed for 41 days on a diet deficient in potassium, but otherwise adequate,[3] were studied with electron microscopy; nearly all the myofibrils in the hearts of these rats were found to be somewhat slacker than usual, with the result that, in addition to the Z and M lines, the I and H bands were clearly recognizable. After long-continued potassium deficiency, two changes occurred. In some cells, there was severe edema with destruction of the myofibrils. Although some mitochondria were usually still well preserved, there was obviously a tendency toward cellular necrosis. In other cells, the contractile substance broke down into an

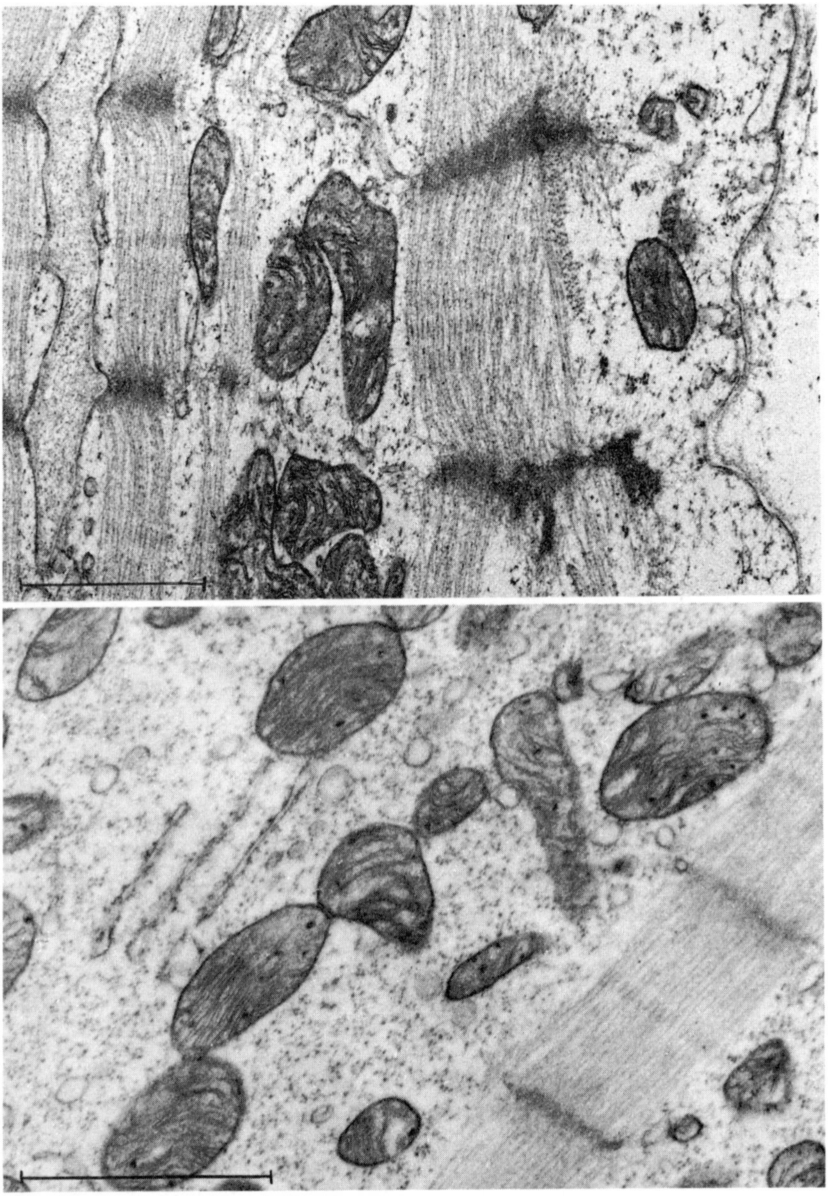

FIGURE 2. Hypertrophic myocardium in two cases of idiopathic hypertrophic subaortic stenosis. (*Top*) Newly formed myofilaments within the subsarcolemmal sarcoplasm. On the left side, a so-called intermediate sarcolemma. (*Bottom*) Ergastoplasmic membranes within the sarcoplasm. × 33,000.

amorphous nonfibrillary mass, and there was an increased number of undifferentiated structures resembling small vacuoles. Even in these cells, there were well-preserved mitochondria. These changes may be referred to as "dedifferentiation."

Perfusion of the coronary vessels with potassium chloride caused cardiac arrest. Other than a slight dilatation of the transverse tubules, the ultrastructure of the myocardium remained unaltered.[28] We observed a pronounced increase in the myocardial concentration of potassium in rats after intraperitoneal (i.p.) injections of hydrocortisone in doses of 10 mg/100 g of body weight daily for 16–23 days, although the serum potassium rose only slightly. After prolonged overdosage with hydrocortisone, the myocardial cells were slightly hypertrophic. The mitochondria contained more granules than usual, and showed signs of increased osmotic activity: The cristae of the mitochondria were densely packed together and often showed concentric layering, but beneath the external membrane there were often patches of low density which developed into large vacuoles. Despite this marginal vacuolization, the cristae of the mitochondria remained visible for a considerable time, forming coherent packages that still contained mitochondrial granules.[6] These findings were unlike the changes seen under conditions of hypoxia, in which marginal mitochondrial swelling and membrane destruction were associated with loss of granules.[8,15] After administration of aldosterone, there was some loss of potassium in the myocardium, accompanied by a rise in the sodium concentration, but the mitochondrial granules nevertheless increased in number.[6] Prolonged osmotic stress, produced by daily i.p. injections of a 25% solution of sodium phosphate (NaH_2PO_4), caused wasting with atrophy of the myocardial cells. The rats finally developed uremia, and microthrombi appeared in the myocardial capillaries.[6]

If calcium was removed by perfusion with potassium citrate, the ultrastructure of the myocardium was not too affected, with only the mitochondria losing their granules and the intercalated discs rupturing at many points, as noted previously.[4,8]

Disorders of Myocardial Energy Exchange

The term "hypoxidosis"[29] is used to define all disturbances of oxidation processes within the cell. Three types can be distinguished: hypoxidosis caused by enzyme failure, hypoxidosis caused by hypoxia, and hypoxidosis caused by substrate deficiency.

Dysenzymatic hypoxidosis of the myocardium caused by phosphorus poisoning led to dilatation of the endoplasmic reticulum and severe mitochondrial swelling. The mitochondrial granules disappeared, and fat droplets became numerous.[3]

Lack of oxygen caused by a brief stay in a low-pressure (hypobaric) chamber revealed so-called hypoxic changes in the myocardium of the rabbit[30] and of the rat.[31] There was a loss of glycogen, and cell edema with pronounced dilatation of the endoplasmic reticulum, mitochondrial swelling, and shrinkage (zonal supercontractions), relaxation, or splitting of the myofibrils. The capillaries were greatly narrowed, or even blocked by edematous swelling of their endothelial cells (FIGURE 3). But not all of the endothelial cells were involved by the edema: Swollen cells and unaffected cells could be found side by side. The endothelial edema persisted for a considerable time and was still present 24 hours after the rats had left the low-pressure chamber.[32] Treatment with

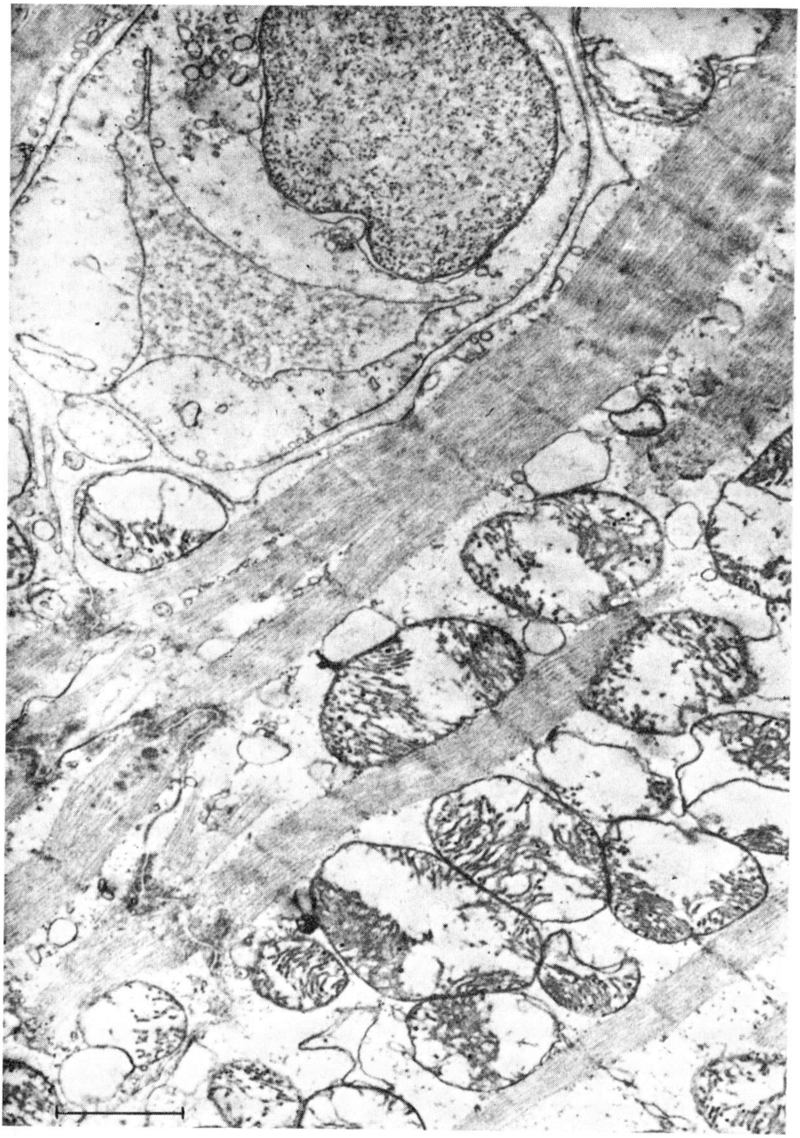

FIGURE 3. Myocardium of the rat after exposure to low atmospheric pressure at an altitude of 30,000 ft for 30 minutes. So-called hypoxic changes of the myocardial cells: clearing of the sarcoplasm, swelling of the endoplasmic reticulum, and swelling of the mitochondria with marginal destruction of their cristae. In the left upper corner there is edematous swelling of the endothelium of a capillary, causing marked narrowing of the lumen. × 17,000.

dipyridamole (Persantin®) § in therapeutic doses immediately before putting the rats into the low-pressure chamber reduced these hypoxic changes;[31,33] metaproterenol prevented them almost entirely.[7,31] The "protective effect" of these drugs on the myocardium is presumably indirect, because electron microscopical studies have shown that after pretreatment with dipyridamole, there was very little edema of the capillary endothelium, and after treatment with metaproterenol, edema was almost totally absent, even after repeated exposures to low pressures.[7,31-34]

To clarify the pathogenesis of the so-called hypoxic changes, further work in isolated empty beating hearts of rats (Langendorff-hearts) was carried out in collaboration with Professor Lochner and Doctor Arnold of the Physiologisches Institut der Universität Düsseldorf. Perfusion of the coronary system with Krebs-Henseleit solution[35] equilibrated with 95% O_2 and 5% CO_2 ("basic perfusion") did not change the ultrastructure of the myocardium. These findings are in accord with previous results of Lindner and Wellensiek.[36] After anoxic perfusion of the coronary arteries (hypoxidosis by hypoxia), the myocardium of the isolated heart, still beating, but empty of blood and kept in oxygen-free surroundings, showed no ultrastructural changes except loss of mitochondrial granules (FIGURE 4).[28] This may mean that the lack of oxygen cannot be the only cause of the so-called hypoxic changes; therefore, other conditions were examined. After perfusion with glucose-free fluid (hypoxidosis by substrate deficiency), the ultrastructure again remained quite normal; even the mitochondrial granules were still present, and the only change was the disappearance of most of the fat droplets (FIGURE 5, top).[37]

Hypercapnia (hypercarbia), induced by equilibrating the perfusion fluid with 80% O_2 and 20% CO_2, caused only very mild changes, such as slight clearing of the sarcoplasm, slight dilatation of the endoplasmic reticulum, and some reduction of the mitochondrial granules (FIGURE 6, top). When the perfusion fluid was equilibrated with 100% CO_2 the mitchondrial granules disappeared, just as they did in simple anoxia.[38] Interruption of coronary perfusion, such as in general or diffuse myocardial ischemia, led to cardiac arrest. In addition, electron microscopy revealed only very mild changes, such as slight clearing of the sarcoplasm, mild dilatation of the endoplasmatic reticulum, and slight clearing of the mitochondrial matrix in some areas, but total loss of mitochondrial granules. In comparison with the so-called hypoxic lesions following exposure to hypobaric pressure, however, these changes were remarkably mild.[38] The same mild changes were seen in hearts perfused in glucose-free fluid working against an intracardiac pressure of 78 mm Hg (FIGURE 5, bottom).[37]

In the isolated heart, severe so-called hypoxic changes were found only in areas where the capillaries had collapsed (FIGURE 7) or where they had been narrowed or blocked by edema of their endothelial cells. (FIGURE 6, bottom).[34]

In hearts fixed by perfusion with osmium tetroxide, areas remained pale where the capillaries were shut down. By contrast, the other areas of the myocardium, where the capillaries were open, turned black immediately. Under electron microscopical examination, myocardial cells in the pale areas invariably showed severe, so-called hypoxic, changes (FIGURES 6 bottom, and 7).[28] The extent of the pale areas varied according to the experimental conditions; the largest pale areas were seen in hypercapnia.[38] Arnold and colleagues[39] showed that an increase in coronary perfusion pressure had an positive inotropic effect

§ Now spelled Persantine®; distributed by Geigy Pharmaceuticals, Ardsley, N. Y.

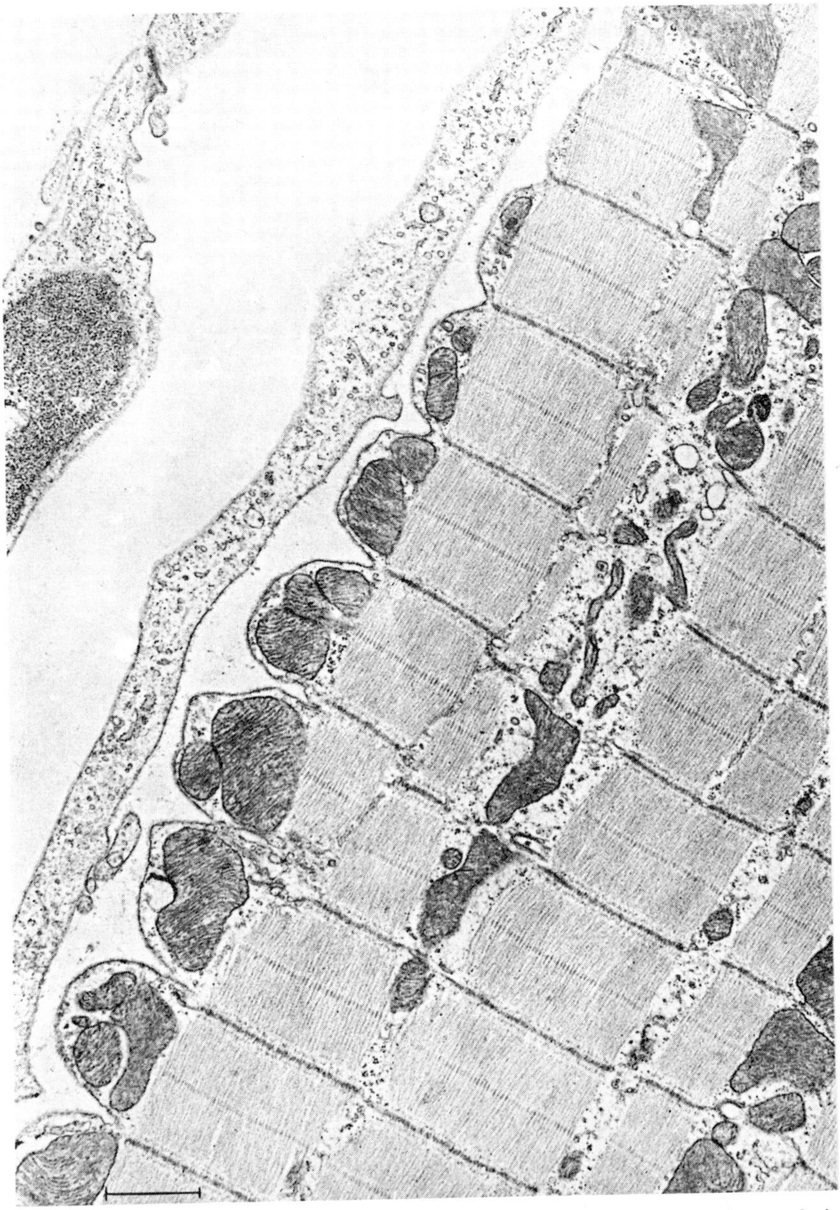

FIGURE 4. Isolated, empty beating heart of the rat (Langendorff-heart) after perfusion without oxygen for 30 minutes. Loss of the granules of the mitochondria, but otherwise no significant changes. On the left side, a well-defined capillary. × 13,000.

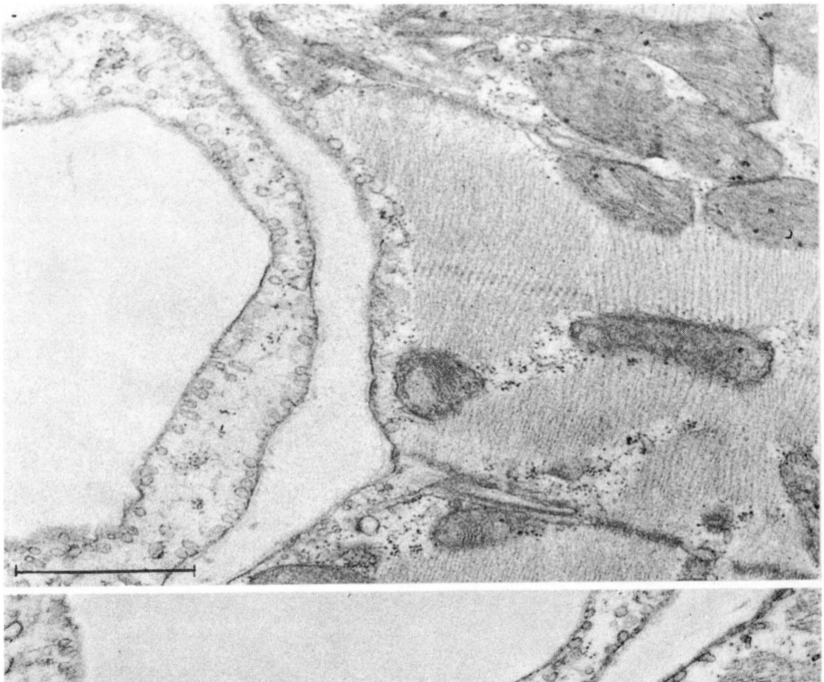

FIGURE 5. (*Top*) Isolated, empty beating heart of the rat after perfusion with glucose-free fluid for 30 minutes. Nearly normal myocardium. On the left side, a well-defined capillary. × 24,000. (*Bottom*) Isolated heart beating against an intracardial pressure of 78 mm Hg after perfusion with glucose-free fluid for 30 minutes. Light clearing of the sarcoplasm and slight spotted clearing of the matrix of the mitochondria. × 24,000.

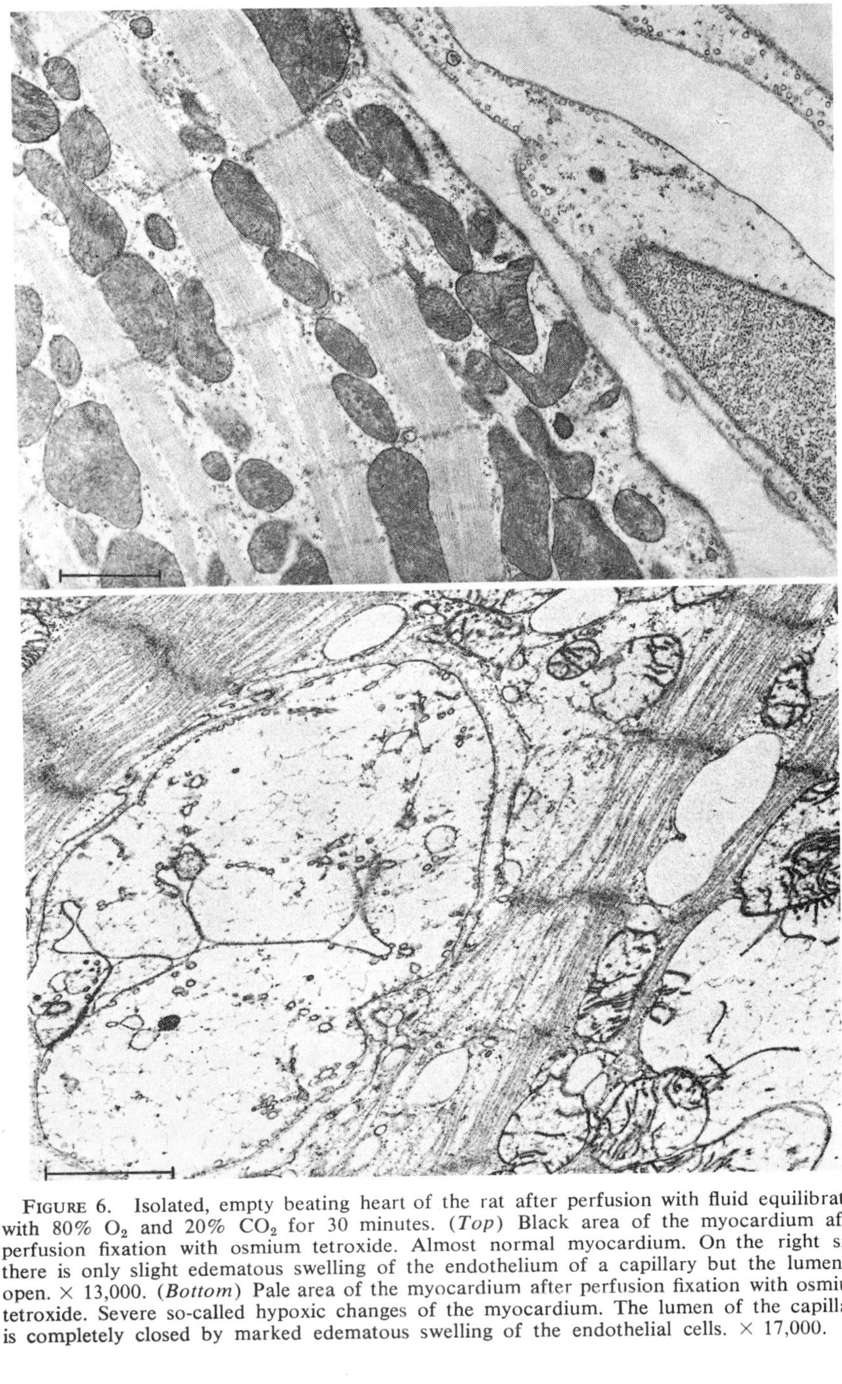

FIGURE 6. Isolated, empty beating heart of the rat after perfusion with fluid equilibrated with 80% O_2 and 20% CO_2 for 30 minutes. (*Top*) Black area of the myocardium after perfusion fixation with osmium tetroxide. Almost normal myocardium. On the right side there is only slight edematous swelling of the endothelium of a capillary but the lumen is open. × 13,000. (*Bottom*) Pale area of the myocardium after perfusion fixation with osmium tetroxide. Severe so-called hypoxic changes of the myocardium. The lumen of the capillary is completely closed by marked edematous swelling of the endothelial cells. × 17,000.

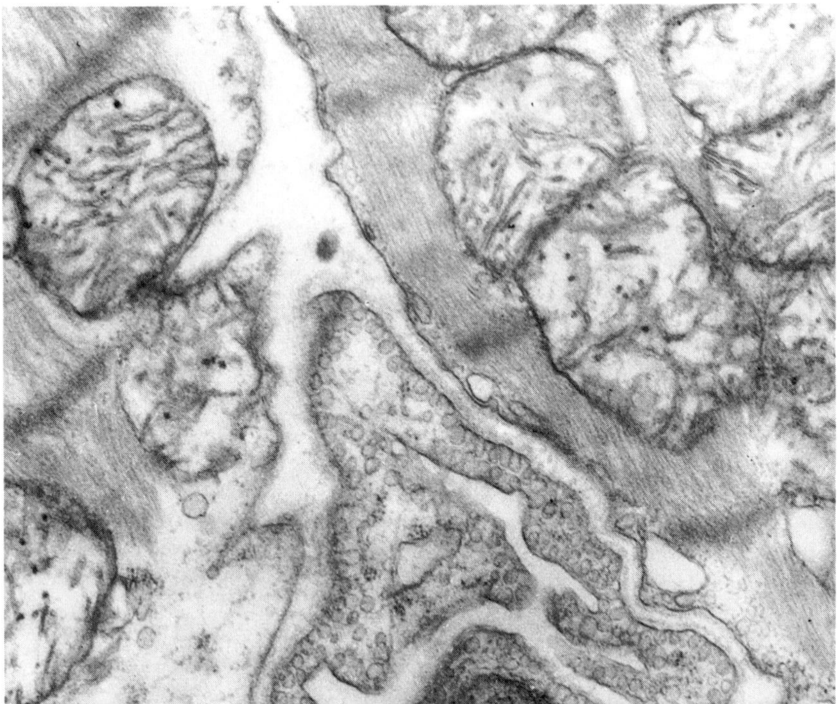

FIGURE 7. Isolated, empty beating heart of the rat after perfusion for 30 minutes with Krebs-Henseleit solution equilibrated with 95% O_2 and 5% CO_2. Pale area of the myocardium after perfusion fixation with osmium tetroxide. Moderate so-called hypoxic changes of the myocardial cells. The capillary is collapsed. × 32,000.

on the heart. In other investigations, as part of the study reported in this paper, the effects of different perfusion pressures were studied. It was found that the pale areas, i.e., the inadequately perfused areas of the myocardium, were most extensive when the perfusion pressure was 40 cc of water. When the pressure was raised to 120 cc of water, the pale areas were quite inconspicuous.

The findings in rats exposed to low atmospheric pressure, with or without pretreatment with dipyridamole or metaproterenol, and the changes in isolated rat hearts make clear that the so-called hypoxic changes of the myocardium—loss of glycogen, edema of the myocardial cells with dilatation of the endoplasmic reticulum, swelling of the mitochondria with loss of mitochondrial granules, and shrinkage and splitting of the myofibrils—depend largely on the state of the blood capillaries. These changes are found wherever the capillaries have collapsed as a result of inadequate perfusion pressures or where they have been narrowed or blocked by endothelial edema. On the other hand, these changes do not occur, even in the presence of diffuse myocardial anoxia, if the capillaries are kept well filled and patent. From these findings one may conclude that the so-called hypoxic lesions, occurring in hearts that are still beating, are really caused by ischemia at the capillary level. Whenever capillary flow ceases, in addition to oxygen deficiency, all other physiological substrates are unavailable to the myocardium. At the same time, acid metabolites accumulate in the nonperfused tissue, owing to the absence of the normal "flushing effect." Furthermore, this process is complicated by the important role of other factors, such as oxygen requirements, (which depend on the rate of cell metabolism), work load, temperature, and perfusion pressures. Thus, the so-called hypoxic lesions are the result of a complex of conditions, including hypoxia or anoxia.

References

1. LINZBACH, A. J. 1947. Mikrometrische und histologische Analyse hypertropher menschlicher Herzen. Virchow. Arch. Path. Anat. **314**: 574–594.
2. LINZBACH, A. J. 1956. Uber das Längenwachstum der Herzmuskelfasern und ihre Kerne in Beziehung zur Herzdilatation. Virchow. Arch. Path. Anat. **328**: 165–181.
3. POCHE, R. 1958. Submikroskopische Beiträge zur Pathologie der Herzmuskelzelle bei Phosphorvergiftung, Hypertrophie, Atrophie und Kaliummangel. Virchow. Arch. Path. Anat. **331**: 165–248.
4. POCHE, R. 1960. Die submikroskopische Morphologie des Herzmuskels unter pathologischen Bedingungen. Acta Tertii Europaei de Cordis Scientia Conventus, Roma, Pars prior: 99–109. Excerpta Medica. Amsterdam, The Netherlands.
5. MEESSEN, H. & R. POCHE. 1963. Pathomorphologie des Myokard. *In* Das Herz des Menschen. W. Bargmann & W. Doerr, Eds. **2**: 644–734. Thieme. Stuttgart, Germany.
6. NIENHAUS, H., R. POCHE & E. REIMOLD. 1963. Elektrolytverschiebungen, histologische Veränderungen der Organe und Ultrastruktur des Herzmuskels nach Belastung mit Cortisol, Aldosteron und primärem Natriumphosphat bei der Ratte. Virchow. Arch. Path. Anat. **337**: 245–269.
7. HAUSAMEN, T.-U. & R. POCHE. 1965. Elektronenmikroskopische Untersuchungen über die Wirkung von Alupent auf die Ultrastruktur des Herzmuskels der Ratte. Virchow. Arch. Path. Anat. **339**: 225–233.
8. LÖHR, B., H. MEESSEN & R. POCHE. 1960. Elektronenmikroskopische Untersuchungen des Herzmuskels vom Hund bei experimentellem Herzstillstand durch Kaliumcitrat und Anoxie. Arch. Kreislaufforsch. **33**: 108–137.
9. HOELSCHER, B., H. O. JUST & H. J. MERKER. 1961. Studies by electron microscope on various forms of induced cardiac arrest in dog and rabbit. Surgery **49**: 492–499.
10. ROSS, JR., J., J. W. GILBERT, JR., E. H. SHARP & A. G. MORROW. 1958. Elective cardiac arrest during total body perfusion: The relationship of elevated intracardiac pressures during arrest to subsequent myocardial function and pathologic pulmonary changes J. Thorac. Cardiov. Surg. **36**: 534–543.

11. POCHE, R. & D. MÖNKEMEIER. 1962. Quantitative morphologische Untersuchungen über das Verhältnis Mitochondrien: Myofibrillen in den Herzmuskelzellen bei Hungeratrophie und im Winterschlaf. Virchow. Arch. Path. Anat. **335**: 271–281.
12. LINZBACH, A. J. 1948. Herzhypertrophie und kritisches Herzgewicht. Klin. Wschr. **26**: 459–463.
13. SCHOENMACKERS, J. 1958. Vergleichende quantitative Untersuchungen über den Faserbestand des Herzens bei Herz- und Herzklappenfehlern sowie Hochdruck. Virchow. Arch. Path. Anat. **331**: 3–22.
14. LINZBACH, A. J. 1950. Die Muskelfaserkonstante und das Wachstumsgesetz der menschlichen Herzkammern. Virchow. Arch. Path. Anat. **318**: 575–618.
15. POCHE, R. & H. G. OHM. 1963. Lichtmikroskopische, histochemische und elektronenmikroskopische Untersuchungen des Herzmuskels vom Menschen nach induziertem Herzstillstand. Arch. Kreislaufforsch. **41**: 86–135.
16. POCHE, R., C. M. DE MELLO MATTOS, H. W. REMBARZ & K. STOEPEL. 1967. Uber das Verhältnis Mitochondrien: Myofibrillen in den Herzmuskelzellen der Ratte bei Druckhypertrophie des Herzens. Virchow. Arch. Path. Anat. **344**: 100–110.
17. POCHE, R. & D. BUSSMANN. 1967. In preparation.
18. SCHMINCKE, A. 1907. Uber linksseitige muskulöse Conusstenose. Deutsch. Med. Wschr. **33**: 2082–2086.
19. BRAUNWALD, E., C. T. LAMBREW, S. D. ROCKOFF, J. ROSS, JR. & A. G. MORROW. 1964. Idiopathic hypertrophic subaortic stenosis. I. A description of the disease based upon an analysis of 64 patients. Circulation **30** (Suppl. 4): 3–119.
20. PEARSE, A. G. E. 1964. The histochemistry and electron microscopy of obstructive cardiomyopathy. Cardiomyopathies. Ciba Foundation Symposium, 1964 : 132–164. J. & A. Churchill, Ltd. London, England.
21. MEESSEN, H. & R. POCHE. 1966. Beiträge zur pathologischen Anatomie der Fallotschen Fehler und zur idiopathischen Herzhypertrophie. Anglo-German Med. Rev. In press.
22. FOLLIS, R. H., E. ORENT-KEILES and E. V. MCCOLLUM. 1942. Production of cardiac and renal lesions in rats by diet extremely deficient in potassium. Amer. J. Path. **18**: 29–39.
23. SMITH, S. G., B. BLACK-SCHAFFER & T. E. LASATER. 1950. Potassium deficiency syndrome in the rat and the dog. Arch. Path. (Chicago) **49**: 185–199.
24. FRENCH, J. E. 1952. A histological study of the heart lesions in potassium-deficient rats. Arch. Path. (Chicago) **53**: 485–496.
25. GRUNDNER-CULEMANN, A. 1952. Experimentelle und morphologische Untersuchungen über Veränderungen des Herzmuskels von Ratten bei Kalium-Mangelernährung. Arch. Kreislaufforsch. **18**: 185–210.
26. MACPHERSON, C. R. 1956. Myocardial necrosis in the potassium-depleted rat: A reassessment. Brit. J. Exp. Path. **37**: 179–285.
27. SCHRADER, G. A., C. O. PRICKETT and W. D. SALMON. 1937. Symptomatology and pathology of potassium and magnesium deficiencies in rat. J. Nutr. **14**: 85–109.
28. POCHE, R., G. ARNOLD, H.-W. REMBARZ & H. NIER. 1967. Uber den Einfluss des Sauerstoffmangels auf die Ultrastruktur des Herzmuskels im stillgestellten und im leerschlagenden isolierten Herzen der Ratte. In press.
29. STRUGHOLD, H. 1944. Hypoxydose. Klin. Wschr. **22**: 221–222.
30. MÖLBERT, E. 1957. Die Herzmuskelzelle nach akuter Oxydationshemmung im elektronenmikroskopischen Bild. Beitr. Path. Anat. **118**: 421–435.
31. POCHE, R. 1965. Elektronenmikroskopische Untersuchungen über die Veränderungen des Herzmuskels der Ratte nach Underdruck und ihre Beeinflussung durch Persantin und Alupent. Zbl. Allg. Path. **108**: 128–129.
32. HAUSAMEN, T.-U. & R. POCHE. 1965. Die Ultrastruktur des Herzmuskels der Ratte nach einmaligen und wiederholten Unterdruckversuchen. Virchow. Arch. Path. Anat. **339**: 212–224.
33. POCHE, R. & T.-U. HAUSAMEN. 1965. Uber den Einfluss von Persantin auf die Ultrastruktur des Herzmuskels der Ratte bei Uberdosierung und im Unterdruckversuch. Virchow. Arch. Path. Anat. **339**: 234–244.
34. POCHE, R. 1965. Uber die Bedeutung der Blutkapillaren für die herdförmige Anordnung von sogenannten hypoxischen Herzmuskelveränderungen. Verh. Deutsch. Ges. Path. **49**: 219–223.
35. KREBS, H. A. & K. HENSELEIT. 1932. Untersuchungen über die Harnstoffbildung im Tierkörper. Hoppe-Seyler. Z. Physiol. Chem. **210**: 33–66.
36. LINDNER, E. & H.-J. WELLENSIEK. 1959. Beitrag zur Morphologie des Zellstoffwechsels am Herzmuskel. Verh. Anat. Ges. **55**: 260–267.

37. Poche, R. & G. Arnold. 1967. Physiologische und elektronenmikroskopische Untersuchungen des isolierten Herzens der Ratte bei glukosefreier Perfusion. In preparation.
38. Poche, R., G. Arnold & H. Nier. 1967. Elektronenmikroskopische Untersuchungen des isolierten Herzmuskels der Ratte bei diffuser Ischämie und Hyperkapnie. In preparation.
39. Arnold, G., F. Kosche, K. Zinganell & W. Lochner. 1966. Beeinflussung des O_2-Verbrauches des Herzens durch den coronaren Perfusionsdruck. Pflüger. Arch. Ges. Physiol. **289:** 54.

ELECTRON MICROSCOPICAL STUDIES ON EXPERIMENTAL ISCHEMIC LESIONS OF THE HEART*

Gerhard Korb and Vladimir Totović

Department of Pathology, University of Marburg
Marburg, Germany

Electron microscopical alterations of the myocardium during or following an ischemia may be investigated by any one of the following three experimental methods: (1) permanent ligation of a coronary artery branch, (2) temporary ligation of a coronary artery branch, and (3) cardiac arrest without coronary perfusion. Since a report on the effects of a temporary ischemia on the myocardium is given by Dr. R. B. Jennings in this monograph, and since cardiac arrest is a special case—in which not only the ischemic but also other factors, such as body temperature and the method used to cause the arrest, are of importance—we should like to concentrate on the electron microscopical findings during and following the development of an experimental infarct.

Material and Methods

The experiments were performed on cats under pentobarbital sodium (Nembutal®)† narcosis with mechanically aided respiration. The anterior descending branch of the left coronary artery and its accompanying vein were ligated immediately next to the left auricle. The animals were sacrificed and the hearts removed for study at different intervals between 30 minutes and five days after the ligation.

In each case, five minutes before the hearts were removed, a 1% solution of acridine orange in phosphate buffer (pH 7.4 at 37° C) was injected intravenously at a dosage of 0.5 ml/kg of body weight. This intravital staining method colored the normal myocardium orange-brown, whereas the ischemic part was not affected (Korb *et al.,* 1965). Thus, it was possible to distinguish accurately between ischemic and nonischemic myocardium.

Tissue samples taken from the center and periphery of the ischemic zone were fixed with buffered osmic acid partly according to the methods described by Caulfield (1957) and Millonig (1962), embedded in Vestopal W, and sectioned on a Porter-Blum ultramicrotome. The sections were stained with lead citrate according to the method described by Reynolds (1963). A Siemens Elmiscop I was used for observation.

Results

Results of the investigation show that an ischemia in the heart-muscle cells can cause two forms of necrobiosis, the first form occurring mainly in the center of the ischemic zone and the second at its periphery.

Necrobiosis in the center of the ischemic zone is apparent 30 minutes after the ligation. As a rule, the muscle cells show a marked depletion of glycogen, a slight swelling of the mitochondria, and a dilation of parts of the sarcoplasmic reticulum, particularly of the longitudinal system (FIGURE 1). Later, an increas-

* The experiments reported in this paper were supported by a grant from the Deutsche Forschungsgemeinschaft.

† Distributed by Abbott Laboratories, North Chicago, Ill.

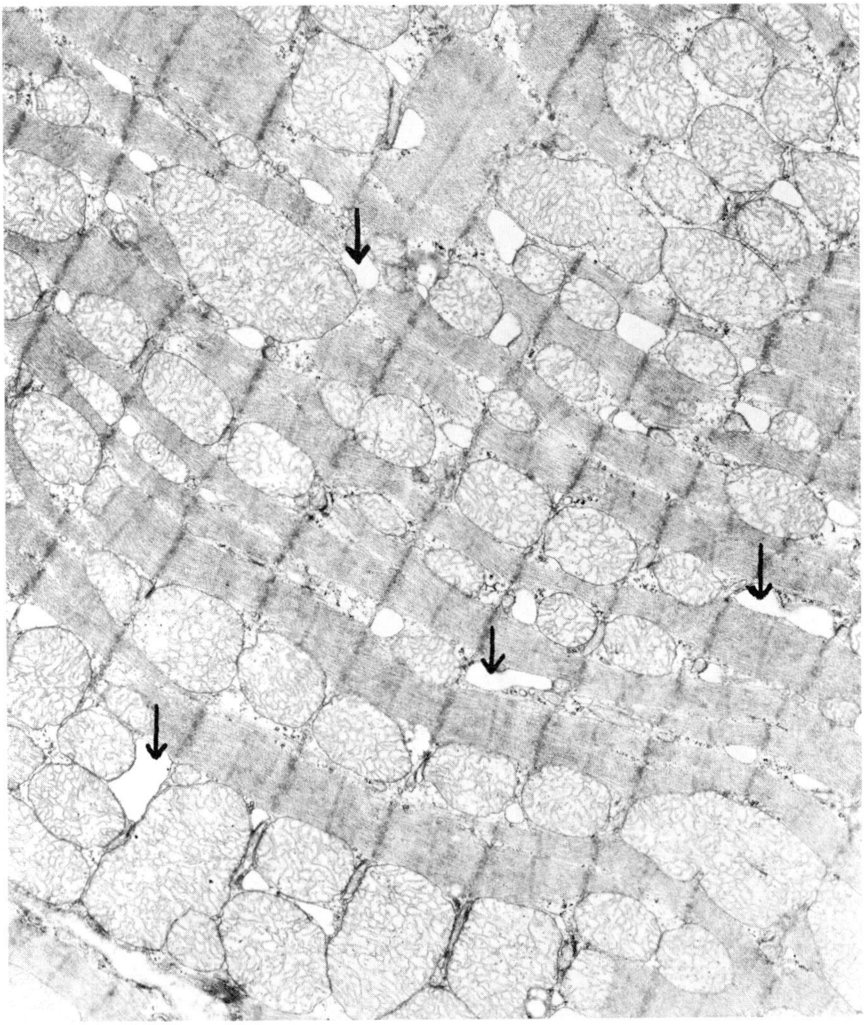

FIGURE 1. Thirty minutes after occlusion. Center of the ischemic area. The glycogen concentration of the muscle cell is diminished. Parts of the sarcoplasmic reticulum are dilated (arrows). Some of the mitochondria show a slight swelling. × 10,500.

ing relaxation of the myofibrils is observed, and I bands of varying width become visible. During the next few hours, the mitochondria show a decrease in the electron density of the matrix and a partial disappearance of the cristae. Frequently, small dense bodies appear inside the mitochondria (FIGURE 2). We cannot decide whether these are calcium deposits, as it is often supposed, or condensed mitochondrial constituents. In the nuclei of the muscle cells, condensation and margination of the nucleoplasm become apparent during these first hours after ligation. At the same time, a distinct edema can be seen in the cells. Some of the cells show a diffuse edema, occasionally combined with a separation of the myofibrils and a destruction of the myofilaments beginning in the I bands (FIGURE 3). Other cells show a localized edema that can cause an uplifting of the sarcolemma from the Z lines. The resulting spaces contain somewhat regressively altered mitochondria of various sizes. At such places a rupture of the sarcolemma can occur, with the result that cell organelles may escape into the interstitial space (FIGURE 4).

After five to six hours, large and irregular edematous spaces are present within the muscle cells. Some of the mitochondria are disintegrating and show

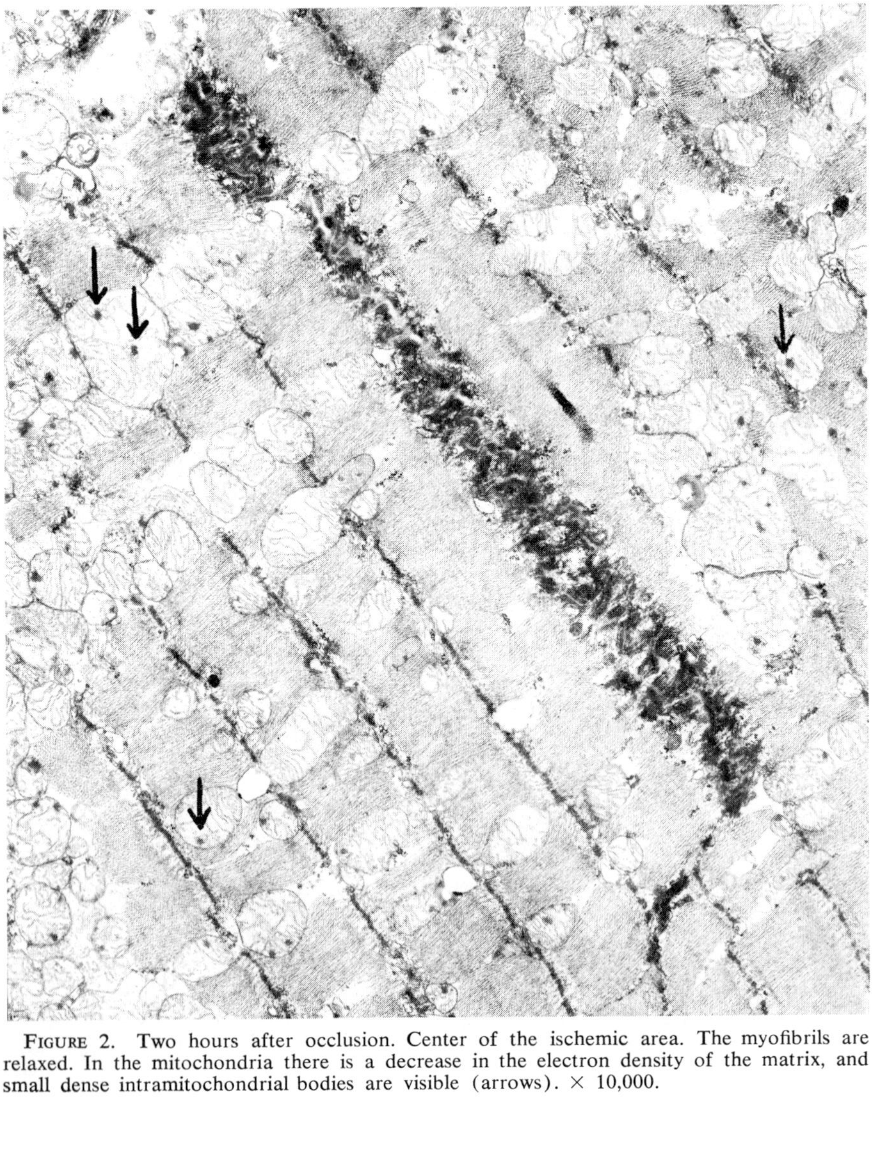

FIGURE 2. Two hours after occlusion. Center of the ischemic area. The myofibrils are relaxed. In the mitochondria there is a decrease in the electron density of the matrix, and small dense intramitochondrial bodies are visible (arrows). × 10,000.

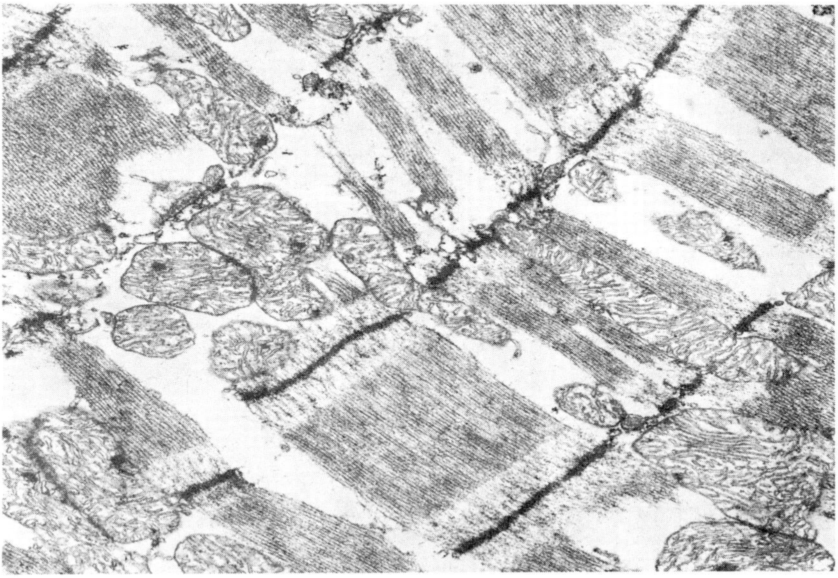

FIGURE 3. Four hours after occlusion. Center of the ischemic area. Diffuse intracellular edema, with separation of the myofibrils. Here and there a beginning destruction of the myofilaments can be seen, especially in the region of the I bands. × 15,000.

ruptures of the limiting membrane. Others are conspicuously small and condensed, so that the picture corresponds to a mitochondrial pycnosis (Wachstein & Besen, 1964). Dilated tubules of the sarcoplasmic reticulum are seldom present (FIGURES 5). For the next few hours the findings remain relatively constant. On the other hand, the alterations after more than 12–24 hours become increasingly less uniform. Some of the highly edematous cells are disintegrating (FIGURE 6), but other cells seem to be condensed and contain numerous vacuoles or, after a reduction in the number of mitochondria, show a disorganization of the myofilament structure with ruptured Z lines. After prolonged ischemia one finds cells that are evidently homogenized, since they show hardly any structures (FIGURE 7). Cells with the variety of alterations mentioned can be found right next to each other.

Thus, necrobiosis in the center of the ischemic zone is characterized essentially by an early depletion of the glycogen in the cells, a relaxation of the myofibrils, and, over a longer period of time, by an extreme intracellular edema, with dilated tubules of the sarcoplasmic reticulum and a swelling of the mitochondria. Some of the damaged cells disintegrate in connection with sarcolemmic ruptures. These alterations, which have been described in their essentials by other authors (Bryant *et al.,* 1958; Caulfield & Klionsky, 1959; Hecht *et al.,* 1961; David & Hecht, 1963; Jennings *et al.,* 1965), correspond to findings as a result of the development of cytolysis not only in the heart (Lindner & Wellensiek, 1958; Korb, 1965), but also in other organs, for example the brain (Hager, 1964), the liver (Cossel, 1966), and the kidney (Totović, 1966). In addition, there is a certain agreement with findings as a result of early changes during postmortem autolysis (Bryant *et al.,* 1958; David & David, 1965;

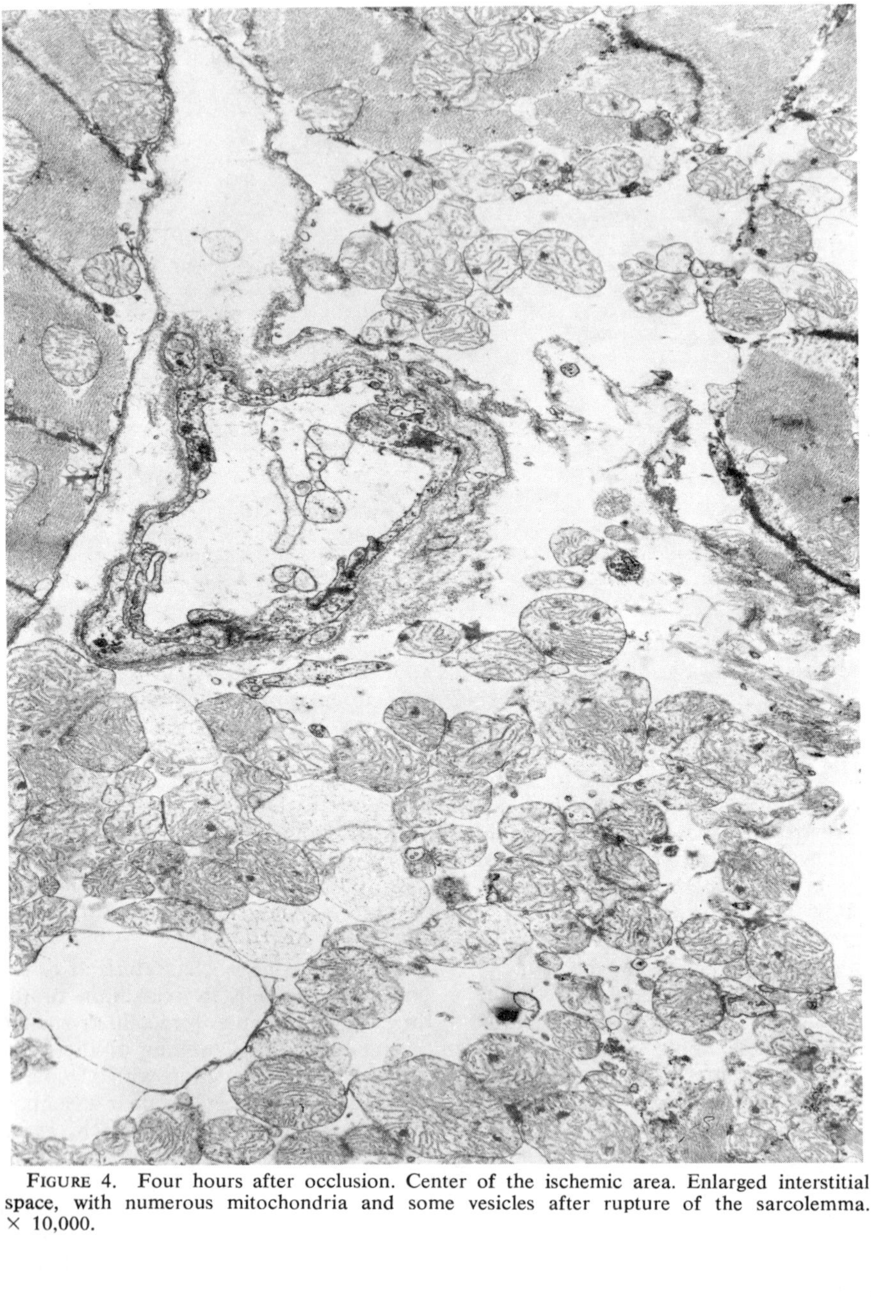

FIGURE 4. Four hours after occlusion. Center of the ischemic area. Enlarged interstitial space, with numerous mitochondria and some vesicles after rupture of the sarcolemma. × 10,000.

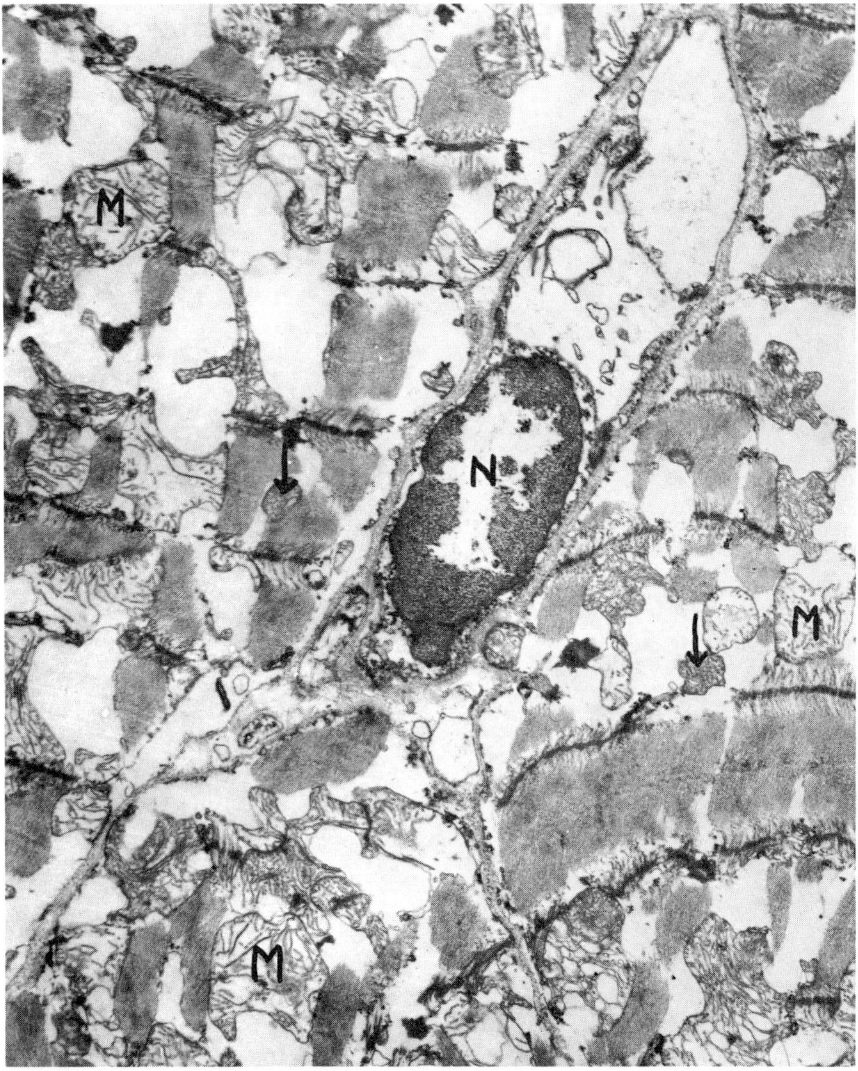

FIGURE 5. Four hours after occlusion. Center of the ischemic area. Irregular edematous spaces are present within the muscle cells. The mitochondria (M) are partially disorganized. The limiting membrane occasionally is disrupted. Some of the mitochondria are small and dense (arrows). The nucleus (N) of an endothelial cell shows condensation and margination of the nucleoplasm. × 10,000.

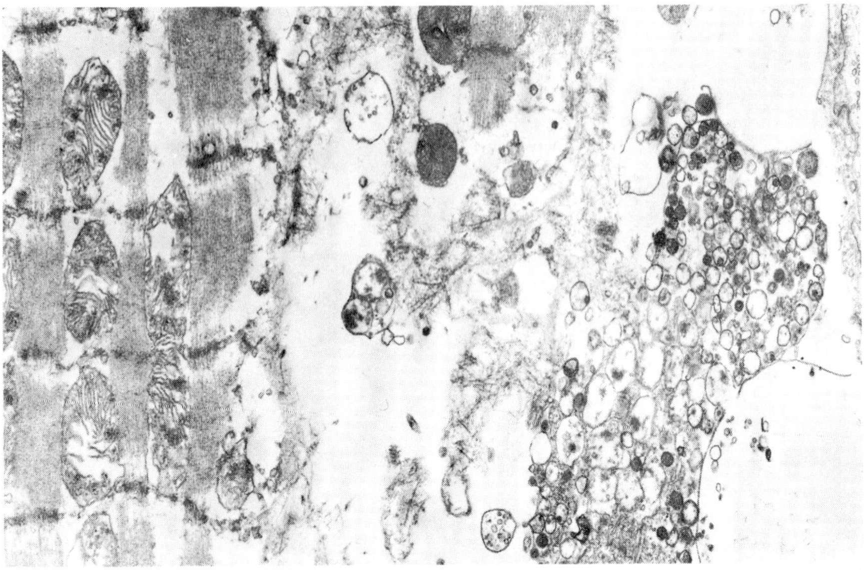

FIGURE 6. Five days after occlusion. Center of the ischemic area. Disintegrating muscle cell. × 9,000.

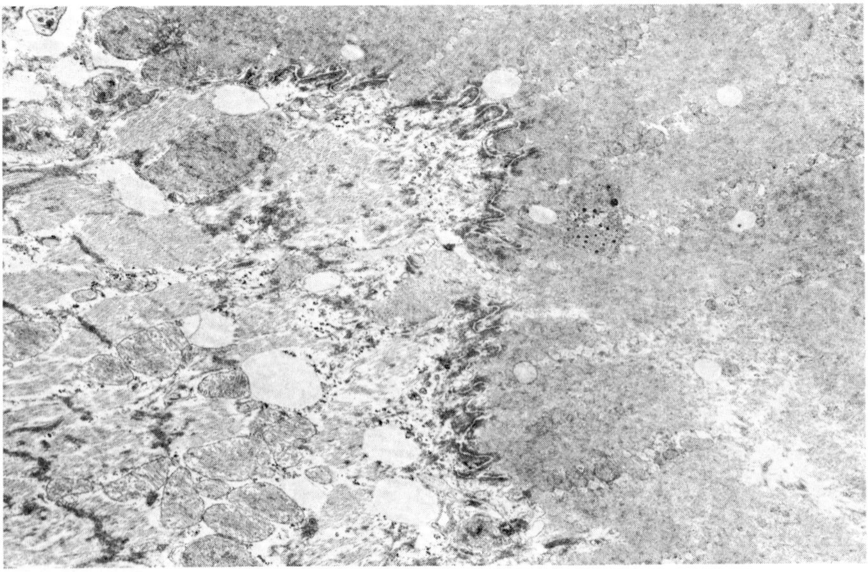

FIGURE 7. Five days after occlusion. Center of the ischemic area. Two damaged muscle cells, with disorganization of the myofilament structure (left side) and a diffuse homogenization (right side). × 8,000.

Wedell *et al.,* 1965). Only after prolonged ischemia does one find diffuse homogenization, such as that typical for a coagulation necrosis.

Necrobiosis at the periphery of the ischemic zone is also marked by an early depletion of the glycogen in the cell. In addition, there are areas in the muscle cells where the myofibrils are extremely contracted. These zones are arranged irregularly or regularly within the cells. This finding is in agreement with the frequently described "hyaline transversal bands" or "transversal contraction bands" (Büchner, 1933–1934; Saram, 1957; Molnar *et al.*, 1962; Poche & Ohm, 1963; Sommers & Jennings, 1964; Herdson *et al.,* 1965; Korb, 1965; Krug & Korb, 1966). Occasionally, such strikingly contracted zones lie near intercalated disks. The minimal presence of mitochondria in the interfibrillary spaces in this case is somewhat similar to findings in the so-called "zonal lesions" after hemorrhagic shock, described by Martin & Hackel (1966). In other portions of the injured muscle cells, a relaxation of the myofibrils occurs, as well as a distinct edema. Some of the mitochondria are swollen; dense intramitochondrial bodies are seldom seen. In the contracted zones, condensation and homogenization take place gradually (FIGURE 8). Six hours after the ligation, the edema is intensified in the noncontracted portions; at the same time there is a beginning disorganization of the myofilaments and mitochondria. After a few days of ischemia, a decrease in the number of organelles becomes noticeable in the noncontracted parts of the cells. The mitochondria still present are usually condensed (FIGURE 9).

A high degree of partial contraction of the myofibrils is notable at an early stage of ischemia in the peripheral zone of the necrobiosis. Because these contracted bands are usually found at the point of transition from contractile to noncontractile musculature, several investigators have theorized that mechanical factors play a part in the formation of the bands (Büchner, 1932; Sommers & Jennings, 1964). At a later stage of the ischemia, a change to a partially coagulative necrosis is observed; this finding was expected on the basis of early investigations with the light microscope (Büchner & von Lucadou, 1934; Grundmann, 1951; Saram, 1957). After prolonged ischemia, a distinct edema and, eventually, a disintegration of the cell organelles occur in the noncontracted portions following a relaxation of the myofibrils. We have the impression that peripheral-zone necrobiosis is similar to that described by Mölbert (1957) in low-pressure experiments. It appears that partial coagulation and lysis take place side by side in the damaged cells, a phenomenon previously mentioned by other authors (Majno *et al.,* 1960; David, 1965).

In addition to alterations in the muscle cells, ischemia also causes changes in the capillaries. Although the endothelial cells show almost normal structure, albeit with a distinct micropinocytosis, up to 30 minutes after the ligation, shortly thereafter an intracellular edema is observed, accompanied by a swelling of the mitochondria. After several hours of ischemia there are vesicles of varying sizes in the cytoplasm of the endothelial cells, as well as in the capillary lumen (FIGURE 10). After five to six hours, one sees a destruction of numerous capillaries, which is the beginning of a disintegration into fragments. These capillary alterations are characteristic of severe anoxia; they are found in organs other than the heart, as has frequently been described (Miller, 1958; David & Hecht, 1961; Hills, 1964; Kisch, 1965; Niden & Schulz, 1965; Poche, 1965).

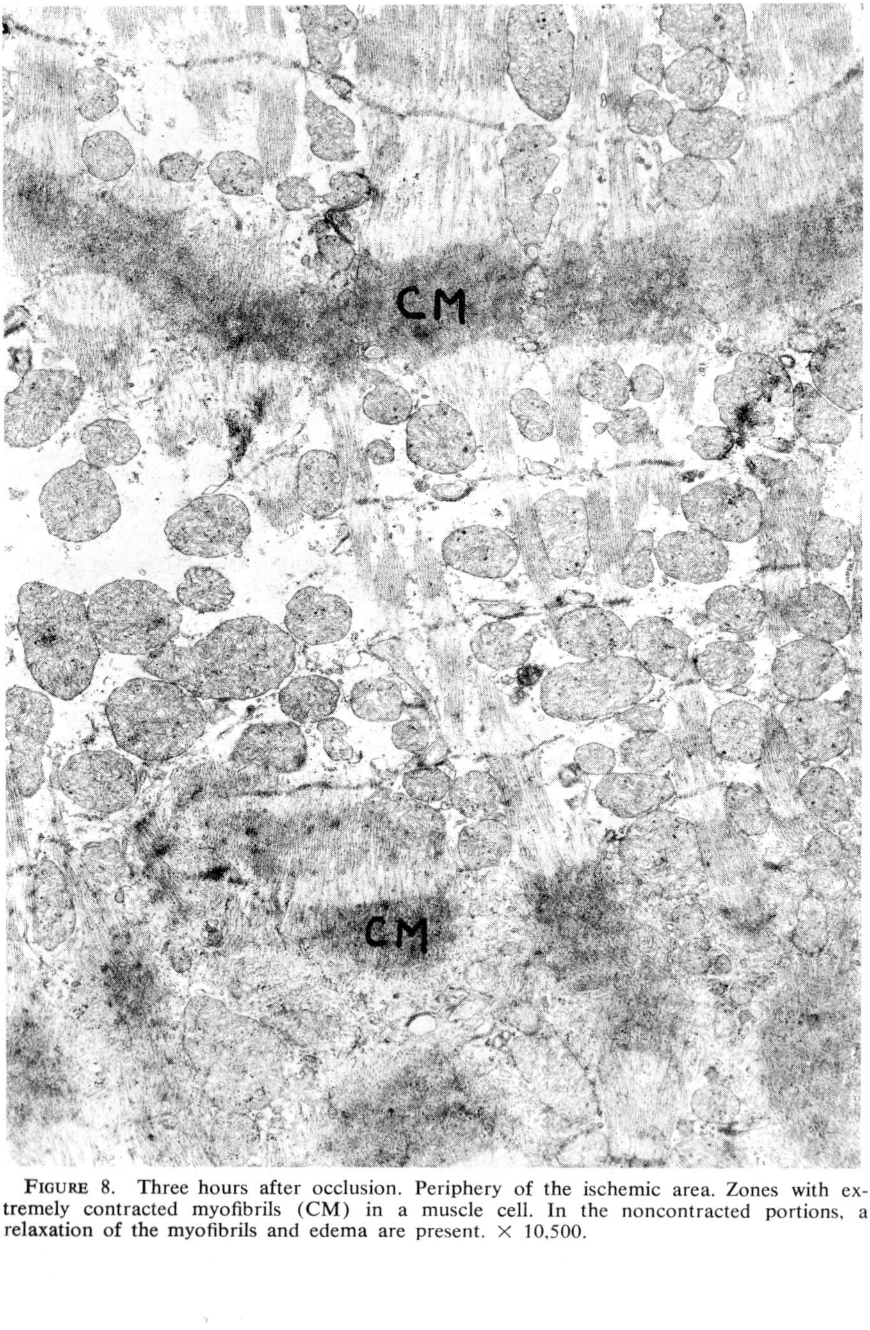

FIGURE 8. Three hours after occlusion. Periphery of the ischemic area. Zones with extremely contracted myofibrils (CM) in a muscle cell. In the noncontracted portions, a relaxation of the myofibrils and edema are present. × 10,500.

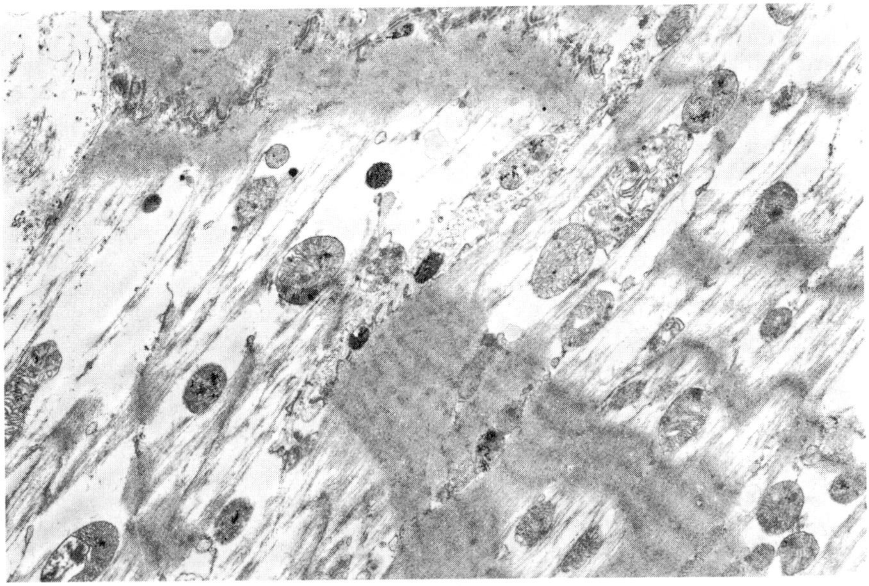

FIGURE 9. Five days after occlusion. Periphery of the ischemic area. Necrotic muscle cell, with condensed, homogenized, and disintegrating zones. × 8,000.

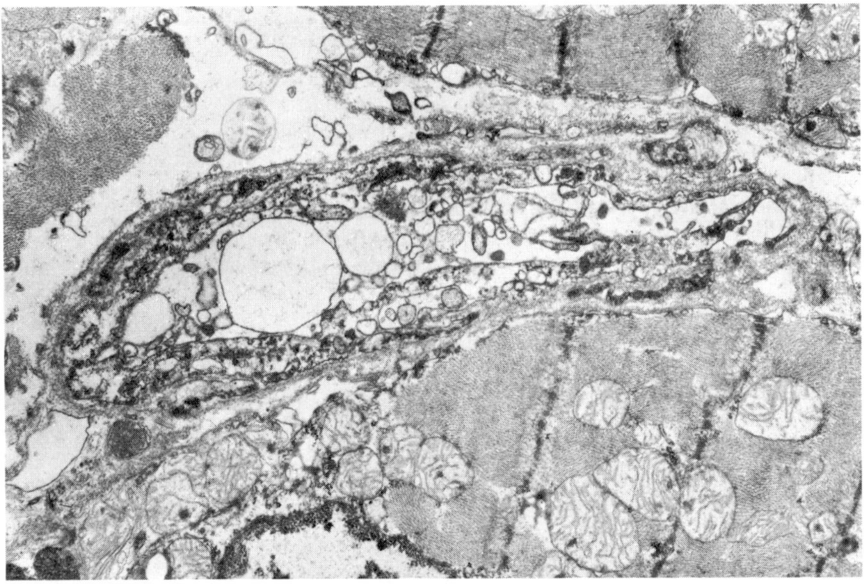

FIGURE 10. Four hours after occlusion. Center of the ischemic area. Capillary with vesicles of various size in the cytoplasm of the endothelial cells as well as in the lumen. × 9,000.

Conclusions

Electron microscopical findings at the center of an experimental ischemic infarct initially show that, apart from some small details and the changes in capillary structure, alterations in the muscle cells are characterized by a distinct intracellular edema, with dilated tubules of the sarcoplasmic reticulum and a swelling of the mitochondria. Thus, a kind of hydropic necrobiosis (Totović, 1966) is present, which is similar to the early alterations during postmortem autolysis. Subsequently, either a cytolysis or a transition to a coagulation necrosis can occur. At the periphery of the ischemia, on the other hand, a partial coagulation is observed in the muscle cells quite early; this apparently takes place in zones of strongly contracted myofibrils. In other portions of the cell, edema occurs, followed by a disorganization of the cell organelles. Thus, partial coagulation and lysis can be seen in a single damaged cell.

Both areas of necrobiosis show a distinct edema *and* a coagulation effect, but in the center of the ischemic zone, the intracellular edema and its effects predominate over a longer period of time, and the transition to coagulation occurs only after several hours, whereas at the periphery, edema and coagulation develop simultaneously in the injured cells. The difference between the development of necrobiosis in the center and at the periphery of ischemic infarcts was noted by several researchers on the basis of light microscopical investigations (Müller, 1938; Sheehan & Davis, 1958; Letterer, 1959). The reason for this difference has not been determined, and probably cannot be by electron microscopical studies alone. It can, however, be assumed that the influx of blood plasma constituents from the surrounding nonischemic myocardium into the damaged area (Schürmann, 1936; Kent, 1966; Krug & Korb, 1966) is decisively involved in causing the difference.

The electron microscopical investigations conducted to date on the ischemically damaged myocardium have undoubtedly improved our understanding of previously reported light microscopical observations, and have considerably increased our knowledge of the morphological alterations that occur during the development of an experimental cardiac infarct. However, our findings raise new questions, the answers to which must still be found: Why in a damaged cell do some of the mitochondria swell and then disintegrate, whereas others become small and dense or retain a normal appearance, even after several hours of ischemia? Why is there seldom a uniform disintegration of the myofilaments, and why are the actin filaments usually altered sooner than the myosin filaments? How can single injury cause both cytolysis and coagulation necrosis? Perhaps the most important question has been posed to date only by Jennings and his colleagues (1963): Why at no time during the development of an infarct necrosis do all the cells show the same alterations under electron microscopical examination? One is repeatedly surprised and confused less by the nature of the alteration than by the variation in its extent from cell to cell, with the result that it is almost impossible to determine the beginning of the irreversible phase of the necrobiosis in a large area. Thus, in spite of numerous electron microscopical studies, a series of morphological findings in ischemic myocardial necrosis remains difficult to evaluate and awaits explanation.

Acknowledgments

We wish to thank Mrs. Anneliese Bartelmess for her technical assistance and Mr. Heinz Staubitz for the photographic reproductions.

References

BRYANT, R. E., W. A. THOMAS & R. M. O. O'NEAL. 1958. An electron microscopic study of myocardial ischemia in the rat. Circ. Res. **6**: 699–709.

BÜCHNER, F. 1932. Die Rolle des Herzmuskels bei der Angina pectoris. Beitr. Path. Anat. **89**: 644–667.

BÜCHNER, F. 1933–1934. Das morphologische Substrat der Angina pectoris im Tierexperiment. Beitr. Path. Anat. **92**: 311–328.

BÜCHNER, F. & W. VON LUCADOU. 1934. Elektrokardiographische Veränderungen und disseminierte Nekrosen des Herzmuskels bei experimenteller Coronarinsuffizienz. Beitr. Path. Anat. **93**: 169–197.

CAULFIELD, J. B. 1957. Effects of varying vehicle for OsO_4 in tissue fixation. J. Biophys. Biochem. Cytol. **3**: 827–830.

CAULFIELD, J. B. & B. KLIONSKY. 1959. Myocardial ischemia and early infarction. An electron microscopic study. Amer. J. Path. **35**: 489–523.

COSSEL, L. 1966. Elektronenmikroskopische Befunde beim intravitalen Untergang von Leberzellen. (Beitrag zur Kenntnis von Kolliquations- und Koagulationsnekrose) Beitr. Path. Anat. **133**: 156–185.

DAVID, H. 1965. Sterben und Tod der Zelle. Monatsber. Deutsch. Akad. Wiss. **7**: 452–463.

DAVID, H. & S. DAVID. 1965. Submikroskopische Strukturveränderungen der Skelettmuskulatur während der postmortalen Autolyse. Acta Biol. Med. German. **14**: 423–435.

DAVID, H. & A. HECHT. 1961. Submikroskopische Strukturveränderungen der Herzmuskelkapillaren im Infarktgebiet. Zbl. Allg. Path. **103**: 68–73.

DAVID, H. & A. HECHT. 1963. Elektronenmikroskopische Befunde an den Herzmuskelzellen der Ratte in späten Stadien des experimentellen Herzinfarktes. Z. Ges. Inn. Med. **18**: 251–257.

GRUNDMANN, E. 1951. Histologische Untersuchungen über die Wirkungen experimentellen Sauerstoffmangels auf das Katzenherz. Beitr. Path. Anat. **111**: 36–76.

HAGER, H. 1964. Die feinere Cytologie und Cytopathologie des Nervensystems. Veröff. Morph. Path. Heft 67. G. Fischer, Stuttgart, Germany.

HECHT, A., G. KORB & H. DAVID. 1961. Vergleichende histochemische, fluoreszenzmikroskopische und elektronenoptische Untersuchungen zur Frühdiagnose des Herzinfarktes bei der Ratte. Virchow. Arch. Path. Anat. **334**: 267–284.

HERDSON, P. B., H. M. SOMMERS & R. B. JENNINGS. 1965. A comparative study of the fine structure of normal and ischemic dog myocardium with special reference to early changes following temporary occlusion of a coronary artery. Amer. J. Path. **46**: 367–386.

HILLS, C. P. 1964. Ultrastructural changes in the capillary bed of the rat cerebral cortex in anoxic-ischemic brain lesions. Amer. J. Path. **44**: 531–551.

JENNINGS, R. B., J. H. BAUM & P. B. HERDSON. 1965. Fine structural changes in myocardial ischemic injury. Arch. Path. (Chicago) **79**: 135–143.

JENNINGS, R. B., J. P. KALTENBACH, H. M. SOMMERS, G. G. BAHR & W. B. WARTMAN. 1963. Studies of the dying myocardial cell. *In* The Etiology of Myocardial Infarction. T. W. James & J. W. Keyes, Eds. : 189–204. J. & A. Churchill Ltd. London, England.

KENT, S. J. 1966. Intracellular plasma proteins: A manifestation of cell injury in experimentally produced myocardial ischemia in the dog. Amer. J. Path. **48**: 31a–32a.

KISCH, B. 1965. Electron microscopy of capillary hemorrhage. I. Post hypoxemia hemorrhage in the lungs. Exp. Med. Surg. **23**: 117–126.

KORB, G. 1965. Elektronenmikroskopische Untersuchungen zur Aludrin (Isoproterenolsulfat)-Schädigung des Herzmuskels. Virchow. Arch. Path. Anat. **339**: 136–150.

KORB, G., A. KRUG & H. BECHTELSHEIMER. 1965. Fluorochromierungsstudien zur Darstellung der normalen und gestörten Herzmuskeldurchblutung in Schnittpräparaten. Beitr. Path. Anat. **131**: 281–289.

KRUG, A. & G. KORB. 1966. Durchblutungsstörungen und histologische sowie enzymhistochemische Frühveränderungen am Katzenherzen nach temporärer Unterbindung von Coronargefässen. Beitr. Path. Anat. **134**: 29–51.

LETTERER, E. 1959. Allgemeine Pathologie. : 158. G. Thieme. Leipzig, Germany.

LINDNER, E. & H. J. WELLENSIEK. 1958. Elektronenmikroskopische Untersuchungen an Langendorff-Herzen unter normalen und abnormalen Bedingungen. 4. Internat. Kongr. Elektronenmikroskopie (Berlin). **2**: 326–327. Springer. Berlin, Germany.

MAJNO, G., M. LA GATTUTA & T. E. THOMPSON. 1960. Cellular death and necrosis: Chemical, physical and morphologic changes in the rat liver. Virchow. Arch. Path. Anat. **333**: 421–465.

MARTIN, JR., A. M. & D. B. HACKEL. 1966. An electron microscopic study of the progression of myocardial lesions in the dog after hemorrhagic shock. Lab. Invest. **15:** 243–260.

MILLER, F. 1958. Orthologie und Pathologie der Zelle im elektronenmikroskopischen Bild. Verh. Deutsch. Ges. Path. **42:** 261–332.

MILLONIG, G. 1962. Further observations on a phosphate buffer for osmium solutions in fixation. Proc. of Vth Internat. Congr. on Electron Microscopy, Philadelphia. S. S. Breese, Ed. Vol. **2:** 8. Academic Press, Inc. New York, N. Y.

MÖLBERT, E. 1957. Die Herzmuskelzelle nach akuter Oxydationshemmung im elektronenmikroskopischen Bild. Beitr. Path. Anat. **118:** 421–435.

MOLNAR, Z., K. LARSEN & B. SPARGO. 1962. Cardiac changes in the potassium-depleted rat. Arch. Path. (Chicago) **74:** 339–347.

MÜLLER, R. 1938. Über feinere, gewebliche Veränderungen bei der Gerinnungsnekrose und Autolyse, untersucht am Niereninfarkt. Frankfurt. Z. Path. **52:** 433–447.

NIDEN, A. H. & H. SCHULZ. 1965. The ultrastructural effects of carbon monoxide inhalation on the rat lung. Virchow. Arch. Path. Anat. **329:** 283–292.

POCHE, R. 1965. Über die Bedeutung der Blutkapillaren für die herdförmige Anordnung von sogenannten hypoxischen Herzmuskelveränderungen. Verh. Deutsch. Ges. Path. **49:** 219–223.

POCHE, R. & H. G. OHM. 1963. Lichtmikroskopische, histochemische und elektronenmikroskopische Untersuchungen des Herzmuskels von Menschen nach induziertem Herzstillstand. Arch. Kreislaufforsch. **41:** 86–135.

REYNOLDS, E. S. 1963. The use of lead citrate at high pH as an electron-opaque stain in electron microscopy. J. Cell. Biol. **17:** 208–212.

SARAM, M. 1957. Über die azelluläre Entstehung von Narben bei Durchblutungsstörungen im Herzmuskel. Beitr. Path. Anat. **118:** 275–291.

SCHURMANN, P. 1936. Über die Entstehung der Infarktnekrose. Verh. Deutsch. Ges. Path. **29:** 234–244.

SHEEHAN, H. L. & J. C. DAVIS. 1958. Complete permanent renal ischemia. J. Path. Bact. **76:** 569–587.

SOMMERS, H. M. & R. B. JENNINGS. 1964. Experimental acute myocardial infarction. Histologic and histochemical studies of early myocardial infarcts induced by temporary and permanent occlusion of a coronary artery. Lab. Invest. **13:** 1491–1503.

TOTOVIĆ, V. 1966. Elektronenmikroskopische Untersuchungen über das Verhalten der Hauptstückepithelien beim experimentellen Niereninfarkt der Ratte. Virchow. Arch. Path. Anat. **340:** 251–269.

WACHSTEIN, M. & M. BESEN. 1964. Electron microscopy of renal coagulative necrosis due to DL-serine, with special reference to mitochondrial pycnosis. Amer. J. Path. **44:** 383–400.

WEDELL, J., H. J. MERKER & D. NEUBERT. 1965. Mitochondrienstruktur und Atmungskettenphosphorylierung im Herzmuskel nach vollständiger Kreislaufunterbrechung. Virchow. Arch. Path. Anat. **338:** 355–370.

Part II. Cardiopathies and Factors Influencing Myocardial Degeneration

ISCHEMIC INJURY OF MYOCARDIUM*

Robert B. Jennings, Herbert M. Sommers,
Peter B. Herdson, and John P. Kaltenbach
Department of Pathology, Northwestern University Medical School, Chicago, Ill.

The sudden onset of ischemia in myocardium is followed within a few seconds by a series of striking functional changes: The area becomes cyanotic; cooler; hydrogen accumulates; electrocardiographic changes appear; and, within 30 to 60 seconds, contraction ceases in the affected myocardium. These changes within the ischemic focus are directly related to the development of local anoxia, which causes the affected cells to shift from an aerobic to an anaerobic form of metabolism, resulting in a substantial decrease in energy production. Although injured and nonfunctional, these severely ischemic, markedly anoxic cells are viable and survive for a period of time. Early restoration of the coronary blood flow to an ischemic focus is followed by almost instantaneous restoration of aerobic metabolism and contractile function. However, if the period of ischemia is more prolonged, restoration of the blood supply is not followed by restoration of function, since the affected cells are either dying or dead. The severely ischemic viable cells are *reversibly injured,* whereas the severely ischemic dead cells are *irreversibly injured.* Our chief interest has been in determining what event or series of events within the cells dictates the onset of irreversible injury.[1]

Our studies are predicated on the assumption that intracellular events discoverable by direct analysis of the tissue lead to the development of the irreversible state. Tissue known to be severely ischemic and fairly uniformly injured is required for analysis in direct studies of early changes in structure and/or function during ischemic injury. One must be able to identify and sample the affected tissue even though it appears normal upon gross examination. We have found that the posterior papillary muscle is an area of maximum ischemia in the large posterolateral infarct resulting from high occlusion of the circumflex branch of the left coronary artery in the dog heart.[2] The posterior papillary muscle is easily identified, and the upper two-thirds of the muscle are uniformly injured in those dogs in which the cyanosis extends to the apex of the heart posteriorly. The muscle is ultimately almost completely replaced by scar tissue. The anterior superior portion of the septum of the left ventricle is not involved in this infarct; therefore it is used as a source of nonischemic control tissue.

Timing of Onset of Irreversibility

In order to determine the timing of the onset of irreversible injury, a series of experiments was performed on dogs in which the circumflex branch of the left coronary artery was occluded with a Goldblatt clamp for periods of five to 60 minutes, following which the clamp was opened and blood flow restored to the ischemic myocardium. The dogs were killed two to 40 days later, and the

* The work reported in this paper was supported in part by grants from the Chicago Heart Association and the National Heart Institute, United States Public Health Service, no. HE-08729.

posterior papillary muscle was studied for evidence of overt necrosis or scarring.[3,4]

TABLE 1 summarizes data of relatively crude histological estimates of the proportion of dead cells in the posterior papillary muscle after various periods of occlusion of the circumflex artery. No dead cells were noted following periods of ischemia up to 18 minutes, but more and more dead cells were observed as the period of ischemia was prolonged, until almost the entire posterior papillary muscle was dead after 60 minutes of occlusion. We have not studied the effects of more than 60 minutes of temporary ischemia because the presence of hemorrhage within the muscle at this and greater time intervals indicated that the vascular system was no longer intact, and conditions of temporary ischemia were no longer possible.

Dead cells were first observed in the posterior papillary muscle after about 20 minutes of ischemia, These cells were scattered randomly throughout the muscle, were never abundant, and were present only in about 50% of the dogs. Occasionally these necrotic cells were calcified in a granular pattern.[5]

The results of these experiments indicate that cells of the posterior papillary muscle are reversibly injured for the first 15 to 18 minutes of ischemia, that the first cells die after 20 to 25 minutes of ischemia, that about 50% of the cells are irreversibly injured after 40 minutes, and that most of the cells are dead following 60 minutes of ischemia.

STRUCTURAL CHANGES IN CELLS IRREVERSIBLY INJURED BY ISCHEMIA

Permanent Ischemia

No changes in the structure of irreversibly injured cells in the center of the posterior papillary muscle following 60 minutes of ischemia are detectable by routine techniques of light microscopy. FIGURE 1 shows that these ischemic

TABLE 1

RELATIONSHIP OF THE PERIOD OF ISCHEMIA TO THE AMOUNT OF NECROSIS FOUND IN THE POSTERIOR PAPILLARY MUSCLE ONE TO SEVEN DAYS AFTER TEMPORARY OCCLUSION OF THE CIRCUMFLEX BRANCH OF THE LEFT CORONARY ARTERY NEAR ITS ORIGIN*

Minutes Circumflex Artery Occluded	No. of Dogs	Average Percentage of Necrosis in Posterior Papillary Muscle
0– 9	8	0
10–14	3	0
15–19	3	0
20–24	25	<4.0†
25–29	7	17.0
30–34	4	42.0
35–39	0	—
40–44	4	57.5
45–49	2	56.5
50–54	3	81.7
55–60	2	72.5

* Modified from Jennings *et al.*[3]

† The data for the 20-to-24-minute time interval come from a series of 43 dogs comprising the untreated control group of an experiment designed to test the effect of various drugs on reducing the incidence of ventricular fibrillation after a 20-minute period of temporary occlusion.[4] Only 58% of the dogs in this control series developed necrosis. The extent of the necrosis varied from <0.5 to 4%.

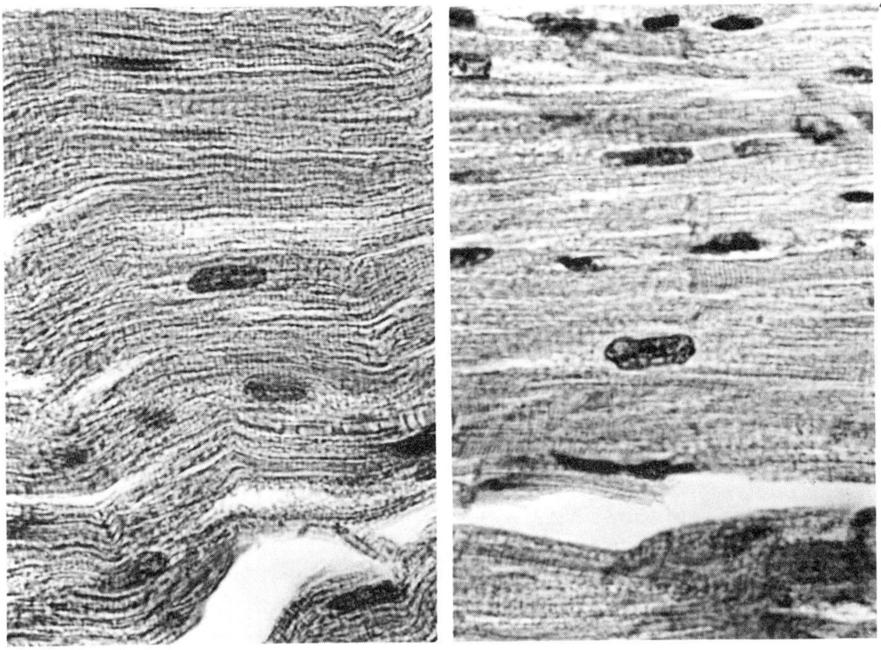

FIGURE 1. Comparison of light microscopical appearances of portions of the posterior papillary (left) and anterior papillary (right) muscles following occlusion of the circumflex branch of the left coronary artery for 60 minutes. The appearances are virtually indistinguishable. Stain: hematoxylin and eosin. × 1,000.

cells are indistinguishable from cells of the nonischemic left ventricle.† Special techniques demonstrate the discrete loss of glycogen and vague changes in the density of the affected fibers.[5]

Electron microscopy, on the other hand, shows uniform, readily recognizable changes in the architecture of irreversibly injured cells following 60 minutes of ischemia (FIGURES 2 and 3). The affected cells show relaxation of myofibrils with the appearance of prominent I bands, virtual absence of glycogen, margination of nuclear chromatin, and prominent abnormalities in mitochondrial structure. The mitochondria show a decrease in matrix density, appear enlarged, and contain dense granules. Most of these changes are present in some cells of the posterior papillary muscle following 30 minutes of ischemia, but are more diffuse and prominent after 60 minutes.[6]

Temporary Ischemia

Prominent changes are detectable by light microscopy in the architecture of cells that have been irreversibly injured by 40 minutes of ischemia and then exposed to freely flowing arterial blood for 20 minutes (FIGURE 4).[3, 5] The affected cells show a disruption of the regular myofibrillar pattern and the presence of prominent contraction bands. These structural changes involve the entire cell and are not focal or zonal in nature.[7] The myofibers are widely separated and show a loss in stainable glycogen, in addition to the presence of

† Frequently the edges of the infarct can be identified by cells showing contraction bands, but these are not always present at the end of one hour.

a diffuse amylase-fast periodic acid-Schiff reaction in the affected cells.[5]

Electron microscopy of such tissue shows equally striking changes, characterized by the appearance of widespread contraction bands, together with disruption of the sarcolemma, translocation and disorganization of mitochondria (FIGURE 5), and the appearance of large dense intramitochondrial granules.[8]

It seems probable that the contraction bands are produced in the irreversibly injured cells by the contractile force of the surrounding functioning myocardial fibers. Our findings indicate that cell death is a prerequisite for such changes to occur, inasmuch as they do not appear following restoration of blood flow to cells injured by periods of ischemia lasting less than 20 minutes.

Electrolyte Changes in Myocardial Cells Irreversibly Injured by Ischemia

Dying and dead myocardial cells eventually assume an electrolyte distribution close to that of the extracellular fluid. Potassium, magnesium, and acid-soluble phosphate leave the cell, whereas sodium, chloride, and water accumulate.[9, 10] One of the puzzles about the early phases of irreversible injury concerns the fact that it takes about eight to 12 hours for the potassium in the infarct to equilibrate with the extracellular fluid. Experiments utilizing transient ischemia showed that slowed diffusion was the most likely cause of this phenomenon; it was possible to produce the electrolyte milieu of dead cells simply by killing them with 40 minutes of ischemia and exposing them to 20 minutes of restored arterial flow.[9]

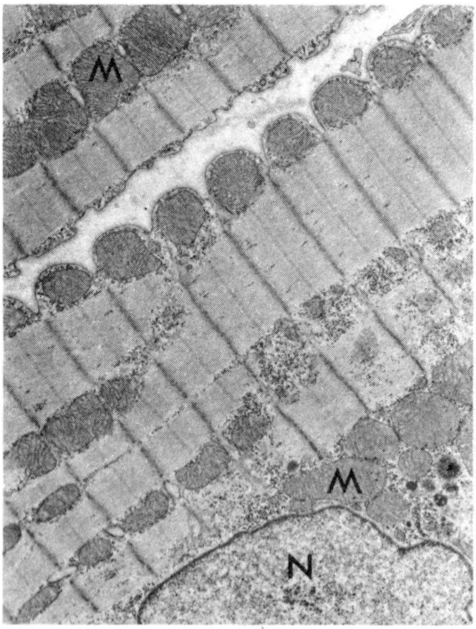

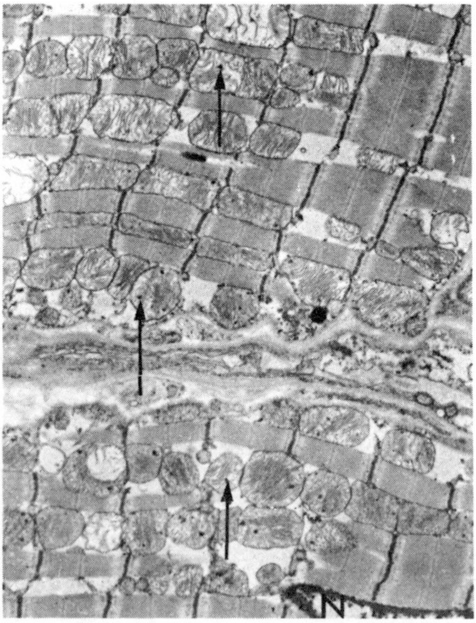

FIGURE 2. (*Left*) Control myocardium. N = nucleus; M = mitochondria. Osmium-fixed, Epon-embedded. × 7,000. (Reprinted with the permission of Laboratory Investigation.)

FIGURE 3. (*Right*) Myocardium showing marked abnormalities, following 60 minutes of ischemia. The fibrils are markedly relaxed, and many mitochondria show decreased matrix density. Arrows denote prominent intramitochondrial granules. Osmium-fixed, Epon-embedded. × 6,000.

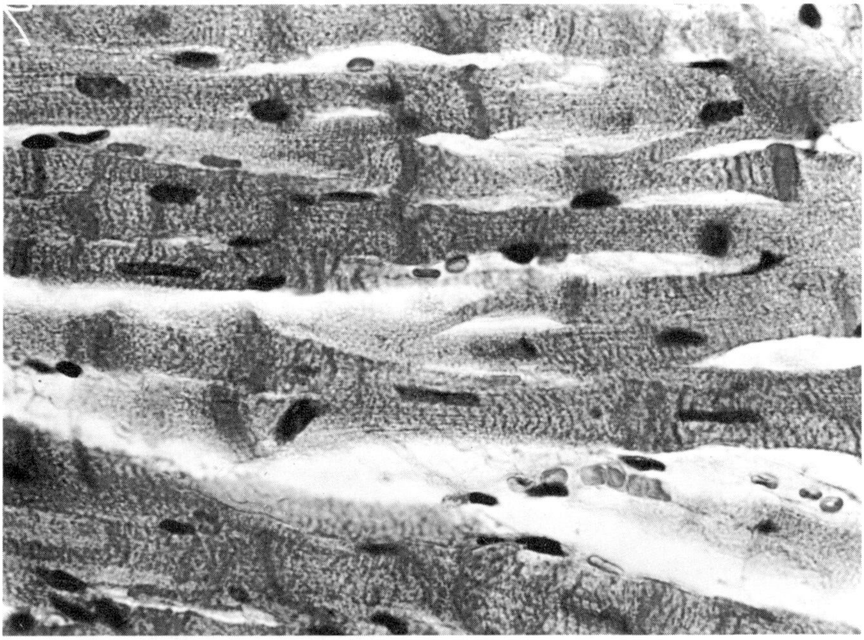

FIGURE 4. Light microscopical appearances of portions of the posterior papillary muscle after 40 minutes of temporary ischemia followed by 20 minutes of restored blood flow. Contraction bands are obvious. Stain: hematoxylin and eosin. × 970.

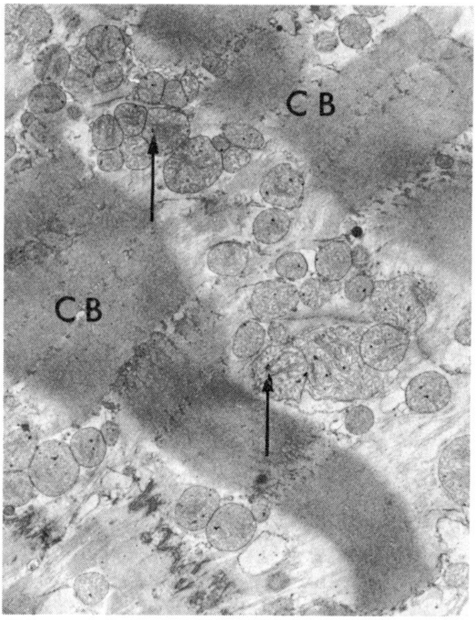

FIGURE 5. Myocardium after 40 minutes of temporary ischemia followed by 20 minutes of restored blood flow. Arrows denote prominent intramitochondrial granules. CB = contraction bands. Osmium-fixed, Epon-embedded. × 6,000.

Other ions, such as calcium, may accumulate within the infarct. The mitochondrial granules previously described probably represent aggregates containing calcium. Moreover, histochemically detectable calcium is prominent throughout many infarcts produced by temporary ischemia, and when first deposited, is found in what appears to be a mitochondrial location.[5]

Metabolic Changes Occurring *in Vivo* in an Area of Ischemia

Although aerobic metabolism is a highly efficient process, some energy is not converted to adenosine triphosphate (ATP), but is released as heat. For this reason, organs composed chiefly of cells dependent on aerobic metabolism, such as the heart, liver, and kidney, are warmer than the circulating blood. The development of small, sensitive implantable thermistors has made it possible to follow, indirectly but continuously, changes in myocardial metabolism *in vivo,* by measuring changes in the temperature of the ischemic and nonischemic myocardium. We have used this technique to monitor the tem-

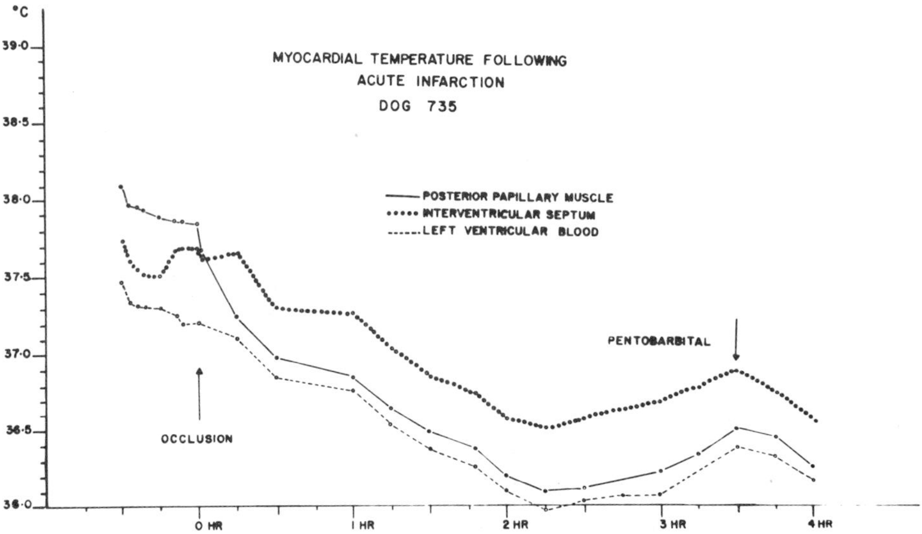

FIGURE 6. Temperature changes in a dog (no. 735) following permanent occlusion of the circumflex branch of the left coronary artery. Note that the blood temperature decreased from 37.5 to 36° C during the first 165 minutes after implantation of the thermistor; the temperature of the interventricular septum (control or nonischemic left ventricle) also decreased 1.5° C but remained 0.5° C warmer than the arterial blood throughout the experimental period. The initial sag in the temperature of the septum during the early part of the equilibration (control) period is an artifact caused by inadequate fixation of the thermistor in this area of the myocardium. The temperature of the posterior papillary muscle was 0.66° C warmer than the arterial blood during the preocclusion equilibration period, but decreased 0.51° C to a level only 0.15° C warmer than the blood within ten minutes after the artery was occluded. This is a decrease of 77% in the preocclusion temperature difference to a value only 23% of normal. Most of the decrease in this positive temperature differential occurred in the first two to four minutes, and there was little further decrease after ten minutes of ischemia. Supplementary pentobarbital always resulted in a drop in temperature of all three sites. (Reprinted with the permission of Laboratory Investigation.)

TABLE 2

TEMPERATURE DIFFERENTIALS BETWEEN THE MYOCARDIUM AND BLOOD IN DOGS WITH PERMANENT OCCLUSIONS OF THE CIRCUMFLEX BRANCH OF THE LEFT CORONARY ARTERY*

	Temperature Differentials (° C) Recorded†					
	0 min	2 min	4 min	10 min	30 min	60 min
Five control animals						
Posterior papillary muscle	0.38	0.37	0.38	0.38	0.38	0.37
Anterior septum	0.40	0.37	0.39	0.40	0.38	0.38
Ten experimental animals						
Posterior papillary muscle	0.45	0.27 (—41%)	0.18 (—59%)	0.16 (—62%)	0.17 (—62%)	0.14 (—66%)
Anterior septum	0.38	0.37	0.38	0.38	0.40	0.37

* From Sommers *et al.*[11] Reprinted with the permission of Laboratory Investigation.

† All values are means and were obtained for each myocardial site at each time interval by subtracting the temperature of the blood from the temperature of the posterior papillary muscle or the anterior septum. The percentages given under the experimental data represent the magnitude of the decrease in the temperature differential between the posterior papillary muscle and the blood from the control value to the experimental value at each time interval. These percentages are obtained by the following calculation: $100\% - [(a/b) \times 100] =$ percentage decrease in temperature differential, where a = the observed temperature difference between the posterior papillary muscle and the blood after ischemia and b = the average preocclusion temperature difference between the posterior papillary muscle and the blood. This calculation is based on the fact that the positive temperature differential between an area of the myocardium (in which a thermistor is placed) and the arterial blood remains constant over the duration of the experimental period. The decrease in temperature noted in the ischemic myocardium of dogs with infarcts was significant ($p < 0.001$) by a two-tailed paired t-test.

peratures of normal and ischemic tissue and the blood in the left ventricle following permanent and temporary ischemia.

During the course of our experiments, we found that the body and heart temperatures of dogs under pentobarbital anesthesia changed continuously over a range of as much as 2° C during the experimental period (see FIGURE 6). The temperature of the left ventricular myocardium also varied slightly from one region to another; but, as long as each implanted thermistor remained steady in its site, the temperature differential between each region of the warmer myocardium and the cooler blood in the left ventricle remained constant.

Permanent Ischemia

FIGURE 6 shows the typical temperature changes in the heart of a dog subjected to a permanent occlusion of the circumflex branch of the left coronary artery. The temperature in the posterior papillary muscle fell rapidly for the first six minutes following occlusion, and then declined slightly over the remaining observation period of four hours. TABLE 2 summarizes results of experiments in which temperatures were monitored in the anterior septum, posterior papillary muscle, and blood of the left ventricle in five control dogs and ten dogs subjected to permanent occlusion of the circumflex branch of the left coronary artery. The positive temperature differential between the posterior papillary muscle (ischemic myocardium) and the arterial blood decreased an average of 41% within two minutes following coronary occlusion and an average of 59% after four minutes. Over the next 56 minutes, only a slight further drop in temperature was noted. The fall in temperature of the ischemic myocardium is believed to reflect the decreased heat production by the predominantly anaerobic metabolism of the ischemic tissue.[11] The temperature differential between the nonischemic septum and the arterial blood remained constant throughout the experiment.

The decrease in the temperature of the ischemic myocardium following coronary occlusion correlated closely with the appearance of cyanosis, the development of electrocardiographic changes, and the cessation of contraction. Interestingly, there was no significant further alteration in the temperature differential between ischemic myocardium and blood when severely ischemic cells passed from the phase of reversible to irreversible injury; as shown in FIGURE 6, temperature differences recorded after four and ten minutes of ischemia were similar to those seen after 30 and 60 minutes.

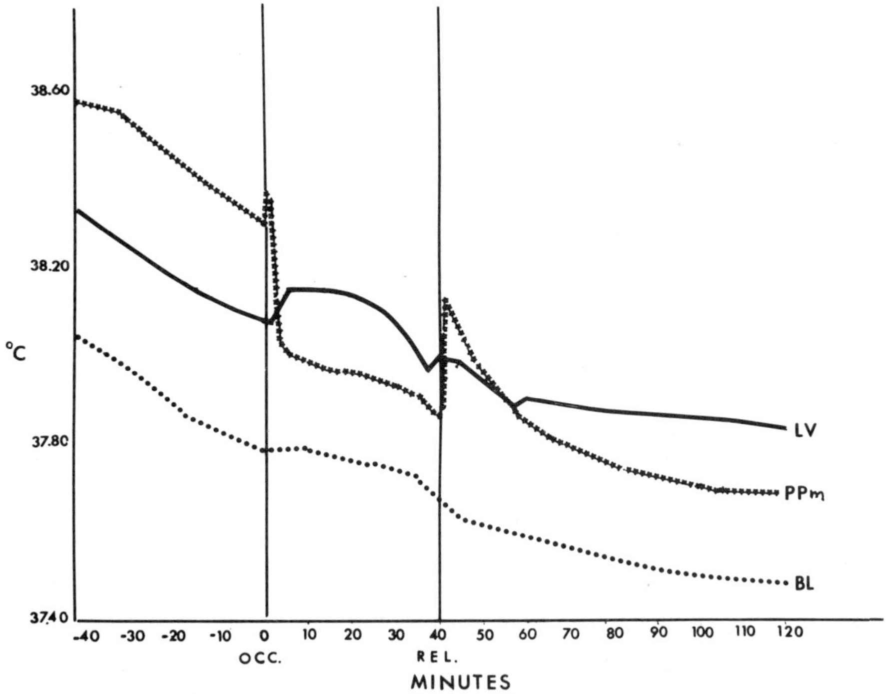

FIGURE 7. Temperature changes in a dog (no. 1014) subjected to a temporary occlusion of the circumflex branch of the left coronary artery for 40 minutes. Throughout the equilibration period the posterior papillary muscle (PPm) was 0.54° C warmer than the arterial blood (BL). Note that its temperature slightly increased immediately after coronary occlusion and then decreased 63% to a temperature differential of + 0.20° C {100 − [(0.20/0.54) × 100] = 63%}. Following release of the occlusion and restoration of the arterial circulation to the ischemic myocardium, the temperature of the posterior papillary muscle rapidly rose 0.55° C to the temperature differential recorded before occlusion, and then fell slowly again to the depressed level noted during occlusion. The slight increase in the temperature of the nonischemic left ventricle (LV) during the period of occlusion was noted in several dogs in this experimental series. FIGURES 8 and 9 show the gross appearance of the infarct.

Temporary Ischemia

We recently completed a series of experiments in which the temperatures of the myocardium and arterial blood were monitored in dogs subjected to a temporary occlusion of the circumflex branch of the left coronary artery for 40 minutes.[12] This period of ischemia is sufficient to kill approximately 50% of the cells in the posterior papillary muscle; the thermistor, therefore, was sometimes in an area of irreversible ischemic injury and sometimes in an area of reversible ischemic injury. Dogs surviving release of the coronary occlusion without developing ventricular fibrillation were allowed to live for two to five months before the relationship of the thermistor in the posterior papillary muscle to the area of fibrosis induced by the episode of ischemia was studied. In all of these experiments, there was the expected abrupt fall in the temperature of the ischemic posterior papillary muscle after occlusion. Following release of the coronary occlusion, those dogs in which the thermistor had been implanted in an area of irreversible cell injury—as indicated by prominent scarring in the posterior papillary muscle—showed a striking increase in the temperature of the ischemic tissue. This temperature increase reached a maximum between three to five minutes following release and then slowly returned to the depressed temperature noted during the period of ischemia. FIGURE 7 shows the typical temperature changes in the heart of a dog subjected to a temporary occlusion of the circumflex branch of the left coronary artery; FIGURES 8 and 9 show the scarred posterior papillary muscle of this dog at autopsy five months later.

In those animals in which the thermistor was in an area of reversible cell injury, the temperature of the ischemic myocardium slowly returned to its preocclusion level over a period of between ten and 20 minutes following release of the occlusion, and then remained at this normal level.

The abrupt increase in temperature in the previously ischemic, irreversibly injured myocardium is believed to be caused by excess heat production associated with uncoupling of oxidative phosphorylation or with sudden uncontrolled respiration in the cells of the injured posterior papillary muscle. An alternative explanation for these temparature changes is that the temperature of the irreversibly injured area rises because of an increase in the temperature of the blood entering the ischemic focus and not because of any local metabolic changes. In this instance, the increase in blood temperature presumably would be caused by heat produced during a brief period of rapid respiration in the reversibly injured cells on the periphery of the infarct. Of these two possibilities, the former seems most likely, because the reversible cell injury was found to be associated with a slow rather than quick return in myocardial temperature to the preocclusion level.

These speculations about the causes of the increase in temperature in the irreversibly injured cells assume that the vessels in the ischemic tissue are not damaged sufficiently to impede the reactive hyperemia known to develop in this infarct with restoration of the arterial flow.[3] Neither light nor electron microscopy has shown any evidence of a vascular lesion or thrombosis in this infarct.[5,6,8] If arterial flow is slowed through the posterior papillary muscle, then a brief period of normal respiration with a depressed flow of cooler arterial blood also could produce these changes.

Mitochondrial Failure and the Irreversible State

Lack of knowledge of the control and integration of reactions within well-

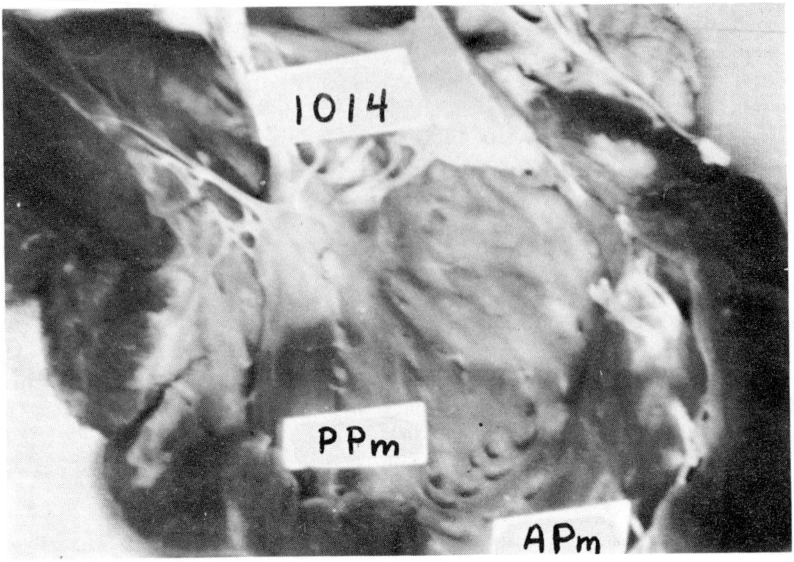

FIGURE 8. Scar involving the upper one-half of the posterior papillary muscle (PPm) and adjacent endocardial surface of the posterolateral wall of the left ventricle. Note the uninvolved anterior papillary muscle (APm). Dog (no. 1014) sacrificed 146 days following coronary occlusion.

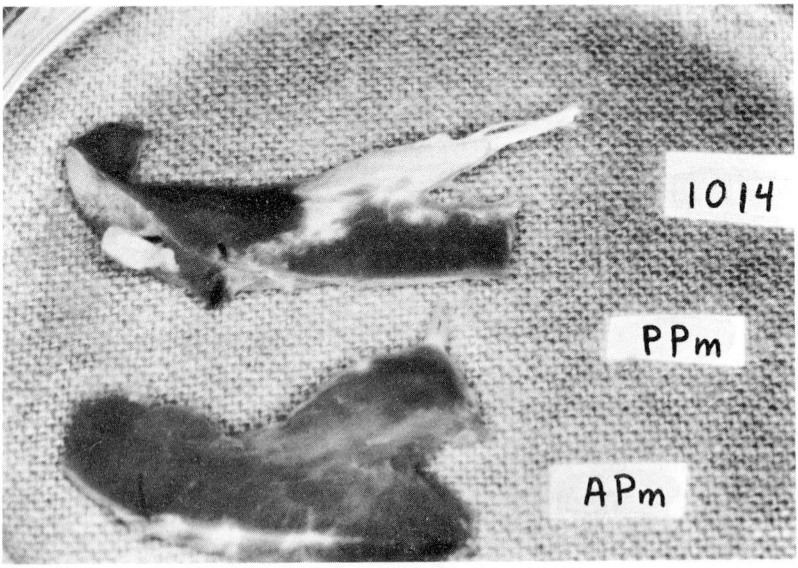

FIGURE 9. Sections taken through the posterior (PPm) and anterior papillary (APm) muscles and adjacent left ventricular wall of dog no. 1014. The infarct involves much of the subendocardial portion of the posteriolateral wall of the left ventricle, and includes most of the posterior papillary muscle. The thermistor tract is noted extending obliquely through the left ventricular wall.

differentiated cells makes it difficult to establish a hypothesis concerning what events occur within ischemic myocardial cells to cause them to enter a state of irreversible injury. It seems likely that the injured cells die when the energy level within them decreases to a point no longer compatible with the maintenance of their integrity. If this theory is correct, one might expect cell death to occur when supplies of glycogen are exhausted or when the pH of the area decreases below some limiting value because of lactic acid accumulation. We have suggested in the past that increased permeability of cells might lead to the loss of vital cofactors, and eventually to the development of the irreversible state.[1,13]

A currently attractive hypothesis, supported by several lines of evidence, is that mitochondrial damage may be the critical feature in the genesis of the irreversible state. The fact that myocardium is almost completely dependent on aerobic (i.e., mitochondrial) metabolism for the production of energy suggests that mitochondrial damage could have far-reaching deleterious consequences. More direct evidence that a mitochondrial deficiency of some sort may be involved comes from the observation that homogenates of ischemic myocardium show a decreased capacity to metabolize glucose to carbon dioxide and water after 30 to 60 minutes of ischemia.[13] Since the mitochondria are the organelles in which most of the carbon dioxide and water are formed during aerobic glycolysis in the dog heart, mitochondrial failure is a likely cause of the deficient oxygen consumption and phosphorylation observed in this system. A third and particularly important line of evidence comes from electron microscopy: Changes in the fine structure of mitochondria are a prominent feature of cells that have entered the irreversible state. The typical appearances of mitochondria within normal (FIGURE 2), reversibly injured (FIGURE 10), and irreversibly injured cells (FIGURE 3) are shown. The disorganized cristae, clear matrix, and dense bodies are characteristic and uniform features of the mitochondria of cells

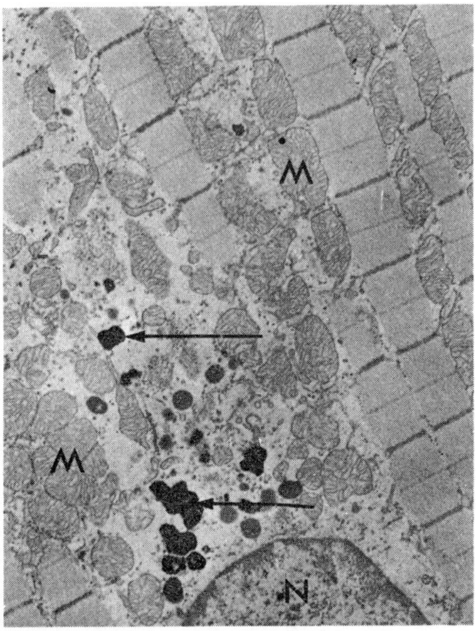

FIGURE 10. Myocardium showing minimal changes, following temporary ischemia for 15 minutes. Arrows denote lipofuscin granules. N = nucleus; M = mitochondria. Osmium-fixed, Epon-embedded. × 7,000.

that have just entered the irreversible state. These changes do not appear in reversibly injured cells, although the matrix of the mitochondria of such cells may be slightly less dense.

If mitochondrial damage is a critical feature of the development of irreversibility, then mitochondria isolated from cells that have recently entered the irreversible state should show a defective capacity to metabolize a representative mitochondrial substrate, such as α-ketoglutarate, when compared with mitochondria isolated from the left ventricle of the same dog, or from the left ventricle and posterior papillary muscle of sham-operated controls. TABLE 3 presents data from manometric studies with a fortified medium designed to insure maximum metabolism; results demonstrate that mitochondria isolated from irreversibly injured cells have little or no capacity to metabolize α-ketoglutarate, whereas mitochondria isolated from reversibly injured cells show a 50% reduction in oxidative and phosphorylative capacity.[14]

The evidence from the manometric experiments with α-ketoglutarate encouraged us to develop techniques for the assessment of several parameters of

TABLE 3

COMPARISON OF MITOCHONDRIAL METABOLISM IN SEVERELY ISCHEMIC VIABLE AND NONVIABLE MYOCARDIAL CELLS AND NONISCHEMIC LEFT VENTRICLE CELLS IN DOGS*

Period of Ischemia†	No. of Dogs	$Q^{N}_{O_2}$	$Q^{N}_{\sim P}$
15 minutes (viable)			
Posterior papillary muscle	4	150 ± 26.0	23.8 ± 5.8
Left ventricle	4	349 ± 57.1	61.4 ± 4.6
120 minutes (nonviable)			
Posterior papillary muscle	4	27 ± 6.6	0.1 ± 0.06
Left ventricle	7	274 ± 21.1	57.4 ± 7.0

* All values are means ± standard error. Mitochondria isolated in a medium containing 0.1 M potassium phosphate buffer (pH 7.4), 10^{-4} M EDTA (ethylenediaminetetraacetic acid), 0.225 M mannitol, and 0.076 M sucrose. Warburg flasks with a volume of 15 ml and a single side arm were used; incubation temperature was 37° C. The flasks contained nicotinaminde, nicotinamide adenine dinucleotide (NAD), potassium fluoride, potassium chloride, potassium phosphate (pH 7.4), malonate, hexokinase, adenosine diphosphate (ADP), and magnesium chloride. The side arm contained glucose and 20 micromoles of α-ketoglutarate, which was added as late as possible to avoid autooxidation; 0.25–0.35 mg of mitochondrial nitrogen was added to each flask. Oxygen uptakes for $Q^{N}_{O_2}$ are from a 20-minute analysis obtained between 20 and 40 minutes of incubation. Oxygen uptakes were confirmed by measurements of α-ketoglutarate utilization; phosphorylation values were confirmed by enzymatic determination of the amount of glucose 6-phosphate formed.

$Q^{N}_{O_2}$ = microliters of oxygen utilized per milligram of mitochondrial nitrogen per hour.

$Q^{N}_{\sim P}$ = micromoles of apparent inorganic phosphate lost from the medium per milligram of mitochondrial nitrogen per hour.

The values for mitochondria isolated from the posterior papillary muscle and the left ventricle of sham-operated controls were not significantly different from the values reported for mitochondria isolated from nonischemic left ventricle.

† The posterior papillary muscle values are significantly different from the left ventricle values: $p < 0.01$ at 15 minutes and $p < 0.001$ at 120 minutes, using the t-test for paired experiments.

TABLE 4

COMPARISON OF RESPIRATORY CONTROL RATIOS AND FUNCTIONAL CAPACITY OF MITOCHONDRIA ISOLATED FOR ISCHEMIC VIABLE AND NONVIABLE MYOCARDIAL CELLS AND NONISCHEMIC LEFT VENTRICLE CELLS OF DOGS WITH AND WITHOUT INFARCTS*

Minutes of Ischemia	No. of Dogs	Respiratory Control Ratio†		Rate of State 3 Respiration‡		$^{14}CO_2$ Production from Pyruvate-3-^{14}C§	
		PPm	LV	PPm	LV	PPm	LV
Dogs without infarcts (control)							
0	4	5.8	5.0	912	837	0.054	0.063
Dogs with infarcts							
Viable							
15	3	5.8	4.5	343¶	840	0.021	0.072
Nonviable							
60	3	0.0	5.7	48¶	639	0.005	0.060
120	1	0.0	4.2	12	666	0.001	0.060
240	1	0.0	7.2	16	912	—	—

* Mitochondria were isolated in a medium containing 0.15 M KCl and 0.002 M EDTA (ethylenediaminetetraacetic acid) and were suspended in 0.18 M KCl.[18] The reaction chamber of the Gilson Model KM oxygraph contained 4 mM potassium phosphate buffer (pH 7.4), 0.2–0.4 mg of mitchondrial nitrogen, 100 μM pyruvate-3-^{14}C, 3.2 mM adenosine diphosphate (ADP), and variable quantities of 0.15 M KCl. No magnesium was used. PPm = posterior papillary muscle; LV = nonischemic left ventricle.

† Respiratory control ratio (RCR) =

$$\frac{\text{rate of respiration with substrate and phosphate acceptor present}}{\text{rate of respiration with substrate but no phosphate acceptor}}$$

‡ Rate of respiration with complete system (State 3),[19] expressed in millimicroatoms of oxygen per milligram of mitochondrial nitrogen per minute.

§ Expressed as micromoles of pyruvate-3-^{14}C completely oxidized to carbon dioxide-^{14}C and water per milligram of mitochondrial nitrogen per minute. These data assess the integrity of the Krebs cycle, since two and one-half circuits of the cycle are required to release carbon dioxide-^{14}C from the ^{14}C-labeled number 3 carbon atom of pyruvate.

¶ These posterior papillary muscle values are significantly different from those of the left ventricle, using the t-test for paired experiments.

mitochondrial intactness on the limited number of mitochondria that can be isolated from the 500–1000 mg of posterior papillary muscle available for analysis. In addition, techniques for correlating the fine structure and metabolic capacity of the isolated mitochondria were adopted from those used to isolate particulates from liver.[15] Since preliminary data in our laboratory[16] had confirmed the observations of Deshpande and co-workers[17] that mitochondria isolated in 0.18 M KCl appeared to be better preserved than those isolated in sucrose, we adapted their technique for isolation of mitochondria and Von Korff's polarographic methods[18] for assessing the metabolism of pyruvate. In addition, we developed a technique for measuring substrate utilization by measuring carbon dioxide-^{14}C production from ^{14}C-labeled substrates in the oxygraph.

The results of these studies with polaragraphic techniques are presented in TABLE 4. Once again, there was about a 50% reduction in the capacity of mitochondria isolated from severely ischemic but viable cells to metabolize a representative substrate (in this case, pyruvate). But the respiratory control ratio (RCR‡)[19] of the mitochondria isolated from the posterior papillary muscle

‡ $$\text{RCR} = \frac{\text{rate of respiration with substrate and phosphate acceptor present}}{\text{rate of respiration with substrate but no phosphate acceptor}}$$

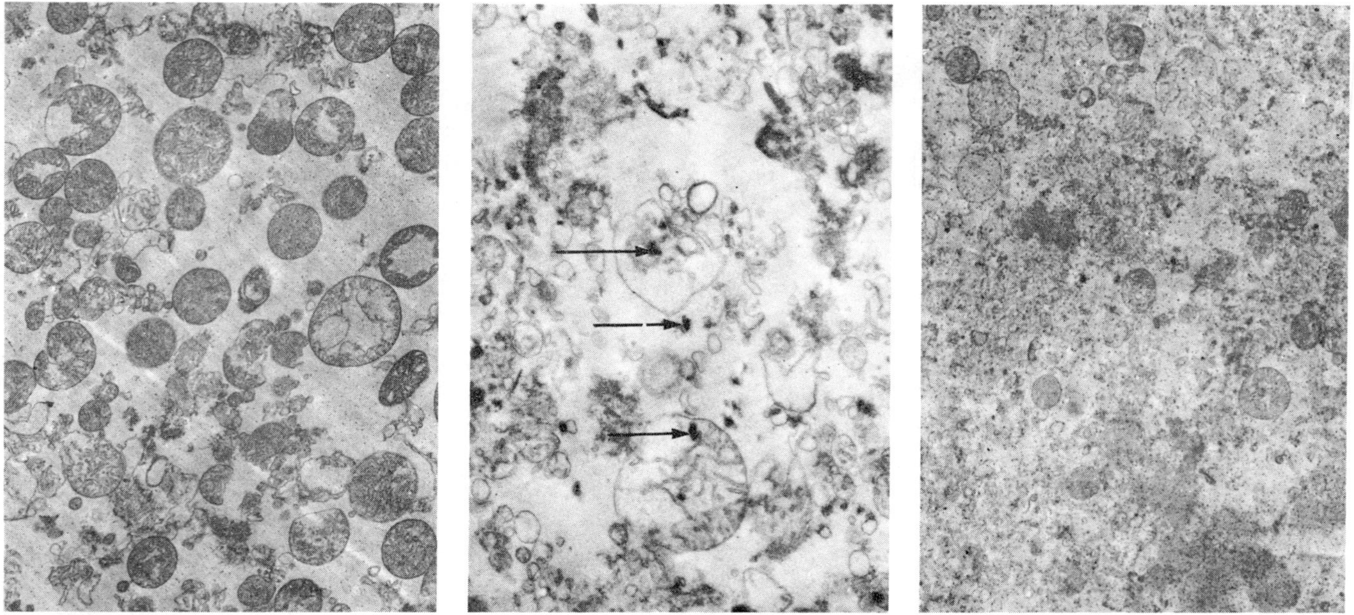

FIGURES 11, 12, and 13 show mitochondrial fractions from various portions of myocardium following occlusion of the circumflex branch of the left coronary artery. Prepared in 0.18 M KCl and 0.002 M EDTA (ethylenediaminetetraacetic acid), and suspended in 0.1 M KCl, then osmium-fixed and Epon-embedded.

FIGURE 11. (*Left*) From nonischemic left ventricle (control) following occlusion for 60 minutes. × 5,000.

FIGURE 12. (*Center*) From the posterior papillary muscle following ischemia for 60 minutes. Arrows denote dense granules, both within mitochondria and lying free. × 10,000.

FIGURE 13. (*Right*) From the posterior papillary muscle following ischemia for 240 minutes. × 5,000.

was similar to that of mitochondria isolated from the left ventricle; this finding suggests that whatever mitochondria were functioning in this preparation were functioning normally, although some material in the mitochondrial pellet was functioning at a decreased rate, if at all. As in the manometric experiments with α-ketoglutarate, the mitochondria isolated from severely ischemic dead cells, whether at 60, 120, or 240 minutes, were unable to metabolize the substrate, and exhibited neither respiratory nor substrate control.

Electron microscopy of aliquots of the preparations listed in TABLE 4 showed that mitochondria isolated from the posterior papillary muscle following 15 minutes of ischemia were indstinguishable from those isolated from the non-ischemic left ventricle of the same dogs or from sham-operated animals. In contrast, the pellets isolated from the irreversibly injured posterior papillary muscle after 60 or more minutes of ischemia showed mostly fragmented mitochondrial membranes, myofibrillar and cytoplasmic debris, and only a few intact mitochondria (FIGURES 11, 12, and 13).

We concluded from these studies that mitochondria of the irreversibly injured cells were more fragile than those in normal myocardium, and that they disintegrated during the considerable trauma required to separate mitochondria from myocardial cells by homogenization. Since intact mitochondria are required for metabolism of pyruvate,[20,21] it seemed likely that the deficient metabolism observed was a result of fragmentation. It was of interest that succinate, which is oxidized in a membrane-bound enzyme system, was metabolized by the mitochondrial pellets of the irreversibly injured cells. This finding was not unexpected, because mitochondrial membranes fragmented by sonication also will metabolize succinate.[20]

Recent experiments, however, indicate that fragmentation is not the only cause of the deficient metabolism. We have been able to isolate intact but nonfunctional mitochondria from myocardial clls injured by 60 minutes of ischemia (FIGURES 14 and 15). These mitochondria metabolize little or no pyruvate, and show a diminished capacity to metabolize succinate.[22] They are very similar to those noted in the tissue and show prominent dense granules. The intact mitochondria are obtained by briefly digesting the myosin of a cold mince of myocardium with a proteolytic enzyme called Nagarse® (*Bacillus subtilus* alkaline proteinase).§ This enzyme seems to have no effect on the mitochondria, but softens the tissue sufficiently so that much less force is required to liberate mitochondria from the muscle.[23-25] The fine structure of mitochondria from normal left ventricle is well preserved and similar to that seen when these organelles are isolated from normal left ventricle in 0.18 M KCl. Moreover, the Nagarse® preparations contain very little debris and consist chiefly of intact mitochondria. These preparations show higher (State 3) rates of respiration[19] and higher respiratory and substrate control ratios than mitchondria isolated from myocardium by other techniques.

Results of the studies presented in this section show that mitochondrial damage occurs early in cells subjected to ischemic injury, but yield little knowledge about any of the defects within the mitochondria which might interfere with their capacity to metabolize. Mitochondria contain a very complex, highly organized multienzyme system, and among the many possible causes of deficient function are spatial disorganization of mitochondrial enzymes, inactivation of mitochondrial enzymes, loss of essential cofactors, and maldistribution of essential anions or cations within the mitochondrion.

§ Distributed by Enzyme Development Corporation, New York, N. Y.

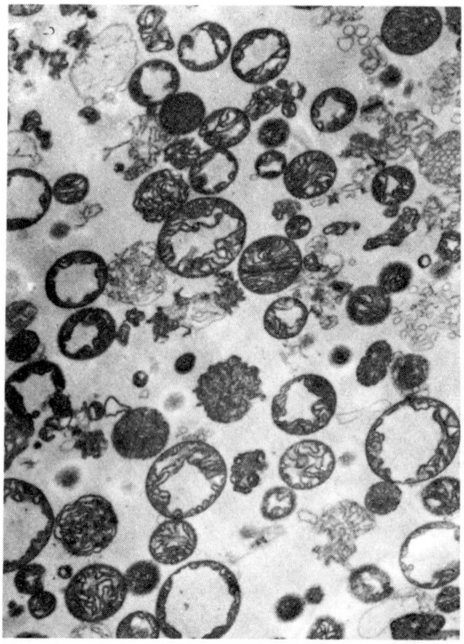

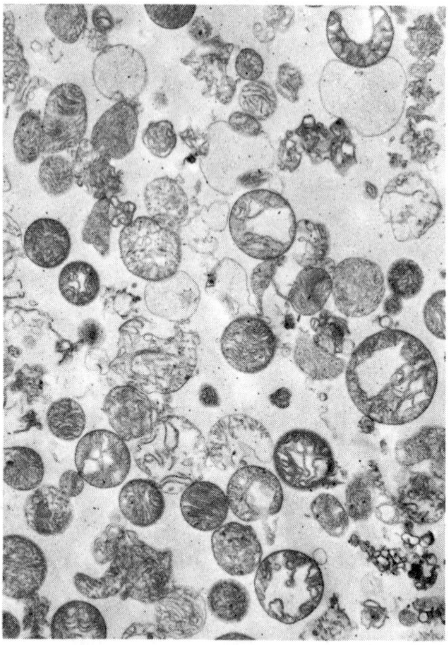

FIGURES 14 and 15 show mitochondrial fractions from the myocardium following occlusion of the circumflex branch of the left coronary artery. Prepared by the Nargarse® procedure in dog no. 1071. Mitochondria isolated from the posterior papillary muscle oxidized 0.01 micromoles of pyruvate-3-^{14}C per milligram of mitochondrial nitrogen per minute to carbon dioxide and water; mitochondria isolated from the nonischemic left ventricle oxidized 0.25 micromoles. The adenosine diphosphate (ADP) to oxygen ratio of mitochondria from the left ventricle was 2.8; the maximum rate of State 3 respiration was 3,921 millimicroatoms of oxygen per milligram of nitrogen per minute; the respiratory control ratio was 18.5. The mitochondria from the posterior papillary muscle exhibited no respiratory control, and essentially no oxygen uptake.

FIGURE 14. (*Left*) From nonischemic left ventricle (control) following occlusion for 60 minutes. × 5,000.

FIGURE 15. (*Right*) From the posterior papillary muscle following ischemia for 60 minutes. × 5,000.

The possibility that alterations in mitochondrial electrolyte distribution may cause the altered metabolism is currently under investigation. The granules that are so uniformly present in the mitochondria of irreversibly injured cells are believed to contain calcium and phosphate, and perhaps magnesium.[26] The facts that calcium inhibits oxidative phosphorylation,[27] and that magnesium and phosphate are essential cofactors in mitochondrial metabolism, together with the fact that excess calcium is noted in some other severely damaged cellular systems,[28,29] are significant, but no definitive data have been obtained to date to establish this hypothesis.

The results of these experiments on the metabolic capabilities of mitochondria isolated from cells injured by ischemia support the concept that mitochondrial failure may play a significant role in the genesis of the irreversible state. The exact cause of the observed failure in mitochondrial metabolism is unknown.

ACKNOWLEDGMENTS

We gratefully acknowledge the technical assistance of Miss. M. L. Hill, Miss A. Hoos, Mrs. C. Moore, Miss M. Moulton, and Mrs. S. Safavi.

REFERENCES

1. JENNINGS, R. B., J. P. KALTENBACH, H. M. SOMMERS, G. F. BAHR & W. B. WARTMAN. 1963. Studies of the Dying Myocardial Cell in the Etiology of Myocardial Infarction. T. N. James & J. W. Keyes, Eds. : 189–204. Little, Brown & Co. Boston, Mass.
2. JENNINGS, R. B., W. B. WARTMAN & Z. E. ZUDYK. 1957. Production of an area of homogeneous myocardial infarction in the dog. Arch. Path. (Chicago) **63**: 580.
3. JENNINGS, R. B., H. M. SOMMERS, G. A. SMYTH, H. A. FLACK, H. LINN & Z. E. ZUDYK. 1960. Myocardial necrosis induced by temporary occlusion of a coronary artery in the dog. Arch. Path. (Chicago) **70**: 68.
4. SOMMERS, H. M. 1966. The effect of reserpine and propranolol on spontaneous ventricular fibrillation and myocardial necrosis following transient coronary artery occlusion. Fed. Proc. **25**: 666.
5. SOMMERS, H. M. & R. B. JENNINGS. 1964. Experimental acute myocardial infarction. Histologic and histochemical studies of early myocardial infarcts induced by temporary or permanent occlusion of a coronary artery. Lab. Invest. **13**: 149.
6. JENNINGS, R. B., J. H. BAUM & P. B. HERDSON. 1965. Fine structural changes in myocardial ischemic injury. Arch. Path. (Chicago) **79**: 135.
7. MARTIN, JR., A. M. & D. B. HACKEL. 1966. An electron microscopic study of the progression of myocardial lesions in the dog after hemorrhage shock. Lab. Invest. **15**: 243.
8. HERDSON, P. B., R. B. JENNINGS & H. M. SOMMERS. 1965. A comparative study of the fine structure of normal and ischemic dog myocardium with special reference to early changes following temporary occlusion of a coronary artery. Amer. J. Path. **46**: 367.
9. JENNINGS, R. B., H. M. SOMMERS, J. P. KALTENBACH & J. J. WEST. 1964. Electrolyte alterations in acute myocardial ischemic injury. Circ. Res. **14**: 260.
10. JENNINGS, R. B., H. M. SOMMERS & J. P. KALTENBACH. 1965. Cell death: electrolyte alterations in injured and dying myocardial cells. *In* Electrolytes and Cardiovascular Diseases. E. Bajusz, Ed. : 192–203. S. Karger. Basel, Switzerland.
11. SOMMERS, H. M., H. U. WESSEL & R. B. JENNINGS. 1966. Myocardial temperature changes in acute experimental infarction. Lab. Invest. **15**: 1982.
12. SOMMERS, H. M. & R. B. JENNINGS. 1967. Myocardial temperature following transient ischemia with necrosis (abstr.) Amer. J. Path. In press.
13. KALTENBACH, J. P. & R. B. JENNINGS. 1960. Metabolism of ischemic cardiac muscle. Circ. Res. **8**: 207.
14. JENNINGS, R. B., J. P. KALTENBACH & P. B. HERDSON. 1966. Mitochondrial metabolism in ischemic injury. Fed. Proc. **25**: 476.
15. HERDSON, P. B. & J. P. KALTENBACH. 1965. Electron microscope studies on enzyme activity and the isolation of thiohydantoin-induced myelin figures in rat liver. J. Cell Biol. **25**: 485.
16. HERDSON, P. B. & R. B. JENNINGS. 1965. Unpublished observation.
17. DESHPANDE, P. O., D. D. HICKMAN & R. W. VON KORFF. 1961. Morphology of isolated rabbit heart muscle mitochondria and the oxidation of extramitochondrial reduced diphosphopyridine nucleotide. J. Biophys. Biochem. Cytol. **11**: 77.
18. VON KORFF, R. W. 1965. Metabolic characteristics of isolated rabbit heart mitochondria. J. Biol. Chem. **240**: 1351.
19. CHANCE, B. & G. R. WILLIAMS. 1956. The respiratory chain and oxidative phosphorylation. Advances Enzymol. **17**: 65.
20. McMURRAY, W. C., G. F. MALEY & H. A. LARDY. 1958. Oxidative phosphorylation by sonic extracts of mitochondria. J. Biol. Chem. **230**: 219.
21. MIYAHARA, J. T. & R. KARLER. 1965. Effect of salicylate on oxidative phosphorylation and respiration of mitochondrial fragments. Biochem. J. **97**: 194.
22. JENNINGS, R. B., P. B. HERDSON, H. M. SOMMERS & M. L. HILL. 1967. Mitochondrial metabolism in ischemic injury. In preparation.
23. CHANCE, B. & B. HAGIHARA. 1963. Direct spectroscopic measurements of interaction of components of the respiratory chain with ATP, ADP, phosphate, and uncoupling agents. *In* Proc. Fifth Intern. Congr. Biochem. **V**: 3.

24. DAVIS, R. J. 1965. On the oxidation of acetate and pyruvate by guinea-pig heart sacrosomes. Biochem. Biophys. Acta **96:** 217.
25. CHIDSEY, C. A., E. C. WEINBACH, P. E. POOL & A. G. MORROW. 1966. Biochemical studies of energy production in the failing human heart. J. Clin. Invest. **45:** 40.
26. LEHNINGER, A. L. 1964. The Mitochondrion. : 263. W. A. Benjamin, Inc. New York, N. Y.
27. SLATER, E. C. & K. W. CLELAND. 1953. The effect of calcium on the respiratory and phosphorylative activities of heart-muscle sarcosomes. Biochem. J. **55:** 566.
28. JUDAH, J. D. 1962. Action of antihistamine and other drugs on ion and water movements in cells and mitochondria. Fed. Proc. **21:** 1097.
29. REYNOLDS, E. S., R. E. THIERS & B. L. VALLEE. 1962. Mitochondrial function and metal content in carbon tetrachloride poisoning. J. Biol. Chem **237:** 3546.

MECHANISMS IN THE DEVELOPMENT OF MYOCARDIAL LESIONS IN HEMORRHAGIC SHOCK*

Arthur M. Martin, Jr., Donald B. Hackel,† Mark L. Entman, M. Paul Capp, and Madison S. Spach

Departments of Pathology, Medicine, Radiology, and Pediatrics Duke University Medical Center, Durham, N. C.

Many investigations have shown that the heart plays an important role in the evolution of the irreversible state of hemorrhagic shock.[1-4] Early in the course of experimental hemorrhagic shock the heart sustains anatomical damage, namely, subendocardial hemorrhage and necrosis,[5] and "zonal" lesions,[6-8] which could contribute to the development of impaired cardiac function. It is the purpose of this paper to describe and discuss certain factors in hemorrhagic shock which may be important in the etiology of myocardial lesions, especially the "zonal" lesions. The principles of laboratory animal care, as promulgated by the National Society for Medical Research, have been observed.

Pathological Anatomy of the Heart

Previous investigations of hemorrhagic shock have shown that one of the more frequent pathological findings is the presence of areas of hemorrhage and necrosis in the subendocardial regions of the heart, especially in the papillary muscles of the left ventricle and in the middle portion of the interventricular septum.[5] The severity of these changes is variable, but is related to the duration of shock and the interval of survival. Both the hemorrhage and necrosis are usually of sufficient extent to be visible upon gross examination. Other investigations have shown that similar pathological findings are present following isoproterenol[9] or noradrenaline[10] infusion, cervical sympathetic ganglion stimulation,[11] trauma,[12] and dextran[13] administration.

Of more recent interest has been the demonstration in dog hearts of a characteristic type of microscopical damage referred to as "zonal" lesions[6-8] (FIGURE 1).

Enzymatic histochemical stains (succinic dehydrogenase) of longitudinal sections under light microscopy[6] have shown that this type of lesion is a swollen transverse band in the myofiber of decreased or absent enzymatic activity, approximately 10–20 μ in length, bordered on each side by zones of increased enzymatic activity. The portions of the myofiber between consecutive lesions appear normal. These lesions may be seen with some difficulty in sections stained with hematoxylin-eosin, and especially in sections stained with phosphotungstic acid-hematoxylin. With these stains, the zonal lesions are found to be located predominantly at intercalated discs.

Electron microscopical studies of the zonal lesions[7,8] (FIGURE 2) have shown that they are areas of intense contraction adjacent to an intercalated disc; the contraction causes marked disruption of sarcomeres, with displacement of myofilaments and translocation of mitochondria. This translocation of mitochondria accounts for the staining pattern seen with succinic dehydrogenase. The sarcolemma overlying these areas is markedly scalloped, but intact, and

* The investigations reported in this paper were supported by United States Public Health Service research grants nos. HE-05875, HE-09566, HE-10179, and HE-3549.

† Recipient of a United States Public Health Service career research award no. HE-K6-14188.

this portion of the myocyte is swollen. The ultrastructure of the remainder of these damaged myocytes appears normal. Usually the damage involves the ends of both myocytes at an intercalated disc. In this situation, the intercalated disc appears unaltered. However, when the damage involves only one of the myocytes, the intercalated disc may be markedly distorted, resulting in herniations into the adjacent uncontracted myocyte.

The myocardial zonal lesion is a consistent finding in dogs in hemorrhagic shock. Although the lesions are microscopical, they are widely distributed throughout the heart, primarily in the subendocardial areas, and in the papillary muscles of both the right and left ventricles. The areas of involvement are usually more extensive than either subendocardial hemorrhage or necrosis. Unlike necrosis, zonal lesions are potentially reversible. In animals surviving for two or three weeks following one hour of severe hemorrhagic shock, residual changes are sparse. Even under electron microscopical examination, very few myocytes show any evidence of a previous zonal lesion.

Pathophysiology and Metabolism of the Heart

The cardiac response to hemorrhagic shock is mediated primarily via the sympatheticoadrenal system. Increased sympathetic activity produces positive

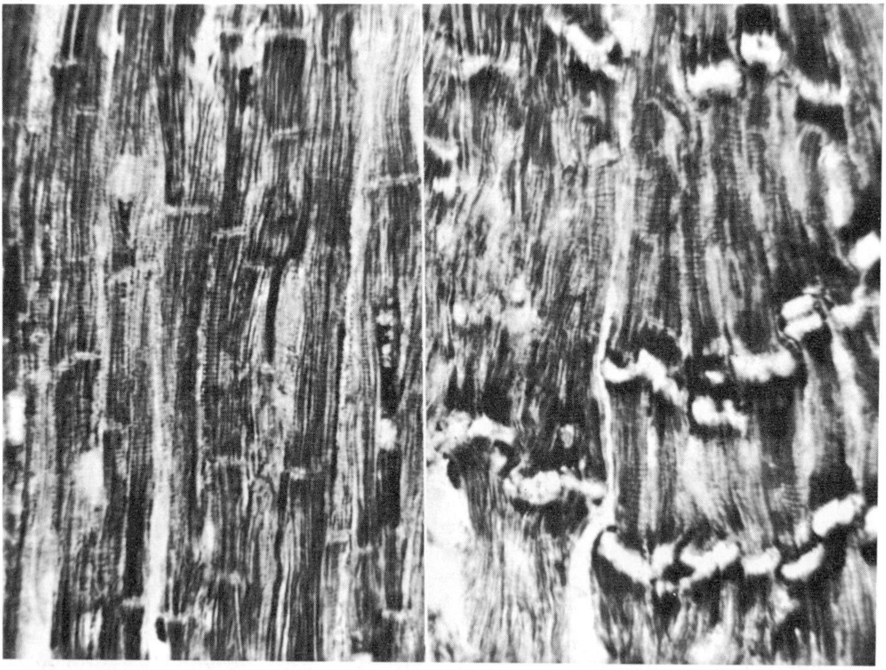

FIGURE 1. Longitudinal sections of the septal papillary muscle of the right ventricle (*Left*) Normal dog. Note the absence of activity in the regions of nuclei and decreased activity at intercalated discs. Activity is present only in mitochondria. (*Right*) Dog in shock. Note the central clear zones bordered on each side by the dark zones characteristic of the zonal lesions. Stain: succinic dehydrogenase. Photograph reproduced by permission of the United States Army. × 500.

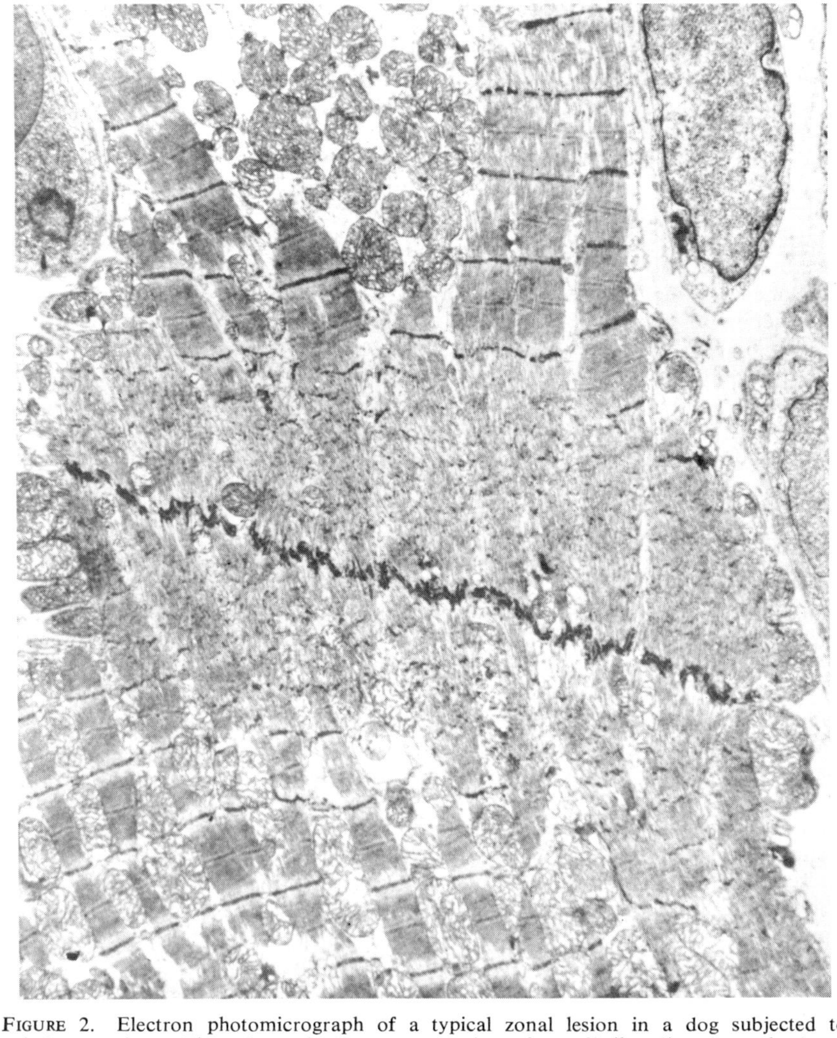

FIGURE 2. Electron photomicrograph of a typical zonal lesion in a dog subjected to shock for one hour. There is marked supercontraction of myofibrils adjacent to the intercalated disc, with fragmentation of Z bands and distortion and displacement of myofilaments. The myofiber is swollen at the position of the intercalated disc, and the sarcolemma is tightly scalloped. Most of the mitochondria are absent from the contracted zone, and are tightly packed between the adjacent, more normal myofibrils. Photograph used by permission of the United States Army. × 5,000.

chronotropic and inotropic stimulation in an attempt to compensate for the decreasing cardiac output. These stimuli, together, with the marked decrease in venous return, lead initially to an increased force of contraction,[3,14] followed by a pronounced tachycardia and decreased ventricular volumes.[15,16] Coronary blood flow is decreased, even though there is vasodilatation of the coronary arteries, with a greater percentage of the cardiac output now supplying the myocardium.[17-19] The percentage of oxygen extraction increases to compensate for this decreased blood flow, as well as to meet the increased demands for oxygen caused by increased sympathetic activity.[20]

One of the interesting findings in hemorrhagic shock is the alteration of myocardial metabolism.[17,19] Normally, the myocardium extracts about 40–60% of the arterial pyruvate. During shock, this pyruvate extraction decreases until a negative arteriovenous difference across the myocardium develops, with the result that the concentration of pyruvate is greater in the coronary sinus blood than in arterial blood; this phenomenon occurs in the presence of a rising arterial pyruvate level. The negative myocardial extraction of pyruvate will revert toward normal following transfusion, provided the animal has not developed irreversibility.[21] Once the animal has entered an irreversible state, this metabolic change becomes refractory to transfusion. A similar decrease occurs in myocardial lactate extraction, although the arteriovenous difference usually remains positive.

As the state of severe hemorrhagic shock progresses, acute progressive cardiac failure develops.[2] This failure is refractory to transfusion, and an irreversible state of shock occurs, leading to death of the experimental animal.

Prevention of Myocardial Damage

Previous studies have shown that myocardial zonal lesions can be prevented by elimination of tachycardia[22] or by beta-sympathetic blockade[23] during shock. Dogs with surgically produced complete heart block do not develop significant myocardial damage even when subjected to three hours of severe hemorrhagic shock. However, the abnormalities in myocardial metabolism, namely, increased oxygen extraction and decreased lactate and pyruvate extraction, occur to the same extent as in normal dogs subjected to shock (TABLE 1). If, on the other hand, tachycardia is produced in the heart-block dogs with a pacemaker, marked zonal lesions will be present following one hour of shock. Tachycardia alone, at a rate normally seen in our dogs during shock (150–180 beats per minute), will not produce significant myocardial damage in a normovolemic animal.

Beta-sympathetic blockade with pronethalol (Alderlin®)‡ also will prevent the development of marked myocardial damage if the dogs are treated with this drug prior to and at 30-minute intervals throughout the period of hemorrhagic shock.[23] Pronethalol will not prevent the development of zonal lesions if given only after shock has already been produced. Alpha-sympathetic blockade with phentolamine (Regitine®)§ has no effect in protecting the myocardium from damage during hemorrhagic shock.[24]

Biplane cineangiocardiography has shown that both complete heart block and beta-sympathetic blockade result in increased ventricular volumes during hemorrhagic shock as compared with normal untreated dogs in shock. In a group of three dogs with complete heart block,[25] cineangiocardiograms were taken during a control period, following the 30-minute bleeding period, and at hourly intervals during three hours of hemorrhagic shock at a mean arterial pressure of 35 mm. Hg. TABLE 2 presents the cardiodynamic values recorded during this experiment. For each time period, cineangiocardiograms were obtained at the idioventricular heart-block rate (26–38 beats per minute), and

‡ Distributed by Ayerst Laboratories, New York, N. Y.

§ Distributed by Ciba Pharmaceutical Products, Inc., Summit, N. J.

TABLE 1

MYOCARDIAL METABOLISM IN HEMORRHAGIC SHOCK*

	Blood Pressure (mm Hg)	Heart Rate (beats/min.)	Oxygen Extraction (%)†	Pyruvate Extraction (%)†	Lactate Extraction (%)†	Arterial Pyruvate (mg/100 ml)	Arterial Lactate (mg/100 ml)	Zonal Lesions‡
Control (pre-shock)								
Normal	112	85	73	55	45	1.39	14.6	
Heart block	80	38	73	56	36	1.36	12.8	
Heart block with tachycardia	101	30	77	55	32	1.82	11.9	
Normovolemic§	121	50	59	60	51	1.16	10.4	
One hour of Shock								
Normal	34	163	91	—10	7	2.79	82.0	
Heart block	35	43	90	— 6	7	2.13	61.1	
Heart block with tachycardia	36	180	91	—16	—2	2.45	84.7	
Normovolemic§	135	183	76	49	38	1.16	12.0	
Recovery (post-shock)								
Normal	91	133	72	21	16	5.00	16.3	4+
Heart block	95	43	78	32	32	1.79	32.3	0 to ±
Heart block with tachycardia	91	45	52	22	20	3.45	40.9	4+
Normovolemic§	138	97	77	54	50	1.28	13.4	0 to ±

* All values are means for four dogs in each group.
† Percentage of myocardial extraction:

$$\frac{\text{arterial concentration} - \text{venous concentration}}{\text{arterial concentration}} \times 100$$

‡ Rough estimation of severity of lesions from 0 (absent) to 4+ (most severe).
§ Normal (no heart block) dogs subjected to one hour of tachycardia but no shock.

TABLE 2

CARDIODYNAMIC VALUES DURING THREE HOURS OF HEMORRHAGIC SHOCK WITH HEART BLOCK AND INTERMITTENT TACHYCARDIA*

	Left Ventricular Pressure (mm Hg)		Aortic Pressure (mm Hg)		Left Ventricular Volumes (ml)			Heart Rate (beats/min)	Cardiac Output (liters/min)
	Systolic	Diastolic	Systolic	Diastolic	End-Diastole	End-Systole	Stroke Volume		
Control (pre-shock)									
Heart block	154	8	154	76	77.9	18.3	59.6	32	1.84
+ Tachycardia	128	0.5	128	96	38.0	16.4	21.6	160	3.43
Early shock									
Heart block	60	—5	60	23	22.6	8.2	14.4	28	0.40
+ Tachycardia	54	—3	54	28	18.4	10.3	8.1	158	1.28
One hour of shock									
Heart block	79	—4	79	22	25.1	7.1	18.0	31	0.57
+ Tachycardia	55	—7	55	25	16.0	7.7	8.3	159	1.31
Two hours of shock									
Heart block	86	—6	86	18	24.7	5.4	19.3	26	0.49
+ Tachycardia	59	—6	59	24	15.4	6.8	8.6	159	1.38
Three hours of shock									
Heart block	75	—6	75	21	25.0	6.4	18.6	30	0.56
+ Tachycardia	61	—5	61	24	16.9	7.6	9.3	160	1.49
Post-transfusion									
Heart block	135	8	135	41	59.9	18.8	41.1	38	1.60
+ Tachycardia	123	2	123	62	29.4	11.6	17.8	158	2.83

* All values are means for three dogs.

then repeated five minutes following the onset of tachycardia (at a mean rate of 160 beats per minutes) produced with an internal electrode catheter in the right ventricle connected to a Grass stimulator. The pacemaker was turned off immediately following each tachycardia cineangiocardiogram, and the animal was allowed to continue in shock at its idioventricular heart-block rate. As shown in FIGURE 3, end-diastolic volumes decrease ($p < 0.001$) with tachycardia during shock, and end-systolic volumes increase ($p < 0.001$). TABLE 3 presents the cardiodynamic values of the dog shown in FIGURE 3.

Biplane cineangiocardiograms were obtained during shock in four normal dogs before and after the administration of a blocking dose of pronethalol (170 mg/m^2 of body surface).[26] TABLE 4 presents the cardiodynamic values recorded during this experiment. Prior to the pronethalol dose, the mean end-diastolic volume during shock was 15.1 ml, and the mean end-systolic volume was 8.3 ml. Five minutes following the pronethalol dose, the mean end-diastolic volume had increased to 25.6 ml, and the mean end-systolic volume had increased to 16.5 ml (FIGURE 4). Both changes are highly significant ($p < 0.001$). As noted in TABLES 4 and 5, cardiac output during the two periods was essen-

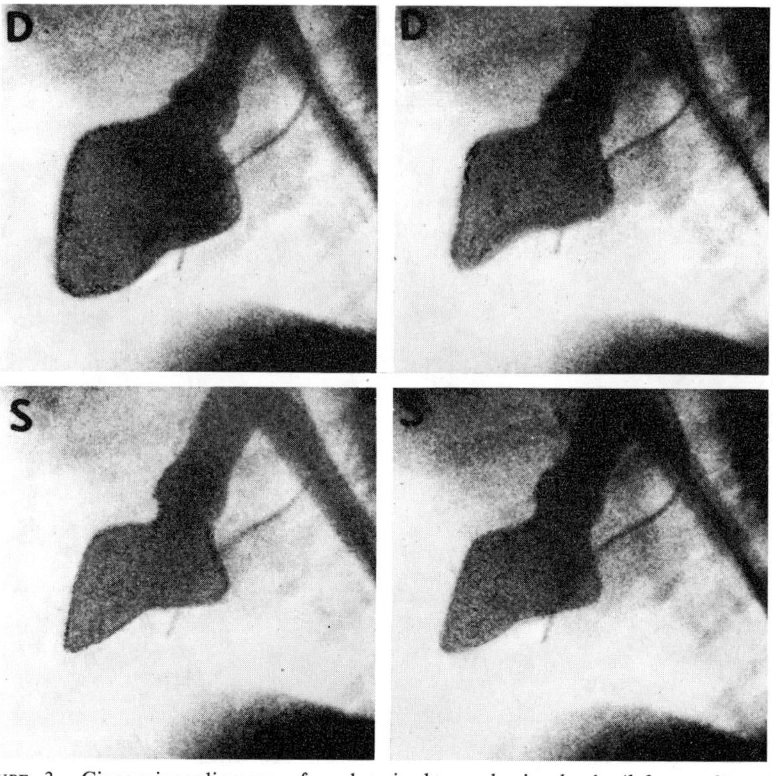

FIGURE 3. Cineangiocardiogram of a dog in hemorrhagic shock (left panel) and in tachycardia during shock (right panel) at end-diastole (D) and end-systole (S). Right anterior oblique view. Cardiodynamic values are given in TABLE 3. Photograph used by permission of the United States Army. One-third actual size.

TABLE 3

CARDIODYNAMIC VALUES OF A DOG WITH HEART BLOCK IN HEMORRHAGIC SHOCK

	Heart Block	Heart Block plus Tachycardia
End-diastolic volume (ml)	28.3	19.9
End-systolic volume (ml)	10.6	12.8
Stroke Volume (ml)	17.7	7.1
Heart rate (beats/min)	22	160
Cardiac output (liters/min)	0.45	1.14
Blood pressure (mm Hg)		
Left Ventricle	60/—4	58/—6
Aortic	60/23	58/31

TABLE 4

EFFECT OF PRONETHALOL ON VENTRICULAR VOLUMES DURING HEMORRHAGIC SHOCK*

	Left Ventricular Volumes (ml)			Heart Rate (beats/min)	Cardiac Output (liters/min)
	End-Diastole	End-Systole	Stroke Volume		
Control (pre-shock)	49.9	28.1	21.8	94	1.94
Shock	15.1	8.3	6.8	140	0.95
Shock with pronethalol	25.6	16.5	9.1	116	0.98

* All values are means for four dogs.

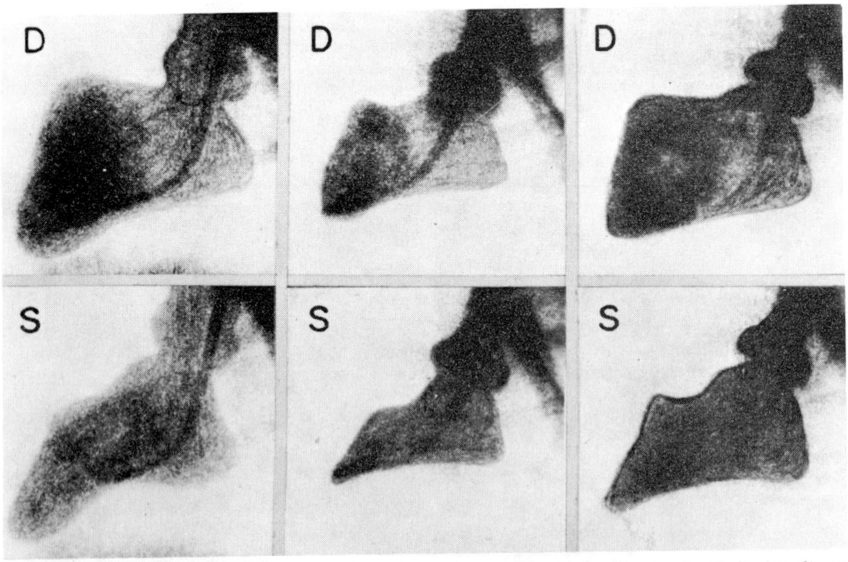

FIGURE 4. Cineangiocardiogram of a dog prior to hemorrhagic shock (left panel) and during shock before (center panel) and after (right panel) treatment with pronethalol. End-diastole (D) and end-systole (S). Right anterior oblique view. Cardiodynamic values are given in TABLE 5. Photograph used by permission of the United States Army. One-third actual size.

TABLE 5

EFFECT OF PRONETHALOL ON CARDIODYNAMIC VALUES OF A DOG IN HEMORRHAGIC SHOCK

	Control	Shock	Shock with Pronethalol*
End-diastolic volume (ml)	31.4	14.9	27.2
End-systolic volume (ml)	20.6	7.5	19.8
Stroke volume (ml)	10.8	7.4	7.4
Heart rate (beats/min)	118	136	109
Cardiac output (liters/min)	1.26	0.98	0.82

* Pronethalol administered after 15 minutes of shock at a dose of 170 mg/m^2 of body surface.

tially unchanged. The heart rate usually decreases when pronethalol is given to a dog in shock; in other experiments, however, the heart was paced at the original shock heart rate following pronethalol administration, and increases in ventricular volumes still occurred.

Recent studies[27] have enabled us to assess separately the role of cardiac versus extracardiac factors in the production of zonal lesions. The cardiopulmonary and systemic circulations were separated *in vivo* by ligating the superior and inferior vena cavas and ascending aorta, and the blood volumes, flows, and pressures of each were regulated separately with an extracorporeal pump-oxygenator. Blood flow in the systemic circulation was drained from the vena cavas and returned via one carotid and one femoral artery. Blood flow in the cardiopulmonary circulation was drained from a cannula ligated in the ascending aorta via the left subclavian artery, and returned to the right atrium. Blood from both circulations was allowed to mix in a common reservoir in the external circulation. Under these conditions, hypovolemic hypotension could be produced in one circulation while normal blood volumes, flows, and pressures were maintained in the other. All blood pressures (arterial, venous, and left ventricular) and flows, as well as an electrocardiogram, were monitored continuously. Arterial, coronary sinus, and oxygenator blood samples were analyzed for blood gases, pH, hematocrit, and the myocardial extraction of lactate, pyruvate, and glucose to document the adequacy of the method used in producing "regional shock." The period of "regional shock" was 60–90 minutes, following which the animals were sacrificed and autopsied to determine the extent of damage to the heart. Gross and microscopical examinations of all organs were performed.

Marked myocardial zonal lesions were produced when the heart was "in shock," but very few zonal lesions developed when only the systemic circulation was "in shock." TABLE 6 illustrates the differences in blood analyses between the two groups.

As noted previously, the sympathetic nervous system has a role in the production of myocardial zonal lesions in shock. Total blockade of beta-sympathetic stimulation with pronethalol will prevent development of these lesions. However, bilateral stellate ganglionectomy has no effect in preventing the zonal lesions. Infusions of large doses of adrenaline, noradrenaline, or isoproterenol to the intact dog not in shock does not produce zonal lesions. If, on the other hand, an infusion of one of these agents is given during the period of "heart shock" in the "separate circulation" studies, there is an increase in the severity of zonal lesions.

TABLE 6

BLOOD ANALYSES DURING "SEPARATE CIRCULATION" STUDIES*

	Heart in Shock, Body Normal		Body in Shock, Heart Normal	
	Control	Shock	Control	Shock
Oxygen concentration†				
Arterial	13.03 ± 2.21	13.68 ± 3.34	14.78 ± 0.98	12.67 ± 2.41
Pump-oxygenator	15.32 ± 1.24	15.62 ± 1.87	16.62 ± 0.45	16.32 ± 2.25
Coronary sinus	4.88 ± 1.94	2.80¶ ± 1.12	6.20 ± 3.29	3.15 ± 2.67
Oxygen extraction§	62.0 ±15.4	80.2¶ ± 4.0	57.6 ±22.3	75.6 ±15.1
Lactate concentration‡				
Arterial	40.5 ± 7.4	41.6 ±16.6	31.0 ±10.2	54.9¶ ±12.5
Coronary sinus	35.1 ± 6.6	32.9 ±14.2	24.7 ±12.0	53.8¶ ±15.8
Lactate extraction§	12.3 ±14.6	21.1 ±13.4	20.3 ±15.4	1.9¶ ±14.0
Pyruvate concentration‡				
Arterial	2.18 ± 0.56	2.21 ± 1.07	2.18 ± 0.23	1.74¶ ± 0.40
Coronary sinus	1.65 ± 0.71	1.95 ± 1.06	1.54 ± 0.73	1.45 ± 0.17
Pyruvate extraction§	24.6 ±26.3	11.9 ±18.8	30.6 ±36.2	23.0 ± 5.4

* All values are means; seven dogs were included in the heart in shock, body normal group; six dogs were included in the body in shock, heart normal group.

† Top number, ml/100 ml; bottom number, standard deviation.

‡ Top number, mg/100 ml; bottom number, standard deviation.

§ Top number, percentage of myocardial extraction; bottom number, standard deviation. Percentage of myocardial extraction:

$$\frac{\text{arterial concentration} - \text{venous concentration}}{\text{arterial concentration}} \times 100$$

¶ Significant changes ($p < 0.01$).

Conclusions

These studies have dealt with the etiology of the myocardial zonal lesions seen in experimental hemorrhagic shock. The findings support the hypothesis that the heart itself may be responsible for its own damage during hemorrhagic shock. Important in this regard are the compensatory mechanisms that result in tachycardia, decreased ventricular volumes, and an increased positive inotropic response. Although these responses are regulated by the sympathetic nervous system, sympathetic stimulation alone will not produce zonal lesions in the absence of shock, but may contribute to the severity of cardiac lesions during shock.

Exactly which insult causes the zonal lesions is not known. The possibility that subendocardial ischemia may contribute to the development of these lesions cannot be excluded. However, the present studies indicate that mechanical forces may have a more direct role in their production. The heart is small and beats rapidly and vigorously; the result could be mechanical trauma to the subendocardial regions.

References

1. COOLEY, J. C. & C. L. MCINTOSH. 1963. Myocardial contractile force in experimental hemorrhagic shock. Arch. Surg. (Chicago) **87:** 330–340.
2. CROWELL, J. W. & A. C. GUYTON. 1962. Further evidence favoring a cardiac mechanism in irreversible hemorrhagic shock. Amer. J. Physiol. **203:** 248–252.
3. GLAVIANO, V. V. & M. A. KLOUDA. 1965. Myocardial catecholamines and stimulation of the stellate ganglion in hemorrhagic shock. Amer. J. Physiol. **209:** 751–756.
4. GOMEZ, O. A. & W. F. HAMILTON. 1964. Functional cardiac deterioration during development of hemorrhagic circulatory deficiency. Circ. Res. **14:** 327–336.
5. HACKEL, D. B. & B. N. CATCHPOLE. 1958. Pathologic and electrocardiographic effects of hemorrhagic shock in dogs treated with l-norepinephrine. Lab. Invest. **7:** 358–368.
6. MARTIN, JR., A. M. & D. B. HACKEL. 1963. The myocardium of the dog in hemorrhagic shock. Lab. Invest. **12:** 77–91.
7. MARTIN, JR., A. M., D. B. HACKEL & S. M. KURTZ. 1964. The ultrastructure of zonal lesions of the myocardium in hemorrhagic shock. Amer. J. Path. **44:** 127–140.
8. MARTIN, JR., A.M. & D. B. HACKEL. 1966. An electron microscopic study of the progression of myocardial lesions in the dog after hemorrhagic shock. Lab. Invest. **15:** 243–260.
9. FERRANS, V. J., R. G. HIBBS, W. C. BLACK & D. G. WEILBAECHER. 1964. Isoproterenol-induced myocardial necrosis. Amer. Heart J. **68:** 71–90.
10. SZAKÁCS, J. E. & A. CANNON. 1958. l-Norepinephrine myocarditis. Amer. J. Clin. Path. **30:** 425–434.
11. KAYE, M. P., R. H. MCDONALD & W. C. RANDALL. 1961. Systolic hypertension and subendocardial hemorrhages produced by electrical stimulation of the stellate ganglion. Circ. Res. **9:** 1164–1170.
12. LIGHT, JR., F. W. & S. C. BENBROOK. 1958. Subendocardial hemorrhages of the left ventricle following trauma in goats. Arch. Path. (Chicago) **65:** 407–414.
13. BEHRMANN, V. G. & F. W. HARTMAN. 1955. Effects of plasma expanders upon capillary resistance. Lab. Invest. **4:** 190–205.
14. WALTON, R. P., J. A. RICHARDSON, R. P. WALTON, JR. & W. L. THOMPSON. 1959. Sympathetic influences during hemorrhagic hypotension. Amer. J. Physiol. **197:** 223–230.
15. BRISTOW, J. D., R. E. FERGUSON, F. MINTZ & E. RAPAPORT. 1963. Thermodilution studies of ventricular volume changes due to isoproterenol and bleeding. J. Appl. Physiol. **18:** 129–133.
16. HAMILTON, JR., W. F., P. DOW & W. F. HAMILTON. 1950. Measurement of volume of dogs heart by x-ray. Effect of hemorrhage, of epinephrine infusion and of buffer nerve section. Amer. J. Physiol. **161:** 466–472.
17. EDWARDS, W. S., A. SIEGAL & R. J. BING. 1954. Studies on myocardial metabolism: III. Coronary blood flow, myocardial oxygen consumption, and carbohydrate metabolism in experimental hemorrhagic shock. J. Clin. Invest. **33:** 1646–1661.
18. GREGG, D. E. Hemodynamic factors in shock. 1962. *In* Shock-Pathogenesis and Therapy. K. D. Bock, Ed. : 50–60. Academic Press, Inc. New York.
19. HACKEL, D. B. & W. T. GOODALE. 1955. Effects of hemorrhagic shock on the heart and circulation of intact dogs. Circulation **11:** 628–634.
20. GRANATA, L., R. A. OLSSON, A. HUVOS & D. E. GREGG. 1965. Coronary inflow and oxygen usage following cardiac sympathetic nerve stimulation in unanesthetized dogs. Circ. Res. **16:** 114–120.
21. HACKEL, D. B. & R. BREITENECKER. 1963. Time factor in reversibility of myocardial metabolic changes in hemorrhagic shock. Proc. Soc. Exp. Biol. Med. **113:** 534–537.
22. HACKEL, D. B., A. M. MARTIN, JR., M. S. SPACH & H. O. SIEKER. 1964. Hemorrhagic shock in dogs. Relation of hemodynamic and metabolic changes to myocardial lesions. Arch. Path. (Chicago) **77:** 575–581.

23. ENTMAN, M., D. B. HACKEL, A. M. MARTIN, E. MIKAT & J. CHANG. 1967 . Prevention of myocardial lesions during hemorrhagic shock in dogs by pronethalol. Arch. Path. (Chicago) **83:** 392–395.
24. Unpublished observations.
25. MARTIN, JR., A. M., D. B. HACKEL, M. P. CAPP, M. S. SPACH & E. MIKAT. Cineangiocardiographic studies of hemorrhagic shock in dogs with complete heart block. To be published.
26. HACKEL, D. B., A. M. MARTIN, JR., M. P. CAPP, M. S. SPACH & E. MIKAT. Cineangiographic studies of the effects of pronethalol on the heart in hemorrhagic shock. To be published.
27. MARTIN, JR., A. M., D. B. HACKEL, J. C. CHANG, M. L. ENTMAN, and E. MIKAT. The role of cardiac and extracardiac factors in the etiology of myocardial zonal lesions in hemorrhagic shock. To be published.

EXPERIMENTAL GRANULOMATOUS MYOCARDITIS: GENESIS AND IMMUNOLOGICAL ASPECTS*

Alexander Laufer and A. Michael Davies

Departments of Pathology and Medical Ecology
Hebrew University–Hadassah Medical School
Jerusalem, Israel

The clinical association of "rheumatism" with disease of the heart was noted by Pitcairn about 180 years ago,[1] and experimental studies aimed at reproducing this type of myocarditis have been in progress for half a century.[2]. Although production of Aschoff bodies (or Aschoff-like bodies) as the morphological expression of human rheumatic heart disease was soon achieved,[3] production of valvular lesions was less frequent.[4]

In attempting to understand the pathogenesis of these myocardial lesions, we were impressed by the similarity of the histological patterns resulting from a wide variety of noxious agents. The main features of this picture are two-fold: myofiber damage, either of displacement and/or necrosis, and a cellular infiltrate consisting mainly of histiocytic- or lymphocytic-type round cells, with rare polymorphonuclear and giant cells. Foci of this type of lesion may be single or scattered, may be found anywhere in the ventricles, and may vary widely in intensity.

Early experiments[5] involving the injection of streptococci, lactobacilli, and *Escherichia coli* into the myocardium produced this type of lesion (FIGURES 1 and 2), and similar results were obtained with staphylococci and *Pseudomonas aeruginosa*.[6,7] In no case were the pathogens found in the myocardial lesions. In other work, proteolytic enzymes were injected into the bloodstream,[8] and streptococci were introduced into the tonsils[9] of experimental animals. Success with the latter method has been confirmed by Ginsburg and his colleagues,[10] who also obtained focal myocardial lesions (but with more extensive muscle damage) by the intratonsillar injection of extracellular streptococcal products. Murphy's classical experiments with repeated subcutaneous injections of streptococci[3] and Rubenstone's and Saphir's direct physical damage to the heart[11] produced the identical pattern of focal myocarditis. To this list of noxious agents may be added viruses of different species,[12] bacterial lipopolysaccharides,[13] toxins such as diphtheria,[14] and parasites such as *Trypanosoma cruzi*[15] which, if they damage the heart, always produce the same pattern.

An identical histological picture is well known in man,[16] associated mainly with acute, generalized bacterial and viral disease[17] but also found in chronic viral and parasitic infections. Jaffe[18] noted a 10% incidence of myocarditis in a series of 5,000 autopsies in Venezuela, associated with both infectious and metabolic diseases. He assumed that there was primary, multicausal damage to the myofiber, the cellular infiltration being secondary. Myocarditis also occurs as a result of heat stroke, burns,[16] and some types of autoimmune disease;[19] this indicates that there must be a specific response to a variety of noxious stimuli.

FIGURE 3 shows the picture of granulomatous myocarditis in a 75-year-old man with a thymoma but without clinical evidence of myasthenia gravis. Another patient, a three-year-old girl, died suddenly two days after the onset

* Supported by United States Public Health Service research grant no. HE-05739 from the National Institutes of Health, Bethesda, Md.

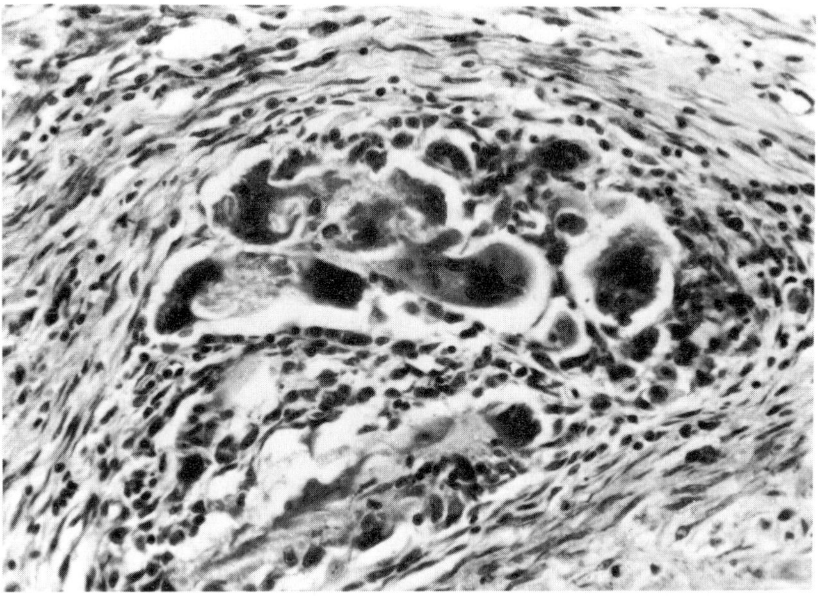

FIGURE 1. Granulomatous myocarditis in a rabbit, seven days after intramyocardial injection of hemolytic streptococcus. Stain: hematoxylin and eosin. × 270.

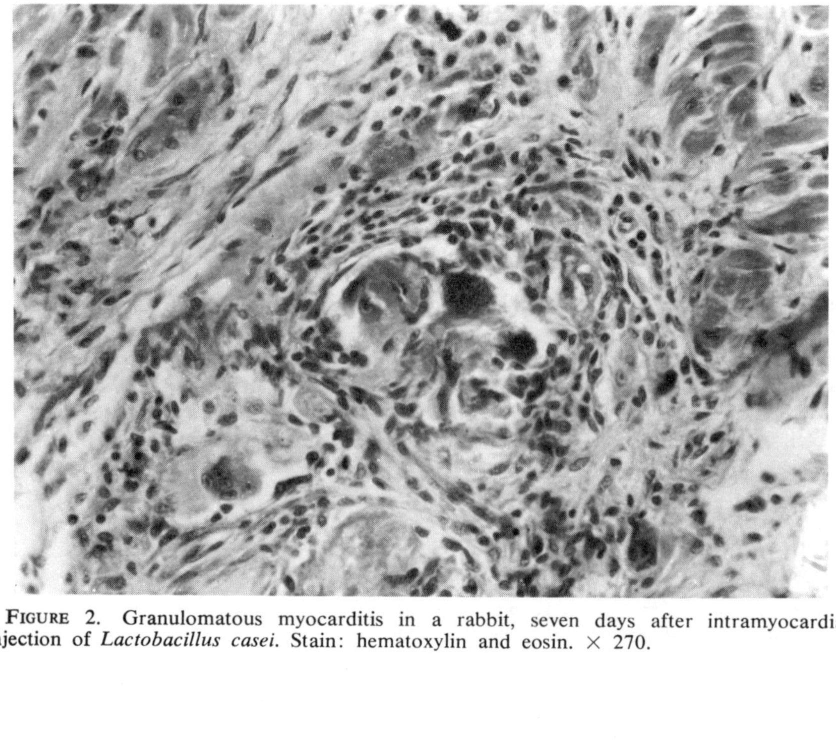

FIGURE 2. Granulomatous myocarditis in a rabbit, seven days after intramyocardial injection of *Lactobacillus casei*. Stain: hematoxylin and eosin. × 270.

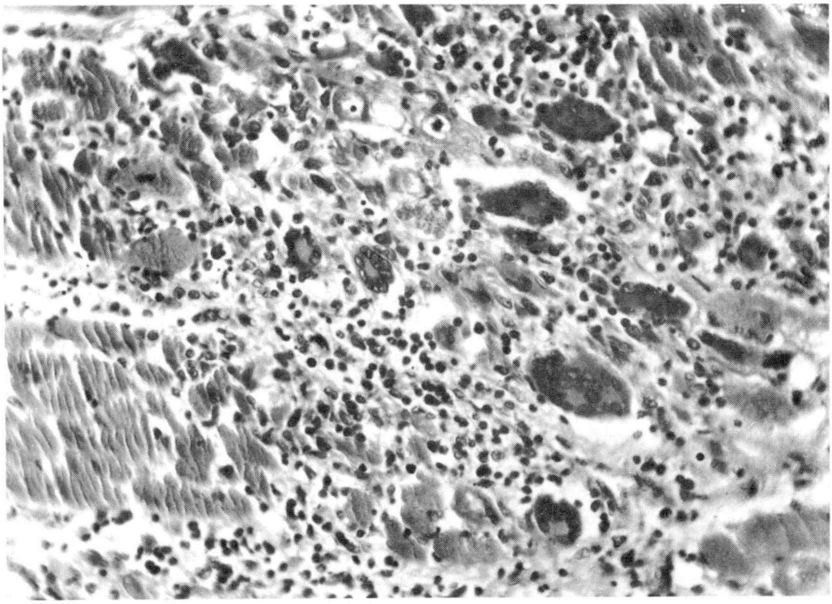

FIGURE 3. Granulomatous myocarditis in a 75-year-old man with thymoma but no clinical evidence of myasthenia gravis. Stain: hematoxylin and eosin. × 270.

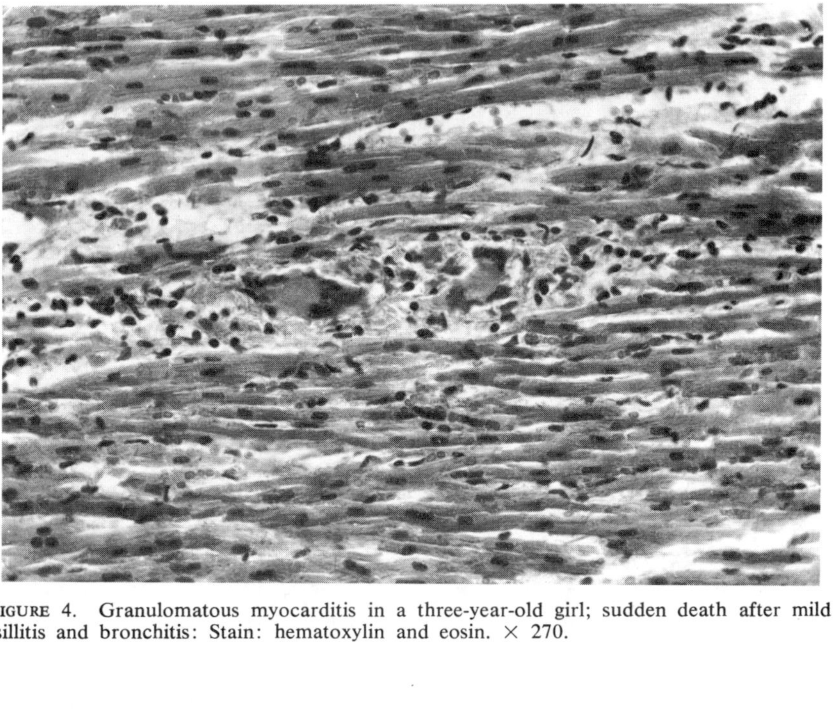

FIGURE 4. Granulomatous myocarditis in a three-year-old girl; sudden death after mild tonsillitis and bronchitis: Stain: hematoxylin and eosin. × 270.

of mild tonsillitis and bronchitis. The granulomatous giant-cell myocarditis discovered at autopsy is shown in FIGURE 4. A third illustrative case from our hospital is that of a one-month-old child with sagittal sinus thrombosis and myocarditis as an unsuspected finding.

Focal myocarditis of the same type as, and presumably of similar etiology to, autoimmune disease in man is produced in experimental animals by injections of extracts of homologous and heterologous heart.[20] The lesions in animals, although of the same basic type, differ in distribution and intensity in different species (FIGURES 5 and 6).

When injected into rabbits, guinea pigs, or rats, with or without Freund's complete adjuvant, heterologous heart extracts cause the production of antibodies, both anti-heart and anti-"species"; lesions of focal myocarditis are more frequent in animals receiving adjuvant (TABLE 1). On the other hand, rats injected with rat heart extracts showed myocarditis without antibody formation; those given the same extracts with Freund's adjuvant showed either antibody formation or myocarditis, but not both.[21] There is a distinct impression that in cases of immunopathological myocarditis, as in allergic encephalitis, the circulating antibody protects against myofiber damage caused, presumably, by sensitized lymphocytes.[22]

Because so many noxious stimuli, widely different in their biological effects, all lead to focal myocarditis of the same morphological type, one is attracted to the idea that the various stimuli trigger a common sequence of events to produce the lesion. It is suggested that the end target in this sequence is the lysosome, itself "triggered" perhaps by mitochondrial damage, with both being affected by, and affecting, changes in cell-wall permeability. This theory and its possible pathways are illustrated in FIGURE 7. There is already some evi-

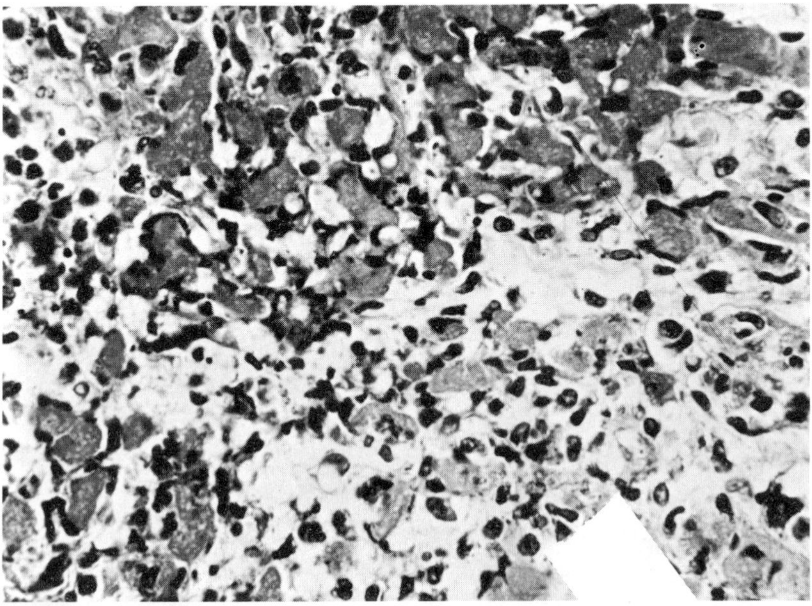

FIGURE 5. Granulomatous myocarditis in a rabbit given six weekly injections of rabbit heart extract with Freund's adjuvant. Note the myofiber necrosis and cellular infiltration. Stain: hematoxylin and eosin. × 500.

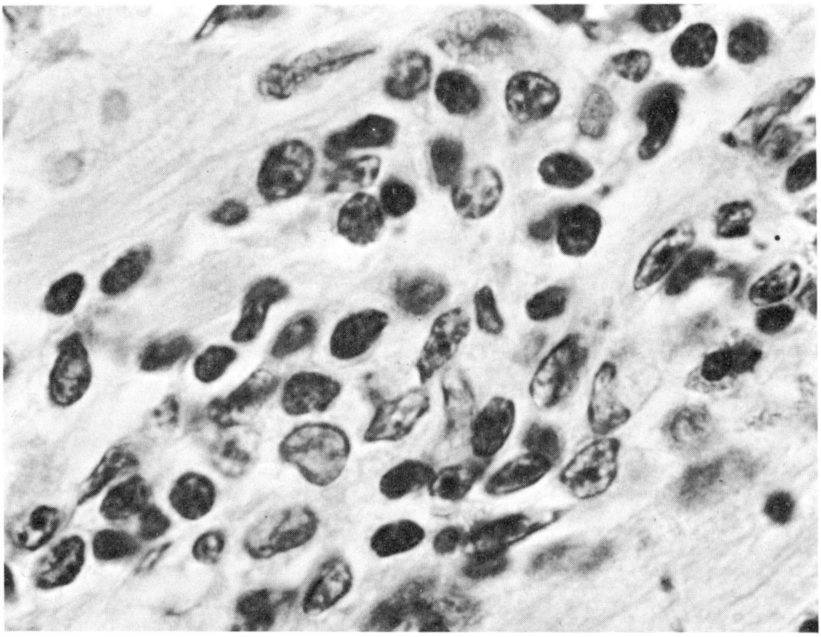

FIGURE 6. Granulomatous myocarditis in a guinea pig given six weekly injections of rabbit heart extract with Freund's adjuvant. Note the cellular infiltrate consisting of histiocytes, lymphoid cells, and a few plasma cells. Stain: hematoxylin and eosin. × 1,300.

TABLE 1

FOCAL MYOCARDITIS AND SPECIFIC ANTIBODY PRODUCTION BY ANIMALS IMMUNIZED WITH EXTRACTS OF HOMOLOGUS AND HETEROLOGOUS HEART

Species	Number of Animals	Immunizing Heart Antigen	Freund's Adjuvant Added	Antibody Production (%)*	Incidence of Myocarditis (%)†
Rabbit	20	Rabbit	Yes	25	20
	10	Rabbit	No	0	0
Rat	24	Rat	Yes	40	12
	67	Rat	No	0	19
Hamster	12	Hamster	Yes	17	40
Rabbit	22	Rat or guinea pig	Yes	100	65
Guinea pig	18	Rabbit	Yes	94	78
Rat	17	Rabbit or guinea pig	No	100	18

* Specific anti-heart antibodies in the passive hemagglutination test at a titer of 1 : 20 or more.

† Animals with focal granulomatous myocarditis graded ++ or more, as defined by Davies *et al.*[13]

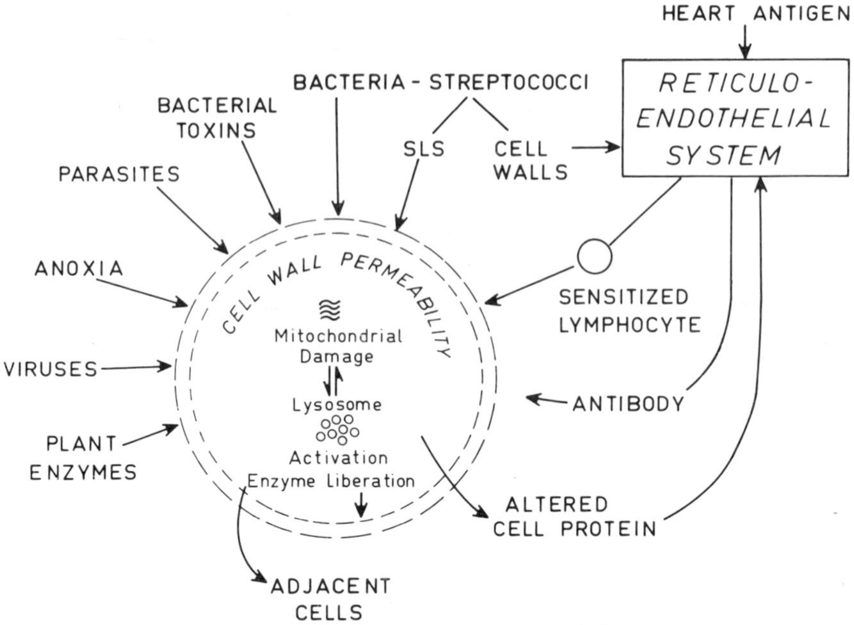

FIGURE 7. Possible pathways of myofiber lesions.

dence, both direct and indirect, to support this theory. First, preliminary electron microscopical studies of the normal rat heart, performed by Dr. Ben-Ishay in our laboratory, confirm the presence of "residual bodies," presumably lysosomes[23] (FIGURE 8). Seven to ten days after a single injection of homologous heart extract, the guinea pig heart shows round-cell infiltration and mitochondrial damage (FIGURE 9). At this stage, lysosomes were not seen, although it must be stressed that these observations are based on the study of a limited number of hearts. Observations of the effect of heterologous antibodies and streptolysin S on tissue cultures of rat heart[24] show that the main lesion is an alteration of cell-wall permeability leading to ionic imbalance, swelling, and bursting (FIGURES 10 and 11). These results are in agreement with what is known about the effect of streptolysins S on membrane permeability in general, and on the lysosome in particular.[25] Moreover, agents known to labilize lysosomes, e.g. bacterial toxins and heteroantibodies, also increase the permeability of other membranes, including those of mitochondria and the cell itself.[26]

The possibility of myofiber damage by hypersensitivity reaction is indicated by the studies of Zvi Marcus in our laboratory. He observed that rat heart cells, cultured *in vitro,* undergo cytolysis when incubated with rabbit lymphocytes sensitized to rat heart extracts; however, when incubated with rat lymphocytes sensitized to rabbit heart extracts, the rat heart cells show emperipolesis† (FIGURE 12).

Further evidence of the role of immunological sensitization comes from experiments with isoproterenol.[27, 28] In rats of the Hebrew University strain,

† "Emperipolesis" is the appearance of lymphocytes within the cytoplasm of other cells (Trowell, O. A. 1958. Int. Rev. Cytol. 7: 235).

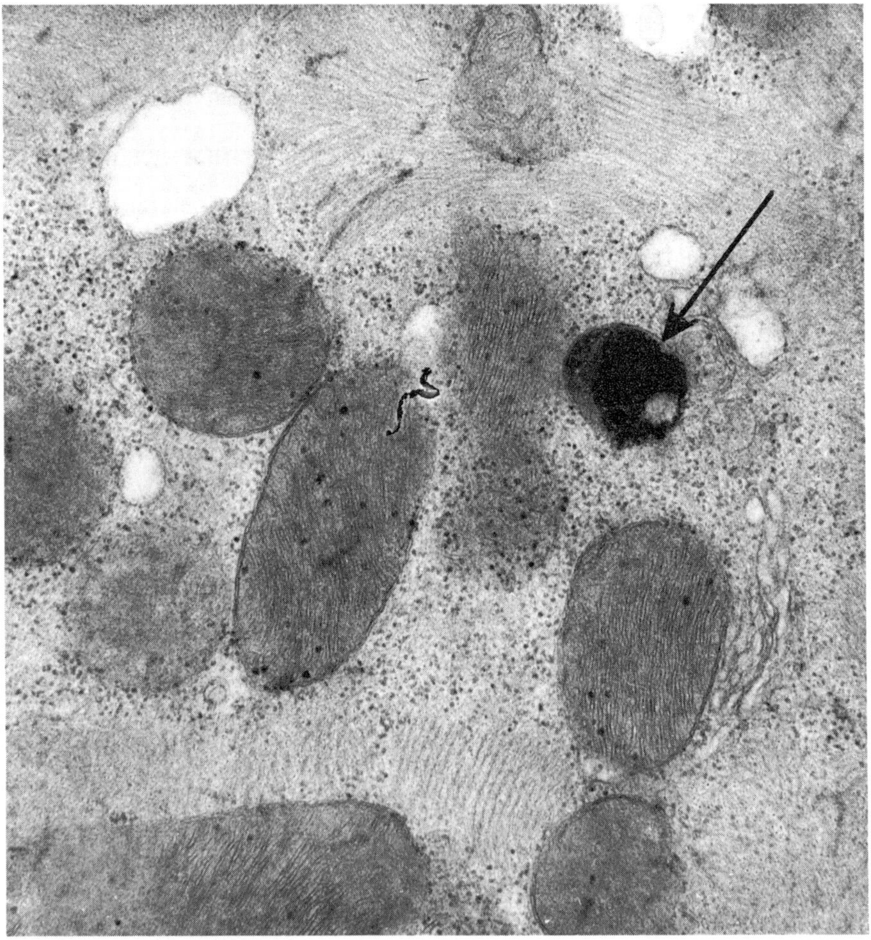

FIGURE 8a. Electron micrograph of normal rat myocardium. Arrow indicates residual body, which is shown in greater detail in FIGURE 8b. × 23,800 (orig. mag. × 28,000).

a single injection of 30–100 mg/kg produces the typical picture of focal necrosis with infiltration after 24 hours (FIGURE 13). The same dose given to rats previously immunized against heart extracts produces a much more severe reaction (FIGURE 14); the effect of homologous heart extracts is greater than that of heterologous, in spite of the low levels of circulating antibody in the former case.[28] Administration of high-titer anti-heart antibody intravenously to rats has no detectable effect on their hearts; when isoproterenol is given, even normal heterologous sera greatly increase the cardiac damage. There are strong parallels between these findings and those seen in cases of thyroiditis, where passive administration of anti-thyroid sera does not affect the thyroid, but the synergistic effect of simultaneous mild direct damage is marked.[29]

On the other hand, Kaplan[30] has demonstrated the binding of globulins from rheumatic fever patients to the sarcolemma and has shown that this involves the fixation of complement.[31] The suggestion that it is the antigen-antibody reaction between sarcolemma and circulating antibody (to heart or to streptococcal membrane[32]) which leads to various changes, such as in permeability,[31] can also be argued conversely, i.e., that cells damaged by other means (e.g. by streptococcal toxins) leak antigen, and it is this that combines with already circulating antibody. The second interpretation is strengthened by the observation that the rise in circulating antibody, in different forms of heart disease in man, follows rather than precedes the myocardial lesions;[33,34] this is also true after surgical procedures.[35]

There are still gaps in the "unitary" theory of myocarditis, but the weight of the evidence points to myofiber permeability changes and lysosomal dam-

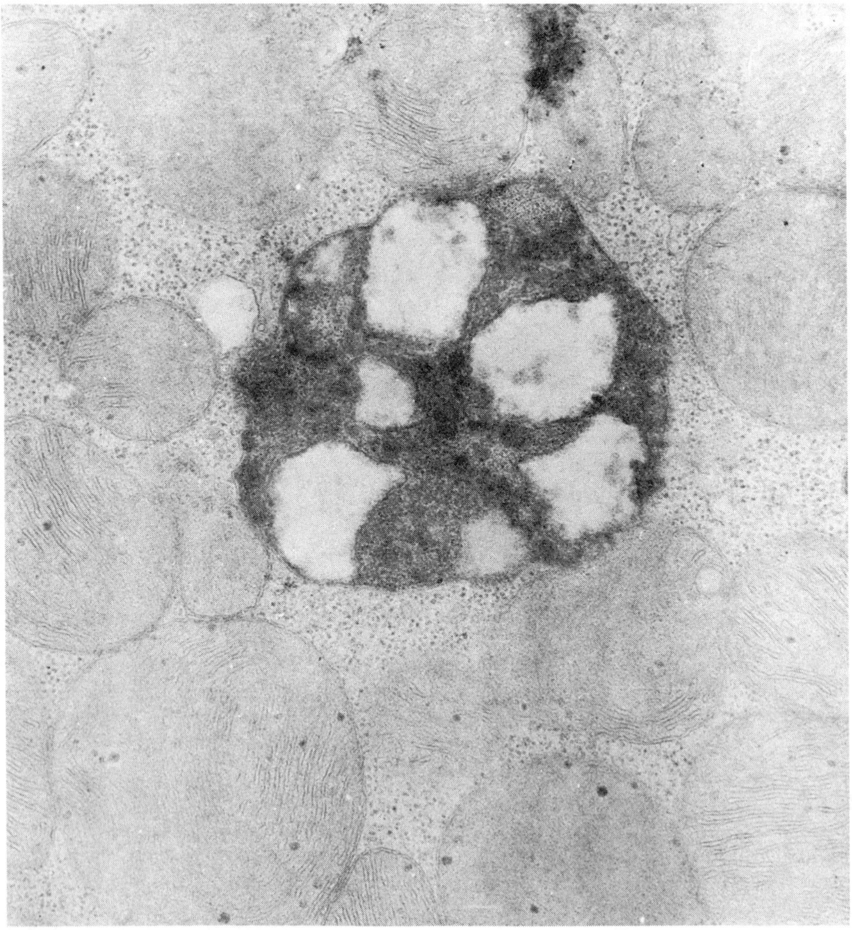

FIGURE 8b. Electron micrograph of a residual body in normal rat myocardium, as shown in FIGURE 8a. × 38,250 (orig. mag. × 45,000).

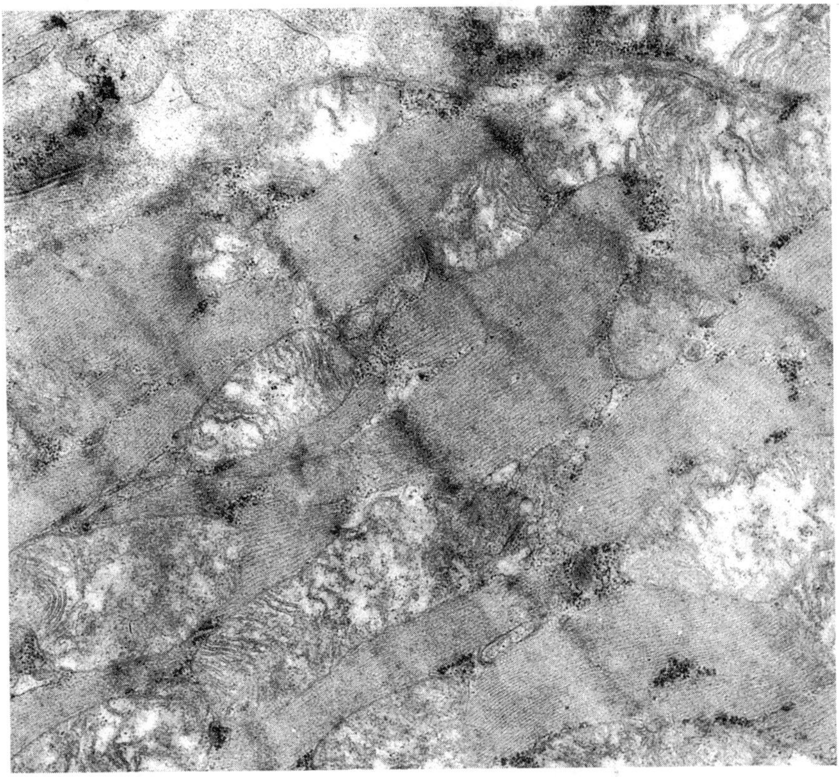

FIGURE 9. Electron micrograph showing diffuse mitochondrial damage in the myocardium of a guinea pig, eight days after a single injection of guinea pig heart extract with Freund's adjuvant. × 16,500 (orig. mag. × 22,000).

age. Weissman has suggested[36] that lysosomes may be involved in the alteration of tissue necessary for the initiation of the autoimmune process;[37] the fact that antigenic change can lead to autoimmune heart disease in animals and man is well established.[13, 33]

Summary

The myocardium may be damaged in many ways, but reacts in very few. The same histological picture that resulted from the intramyocardial injection of bacteria, pathogenic and otherwise, could also be produced by immunization against extracts of heart muscle or by administration of bacterial polysaccharide. Intravenous papain and subcutaneous diphtheria toxin both produce the same type of focal myocarditis, and similar lesions may be seen in "normal" laboratory animals.

The basic lesion is one of microscopical foci of mononuclear cells with or without obvious muscle fiber necrosis. This cellular reaction consists mainly of histiocyte-like cells, lymphocytes, rare eosinophils and polymorphs, and, under certain conditions, multinucleate giant cells. Endocardial and pericardial inflammatory foci have also been detected.

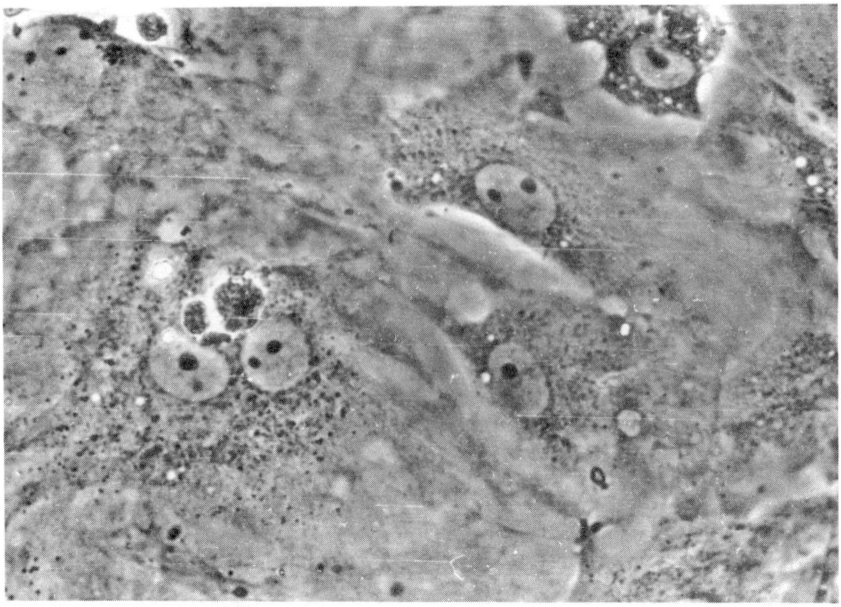

FIGURE 10. Rat heart cells in tissue culture, seventh day. Addition of streptoccocal cell-bound hemolysin at time zero. Note the clarity of cell outlines, nuclei with nucleoli, and degree of granulation. Phase contrast (Zeiss). × 400.

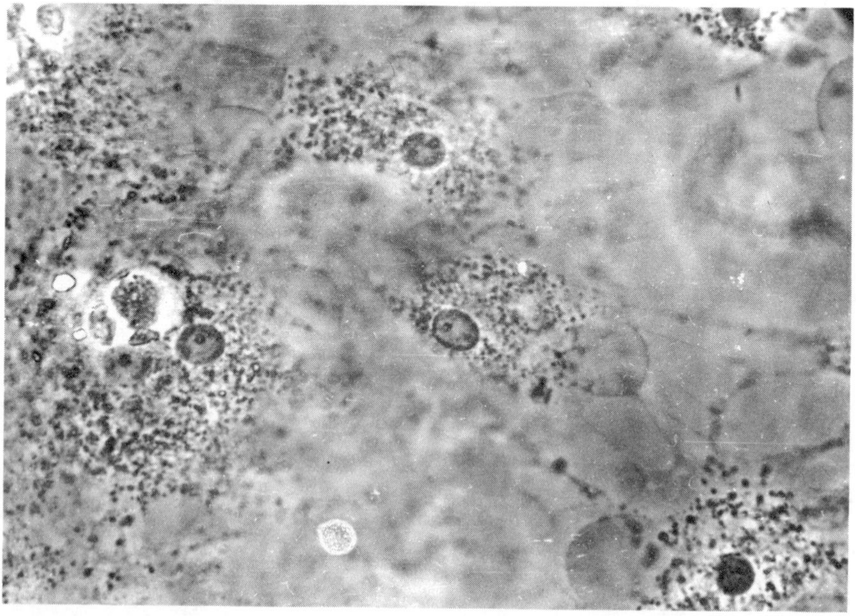

FIGURE 11. Rat heart cells in tissue culture, seventh day. Same field as in FIGURE 10, 20 minutes after the addition of streptoccocal cell-bound hemolysin, with incubation. Note the loss of cell borders, increased granulation, and blebbing. Phase contrast (Zeiss). × 400.

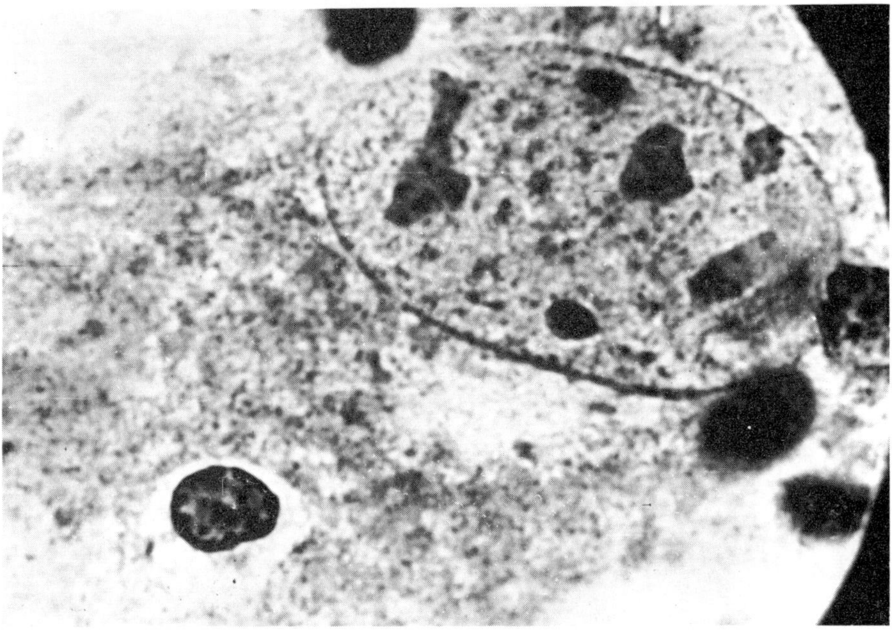

FIGURE 12. Seven-day-old rat heart cell culture incubated with rat lymphocytes sensitized to rabbit heart extract, 48 hours after the addition of the lymphocytes. Note emperipolesis. Stain: Giemsa. × 1,000.

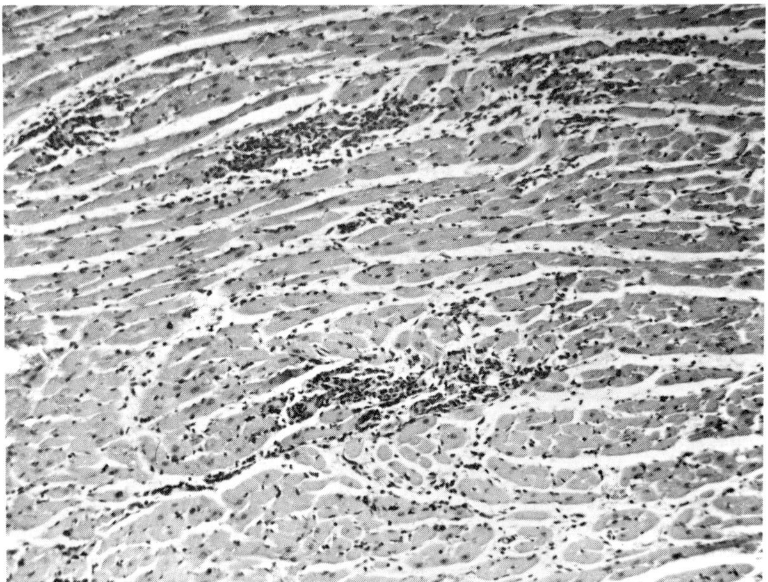

FIGURE 13. Focal myocardial necrosis and infiltration in a nonimmune rat, 24 hours after a single injection of isoproterenol (100 mg/kg). Stain: hematoxylin and eosin. × 110.

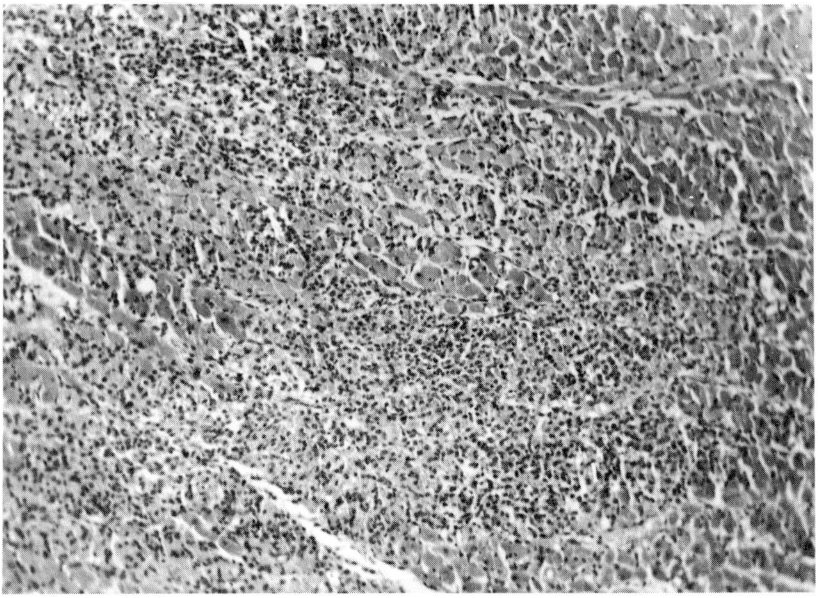

FIGURE 14. Extensive myocardial necrosis and infiltration in a rat previously immunized with rat heart extract, 24 hours after a single injection of isoproterenol (100 mg/kg). Stain: hematoxylin and eosin. × 110.

It is proposed that different noxious stimuli act by different pathways to damage the myofiber and evoke a common sequence of events leading to the histological pattern described. The initial myofiber lesion is, probably, one of increased cell-wall permeability, which leads to electrolyte imbalance and lysosomal damage. A twofold result of this cell disruption would be the extension of the lesion to adjacent cells by direct action of lysosomal enzymes and the production of changed, and therefore antigenically different, cell material. Such antigenic material might serve to sensitize immunologically competent cells, and these, in turn, would damage the cross-reacting antigen of normal myofiber walls. In this way the lesion could be self-perpetuating, even when the initial stimulus ceased and the continued antigenic stimulus led to the production of circulating antiglobulins that would bind to damaged cells.

Specific anti-heart antibodies have been demonstrated in the sera of some of the experimental animals, but there was no correlation between titer and the presence of histological lesions. In some animals the circulating antibodies seemed to exert a protective role, although the evidence from man is that the antibodies are a *result* rather than a *cause* of the myocardial lesion. Passive immunization with homologous or heterologous anti-heart sera does not produce myocardial lesions, although the heterologous sera are cytopathogenic to tissue cultures of the heart. On the other hand, rats actively immunized against heart-muscle extracts show a marked increase in the severity and extent of the myocardial lesions produced by a standard injection of isoproterenol. The same effect is seen with passive transfer of anti-heart antisera, and it seems likely that the specific antibodies become cytotoxic only after the myofiber cell-wall barrier is broken down.

The histological pattern described above is also seen in human myocarditis of widely different, viral and parasitic, known and unknown, etiologies. The association of granulomatous myocarditis with cases of thymoma in man and autoimmune disease in animals lends further support to the proposal of an immunologically mediated lesion.

References

1. WELLS, W. C. 1810. On rheumatism of the heart. Trans. Soc. Improve., Med. Chir. Knowledge (London) **101**: 372.
2. MURPHY, G. E. 1952. Attempts to induce rheumatic fever in experimental animals. *In* Rheumatic Fever. : 150–169. L. Thomas, Ed. University of Minnesota Press. Minneapolis, Minn.
3. MURPHY, G. E. 1964. Experimental and histologic investigation of the nature of rheumatic heart diseases. *In* The Streptococcus, Rheumatic Fever and Glomerulonephritis. J. W. Uhr, Ed. Williams & Wilkins Co. Baltimore, Md.
4. CROMARTIE, W. J. & J. G. CRADDOCK. 1966. Rheumatic-like cardiac lesions in mice. Science **154**: 285.
5. GINSBURG, I., A. LAUFER & S. Z. ROSENBERG. 1960. Cardiac lesions produced in the rabbit by intramyocardial injections of various microorganisms. Brit. J. Exp. Path. **41**: 19.
6. GROSS, P., F. B. COOPER & J. D. PHILLIPS. 1941. The cytologic response of rats and mice to a strain of greening streptococci. Amer. J. Path. **17**: 377.
7. KOIWAI, E. K. 1961. Inflammatory states due to bacterial infection having a histopathological resemblance to the dyscollagenoses. *In* Inflammation and Diseases of Connective Tissue. L. C. Mills & J. H. Moyer, Eds. : 58–66. W. B. Saunders Co. Philadelphia, Pa.
8. KELLNER, A. & T. ROBERTSON. 1954. Selective necrosis of cardiac and skeletal muscle induced experimentally by means of proteolytic enzyme solutions given intravenously. J. Exp. Med. **99**: 387.
9. GLASER, R. J., W. A. THOMAS, S. I. MORSE & J. E. DARNELL. 1956. The incidence and pathogenesis of myocarditis in rabbits after group A streptococcal pharyngeal infections. J. Exp. Med. **103**: 173.
10. GINSBURG, I., N. ZEIRI, Y. H. BOSS, Z. BENTWICH & T. HARRIS. 1967. Organ lesions produced in rabbits following intratonsilar injection of group A streptococci and some of their extracellular products. *In* Proc. Symp. on Present State of Research on Group A. Streptococci, I.C.C. Paris, July, 1966. Excerpta Medica Found. Amsterdam, The Netherlands. In press.
11. RUBENSTONE, A. I. & O. SAPHIR. 1962. Myocardial reactions to induced necrosis and foreign bodies, with particular reference to the role of the Anitschkow cell. Lab. Invest. **11**: 791.
12. MELNICK, J. L. & G. C. GODMAN. 1951. Pathogenesis of coxsackie virus infection. Multiplication of virus and evolution of the muscle lesion in mice. J. Exp. Med. **93**: 247.
13. DAVIES, A. M., I. GERY, ROSENMANN, E. & A. LAUFER. 1963. Endotoxin as adjuvant in autoimmunity to cardiac tissue. Proc. Soc. Exp. Biol. Med. **114**: 520.
14. GUKELBERGER, M. 1936. Neue experimentelle Arbeiten über Beginn und Ausbreitung der diphtheritischen Schädigung des Herzmuskels. Z. Ges. Exp. Med. **97**: 749.
15. LARANJA, F. S., E. DIAS, G. NOBREGA & A. MIRANDA. 1956. Chagas disease. A clinical, epidemiologic and pathological study. Circulation **14**: 1035.
16. GORE, I. & O. SAPHIR. 1947. Myocarditis. A classification of 1402 cases. Amer. Heart J. **34**: 827.
17. BURCH, G. E. & N. P. DEPASQUALE. 1964. Viral myocarditis. *In* Cardiomyopathies. G. E. W. Wolstenholme & M. O'Connor, Eds. : 376. Ciba Found. Symp. J. & A. Churchill. London, England.
18. JAFFE, R. 1946. Myocarditis chronica als selbständiges Krankheitsbild (Entstehung und Pathogenese). Cardiologia (Basel) **10**: 402.
19. GLYNN, L. E. & E. J. HOLBOROW. 1965. Autoimmunity and Disease. : 100. Blackwell Scientific Publ. Oxford, England.
20. GERY, I., A. M. DAVIES & E. LAZAROV. 1964. Immunity and immunotolerance to bovine heart antigens in the rat. Immunology **7**: 182.

21. DAVIES, A. M., A. LAUFER, I. GERY & E. ROSENMANN. 1964. Organ specificity of the heart. III. Circulating antibodies and immunopathological lesions in experimental animals. Arch. Path. (Chicago) **78:** 369.
22. PATERSON, P. Y. 1962. Cellular and humoral immune factors in allergic encephalomyelitis. *In* Proc. 2nd Int. Symp. Immunopath. P. Graber & P. A. Miescher, Eds. : 184. Benno Schwabe. Basel, Switzerland.
23. PALADE, G. E. 1964. Specific granules in arterial muscle cells. J. Cell. Biol. **23:** 151.
24. MARCUS, Z., A. M. DAVIES & I. GINSBURG. 1965. Oxygen stable hemolysin of group A streptococci. V. Effect on rat heart and kidney cells grown in tissue culture. Exp. Molec. Path. **4:** 93.
25. WEISSMAN, G. 1965. Lysosomes. New Eng. J. Med. **273:** 1084.
26. ALLISON, A. C. 1966. The possible role of lysosomes in carcinogenesis. Proc. Roy. Soc. Med. **59:** 868.
27. ROSENMANN, E., E. GAZENFELD, A. LAUFER & A. M. DAVIES. 1964. Isoproterenol-induced myocardial lesions in the immunized and non-immunized rat. I. Histopathological lesions in normal rats. Path. Microbiol. (Basel) **27:** 303.
28. GAZENFELD, E., E. ROSENMANN, A. M. DAVIES & A. LAUFER. 1966. Isoporterenol-induced myocardial lesions in the immunized and non-immunized rat. II. Histopathological lesions after specific immunization. Immunology **10:** 193.
29. ROITT, I. M., H. E. H. JONES & D. DONIACH. 1962. Mechanisms of tissue damage in human and experimental autoimmune thyroiditis. *In* Proc. 2nd Int. Symp. Immunopath. P. Grabar & P. A. Miescher, Eds. : 174. Benno Schwabe. Basel, Switzerland.
30. KAPLAN, M. H. & J. M. CRAIG. 1963. Immunologic studies of heart tissue. VI. Cardiac lesions in rabbits associated with autoantibodies to heart induced by immunization with heterologous heart. J. Immun. **90:** 725.
31. KAPLAN, M. H., R. BOLANDE, L. RAKITA & B. BLAIR. 1964. Presence of bound immunoglobulins and complement in the myocardium in acute rheumatic fever associated with cardiac failure. New Eng. J. Med. **271:** 637.
32. ZABRISKIE, J. B. & E. H. FREIMER. 1966. An immunological relationship between the group A streptococcus and mammalian muscle. J. Exp. Med. **124:** 661.
33. DAVIES, A. M. & I. GERY. 1963. Autoimmunity in heart diseases. Biochem. Clin. **1:** 19.
34. KAPLAN, M. H. 1961. Immunopathologic studies in rheumatic heart disease; concept of autoantibodies to heart in rheumatic fever and post-commissurotomy syndrome. *In* Inflammation and Diseases of Connective Tissue. L. C. Mills & J. H. Moyer, Eds. : 108. W. B. Saunders Co. Philadelphia, Pa.
35. KAPLAN, M. H. 1960. The concept of autoantibodies in rheumatic fever and in the post-commissurotomy state. Ann. N. Y. Acad. Sci. **86:** 974.
36. WEISSMAN, G. 1964. Lysosomes, autoimmune phenomena and diseases of connective tissue. Lancet **ii:** 1373.
37. DUMONDE, D. C. 1965. Tissue-specific antigens. Adv. Immunol. **5:** 245.

SPONTANEOUS, HEREDITARY MYOCARDIAL DEGENERATION AND CONGESTIVE HEART FAILURE IN A STRAIN OF SYRIAN HAMSTERS*

E. Bajusz, J. R. Baker, C. W. Nixon, and F. Homburger
Bio-Research Institute, Cambridge, Mass.

Introduction

Studies on the pathogenesis, therapy, and prevention of congestive heart failure are greatly hindered by the lack of easily reproducible disease models. There is presently no standardized and generally accepted method for the induction of heart failure in laboratory animals, although a number of techniques have been devised.[1-10] Pertinent literature indicates that the type of failure which develops during persistently increased stress produced by overload, when the mechanical demand is enhanced in proportion to the active mass of the heart (e.g. failure caused by aortic stenosis or by aortic valve insufficiency), has been the most intensively investigated because its primary causes are the least complicated and because it can readily be imitated by experimental procedures. Although theoretically an analogous situation prevails when, conversely, the active contractile mass of the heart is diminished (e.g. by an infarct or other degenerative myocardial lesion), this type of failure is difficult to induce experimentally. Studies on dogs, rats, and other laboratory animals suggest that, if the survival time following extreme destruction of the myocardium (by coronary artery ligature or electrocautery) is sufficient, the remaining contractile ventricular mass is able to compensate for the nonfunctioning portion of the heart over a long period.[11-14] In fact, some investigators believe that as little as 15–20% of the total ventricular mass is sufficient to maintain adequate systemic circulation.[15] Nevertheless, it should be noted that a single injury to the heart muscle was produced in all the afore-mentioned studies, whereas spontaneous pathological processes in man often cause intermittent and graded injuries to the myocardium.

The existence in an inbred strain of Syrian hamsters of a genetically transmitted (or conditioned), degenerative cardiomyopathy that terminates in congestive heart failure offers unique opportunities to study the sequence of events leading to cardiac insufficiency and to analyze the importance of extracardiac factors in the mechanism of generalized venous congestion. This hereditary disease, which has a 100% incidence in the pedigreed BIO 14.6 strain of hamsters, is apparently a primary myopathy. The degenerative lesions that occur in all striated muscles are definitely noninflammatory in nature.[16-19] The gross and histopathological abnormalities seen in the middle-aged or older myopathic hamsters, except those of the cardiac and skeletal muscles, are consistent with long-standing passive venous congestion, and this progressive cardiovascular insufficiency may be regarded as the ultimate cause of death.[20]

Although our earlier studies, briefly summarized above, largely characterized the morphogenesis and, at least in some respects, the enzyme histogenesis of the cardiac- and skeletal-muscle lesions of the myopathic animals, several important questions remained unanswered. We were especially interested in estab-

* This work was supported by United States Public Health Service research grant no. HE-09791 (National Heart Institute) and general research support grant no. FR-05525 (Division of Research Facilities and Resources).

lishing the role of myocardial degeneration in the subsequent development of congestive heart failure; hence, during the past two years we have concentrated on the cardiac aspects of the hereditary disease of the BIO 14.6 hamster. This paper, which describes one phase of these investigations, will be concerned with: (1) observations on the incidence of spontaneous mortality in relation to cardiac pathology and congestive heart failure, (2) studies on the evolution and healing of cardiac lesions and their relationship to congestive heart failure, and (3) investigations performed in parabiosed hamsters which have indicated the decisive role of some extracardiac factors in the mechanism of cardiac insufficiency.

Cardiac Pathology and Congestive Heart Failure

Human congestive heart failure is known to have its counterpart in other animal species. Its spontaneous occurrence is best documented in dogs[21,22] and cattle,[23] but sporadic cases have also been observed in cats, horses, sheep, goats, and in a variety of zoo animals. In the dog, mitral insufficiency of undetermined etiology and dirofilariasis ("heartworm disease") are the most common causes of cardiac failure, whereas in cattle the condition is usually caused by high-altitude-induced pulmonary hypertension. Not much is known about the participation of genetic factors in the development of these conditions, although an epidemiological study among dogs presented to a veterinary clinic has indicated that the male cocker spaniel possesses an unusually high susceptibility to acquired cardiac diseases leading to congestive heart failure.[24] In any event, none of these spontaneous heart failures is suitable for serial investigation, large-scale testing of cardioactive compounds, and/or analysis of the sequence of events leading to circulatory insufficiency.

Among the various types of failures, those developing during the course of chronic myocardial disease, especially degenerative cardiomyopathies, have been the least investigated because of the lack of appropriate experimental models. Consequently, nothing definite is known about the relationship between the presence of myocardial degenerative changes and heart failure. It is repeatedly noted in human pathology that a few fibrotic and scarred foci are regularly observed in the hypertrophic and/or dilated failing heart,[25] but their presence is generally regarded as insignificant. An analysis of the progression and healing of myocardial lesions in relation to the development of congestive failure in the myopathic hamster suggests that this conclusion may not be entirely correct.

Materials and Methods

Between October, 1963 and December, 1965, 1,478 untreated myopathic hamsters of the BIO 14.6 strain were closely observed and autopsied after spontaneous death or sacrifice for specific purposes. Hamsters (526) of an unrelated healthy strain (London School of Hygiene: LSH) served as controls. The animals were of both sexes, ranging from 15 to 286 days of age. They were kept under identical and controlled housing conditions and fed according to previously defined specifications.[19] The gross pathological observations as well as the body weight and organ weights (heart, liver, spleen, lungs, kidneys, and adrenals) were regularly recorded. For routine morphological studies, the selected specimens were fixed in Bouin's fluid, Heidenhain's Susa, or formol solution, and the sections were stained with hematoxylin-eosin. In a number of cases, special methods (i.e., periodic acid-Schiff reaction, van Gieson's method, the von Kóssa silver nitrate technique, and Perls' Prussian blue reaction) were used.

The severity of myocardial lesions were assessed on an arbitrary scale of 0 to 4, with 0 designating no lesion; grade 1, mild lesion; grades 2 and 3, moderate lesions; and grade 4, severe lesions. Since the myocardial degeneration in the diseased hamsters is focal in nature, the following criteria provided good insight into the extent of damage: grade 1, 1 to 3 small affected areas, each focus involving not more than 10 adjacent muscle fibers; grade 2, 4 to 6 small and/or not more than 2 larger foci; grade 3, 7 to 12 small and/or 3 to 5 larger foci; grade 4, more than 12 small and/or more than 5 larger foci. In some experimental series, however, more precise information was needed on the relationship between the extent of active (fresh or newly formed) lesions and those showing varying degrees of healing (i.e., connective tissue replacement, fibrosis, and scar formation). Here, the active and healing (or healed) lesions were evaluated individually on the basis of the following criteria: degeneration (myolysis, necrosis, fibrosis, scarring) involving an area of about ten cross-sectioned adjacent muscle fibers was considered as one lesion-unit. Smaller and larger foci of degeneration were approximated in terms of lesion-units with a constant microscopical magnification. The presence of a small linear scar counted as one lesion-unit. Three sections were prepared from each heart at various levels, and the average of the total number of lesion-units was taken to indicate the severity (grade) of fresh (active) and old (healed) involvements, in each case. The severity of the lesion was considered to be grade 1 when the total number of lesion-units did not exceed 3; grade 2, 4–10 units; grade 3, 11–25 units; grade 4, more than 25 units (FIGURE 1).

The exact rating and interpretation of findings concerned with the onset and progression of cardiac hypertrophy in the myopathic hamsters are complicated by the lack of an absolute baseline by which an observed change could be evaluated. The increased body weight caused by the accumulation of edema fluids and congestion of internal organs, on the one hand, and the weight alterations which result from the progressive loss of skeletal muscle and adipose tissues during the different phases of the disease, on the other hand, make it impossible to use the heart weight:body weight ration as a reference base. Furthermore, since the myopathic animals have a growth rate significantly different from that of the LSH-strain hamsters, age could not be used as a basis for comparison. Somewhat more satisfactory data were obtained when heart weight:body length ratios were compared between animals of the BIO 14.6 and LSH strains; here again, however, several factors minimized the significance of any statistical evaluation. Among these factors, two are noteworthy: (1) Even in the healthy LSH hamsters, the changes in the relationship of heart weight to body length are not linear, but this parameter varies considerably during the different phases of postnatal development. (2) During the advanced stages of cardiac failure characterized by extended dilatation of the ventricular and auricular chambers, the heart weight increase in the myopathic animals no longer indicates the presence of hypertrophy of muscle fibers, as judged by morphological criteria. Therefore, the phrases "moderate cardiac hypertrophy" and "marked cardiac hypertrophy" are used in this paper only when the conclusions derived from the heart weight analyses were confirmed by histological observations (thickness of muscular walls, size of muscle cells).

To estimate the severity of congestive heart failure, the degree of generalized edema was assessed and complemented by histopathological studies of the liver, as well as by observations on the presence of pleural effusion and pulmonary congestion. By means of studies on the progression of the various perpiheral manifestations of congestive heart failure, the following scale of grading was established and used in the present investigations:

Mild heart failure (grade 1): a moderate degree of subcutaneous edema restricted to the dependent parts; absence of a measurable amount of exudate in the body cavities; liver enlargement accompanied by dilatation of the centrilobular veins and of the sinusoids, but without structural alterations.

Moderate heart failure (grades 2 and 3): diffuse subcutaneous edema; liver pathology consisting of hemorrhages and necroses around the central veins; pleural effusion (grade 2). The additional occurrence of measurable amounts of exudates in the abdominal and chest cavities (not exceeding a total of 2.5 ml) and of pulmonary congestion was considered to represent a more advanced stage of moderate failure (grade 3). In such cases, the liver pathology was usually diffuse and showed progressive destruction of the parenchymal tissues.

Severe heart failure (grade 4): severe generalized edema involving the subcutaneous areas of the entire body (including the facial parts), together with

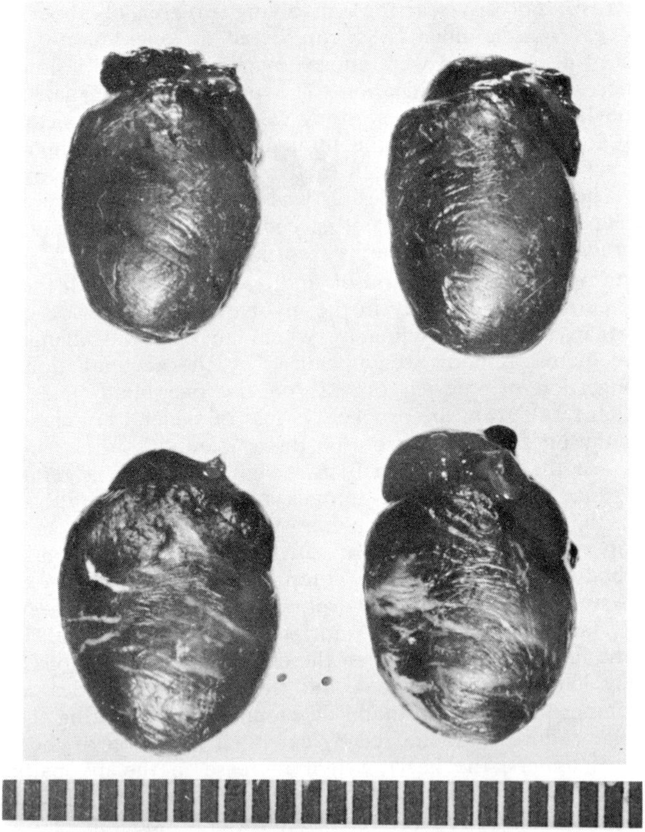

FIGURE 1. Sex-dependent variation in cardiac pathology of 60-day-old BIO 14.6 myopathic hamsters. (*Top*) The hearts of males show no macroscopically visible cardiac damage. (*Bottom*) The hearts of females are already somewhat enlarged, revealing easily visible necrotic and calcified muscle fibers. The hearts with calcified fibers are obviously in an advanced stage of myocardial involvement.

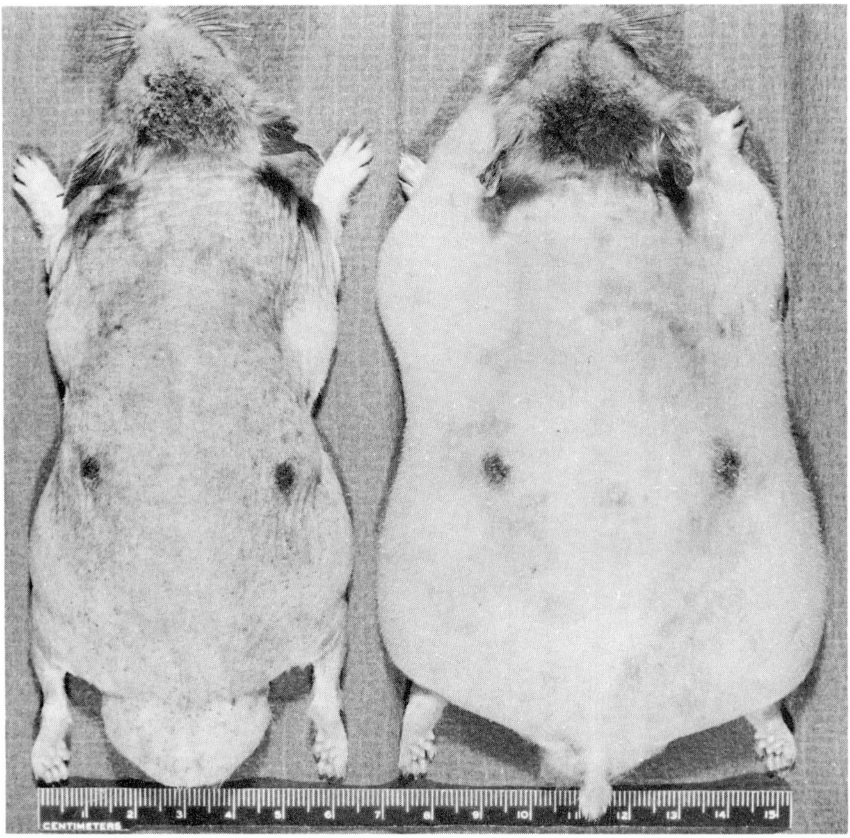

FIGURE 2. Sex-dependent variation in congestive heart failure of 105-day-old BIO 14.6 hamsters. (*Left*) Male hamster with no appreciable degree of subcutaneous edema. (*Right*) Severely edematous female hamster of the same age.

ascites, hydrothorax, and hydropericardium. In such severe cases, the majority of skeletal-muscle groups, especially those of the hind legs and abdominal wall, were markedly swollen. The mesentery of intestines and the pancreas were highly edematous, and the measurable exudates amounted to well over 2.5 ml. There were diffuse necrotic and fibrotic alterations in the liver, and hemosiderin-laden macrophages ("heart-failure cells") were seen in the congested lungs (FIGURE 2).

Results and Discussion

Incidence of Spontaneous Mortality in Relation to Cardiac Pathology and Congestive Heart Failure

In a random sample of 500 myopathic hamsters of both sexes (211 females and 289 males), the spontaneous mortality rate was recorded, and the severity of cardiac pathology and that of congestive heart failure were determined. The results are summarized in TABLE 1.

TABLE 1

RELATIONSHIP BETWEEN AGE, INCIDENCE OF SPONTANEOUS MORTALITY, MYOCARDIAL PATHOLOGY, AND CONGESTIVE HEART FAILURE AT TIME OF DEATH IN 500 MYOPATHIC HAMSTERS

	Age (days)								
	25–45	46–65	66–85	86–105	106–125	126–145	146–165	166–185	186–205	Over 205
Number of deaths	0	3	8	24	109	178	76	43	37	22
Average severity of cardiac pathology (grade: 0–4)	—	3.6	3.8	2.4	1.7	1.6	1.4	1.1	1.3	0.7
Average severity of congestive heart failure (grade: 0–4)	—	—	0.3	2.2	3.1	3.7	3.2	3.6	3.1	3.4

It is evident from the data recorded here that the mortality rate was highest between the 106th and 145th days of age. The first spontaneous death occurred on the 49th day, and the life-span of the oldest survivor was 286 days. It should be noted that this study was initiated after weaning; hence, the mortality prior to the 25th day of age is not included.

The most severe cardiac pathology was found in the animals that died between the 49th and 85 days; thereafter, the severity of heart-muscle lesions declined sharply. This is surprising, since earlier studies had established that the spontaneous disease seen in these hamsters is progressive, and not a single case of regression has been observed.[19]

In order to evaluate the data summarized in TABLE 1, it is important to recall that myocardial lesions have never been observed in the myopathic hamsters before the 25th day of life.[20] Furthermore, the data collected during the past two years indicate that, although the disease affects the hearts of both sexes within the strain, cardiac-muscle pathology occurs earlier in females (on an average, at about 30 days of age) than in males (at about 45 days of age). The incidence of cardiac lesions is 100% in both sexes around the 60th day of age. Between the 60th and 80th days, heart-muscle degeneration is usually more severe in females (even if only nonbreeders are observed) than in males; the females reach the terminal stage of congestive heart failure earlier. Repeated pregnancies further accelerate the onset of the fatal stage when the females clinically exhibit hyperpnea and cyanosis. The average life-span is about 125 days in nonbreeding females and 167 days in males.

From the standpoint of qualitative morphology, the development and healing of cardiac lesions can be summarized as follows: The earliest histologically detectable abnormality in the heart muscle consists of focal myolysis (FIGURE 3), with primary disappearance of sarcoplasm. The formation of small vacuoles, often observed in the initially affected muscle fibers, resembles hydropic vacuolar degeneration. However, in the diseased hamster hearts, the fiber disintegration is marked by a dissolution of myofibrils, so that the sarcoplasm becomes filled with a more or less amorphous material. The myofibrils eventually disappear, and the sarcolemmal remnants are often indistinguishable from the endomysial connective tissue. In fact, these small focal degenerating areas closely resemble the condition usually referred to by pathologists as "spotty myolysis" because it is characterized by the disappearance of muscle fibers of fiber segments. The myolytic foci are randomly distributed throughout the walls of both ventricles and auricles, the intraventricular septum apparently being the least affected. Free muscle nuclei are regularly seen within such early lesions.

As the disease progresses, the number of myolytic foci increases, and, at the same time, another type of lesion also appears in the heart. Here, fibers in various stages of myolysis are intermixed with necrotic muscle cells showing nuclear changes. Such lesions are usually larger than the foci showing only myolysis. Furthermore, although cellular infiltration is absent in the areas affected by myolysis, the degenerating lesions of mixed type are usually filled with masses of cells. The majority of these cells have proved to be sarcolemmal in origin, but occasionally round cells, histiocytes, and fibroblasts are also observed. It is generally believed that cardiac-muscle fibers do not regenerate; nevertheless, the appearance of masses of sarcolemmal nuclei, as is seen in the myopathic hamsters is considered by some investigators as an indication of attempted or abortive regeneration.[26,27]

In more advanced cases, there are focal lesions of various sizes, in different

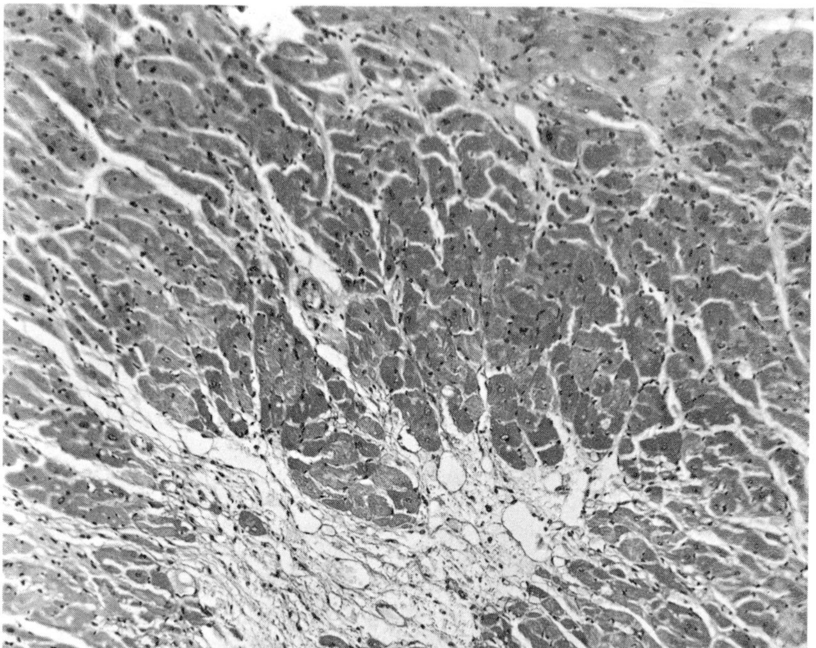

FIGURE 3. Focal myolysis in the heart of a 50-day-old male BIO 14.6 hamster. Stain: hematoxylin-eosin. × 120.

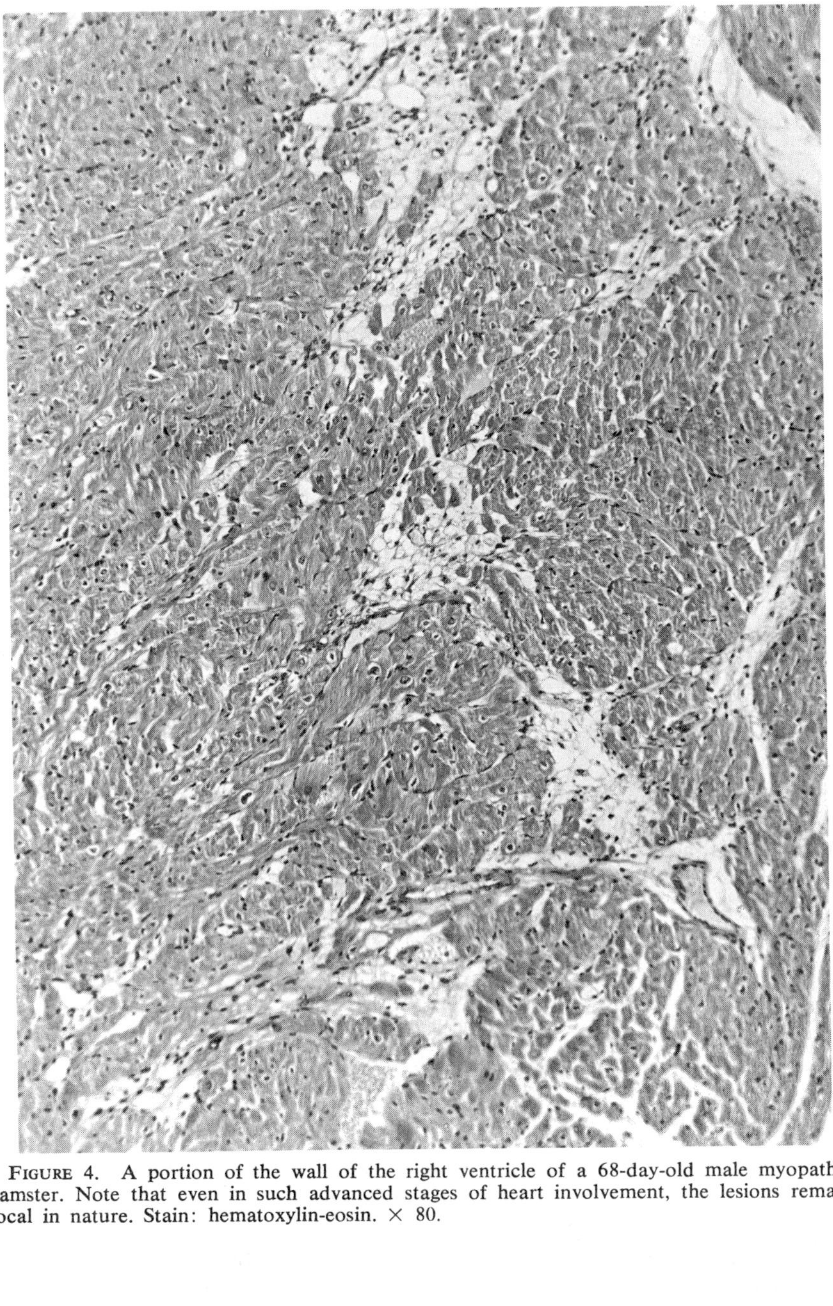

FIGURE 4. A portion of the wall of the right ventricle of a 68-day-old male myopathic hamster. Note that even in such advanced stages of heart involvement, the lesions remain focal in nature. Stain: hematoxylin-eosin. × 80.

stages of evolution. Newly formed and healing lesions are often seen in the same hearts. The disintegrated fibers within the smaller foci are replaced by connective tissue. Larger lesions show histiocytic proliferation, fibroplasia, and increased vascularization; still others exhibit calcification and/or progressive sclerosis. Mineral (calcium phosphate) deposits are not seen in lesions in advanced stages of healing, the end result of which is the formation of a collagenous fibrillar scar (FIGURE 4).

As noted in one of our earlier papers,[20] valvular or endocardial changes are rare, and, although atrial mural thrombi do occur during the late stages of the disease, there is no correlation between the presence or absence of atrial thrombi and the severity of congestive heart failure.

An analysis of the data in TABLE 1, in the light of considerations outlined above, indicates the presence of only active (i.e., newly formed) lesions in the hearts of the three animals that died between th 46th and 65th days. In the 66-to-85-day-old group, about an equal numer of newly formed foci and healing lesions was seen, whereas in the hamsters that died between 86 and 205 days of age, occasional scars were observed in addition to a few fresh and healing lesions.

A moderate to advanced cardiac hypertrophy, accompanied by some dilatation of the ventricular and auricular chambers, was a constant finding in hamsters that died between 86 and 145 days of age. Among the older ones, extreme dilatation was the characteristic finding. The total mass of the heart (as judged by heart weight analysis) in these animals was considerably increased, yet the muscular walls of both ventricles and auricles were thin. In fact, cardiac rupture with hemothorax was the immediate cause of death of almost half (48.8%) of this group.

Among the animals that died prior to 85 days of age, only one showed a moderate degree of congestive heart failure. In this acute case—characterized by severe pulmonary congestion with hydrothorax and hydropericardium, but without liver pathology and subcutaneous edema—the sequence of events did not follow the usual pattern. In the majority of the hamsters that died later, the pathological findings were consistent with long-standing passive venous congestion of moderate to severe intensity. Nevertheless, signs of congestive heart failure were totally absent in 8.3% of the middle-aged or older animals (between 86 and 285 days of age); the cause of death in these cases could not be ascertained. In the older animals, heart-muscle pathology was regularly observed, but several old edematous ones showed no significant heart lesions. This was an unexpected finding, since, as stated earlier in this paper, the incidence of cardiac pathology was constantly 100% in hamsters that died spontaneously or were sacrificed about the 60th day of age. Furthermore, the data in TABLE 1 permit the conclusion that very few animals develop severe myocardial degeneration and die as a result of this condition, while the hearts of all the survivors are only moderately or slightly affected. However, our observations did not support this conclusion, and additional studies were performed to elucidate the reasons for the discrepancies.

Quantitative Aspects of the Evolution and Healing of Myocardial Lesions and Their Relationship to Congestive Heart Failure

In order to gain more information concerning the evolution of the chronic cardiac condition in the myopathic hamster, we have tabulated the data obtained in 250 male hamsters, divided into five age groups of 50 animals each. The effect of natural selection due to spontaneous mortality has been disregarded by including data from sacrificed hamsters only. The observations were evaluated for different aspects of the condition, and the results are summarized in TABLES 2–4.

TABLE 2 shows the distribution and severity of active (fresh or newly formed) myocardial lesions. In the youngest (50-day-old) age group, the majority of fresh lesions were mild to moderate in severity. During the next 20 days, a sudden increase in the intensity of the disease process may have occurred, since 100% of the 70-day-old animals had moderate to severe myocardial lesions. In the older (90-, 120-, and 150-day-old) age groups, the occurrence of severe and moderate lesions gradually decreased, but mild lesions were always present. Active lesions were not seen in 14 to 36% of the two oldest age groups, respectively. Thus, when newly formed lesions appear in the heart muscle during the advanced phases of the disease, they are usually of mild intensity.

TABLE 3 shows the distribution of healing and healed myocardial lesions in the same 250 male hamsters. The data indicate a normal pattern of healing, as might be anticipated on theoretical grounds. Nevertheless, it is difficult to explain the significant number of animals with neither fresh nor old cardiac pathology in the two oldest age groups, since both types of lesions were seen in 100% incidence in the 70- and 90-day-old age groups. Moreover, the average number of fresh lesions per section was 18.7 in the 70-day-old group, whereas only one or two small scars could be detected in about 40% of the three older groups.

These observations suggest that the scar tissue seen during the advanced stages of myocardial involvement is not indicative of the extent of original heart-muscle damage. Although recent experiments performed in other laboratories resulted in similar conclusions,[28,29] this fact is largely neglected in human pathology. The present investigations in the myopathic hamster suggest that the normal healing processes in the heart muscle are significantly influenced by the concurrent development of hypertrophy and dilatation. It is likely that the small focal lesions heal without collagenous scar formation; the loss of muscle bands leads to a collapse of the surrounding hypertrophic fibers upon the interstitium, and, at this stage, the initially affected area can no longer be recognized by routine histological studies.

TABLE 4 indicates the distribution and progression of congestive heart failure in the same hamsters. A correlative evaluation of the data (TABLES 2–4) leaves little doubt that the myocardial degeneration itself is the factor that elicits the sequence of events leading to the development of congestive heart failure in these animals.

Three distinct stages can be distinguished in the evolution of the chronic cardiac condition of the hamster. During the first stage (between the 25th and 65th days of age, approximately), severe degenerative processes affect the heart muscle. The extent of this initial myocardial injury is comparatively uniform and has 100% incidence in both sexes. Nevertheless, this rapidly progressing, acute phase of the condition results in negligible mortality. During the second stage (ranging approximately between the 55th and 85th day), the older lesions are already in various stages of healing, and, at the same time, cardiac hypertrophy and/or dilatation develop. The occurrence of these compensatory phenomena clearly indicates that the damaged hearts are hemodynamically overloaded. In a small percentage of the hamsters (about 6–10%), dilatation

TABLE 2

DISTRIBUTION OF ACTIVE (FRESH) MYOCARDIAL LESIONS OF VARYING INTENSITY IN MALE MYOPATHIC HAMSTERS AT DIFFERENT AGES

Group	Age (days)	Number of Animals	Animals with No Active Lesions (%)	Animals with Active Lesions (%)		
				Mild Lesions (Grade 1)	Moderate Lesions (Grades 2 and 3)	Severe Lesions (Grade 4)
1	50	50	2	54	38	6
2	70	50	0	0	34	66
3	90	50	0	48	36	16
4	120	50	14	66	18	2
5	150	50	36	60	4	0

TABLE 3

DISTRIBUTION OF MYOCARDIAL LESIONS AT VARIOUS STAGES OF HEALING IN MALE MYOPATHIC HAMSTERS AT DIFFERENT AGES

Group	Age (days)	Number of Animals	Animals without Healing or Healed Lesions (%)	Animals with Healing or Healed Lesions (%)		
				Healing Lesions Only	Healing Lesions Plus Scars	Scars Only
1	50	50	58	42	0	0
2	70	50	0	52	46	2
3	90	50	0	30	28	42
4	120	50	8	38	18	36
5	150	50	22	22	12	44

TABLE 4

DISTRIBUTION OF CONGESTIVE HEART FAILURE OF VARYING INTENSITY IN MALE MYOPATHIC HAMSTERS AT DIFFERENT AGES

Group	Age (days)	Number of Animals	Animals without Congestive Failure (%)	Animals with Congestive Failure (%)		
				Mild (Grade 1)	Moderate (Grades 2 and 3)	Severe (Grade 4)
1	50	50	100	0	0	0
2	70	50	96	4	0	0
3	90	50	42	38	16	4
4	120	50	6	20	38	36
5	150	50	8	2	22	68

is seen with no appreciable degree of hypertrophy; these animals develop congestive failure much more rapidly and die earlier than those with compensatory hypertrophy. New lesions appear less frequently in hypertrophied than in non-hypertrophied hearts and, when they do occur in the former, are always of mild intensity. It is possible that, during this phase of the disease, a metabolic adaptation occurs in the heart muscle which makes it less susceptible to the disease process. Among many other possibilities, the increased resistance of hypertrophic fibers to this type of degeneration should also be considered. During the third stage (usually after the 80th day of age), the hypertrophy is overtaken by extended dilatation of the cardiac chambers, and peripheral manifestations of the generalized venous congestion become marked. This progressive circulatory insufficiency is the ultimate cause of death in the majority of cases. It should be reemphasized that the extent of healed damage detectable during the advanced stages of heart failure is no longer indicative of the severity of the original damage.

Studies in Parabiosed Hamsters

Experimental parabiosis, the surgical union of two living animals, is a widely used and valuable technique for the study of any problem involving humoral transmission. Small laboratory rodents are joined by surgical union of skin and abdominal muscular walls; several investigations have shown that there is direct interchange between the parabionts through anastomosis of capillary-sized vessels.[30-32]

Our original purpose in establishing parabioses between myopathic and healthy hamsters was to study whether the genetically conditioned disease in the myopathic animal could be transmitted to the healthy partner. We found that, although such transmission does not occur, parabiosis significantly prolongs the life of the myopathic partner. A further analysis of this prolongation of life, or "protective effect," resulted in some observations that appear to have an important bearing on our findings concerning the relationship of cardiac pathology and congestive heart failure.

Materials and Methods

Surgical parabiosis was performed under pentobarbital anesthesia according to the technique described by Bunster and Meyer.[33] This procedure, briefly, consists of: (1) removal of hair from the right half of one animal and the left half of the other; (2) longitudinal incision of the shaven skin of each from ear to base of tail; (3) union of the ventral edges of the skin incisions with continuous sutures; (4) incision of the abdominal walls from last rib to ilium; (5) union of the four edges of abdominal wall with interrupted sutures (without causing coelio-anastomosis); (6) tying the lateral aspects of the adjacent scapulas of the two animals firmly together with gut; and (7) union of the dorsal edges of the skin incisions. The skin sutures were removed on the 12th postoperative day.

In our series, 356 hamsters of the myopathic strain (BIO 14.6) were joined to 356 hamsters of a healthy strain (LSH); 22 BIO 14.6-BIO 14.6 unions and 16 LSH-LSH unions were also established. The animals were paired by weight and sex. Unless otherwise indicated, the animals were parabiosed between the 25th and 30th day of age (i.e., during the very early phase of the spontaneous disease, when cardiac pathology is not yet present). Losses among these unions were caused primarily by parabiosis intoxication[30,34] and, much less frequently, by infection of the skin and muscle wounds, physical separation, or chronic fighting. These losses amounted to 38.6% and always occurred within three weeks after the operation.

In a number of the experimental unions, surgical intervention on internal organs was performed in one or both partners, e.g. coronary artery ligation, ventricular wall ligation, partial or total adrenalectomy, partial or total nephrectomy, thyroparathyroidectomy, and partial hepatectomy (involving about two-thirds of the total liver mass). This last-mentioned operation consists of liver lobectomy; ligatures are applied to the pedicles of the left lateral and median lobes, which are removed, leaving the associated right lateral and caudal lobes.

The left main coronary artery was ligated about 1 mm below its origin according to a technique described in detail elsewhere.[14] It should be noted that virtually the entire free (lateral) wall of the left ventricle is transformed into a thin scar tissue following this procedure. In another group, the ligature was placed around the ventricles at the level of the lower third of the chambers.

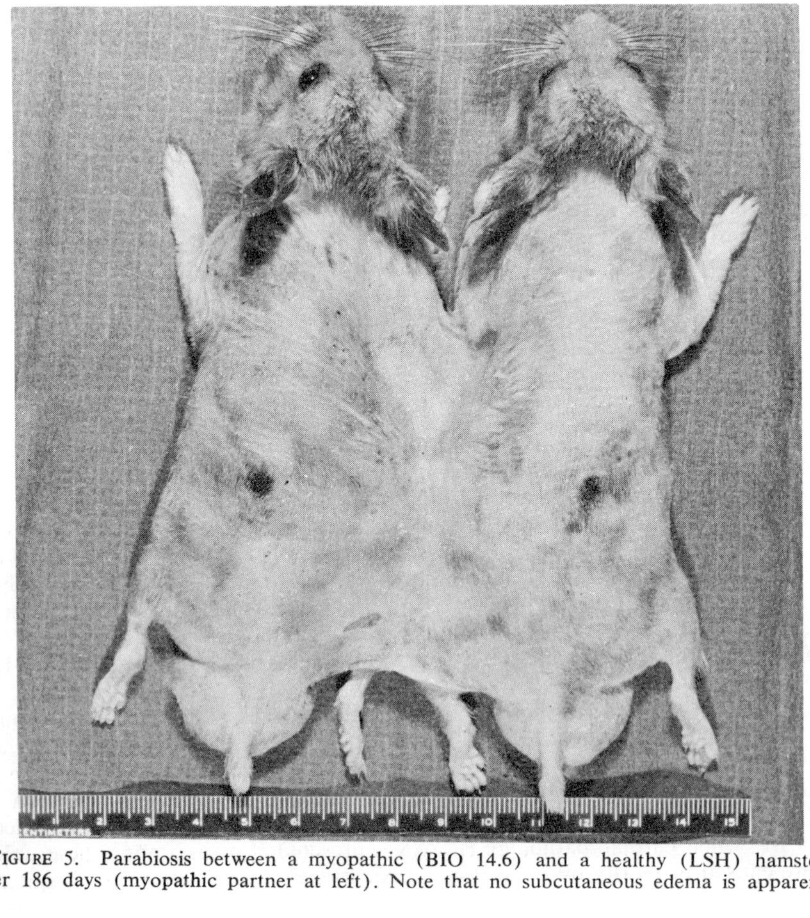

FIGURE 5. Parabiosis between a myopathic (BIO 14.6) and a healthy (LSH) hamster, after 186 days (myopathic partner at left). Note that no subcutaneous edema is apparent.

When both ventricles are firmly ligated, intensive necrosis and suppurating abscess formation occur around the apex. In fact, the whole ligated one-third of the ventricles becomes necrotic, and it was observed that this type of damage reduces the efficiency of cardiac work even more drastically than does coronary artery ligation.[35] All the interventions described above were performed two weeks after parabiosis.

The severity of cardiac-muscle pathology and the degree of congestive heart failure were established in a manner identical to that used in the previous experiments. Histological sections were often prepared from skeletal-muscle specimens also, in order to gain information concerning the effect of parabiosis on the muscle degeneration normally seen in the BIO 14.6 hamster.

Results and Discussion

The effect of parabiosis upon survival time was observed in both BIO 14.6-LSH and BIO 14.6-BIO 14.6 unions. The average life-span was 398 days in the 56 BIO 14.6-LSH pairs, and 96 days in the 16 BIO 14.6-BIO 14.6 pairs. It should be recalled that the average life-span is about 143 days in non-parabiosed BIO 14.6 myopathic males and females. Thus, the union to a healthy animal almost tripled the survival time of the myopathic partner. However, when two myopathic hamsters lived in parabiotic union, the average survival time was significantly shortened.

The observations made at autopsy and the subsequent histopathological studies indicated that parabiosis between a myopathic and a healthy hamster does not alter per se the onset and progression of striated-muscle pathology in the diseased partner, but it does prevent the development of congestive heart failure (FIGURES 5 and 6).

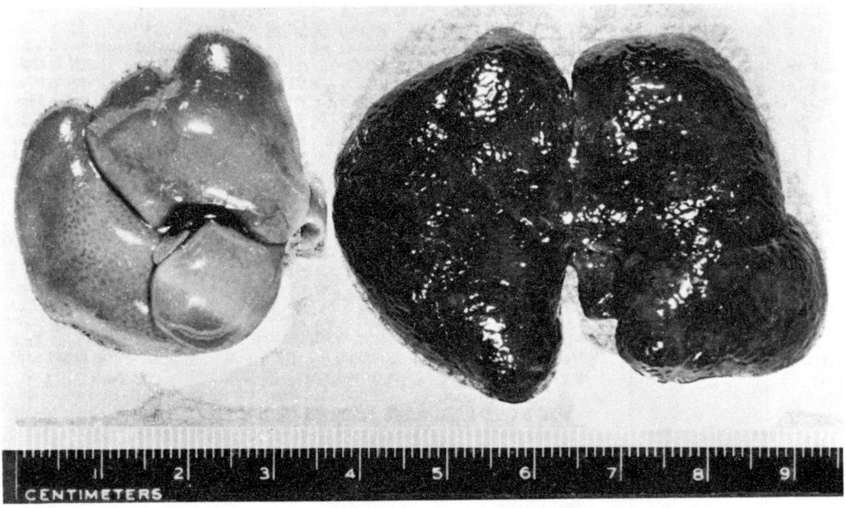

FIGURE 6. Prevention of liver congestion by parabiosis between myopathic and healthy hamsters. (*Left*) Normal liver obtained from the myopathic parabiont shown at left in FIGURE 5. (*Right*) Enlarged and severely congested liver of a nonparabiosed myopathic animal of the same sex. The male hamsters used here for comparison were both 212 days old at the time of autopsy.

TABLE 5

EFFECT OF PARABIOSES OF DIFFERENT DURATIONS BETWEEN MYOPATHIC AND HEALTHY HAMSTERS UPON DEVELOPMENT OF CONGESTIVE HEART FAILURE

Group*	Age of Myopathic Partner at Parabiosis (mean, days)	Duration of Parabiosis (days)†	Congestive Heart Failure: At Start of Experiment‡ Severity (Grades: 0–4)	Congestive Heart Failure: At Start of Experiment‡ Incidence %	Congestive Heart Failure: At 120 Days of Age§ Severity (Grades: 0–4)	Congestive Heart Failure: At 120 Days of Age§ Incidence %
1	27	5	0	0	3.6	100
2	26	10	0	0	3.7	100
3	25	22	0	0	2.3	67
4	27	31	0	0	1.9	67
5	29	45	0	0	0	0
6	29	52	0	0	0	0

* Each experimental group consisted of six pairs of parabiosed hamsters (paired according to weight and sex).

† Following the time period indicated, the animals were surgically separated.

‡ Data of nonparabiosed BIO 14.6 hamsters of corresponding ages.

§ In nonparabiosed, 120-day-old myopathic hamsters, the incidence of congestive heart failure is more than 90%.

TABLE 6

EFFECT OF 45-DAY PARABIOSIS BETWEEN MYOPATHIC HAMSTERS AND HEALTHY HAMSTERS UPON DEVELOPMENT OF CONGESTIVE HEART FAILURE AT DIFFERENT PHASES OF THE DISEASE

		Congestive Heart Failure				
		At Time of Parabiosis†		At Time of Death, or 55 Days after Separation of Parabionts		
Group*	Age of Myopathic Partner at Parabiosis (mean, days)	Severity (Grades: 0–4)	Incidence (%)	Severity (Grades: 0–4)	Incidence (%)	Number of Myopathic Survivors
1	28	0	0	0	0	6
2	34	0	0	0	0	6
3	46	0	0	0.3	17	6
4	58	0–2	67	2.1	34	6
5	76	1–3	100	3.5	100	4
6	96	2–4	100	4.0	100	0
7	103	3–4	100	4.0	100	1

* Each experimental group consisted of six pairs of parabiosed hamsters.

† Approximate estimates based on subjective clinical impressions (e.g. subcutaneous edema, cyanosis) and body weight.

In order to analyze the effect of parabiosis on the occurrence of congestive heart failure, the duration of parabiosis was varied, as indicated in TABLE 5. Each experimental group consisted of six pairs of BIO 14.6-LSH parabionts. Spontaneous mortality occurred only in groups 1 and 2; all survivors were killed on the 120th day of life. The data in TABLE 5 indicate that a parabiotic union for 45 or 52 days is sufficient to prevent the development of congestive heart failure, whereas parabiosis of shorter duration is less effective, or even completely ineffective, in this respect.

In the next experimental series (see TABLE 6), the age of the animals varied at the onset of parabiosis, but the duration of parabiosis was constant (45 days). Thus, 46 days after the establishment of parabiotic unions between myopathic and healthy hamsters, the animals were surgically separated, and the effect of their temporary union upon the cardiac condition was observed.

The data appear to indicate that parabiosis must be performed prior to the 58th day of age in order to achieve a protective effect. It should be noted that the age of the myopathic partner is the decisive factor in this respect. The union of a healthy partner to 58-day or older myopathic (nonedematous or edematous) hamsters had no obvious effect on the progression of congestive heart failure. Comparable results were obtained when this experimental series was repeated with a temporary parabiosis for 55 days, and continuous parabiosis actually shortened the life-span of the 60-to-70-day-old and older myopathic partners.

The cardiac pathology of parabiosed myopathic hamsters was carefully studied and analyzed in comparison with data collected from a large number of nonparabiosed animals of the same sex and age. It was concluded that parabiosis exerts a negligible influence on the onset and progression of myocardial degeneration. In groups of 60-day-old parabiosed and nonparabiosed hamsters, the severity of cardiac lesions was comparable. However, it was noted that only a mild to moderate degree of hypertrophy develops in parabiosed animals, and cardiac dilatation does not occur. Furthermore, and interestingly enough, many healed lesions could easily be recognized in the moderately hypertrophied heart muscle of middle-aged or older parabiosed myopathic animals. This last finding is in sharp contrast with the presence of only occasional scars in the majority of nonparabiosed BIO 14.6 hamsters of comparable age (FIGURES 7 and 8).

Since no other difference could be established in the morphological aspects of cardiac pathology between parabionts and nonparabionts, the following working hypothesis has been advanced: Union to a healthy partner (continuous or temporary when maintained during a critical period) prolongs the life-span of the myopathic partner by preventing the development of congestive heart failure. The presence of only a mild to moderate degree of cardiac hypertrophy and the absence of cardiac dilatation in the myopathic animals suggest that, under these experimental conditions, either the contractile force of the heart muscle is increased or the hemodynamic overload is diminished. This protective effect, in turn, exerts an influence upon the qualitative aspects of the healing of myocardial degeneration. Although newly formed myocardial lesions do occur in "protected" hamsters during a later period of their lives, the lesions are only of mild intensity and do not elicit cardiac insufficiency even if the healthy partner has already been removed.

Studies were also performed on the nature of the protection afforded by parabiosis. Although these investigations are not yet fully conclusive, it is worth noting that the following surgical interventions performed in the healthy

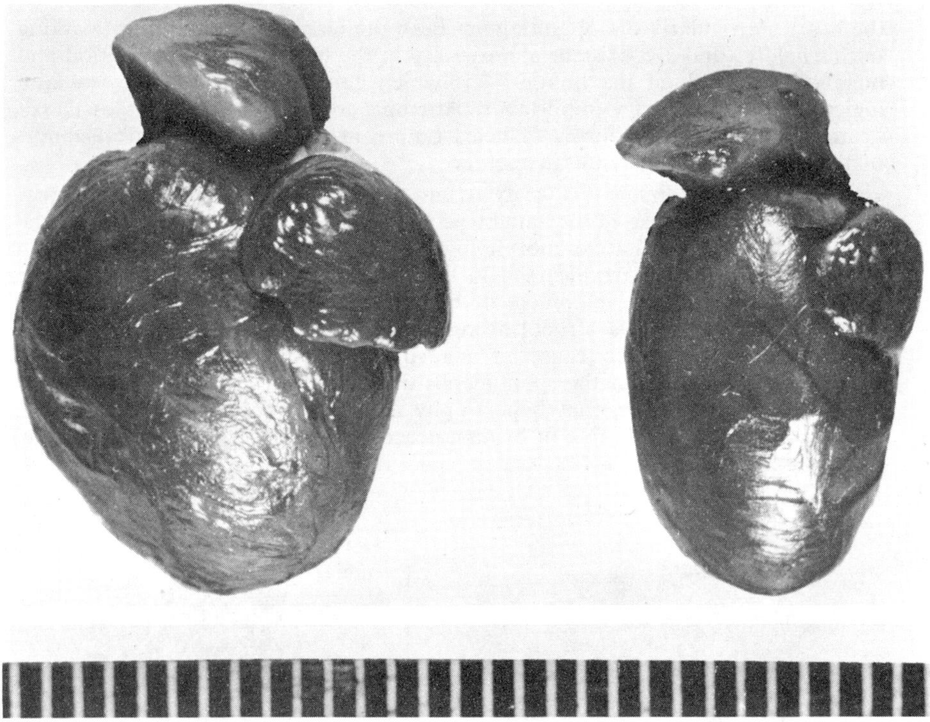

FIGURE 7. Prevention of heart enlargement by parabiosis between myopathic and healthy hamsters. (*Left*) The heart of an 81-day-old nonparabiosed myopathic hamster shows hypertrophy and dilatation. (*Right*) The heart of a parabiosed myopathic hamster of the same sex and age following a 55-day union to a healthy partner.

partner proved to be without any influence: thyroparathyroidectomy, total nephrectomy, left coronary artery ligature, and ventricular wall ligation. Thus, the simple explanation that the two additional kidneys and/or the additional heart in the joined system contribute to, or are primarily responsible for, the maintenance of an adequate circulation appears to be invalid. On the other hand, when partial hepatectomy was performed in both parabionts, or when three adrenals were removed (i.e., two from the healthy and one from the myopathic partner), congestive heart failure developed rapidly in the BIO 14.6 animal. Here again, however, the interventions were effective in eliminating the protection normally exerted by parabiosis only when performed during a critical period.

CONCLUSIONS

Hypothetically, every disorder of cardiac contractility must find its ultimate explanation in a biochemical abnormality. In fact, this hypothesis has motivated a considerable amount of biochemical study on the possible causes of heart failure in man and animals. Despite its appreciable volume, this research has not yet provided insight into the biochemical etiology of contractile failure of the heart. Particularly disappointing has been the inability of any group working in this field to find a consistent abnormality in the biochemical composition and metabolic function of the failing heart which could be considered as an etiological factor of primary importance. Attempts to formulate systems of classification for the various forms of heart failure in terms of biochemical abnormalities have been largely unsatisfactory.

There has been much less analysis and appreciation of the possibility that certain types of cardiac failure might be the result of changes occurring in the quantitative and qualitative morphology of the heart. It has recently been demonstrated that a rearrangement in the normal position of the muscle fibers take place during the development of hypertrophy and dilatation; a theory has been advanced that this structural rearrangement is, from a morphological point of view, the basic cause of inadequate cardiac function.[36] The data collected from a study of the spontaneous disease model of the hamster appear to indicate, furthermore, that hypertrophy and dilatation exert a considerable influence on the ultimate fate of healing processes in the damaged heart muscle,

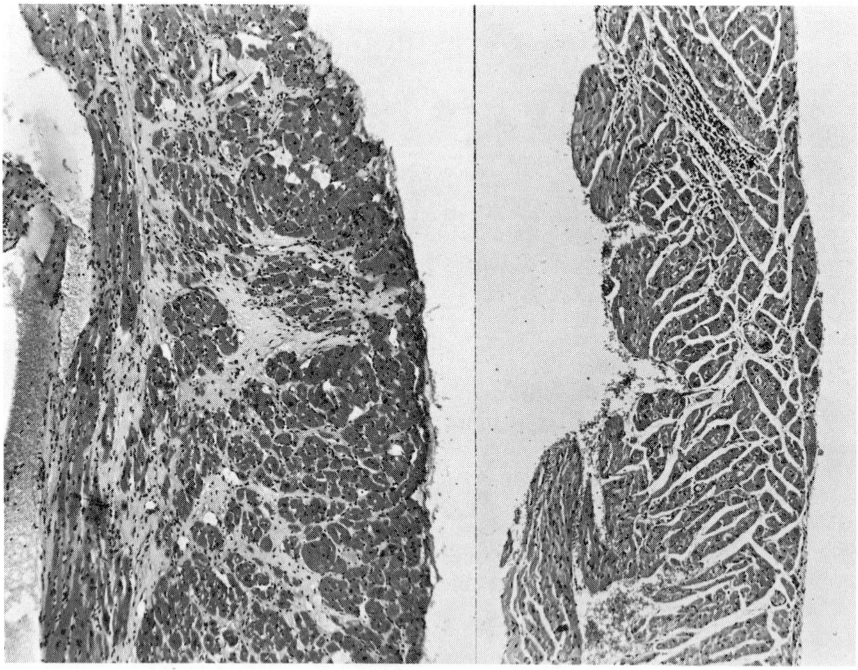

FIGURE 8. (*Left*) Numerous old fibrotic lesions can be seen in heart of the parabiosed, nonedematous myopathic hamster. (*Right*) Only one relatively recent lesion can be recognized in heart of the nonparabiosed, highly edematous myopathic hamster. Note that in the latter animal the wall of the left ventricle is thinner (due to the extended cardiac dilatation) than in the parabiosed animal, in which moderate hypertrophy was present but no dilatation occurred. Both animals were 164 days old at the time of autopsy. Stain: hematoxylin-eosin. × 48 (orig. mag. × 60).

and this, in turn, may result in additional alterations of the normal quantitative anatomy.

As early as 1891, Krehl[37] suggested that the small foci of inflammation, necrosis, and fibrosis or scars, often seen at autopsy in the hypertrophied and dilated hearts of patients with congestive heart failure, may play a role in the development of this condition. However, it is generally believed that such minor structural alterations are unimportant from a functional point of view. Nevertheless, the experimental findings discussed in this paper reveal that minor structural changes are sometimes the only recognizable remnants of an earlier severe myocardial degeneration, and, hence, they may be of etiological significance.

Finally, the demonstration that the development of congestive heart failure can be prevented by parabiosis deserves some discussion. It has long been known that the mammalian heart, even though well supplied with oxygenated blood, loses efficiency when separated from the rest of the body in a heart-lung preparation. The contractile force gradually weakens, thereby leading to a failure which, in some respects, is comparable to chronic congestive heart failure. This mechanical failure has been attributed to denervation of the heart,[38,39] to the loss of metabolic control caused by depletion of hormones,[40] and to the absence of unknown substance(s) normally supplied by the liver.[41,42] Since the contractile force of such a failing heart may be restored to normal if the liver and spleen are returned to the circulatory pathway, it has been concluded that these organs supply a factor with physiological effects closely resembling those of strophanthin.[43-47] Furthermore, a substance (β-palmitoyl lysolecithin) with digitalis-like activity has been isolated from the blood and other tissues of mammals, and this naturally occurring cardioactive principle was found to be present in the highest concentration in the adrenal medulla.[48] If we assume that the protective effect of parabiosis is humoral in nature, the literature data reviewed here may indicate the area(s) toward which future investigations should be directed.

Summary

The existence in an inbred strain of Syrian hamster of a genetically transmitted (or conditioned), degenerative cardiomyopathy that terminates in congestive heart failure offers unique opportunities to study the sequence of events leading to a congested state and to analyze the participation of extracardiac factors in the mechanism of generalized venous congestion. Cardiac insufficiency develops relatively slowly and progressively in these myopathic animals through three distinct stages. During the first stage (approximately between the 25th and 65th days of age), myocardial lesions characterized by spotty myolysis occur; during the second stage (ranging approximately between the 55th and 85th days of age), cardiac hypertrophy and dilatation develop; during the third stage (usually after the 80th day of age), the hypertrophy is overtaken by extended dilatation of the cardiac chambers, and, concurrently, the peripheral manifestations of the heart failure become increasingly marked.

Although the disease affects both sexes within the myopathic strain, cardiac-muscle pathology occurs earlier in females (at about 30 days of age) than in males (at about 45th days of age). The average life-span is about 125 days in nonbreeding females and 167 days in males. The myocardial degeneration is progressive until about the 60th to 70th days of age, and only a few fresh lesions appear in the heart muscle of the older animals. The extent to which lesions can be detected in the heart during the advanced stages of failure is not indicative of the extent of the initial myocardial damage. The rapidly progressing compensatory phenomena (hypertrophy and dilatation) apparently exert a marked influence on the qualitative aspects of healing processes, and the small focal lesions disappear without collagenous scar formation.

Parabiosis between a diseased hamster and a healthy one considerably prolongs the life of the myopathic partner. Such parabiotic union influences neither the onset nor the progression of cardiac- or skeletal-muscle pathology, but it completely prevents the development of generalized venous congestion.

References

1. Armstrong, T. G. 1940. Quart. J. Exp. Physiol. **30**: 263.
2. Barger, A. C., G. S. Richardson & B. B. Roe. 1950. Proc. Soc. Exp. Biol. Med. **73**: 113.
3. Hufnagel, C. A., B. B. Roe & A. C. Barger. 1951. Surgery **29**: 77.
4. Munro, A., O. J. Balchum, J. C. Owens & H. Swan. 1955. Surg. Forum **6**: 204.
5. Veith, F. J. & W. B. Thrower. 1959. Surg. Gynec. Obstet. **109**: 687.
6. Gertler, M. M. 1959. Proc. Soc. Exp. Biol. Med. **102**: 396.
7. Bor, N. B. & A. P. Rieben. 1961. Amer. J. Cardiol. **8**: 41.
8. Imai, H. & R. M. O'Neal. 1961. Arch. Path. (Chicago) **7**: 688.
9. Weil, M. H. & B. S. Miller. 1961. J. Lab. Clin. Med. **57**: 683.
10. Schwartz, A. & K. S. Lee. 1962. Circ. Res. **10**: 321.
11. Donald, D. E. & H. E. Essex. 1954. Amer. J. Physiol. **177**: 477.
12. Bakos, A. C. P. 1950. Circulation **1**: 724.
13. Johns, T. P. N. & B. J. Olson. 1954. Ann. Surg. **140**: 675.
14. Bajusz, E. 1963. Conditioning Factors for Cardiac Necroses. Intercontinental Medical Book Corp. New York, N. Y.
15. Corday, E., R. Spitzler & M. Prinzmetal. 1949. Ann. Intern. Med. **31**: 450.
16. Homburger, F., J. R. Baker, C. W. Nixon & R. Whitney. 1962. Med. Exp. (Basel) **6**: 339.
17. Homburger, F., J. R. Baker, C. W. Nixon, G. Wilgram & J. Harrop. 1965. J. Path. Bact. **89**: 133.
18. Bajusz, E., F. Homburger, J. R. Baker & C. W. Nixon. 1965. Fed. Proc. **24**: 560.
19. Homburger, F., J. R. Baker, G. Wilgram, J. B. Caulfield & C. W. Nixon. 1966. Arch. Path. (Chicago) **81**: 302.
20. Bajusz, E., F. Homburger, J. R. Baker & L. H. Opie. 1966. Ann. N. Y. Acad. Sci. **138**: 213.
21. Wallace, C. W. & W. F. Hamilton. 1962. Circ. Res. **11**: 301.
22. Wallace, C. W. 1965. Ann. N. Y. Acad. Sci. **127**: 570.
23. Hecht, H. H., H. Kuida, R. L. Lange, J. L. Thome & A. M. Brown. 1962. Amer. J. Med. **32**: 171.
24. Detweiler, D. K. 1964. Circulation **30**: 114.
25. Hudson, R. E. B. 1965. Cardiovascular Pathology. **1**. Williams & Wilkins Co. Baltimore, Md.
26. Cannon, P. R., L. E. Fraizer & R. H. Hughes. 1950. Metabolism **1**: 49.
27. French, J. C. 1952. Arch. Path. (Chicago) **53**: 485.
28. Rona, G., C. I. Chappel & D. S. Kahn. 1963. Exp. Molec. Path. **2**: 40.
29. Korb, G. & V. Totovic. 1963. Frankfurt. Z. Path. **73**: 175.
30. Finerty, J. C. 1952. Physiol. Rev. **32**: 277.
31. Florsheim, W. H., N. S. Austin & S. M. Velcoff. 1963. Endocrinology **72**: 817.
32. Hunt, E. L., H. W. Carroll & D. J. Kimelford. 1965. Science **150**: 1747.
33. Bunster, E. & R. K. Meyer. 1933. Anat. Rec. **57**: 339.
34. Hall, C. E. & O. Hall. 1966. *In* Methods and Achievements in Experimental Pathology. E. Bajusz & G. Jasmin, Eds. 1: 585–606. Year Book Medical Publishers, Inc. Chicago, Ill.
35. Zsoter, T. & E. Bajusz. 1962. Cardiologia **40**: 290.
36. Linzbach, A. J. 1960. Amer. J. Cardiol. **5**: 370.
37. Krehl, L. 1891. Deutsche Arch. Klin. Med. **48**: 414.
38. Gremels, H. 1936. Arch. Exp. Path. Pharmakol. **182**: 1.
39. Gollwitzer-Meier, K. & E. Kruger. 1938. Arch. Ges. Physiol. **240**: 89.

40. Gremels, H. 1940. Arch. Exp. Path. Pharmakol. **194:** 629.
41. Pinotti, O. 1941. Arch. Fisiol. **42:** 160.
42. Rein, H. 1942. Klin. Wschr. **21:** 873.
43. Bucherl, E. & H. Rein. 1949. Naturwissenschaften **36:** 260.
44. Rein, H., O. Mertens & E. Bucherl. 1949. Naturwissenschaften **36:** 233.
45. Mertens, O. & H. Rein. 1949. Naturwissenschaften **36:** 237.
46. Kohler, U. 1955–1956. Wiss. Z. Martin-Luther-Universität **5:** 409.
47. Meesmann, W. & J. Schmier. 1956. Pfluegers Archiv. Ges. Physiol. **263:** 304.
48. Hajdu, S., H. Weiss & E. Titus. 1957. J. Pharmacol. Exp. Ther. **120:** 99.

THE RELATIONSHIP OF NUTRITION TO FATTY DEGENERATION OF THE MYOCARDIUM AND KIDNEY*

Peter Rasmussen

Department of Pathology
University of Maryland School of Medicine
Baltimore, Md.

After 24 to 48 hours of starvation, rabbits develop a fatty change of the myocardium and kidney.[1] Fatty degeneration has been described in the muscles of other animals following starvation,[2] and Wittels and Bressler[3] have studied the myocardial fatty change in guinea pigs following starvation and after administration of diphtheria toxin from the standpoint of fatty acid oxidation by the heart. This paper reports the role of another factor acting in the pathogenesis of this acute type of fatty change due to starvation. The occurrence of fatty change is also reported in the kidney, because it parallels the change in the heart.

Materials and Methods

Albino rabbits weighing 1.5–5 kg were maintained on Purina Rabbit Chow, except when starved of water and chow for 24 to 48 hours (acute starvation). Animals were killed with an intravenous (i.v.) injection of 3–4 cc of sodium pentobarbital (50 mg/cc).

Portions of the left ventricle and kidney were fixed in 10% formalin with 1% $CaCl_2$ added. Frozen sections of fresh or formalin-fixed tissue were cut to a thickness of about 10 μ on a cryostat. The sections were placed in 100% propylene glycol for five minutes. They were then stained for lipid with 0.7% oil-red-O in propylene glycol for ten to 15 minutes at 60° C and counterstained with hematoxylin.

Serum triglyceride (TG) levels were measured by the method of Van Handel and Zilversmit.[4] Serum free fatty acid (FFA) levels were measured by the method of Mosinger.[5] For the chemical determination of tissue lipids, a tissue quantity near 0.5 g was homogenized at 0–4° C in enough 0.07 M phosphate buffer (pH 7.0) to make 5 ml.[6] This homogenate was extracted by the method of Folch and his colleagues.[7] The lower phase was dried in an oven at 30° C and redissolved in chloroform. Chemical quantitation of lipids was performed by the method of Amenta.[8] Blood sugars were measured by an *o*-toluidine reaction with a Harleco kit.† When appropriate, Triton® WR-1339‡ (oxyethylated tertiary octylphenol formaldehyde polymer) was injected i.v. in a 12.5% solution, in 0.9% NaCl at a dose of 300 or occasionally 600 mg/kg of body weight. Regular and protamine zinc insulin were injected subcutaneously in doses of 0.3–1 unit/kg. Doses above 1 unit/kg resulted in death from hypoglycemic convulsions.

The amount of lipid in sections of myocardium or kidney was ranked as 0, ±, or +. The level ± denoted a few lipid droplets in cells often scattered in separated high-power fields examined with the light microscope. The level + designated lipid droplets in great numbers in most cells occupying a high-power field and usually in adjacent high-power fields.

* This work was supported by United States Public Health Service research grant no. HE-07040 from the National Institutes of Health, Bethesda, Md.

† Hartman-Leddon Co., Inc., Philadelphia, Pa.

‡ The Triton® was kindly supplied by Winthrop Laboratories, New York, N. Y.

The significance of differences among enumerative data was evaluated by the X^2 test.[9] When the number of animals was small, the X^2 statistic was confirmed by calculating the exact probability.[10] The significance of differences between groups with quantitative data was tested with the Mann-Whitney U-test[11] or the t-test.[9]

RESULTS

Morphological Changes

With acute starvation, oil-red-O-positive lipid droplets (0.5–2 μ) appeared in the cytoplasm of myocardial cells and renal tubular cells of the cortico-medullary junction (CMJ). After 24 hours of starvation, lipid droplets were just visible in the myocardial cells of some rabbits, although many showed none at this time. The numbers of rabbits showing each of the three lipid levels upon examination of hearts and kidneys after 48 hours of starvation are shown in the left-hand portions of FIGURES 1 and 2. The degree of accumulation of lipid was less in the CMJ than in the myocardium. A significant finding in the kidneys was the absence of lipid accumulation in any of the tubular cells of the renal cortex.

The administration of Triton causes an accrual of TG in the blood by preventing the egress of TG from the blood to peripheral adipose tissue stores.[12] Triton also causes significant mobilization of TG from adipose tissue to the blood;[12] it does not appear to influence carbohydrate metabolism.[13] Thus, Triton was given i.v. at the start of the starvation or feeding interval in order to assess whether its effects might influence the development of renal or myocardial neutral lipid accumulation.

FIGURES 1 and 2 (right-hand portions) also illustrate the numbers of animals in the three lipid levels upon examination of hearts and kidneys of fed and starved rabbits given Triton. The distribution of animals with cardiac lipid accumulation was not greatly altered by Triton. However, the accrual of lipid in the CMJ of the kidney was more pronounced in starved rabbits given Triton. In addition, the renal cortical cells developed abundant fatty change after

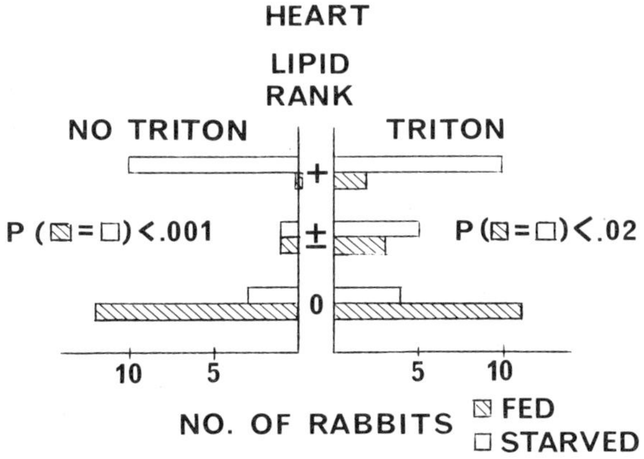

FIGURE 1. Schematic diagram showing the distribution of rabbits according to the level of neutral lipid accumulation in the myocardium, after feeding or starvation for 48 hours, with and without Triton administration.

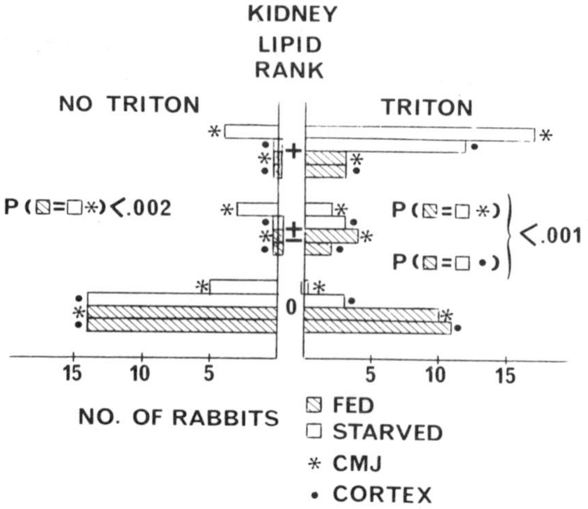

FIGURE 2. Schematic diagram showing the distribution of rabbits according to the level of neutral lipid accumulation in the tubular cells of the cortex and corticomedullary junction of the kidney, after feeding or starvation for 48 hours, with and without Triton administration.

starvation. Among fed rabbits, only a few animals developed significant lipid deposits in the myocardium or in the renal tubules of the cortex or the CMJ. When hepatic lipid content was studied, the numbers of fed and starved animals, with and without Triton, in each of the three lipid ranks generally ran parallel to the findings in the heart and kidney. However, the presence of substantial amounts of lipid in the livers of some fed rabbits blurred the patterns considerably.

Chemical determinations of the qualitative and quantitative nature of the increased myocardial lipid levels after starvation were performed; the results are shown in TABLE 1. Significant elevations were found in the TG and FFA levels. Part of this elevation of the cardiac FFA level after starvation may be caused by the concomitant elevation of the serum FFA level, or by some TG hydrolysis during tissue homogenization. Cholesterol and cholesterol esters were not significantly elevated.

TABLE 1

LEFT VENTRICULAR MYOCARDIAL LIPID LEVELS IN FED AND STARVED RABBITS*

Lipid Class	Lipid Levels (mg/g)	
	Fed Rabbits	Starved Rabbits
Triglyceride	1.43 ± 0.92	3.02 ± 1.27†
Free fatty acids	1.95 ± 1.13	4.30 ± 2.40‡
Cholesterol esters	1.51 ± 0.84	1.73 ± 0.34
Cholesterol	1.81 ± 0.93	2.15 ± 1.48

* All values are means with standard deviation, expressed as milligrams per gram of tissue (wet weight). Starvation period was 48 hours; nine rabbits were in each group.
† p [lipid value (fed) = lipid value (starved)] < 0.01 (t-test).
‡ p [lipid value (fed) = lipid value (starved)] < 0.02 (t-test).

Because of the small quantity of lipid seen in the CMJ of the kidney after starvation, and because of the inordinately high values of serum TG after Triton administration, chemical determinations of renal or cardiac lipids were not attempted under these circumstances. However, the identical morphological characteristics of the cellular lipid accumulations in these instances suggest that these accumulations also are made up of TG and FFA, as in the heart after simple starvation.

Chemical Changes in the Triglyceride, Free Fatty Acid, and Sugar Levels of the Blood

Under conditions of acute starvation, as compared with normal feeding in rabbits, the level of serum TG remained unchanged. The FFA and blood sugar levels were reciprocally changed, with a clear-cut fall in the blood sugar level within 24 hours of the onset of starvation and a doubling of the serum FFA level within 48 hours (TABLES 2 and 3).

In both fed and acutely starved rabbits given Triton, the serum levels of TG rose 20-fold over the serum levels in fed or starved animals not given Triton. Blood sugar levels again showed a significant fall within 24 hours of the onset

TABLE 2

SERUM TRIGLYCERIDE AND FREE FATTY ACID LEVELS IN FED AND STARVED RABBITS WITH AND WITHOUT TRITON ADMINISTRATION*

	Without Triton		With Triton	
Serum Component	Fed Rabbits	Starved Rabbits	Fed Rabbits	Starved Rabbits
Triglyceride (mg/100 ml)	A 80 (8) 25–86	B 93 (8) 47–166	C 2020 (11) 727–2840	D 2340 (8) 1000–3490
Free fatty acids (mEq/L)	E 504 (7) 160–910	F 1313 (8) 869–1970	G 2210 (11) 1951–2305	H 2200 (6) 1841–2317

* In each cell of the table, the mean value is given on the top line, with the number of rabbits given in parentheses. The range of values is given below the mean. Triton was administered i.v. 48 hours before the samples were removed for measurement. The statistical significance of the differences in data for each group of rabbits was computed according to the Mann-Whitney U-test: p (A or B = C or D) < 0.001; p (E = F) < 0.001; and p (F = G or H) < 0.001.

TABLE 3

BLOOD SUGAR LEVELS IN FED AND STARVED RABBITS WITH AND WITHOUT TRITON ADMINISTRATION*

	Blood Sugar Levels (mg/100 ml)					
	Without Triton			With Triton		
	0 hours	24 hours†	48 hours†	0 hours	24 hours†	48 hours
Fed rabbits	112 ± 17	113 ± 18	104 ± 8	107 ± 12	104 ± 10	95 ± 13
Starved rabbits	108 ± 8	77 ± 4	83 ± 6	96 ± 13	80 ± 4	85 ± 6

* All values are means with standard deviations, expressed as milligrams per 100 ml. Six rabbits were in each group.

† p [blood sugar (fed) = blood sugar (starved)] < 0.01 (t-test).

of starvation. The levels of serum FFA in fed and starved animals given Triton were about twice the levels observed after simple starvation (TABLES 2 and 3). A similar but later elevation of serum lipids has been noted in dogs by Scanu and his colleagues.[14]

The Role of Insulin

In order to ascertain whether the relevant factor in inducing cardiac and renal fatty change during starvation was the fall in the blood sugar level or the concomitant fall in the endogenous insulin level, rabbits were injected with regular and protamine zinc insulin at the beginning of the starvation period and 24 hours later. The patterns of blood sugar and FFA level response at 48 hours are shown in TABLE 4. Seven rabbits survived for 48 hours and showed a significant fall in the blood sugar level below that of a group of starved rabbits given only Triton. Serum FFA levels in the starved animals given Triton and insulin were significantly elevated over those in starved animals not given Triton. Six of seven starved rabbits given Triton and insulin showed a clear-cut and substantial fatty degeneration of the myocardium and tubular cells of the renal cortex. With regard to raised lipid levels in the heart, CMJ, and renal cortical cells, the numbers of starved rabbits given Triton and insulin differed significantly from the corresponding distributions among fed rabbits given only Triton. ($p < 0.01$, < 0.01, and < 0.05, respectively). This suggests that a low blood sugar level, rather than a low insulin level, is the significant factor in permitting myocardial and renal fatty change.

TABLE 4

BLOOD SUGAR AND FREE FATTY ACID LEVELS IN STARVED RABBITS WITH AND WITHOUT TRITON AND INSULIN ADMINISTRATION*

Drugs Administered	Blood Sugar Levels† (mg/100 ml)	FFA Levels‡ (mEq/l)
Triton and insulin	40 ± 14 (7)	974 ± 410 (7)
Triton	85 ± 6 (6)	—
No Triton or insulin	—	614 ± 226 (14)

* All values are means with standard deviations. The number of rabbits in each group is given in parentheses. Starvation period was 48 hours.
† p [blood sugar (Triton and insulin) = blood sugar (Triton)] < 0.01 (t-test).
‡ p [FFA (Triton and insulin) = FFA (no Triton or insulin)] < 0.02 (t-test).

DISCUSSION

Investigations have indicated that, under conditions of fasting, the FFA uptake from the blood by an organ such as the heart is directly related to the FFA concentration in the blood.[15] Further studies have shown that TG is synthesized intracellularly from FFA and glycerol.[16] Based on these studies, and on the *in vitro* demonstration of increasing oxidation of FFA by the heart during starvation, Wittels and Bressler[3] have postulated that the myocardial TG accumulation in guinea pigs during starvation is caused by a transient shunting by the heart cell of a temporary excess of FFA into TG.

In addition to its ability to elevate serum TG levels, Triton appears to permit a separation of the usually reciprocal association between blood sugar and blood FFA levels. The data reported here suggest that, independent of the blood FFA level, the recent nutritional state of an animal is related in the development of renal and myocardial fatty change in another way, the mechanism of which is apparently dependent on carbohydrate intake. Thus, most fed rabbits in these experiments did not accumulate lipid (most likely TG) in the myocardium or in renal tubular cells, even when these cells were confronted with high blood levels of FFA, as was the case after Triton administration. In addition, the administration of insulin did not mitigate the renal and cardiac fatty change, which indirectly suggests that carbohydrate availability is a significant factor impeding fatty accumulation in the face of a large supply of FFA. In line with this, Gordon and Cherkes[17] and Olson and Piatnek[18] have indicated that carbohydrate is the preferred substrate for the myocardium and that, in its presence, the heart cell utilizes it rather than fatty acids for energy.

The possibility that Triton, in addition to elevating serum FFA levels, also makes them functionally inaccessible for uptake by heart or kidney appears unlikely in view of the remarkable enhancement of lipid accrual in the tubular cells of the renal cortex in the starved rabbits. Moreover, Scanu and Page[12] have shown in dogs that the FFA in animals given Triton are readily available for uptake by tissues.

The absence of neutral lipid accumulation in the heart and renal cortical tubules of most fed rabbits given Triton suggests that with Triton, despite the abundant supply of blood FFA, the hearts and kidneys of most fed animals with adequate levels of blood sugar do not appreciably pick up otherwise accessible FFA for synthesis to TG. Glucose itself may partially prevent the adaptive changes necessary in certain enzymes for utilization of FFA or their synthesis to TG by maintaining the function of other enzymes utilizing glucose for energy. Such an influence on enzymes would, in effect, function as a block to the uptake of FFA by the myocardium and renal cells. As an example of such a mechanism, Weber and his colleagues[19] have shown a dose-dependent protective effect of glucose against the inhibitory effects of FFA on the function of glukokinase in rat liver.

In the present experiments, the controlling factor of feeding does not appear to be absolute, since a small number of fed rabbits given Triton exhibited substantial fatty change, both in the heart and in tubular cells of the renal cortex (FIGURES 1 and 2).

The significance of an independent permissive effect of feeding on lipid accumulation in the heart and kidney may be speculated on in view of the work of Weber and his colleagues[19] which suggests that fatty acids result in a decreased functioning of the Krebs cycle, which produces the acetyl coenzyme A necessary for the utilization of pyruvate from glucose and the intermediates from the betaoxidation of fatty acids. Thus, a protective effect of glucose might be regulative against surges of FFA mobilization brought on by epinephrine during periods of acute stress. In addition, because the myocardium depends upon fatty acids for energy during periods of reduced glucose availability, the transient storage of fatty acids as TG in the cyptoplasm might represent the mechanism for ensuring the necessary transition of the myocardium and kidney from primarily glucose utilization to fatty acid utilization. Tepperman and Tepperman[20] have suggested a similar hypothesis to explain the storage of lipids in the form of TG rather than fatty acids in adipose tissue.

SUMMARY

Within 48 hours after the onset of starvation, most rabbits accumulate stainable lipid in the myocardium, and many accumulate lipid in renal tubular cells of the CMJ.

The numbers of rabbits accumulating various amounts of lipid in the myocardium with feeding and after 48 hours of starvation is only somewhat affected by the remarkable elevation of the serum FFA level induced by Triton administration, i.e., despite high serum FFA levels, most fed animals do not develop fatty degeneration in the heart. However, Triton greatly enhances the accrual of lipid in the renal tubular cells of the CMJ during starvation, and simultaneously causes the tubular cells of the renal cortex to accumulate lipid. In most animals fed and given Triton, the high serum FFA level does not cause lipid accumulation in renal cortical cells. Thus, a reduced caloric intake, as reflected by lowered blood sugar levels after 24 hours of starvation, appears to be a necessary factor for the use of elevated serum FFA in the synthesis of stainable myocardial and renal tubular cell TG. Exogenous insulin and Triton does not reduce the development of myocardial or renal fatty degeneration in starved rabbits, indirectly suggesting that the low blood glucose level rather than the low serum insulin of starvation is the factor permitting cardiac and renal fatty change with starvation.

Thus, glucose may afford protection against the inhibitory effects of transient surges of FFA on the Krebs cycle. Also, fatty degeneration may represent a protective mechanism against such inhibitory effects of FFA, when glucose becomes unavailable, whereby fatty acids are effectively bound as TG within the cell.

References

1. Rasmussen, P. 1965. Fed. Proc. **24**: 553.
2. Palade, G. E. & G. Schidlowsky. 1958. Anat. Rec. **130**: 352.
3. Wittels, B. & R. Bressler. 1964. Lab. Invest. **13**: 794.
4. Van Handel, E. & D. B. Zilversmit. 1957. J. Lab. Clin. Med. **50**: 152.
5. Mosinger, F. 1964. J. Lipid Res. **5**: 157.
6. Butler, Jr., W. M., M. Maling, M. G. Horning & B. B. Brodie. 1961. J. Lipid Res. **2**: 95.
7. Folch, J., M. Lees & G. H. Sloane Stanley. 1957. J. Biol. Chem. **226**: 497.
8. Amenta, J. S. 1964. J. Lipid Res. **5**: 270.
9. Croxton, F. E. 1953. Elementary Statistics with Applications in Medicine and the Biological Sciences. : 235; 280. Dover Publications, Inc. New York, N. Y.
10. Freeman, G. H. & J. H. Halton. 1951. Biometrika **38**: 141.
11. Diamond, S. 1959. Information and Error. An Introduction to Statistical Analysis. : 248. Basic Books, Inc. New York, N. Y.
12. Scanu, A. & I. H. Page. 1962. J. Clin. Invest. **41**: 495.
13. Scanu, A. & J. M. Szajewski. 1961. Amer. J. Physiol. **201**: 1035.
14. Scanu, A., P. Oriente, J. Szajewski, L. J. McCormick & I. H. Page. 1961. J. Exp. Med. **114**: 279.
15. Ballard, F. B., W. H. Danforth, S. Neagle & R. J. Bing. 1960. J. Clin. Invest. **39**: 717.
16. Kennedy, E. P. 1961. Fed. Proc. **20**: 934.
17. Gordon, R. S. & A. Cherkes. 1956. J. Clin. Invest. **35**: 206.
18. Olson, R. E. & D. A. Piatnek. 1959. Ann. N. Y. Acad. Sci. **72**: 466.
19. Weber, G., H. J. H. Convery, M. A. Lea & N. B. Stamm. 1966. Science **154**: 1357.
20. Tepperman, J. & H. M. Tepperman. 1965. Ann. N. Y. Acad. Sci. **131**: 404.

EXPERIMENTAL INFECTION WITH *TRYPANOSOMA CRUZI* (CHAGAS' DISEASE): A MODEL OF ACUTE AND CHRONIC MYOCARDIOPATHY*

Walter H. Abelmann

Thorndike Memorial Laboratory and the Second and Fourth (Harvard) Medical Services, Boston City Hospital, and the Department of Medicine Harvard Medical School, Boston, Mass.

INTRODUCTION

This paper deals with an experimental model of heart disease with two unique features: first, it closely parallels a human heart disease of considerable clinical importance, and second, it involves both an acute and a chronic phase. Experimental Chagas' disease presents an opportunity to study the possible effects of various factors that have been implicated as modifiers of myocardial disease in man.

Chagas' disease occurs primarily in Central and South American countries, where some 35 million people are exposed to the risk of infection with *Trypanosoma cruzi,* and about 20% are infected.[1] Infected vertebrates have been found throughout the Americas and act as natural hosts. Natural transmission occurs by triatome bugs, which inhabit human dwellings. The bugs ingest trypanosomes by feeding on blood and, in turn, deposit the parasites in their feces upon the skin of their next victim. The parasites enter the new host through a break in the skin or through mucous membrane.

During the acute phase of the disease, trypanosomes are present in the blood. The parasites show a predilection for tissues of mesenchymal origin, such as cardiac muscle. In the myocardium, intracellular leishmanial pseudocysts are formed; they rupture and produce an acute inflammatory reaction and myocardial degeneration, followed by formation of granulomata and interstitial fibrosis. The lesions may be focal or diffuse. In man, the acute phase is generally benign, although occasionally it is accompanied by heart failure; the chronic phase may lead to progressive cardiac hypertrophy, dilatation, and failure, thereby reducing life expectancy.[1-3] Cardiac arrhythmias are frequent, and sudden death is not unusual. Extracardiac manifestations are less common but may be dominant; they are usually related to involvement of visceral smooth muscle and autonomic ganglia, and result in organomegaly such as megaesophagus or megacolon.[4]

Experimental Chagas' myocarditis has been produced in mice,[5-7] in rats,[8-10] and in dogs,[11-14] primarily for the purpose of elucidating the pathophysiology of the disease or to screen potential therapeutic agents. Thus, most experimenters have concentrated upon the acute disease. The chronic disease has been studied in dogs by Laranja and his colleagues[12] and in mice by Pakchanian and Robinson[6] and by Okumura and co-workers.[7]

It is the purpose of the present communication to draw attention to experimental Chagas' disease in mice, of a milder, more chronic form, suitable for use as a model of a myocardiopathy with both an acute and a chronic phase.[15] The effects of both the acute and the chronic disease upon spontaneous activity

* Supported, in part, by grants nos. 1-PO1-HE-10539 and 5-T1-HE-5244 from the National Heart Institute, National Institutes of Health, by United States Public Health Service research grant no. FR-76 from the Division of Research Facilities and Resources, Bethesda, Md., and by the Massachusetts Heart Association, Boston, Mass.

of the animals,[15-16] the effects of elective and of forced exercise upon animals in the acute[16] and subacute phases of the disease, and, finally, the effects of ethanol in the diet will be reported.

Material and Methods

Mice. Male C3H mice were used throughout. The mice were usually inoculated at about one month of age. They were fed standard Purina Rat Chow, except as indicated. The animals were examined and weighed at least once weekly.

The Parasite. One strain of *T. cruzi* (Colombian) was used throughout; it had been passed serially in Harvard Swiss mice. The origin of this strain, its passage history, and the methods of inoculation and of counting of the parasites have been reported in detail previously.[15] Mice were inoculated intraperitoneally, usually with about 10,000 organisms. Parasites in tail blood were counted at weekly intervals.

Spontaneous Activity. Spontaneous activity was measured in activity wheels[15] (FIGURE 1), usually twice a week during a 50-minute period, and expressed as revolutions per minute (rpm).

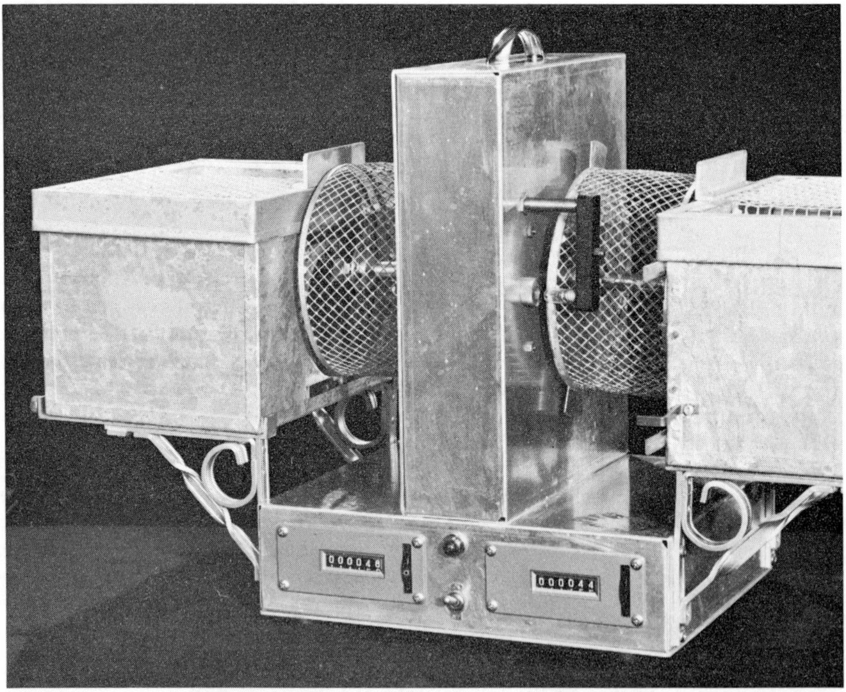

FIGURE 1. Tandem activity wheels. Two phalanges mounted at the periphery of each wheel interrupt a light beam focused on a photocell, which activates a digital counter. Access to the wheel is through a sliding door in the side of the cage. An infected mouse and its control can be tested simultaneously. During measurement of "spontaneous activity," the animal was placed in the drum, and the sliding door was closed. During "mild exercise," the door was kept open.

Mild Exercise. Although spontaneous activity, as noted above, was considered to have at most a negligible effect upon the animal, elective running in the activity cage for 50 minutes four times a week was found to affect heart weight and will be labeled "mild exercise."

Forced Exercise. The form of forced exercise used was swimming in aquaria at 33° C, in groups of six animals, for one hour five times per week.[16]

Pathology. As soon after death as possible, or after the animal was sacrificed with ether, the body weight was recorded. The heart was removed in a standard manner and weighed to the nearest 0.2 mg. After gross examination, portions of the heart and other organs were taken for microscopical study.[15, 16] The degree of cellular infiltration and necrosis of the myocardium was graded as mild (1 +), moderate (2 +), or severe (3 +), and the number of parasitic aggregates per section was counted. The slides were examined by two observers working independently and without knowledge of the identity of the slides. In some series, half of each heart was weighed, dried, and reweighed until weights were stable.

Ethanol Diet. Ethanol was given in a liquid diet, modified after that of Lieber and his associates.[17] The control diet contained 19% of its calories as amino acids, 38% as sucrose, and 42% as fat. In the ethanol diet, sucrose was replaced isocalorically with ethanol to the extent of 14.3% of total calories. Ethanol was introduced into the diet gradually. The animals were inoculated with *T. cruzi* after nine weeks on the special diet.

Results

General Characteristics of the Experimental Disease

Clinical Course of the Disease

Initial passages of the parasite were characterized by the absence of gross evidence of illness during the acute phase. Infection could be demonstrated in all inoculated animals by examination of the peripheral blood for trypanosomes (FIGURE 2). Parasitemia appeared during the second week after inoculation, reached its peak during the fifth week, and had largely subsided 12 weeks after inoculation (FIGURE 3). Occasional motile parasites, however, were demonstrable in the blood as late as eight months after inoculation.

During the acute parasitemic stage of the infection, the animals appeared healthy, grew normally, and maintained their weights. In the third month of infection, ruffling of the fur was noticeable on careful inspection, at times associated with loss of hair. The infected animals gradually took on an appearance of ill health, and, in time, gave evidence of muscle wasting and weakness. Beginning with the third month, the body weights of the infected animals fell significantly below those of the noninfected controls. Animals generally survived the acute myocarditis, but mortality increased gradually in later passages through Harvard Swiss mice, and more rapidly when passages were made through C3H mice.[15]

Pathology in the Acute Phase

Upon gross examination, there was occasional enlargement of the heart, especially of the right atrium and ventricle. This was seen with increasing frequency in subsequent passages.

Microscopical examination revealed myocardial infiltrates, predominantly mononuclear, generally focal, and not limited to any chamber or portion of the myocardium (FIGURE 4). In initial passages, parasites were few and seen only in some hearts (FIGURE 5). With subsequent passages, the lesions became more pronounced; intracellular aggregates of leishmanial forms of *T. cruzi,* degeneration, and necrosis were seen more frequently (FIGURE 6). In some series, predilection of infiltrates for the subepicardial layer of the right ventricle was noted.

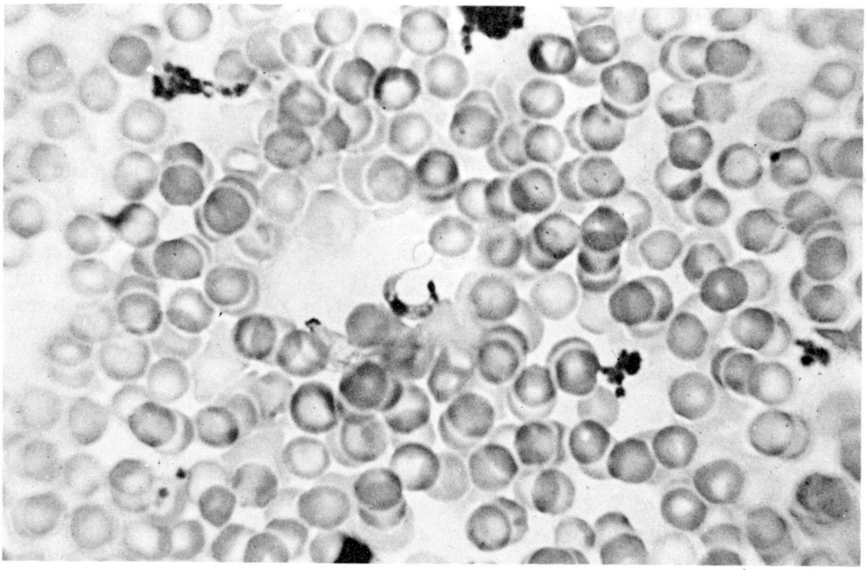

FIGURE 2. *Trypanosoma cruzi* in a smear of peripheral blood from a mouse, 30 days after inoculation. Stain: Giemsa: × 500.

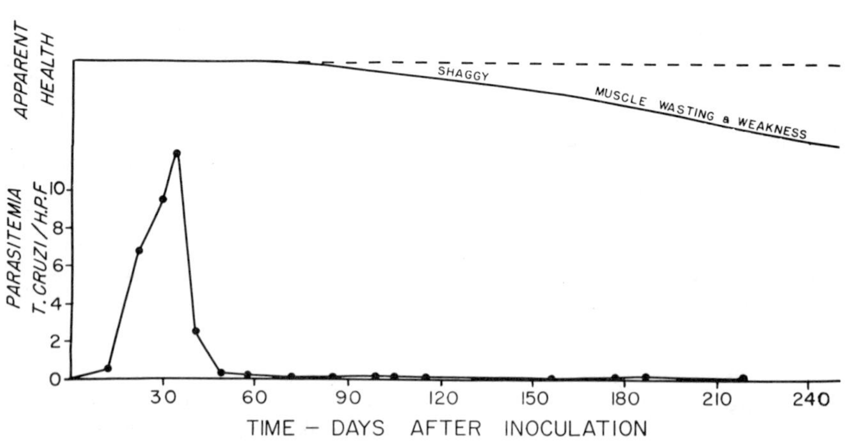

FIGURE 3. Schematic representation of experimental Chagas' disease in the C3H mouse. (*Top*) The clinical course, as measured by apparent health. (*Bottom*) The course of parasitemia, as measured by the number of *T. cruzi* per high-power field (H. P. F.). (After Federici *et al.*[15] Reproduced by permission of the American Journal of Tropical Medicine and Hygiene.)

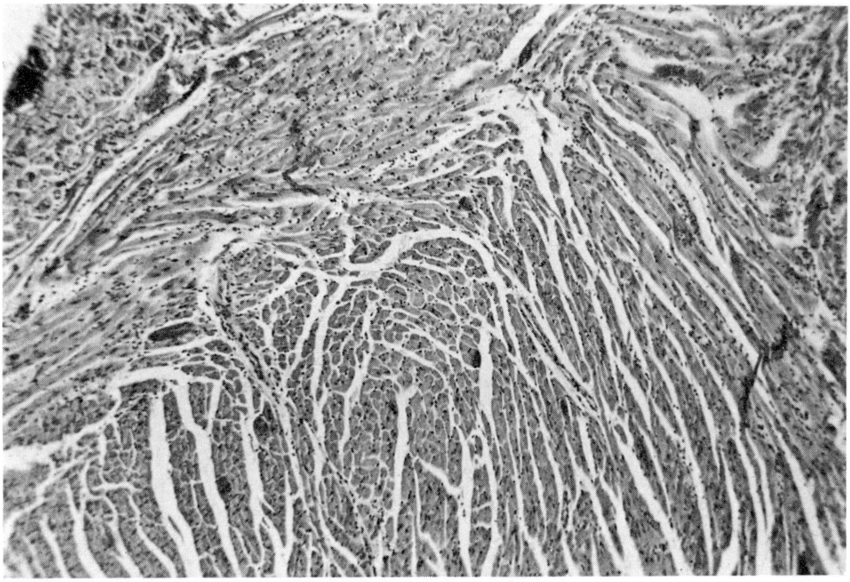

FIGURE 4. Section of myocardium from a mouse, 21 days after inoculation with *T. cruzi*, showing infiltration, with predominantly mononuclear cells and several intracellular aggregates of leishmanial forms of the parasite. Stain: hematoxylin and eosin. × 100.

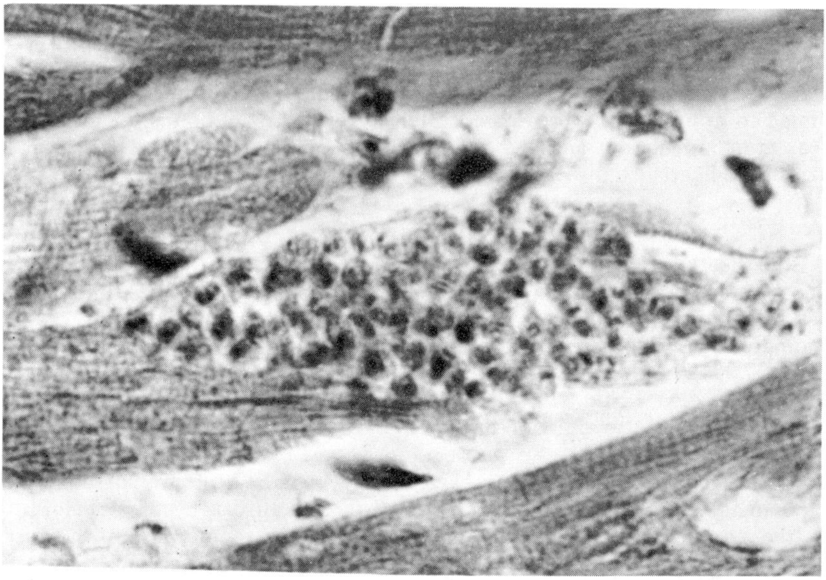

FIGURE 5. Myocardium from a mouse, 49 days after inoculation with *T. cruzi*, showing intracellular leishmanial forms of the parasite. Stain: Giemsa. × 700.

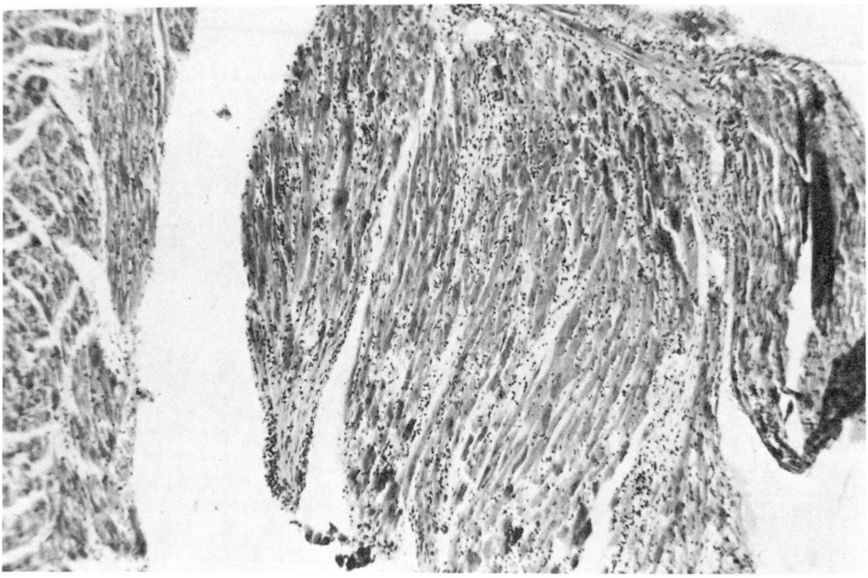

FIGURE 6. Intraventricular septum from a mouse, 50 days after inoculation with *T. cruzi*, showing multifocal infiltration and necrosis. Stain: hematoxylin and eosin. × 100.

Pathology in the Subacute and Chronic Phases

After subsidence of the acute parasitemic stage, gross dilatation of cardiac chambers was seen more frequently. Myocardial infiltrates became progressively more widespread, and foci of degeneration and necrosis became more severe. Five months after inoculation, loose fibrous tissue began to appear and gradually increased in extent (FIGURE 7). Yet, acute infiltrative and necrotic lesions continued to appear and increased in intensity and distribution until more than a year after inoculation (FIGURE 8). Parasites continued to be present in at least half of the hearts examined.

Heart Weight

Both heart weight and heart weight:body weight ratios of infected animals showed an increase over those of the controls, progressive with time. Thus on day 50, the mean heart weight of 15 infected animals was 100.9 ± 11.5 mg, compared with a mean weight in 14 control animals of 91.3 ± 10.1 mg ($p < 0.05$). In the same infected group, the mean heart weight:body weight $\times 10^3$ was 4.61 ± 0.28, 20% higher than the control value of 3.85 ± 0.26 ($p < 0.001$).[16] The ratio of dry to wet weight of the heart was not affected by the infection.

In the subacute stage of the disease, on day 118, the heart weight:body weight ratio in infected animals also exceeded that of controls, by 21% (FIGURE 9). In the chronic phase, between the seventh and 12th months of the disease, heart weight:body weight ratios in the infected animals exceeded those of the controls by 32%.[15] Thus Chagasic myocarditis, whether acute, subacute, or chronic, was associated with an increase in heart weight.

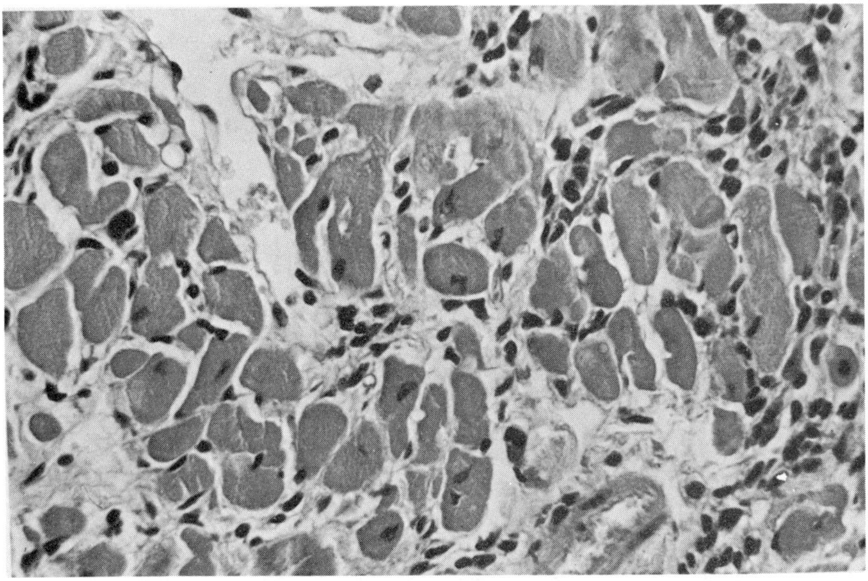

FIGURE 7. Myocardium from a mouse, 178 days after inoculation with *T. cruzi,* showing destruction of myocardium, loose fibrous tissue, and mononuclear infiltrates. Stain: hematoxylin and eosin. × 500.

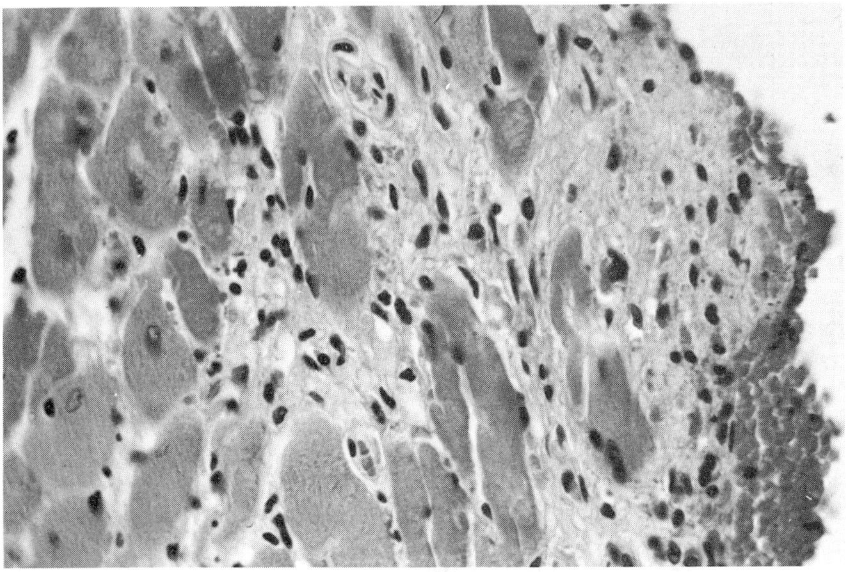

FIGURE 8. Myocardium from a mouse, 232 days after inoculation with *T. cruzi,* showing loss of myocardial cells and replacement by fibrous tissue. Stain: hematoxylin and eosin. × 500.

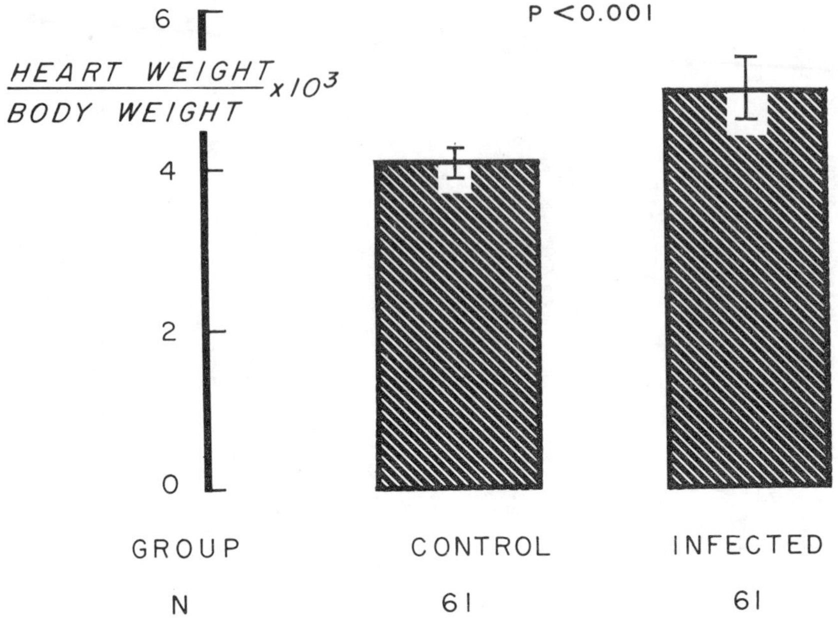

FIGURE 9. Effect of Chagasic myocarditis upon the heart weights of mice sacrificed 118 days after inoculation with *T. cruzi*. Mean values and standard deviations are indicated. N = number of mice in each group.

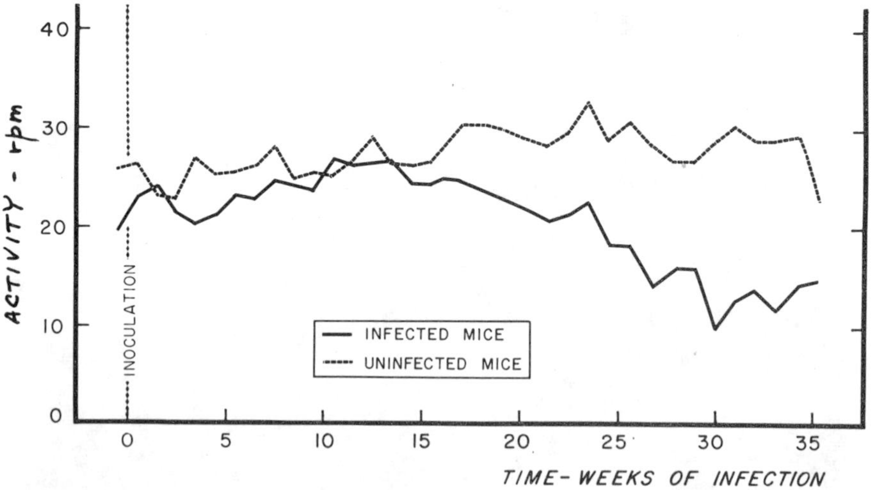

FIGURE 10. Spontaneous activity, in revolutions per minute, of infected mice (solid line) compared with uninfected controls (interrupted line). Data based on at least 12 mice in each group for the first 17 weeks, and at least four mice in each group to the end of the plot. Activity decreased during the acute parasitemic phase and again during the chronic phase of the disease.

Spontaneous Activity during the Acute and Chronic Phases of the Disease

Spontaneous activity in healthy animals (FIGURE 10) showed a gradual increase during the first six weeks of life, then leveled off at about 25–30 rpm. Spontaneous activity was remarkably stable for each animal (coefficient of variation, 8.2%), and variation between mice of this inbred strain was small (coefficient of variation, 5.4%).

Infected animals began to show a significant decrease in spontaneous activity during the fourth week of infection. Activity remained depressed into the sixth week and then recovered, only to decrease again after the 12th week of infection, markedly and progressively after the 15th week. Decreased activity was the first clinical evidence of illness in these animals.

Effects of Forced Exercise during the Acute Phase of the Disease

Uninfected young mice, forced to swim for 300 minutes per week for six weeks and then sacrificed, showed an 8% increase in the heart weight:body weight ratio over that of unexercised uninfected controls ($p < 0.005$) (FIGURE 11.)[16] Animals infected with *T. cruzi* from the 31st passage through Swiss mice and forced to exercise in an identical manner throughout the acute phase of the disease showed a 10% increase in the heart weight-body weight ratio over that of unexercised infected controls ($p < 0.005$). Thus, the combination of acute Chagasic myocarditis and forced exercise produced greater hypertrophy than either factor alone.

The parasitemia of the infected swimmers did not differ from that of infected nonswimming control animals. Four infected swimmers died during the experiment; there was no mortality in the control group. Microscopical examination of the grossly larger hearts of the infected swimmers revealed more diffuse cellular infiltrates and more severe necrosis than were seen in the controls: grade 2.7 vs. grade 2.2 ($p < 0.01$). Although twice as many parasitized cells per section were seen in the exercised animals as in controls (1.3 vs. 0.6), this

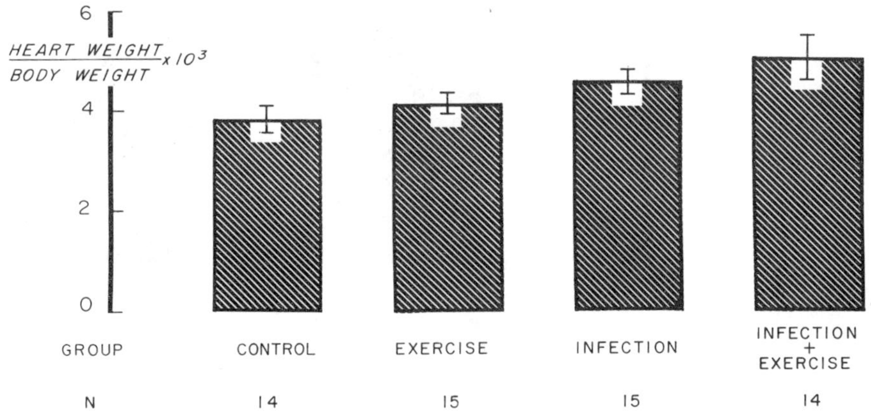

FIGURE 11. Additive effects of forced exercise (swimming for 300 minutes per week for six weeks) and acute myocarditis upon heart weights of mice sacrificed 50 days after inoculation with *T. cruzi*. Mean values and standard deviations are indicated. N = number of mice in each group. (From the data of Elson and Abelmann[16]).

difference was not statistically significant. The ratio of dry to wet heart weight was not affected by swimming.[16] On the whole, forced exercise during the acute disease appeared to have a deleterious effect upon the heart.

Effects of Forced Exercise during the Subacute Phase of the Disease

After inoculation at one month of age with *T. cruzi* from the 36th passage through Swiss mice, 18 mice were forced to swim for 200 minutes per week for 16 weeks. They were sacrificed 118 days after inoculation, in the subacute phase of the disease, and after they had reached maturity.

Seven (39%) of the swimming mice died during the experiment, compared with only one (5.6%) of the infected nonswimming controls. Essentially, exercise during the subacute phase produced the same effect as exercise during the acute phase: The heart weight:body weight ratio increased by 9% ($p < 0.005$) (FIGURE 12). Histologically, the infected animals tended to show more diffuse myocardial infiltration and more severe necrosis than were seen in the earlier experiment. The lesions were not clearly different in the swimming mice.

Whereas spontaneous activity in uninfected animals was not affected by swimming, in infected animals swimming was associated with a progressive decrease in spontaneous activity, which became significant in the 12th week (FIGURE 13).

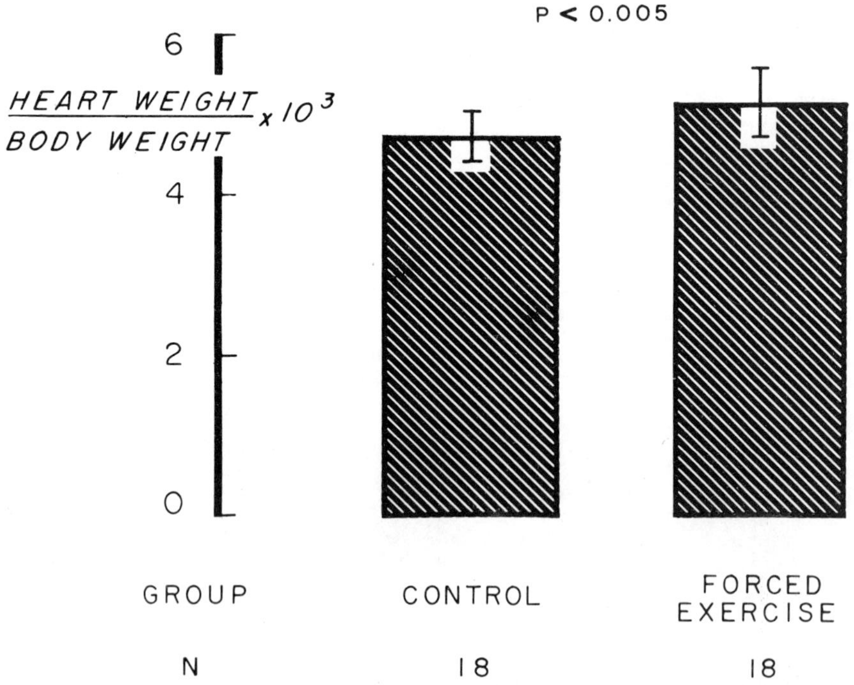

FIGURE 12. Effect of forced exercise (swimming for 200 minutes per week for 16 weeks) upon heart weights of mice sacrificed 118 days after inoculation with *T. cruzi*. Mean values and standard deviations are indicated. N = number of mice in each group.

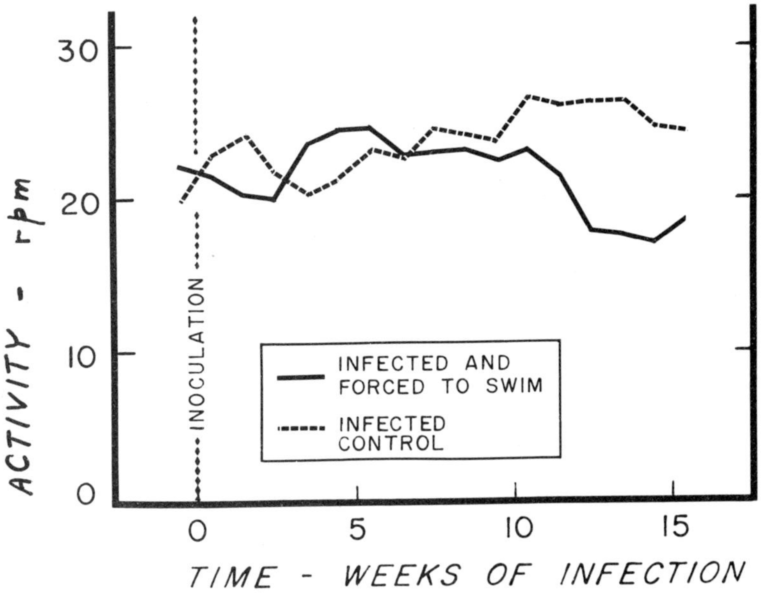

FIGURE 13. Spontaneous activity of 12 infected (solid line) and 12 uninfected mice (dotted line), all of which were forced to swim for 200 minutes per week for 16 weeks. Note that forced exercise in the infected animals was associated with a progressive decrease in spontaneous activity.

Delay of Forced Exercise until after the Acute Parasitemic Stage

As an extension of the preceding experiment, 11 infected mice were forced to swim 200 minutes per week for eight weeks, but commencing only after the parasitemia had all but subsided (day 72). These animals all survived to the end of the experiment, and their mean heart weight:body weight ratio did not exceed that of 11 infected nonexercised animals (4.99 ± 0.27 vs. 5.16 ± 0.36).

Effects of Mild Exercise upon the Acute and Subacute Disease

Elective running in activity cages, 200 minutes per week for 16 weeks, did not affect heart weight in uninfected mice (FIGURE 14). In infected animals, however, this mild exercise throughout the acute and subacute phases of the disease resulted in a small but significant increase in the heart weight:body weight ratio of 6.1% ($p < 0.05$).

Effects of Forced Exercise Preceding Inoculation and Continued during the Acute Disease

When mice were forced to swim 300 minutes per week for eight weeks prior to inoculation and for another eight weeks during infection, nine out of 12 animals died during the acute phase of the disease, compared with zero out of 12 uninfected control animals exercised in an identical manner. The weekly trypanosome counts were unaffected by exercsie.

On day 58 after inoculation, the heart weight:body weight ratio in the infected mice (6.01 ± 0.50) exceeded that of the controls (4.10 ± 0.38) by

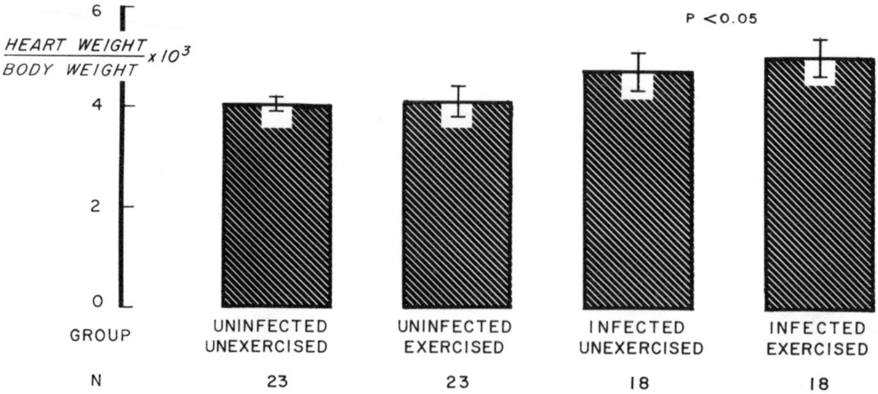

FIGURE 14. Effects of mild exercise (elective running for 200 minutes per week for 16 weeks) upon heart weights of mice with subacute Chagasic myocarditis (day 118). This degree of exercise was insufficient to affect heart weights in uninfected control animals. In the presence of infection, exercise increased heart weight significantly ($p < 0.05$). Mean values and standard deviations are indicated. N = number of mice in each group.

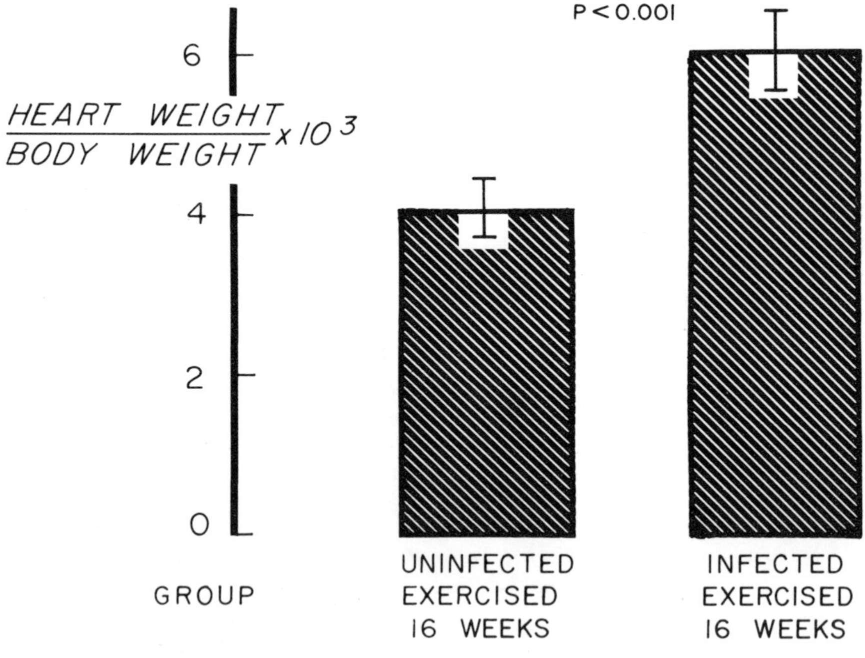

FIGURE 15. Effect of infection with *T. cruzi* upon heart weights of mice exercised (swimming for 300 minutes per week) for eight weeks prior to and eight weeks following inoculation. Mean values and standard deviations are indicated. N = number of mice in each group.

46% ($p < 0.001$) (FIGURE 15). Individual hearts from infected exercised animals—especially those who died early—were remarkable for the severity and diffuseness of myocardial infiltration and necrosis, and for the frequency of parasitic aggregates. Thus, forced exercise preceding infection not only failed to protect the animals from the myocarditis-enhancing effect of forced exercise, but appeared to potentiate this effect.

Effects of Dietary Ethanol upon the Acute Disease

In a recent study, H. Miller and I investigated whether chronic ingestion of alcohol per se could produce myocardial damage. We also wondered whether alcohol could affect the severity and course of an acute infectious myocarditis. The natural aversion of mice to ethanol was overcome by incorporating ethanol in a liquid diet, slightly modified from that described by Lieber and his associates.[17]

Twelve 21-week-old C3H mice, maintained on the control diet for 16 weeks, were inoculated with 9,000 *T. cruzi* after nine weeks. Another 12 mice were placed on the isocaloric ethanol-containing diet and inoculated in an identical manner. All animals were sacrificed 49 days after inoculation.

The two groups did not differ in appearance, body weight, parasitemia level, and mortality. Two animals on the ethanol diet, however, died on the 43rd day of infection with large hearts and ascites, evidently in congestive heart failure, which had not previously been seen in this laboratory in the acute phase of the disease in over 600 mice inoculated. The ethanol-fed group had a mean heart weight of 145.6 ± 19.8 mg, 9.1% greater than that of the control group; its heart weight:body weight ratio (6.43 ± 1.34) exceeded that of the control group by 14.2%. However, neither difference was statistically significant. There was also a tendency for more severe myocardial lesions and a greater number of parasitic aggregates.

DISCUSSION

The studies presented indicate that experimental infection with *T. cruzi* in inbred mice is a model of a myocarditis with acute, subacute, and chronic stages suitable for the study of factors that may modify the disease process.

In the acute and subacute phases of the disease, the level of the animal's activity proved to be a determinant not only of heart weight, but also of the extent of parasitic invasion of the myocardium and of the inflammatory response of the host. In both the acute and the chronic disease, spontaneous activity was found to be significantly decreased. Although the mechanism of this decrease is unknown—it may possibly be a function of the myositis that accompanies the myocarditis[15,16]—it may exert a protective or sparing effect upon the heart.

The enhancing effects of forced exercise upon the myocarditis appeared maximal when exercise was imposed during the acute phase of the disease, but could in turn be enhanced by forced exercise preceding the acute infection.

Stimulated by the prevalence of malnutrition in populations with a high incidence of Chagas' disease, Yaeger and Miller[9,18-20] systematically investigated the effects of specific nutritional deficiencies upon the susceptibility of rats to experimental infection with *T. cruzi*. They reported evidence that acute myocarditis was aggravated by deficiency of thiamine,[9] panthothenic acid,[18] pyridoxine,[19] and lysine.[20] Our studies on the effect of prolonged intake of ethanol, in the absence of any nutritional deficiency, draw attention to yet another factor that may affect the severity and course of acute Chagasic myocarditis.

The myocardial lesions of South American trypanosomiasis have variously been attributed to the parasite itself, to a toxin released by the parasite, to an immune response to the parasite, and to autoimmune reactions.[1,3,4,14] The studies presented here do not shed any light upon the primary pathogenesis of the myocarditis, but they draw attention to a number of factors that may modify the extent and course of the myocarditis.

Although it seems reasonable to extrapolate from this work to Chagas' disease in man, the operation of these factors in other forms of myocarditis remains to be established. However, research in our laboratory[21] has shown that forced exercise also enhances the myocardial replication of Coxsackie virus. The clinical implications of the studies reported have been discussed elsewhere.[22]

It was our initial impression that we were working with a stable strain of *T. cruzi* and, hence, a stable model of a relatively mild myocarditis, suitable for screening of factors that might potentiate the disease. Unfortunately, the parasite became more virulent with repeated passages through mice. There is every reason to believe, however, that other, less virulent strains of *T. cruzi* exist.

A word of caution to the research worker must be added. Laboratory infections of man have been reported.[23] Inasmuch as no cure for Chagas' disease is as yet known, great care must be used in handling the parasites.

Summary and Conclusions

Experimental South American trypanosomiasis *(T. cruzi)* in C3H mice has been studied as a model of a myocardiopathy with both an acute and a chronic phase. A Colombian strain of *T. cruzi* in C3H mice produced a benign parasitemic state lasting about two months, followed by chronic progressive myocarditis associated with cardiac hypertrophy. This model was used to investigate the potential modifying effects of several factors upon the severity and course of the disease.

Spontaneous activity, measured in activity wheels, was significantly decreased during the acute phase of the disease and again during the chronic stage. Forced exercise, in the form of swimming, increased the heart weight and was associated with more severe and more diffuse cellular infiltration and with a greater number of parasites in the myocardium. Ethanol, administered in a liquid diet, tended to aggravate the acute myocardiopathy.

Acknowledgments

The collaboration of Drs. S. H. Elson, E. E. Federici, H. Miller, and F. A. Neva is gratefully acknowledged. Mrs. Elaine V. Fino and Miss Roberta S. Shaftel gave valuable technical assistance.

References

1. World Health Organization. 1960. Chagas' Disease. Report of a study group. Tech. Rep. Ser. **202:** 1–21. Geneva, Switzerland.
2. Laranja, F. S., E. Dias, G. Nobrega & A. Miranda. 1956. Chagas' disease: A clinical, epidemiologic and pathologic study. Circulation **14:** 1035–1060.
3. Rosenbaum, M. B. 1964. Chagasic myocardiopathy. Progr. Cardiov. Dis. **7:** 199–225.
4. Koberle, F. 1961. Patologia y anatomia patologica de la enfermad de Chagas. Bol. Ofic. Sanit. Panamer. **51:** 404–428.
5. Goble, F. C. 1951. Studies on experimental Chagas' disease in mice in relation to chemotherapeutic testing. J. Parasit. **37:** 408–414.

6. PACKCHANIAN, A. & A. ROBINSON. 1958. Electrocardiographic studies in experimental Chagas' disease in mice (*Mus musculus*). Texas Rep. Biol. Med. **16:** 363–379.
7. OKUMURA, M., L. C. M. FRANCA & A. C. NETTO. 1963. Comentarios sobre a patogenia da molestia de Chagas. Especial referencia a infeccao experimental em camundongos. Rev. Hosp. Clin. Fac. Med. S. Paulo **18:** 151–164.
8. KOLODNY, M. H. 1939. Studies on age resistance against trypanosome infections. I. The resistance of rats of different ages to infection with *Trypanosoma cruzi.* Amer. J. Hyg. **29** (Sect. C): 13–24.
9. YEAGER, R. G. & O. N. MILLER. 1960. Effect of malnutrition on susceptibility of rats to *Trypanosoma cruzi.* I. Thiamine deficiency. Exp. Parasit. **9:** 215–222.
10. DE B. COSTA, R. 1964. Hipertrofia cardiaca experimental em ratos Chagasicos e ratos atropinizados. Rev. Inst. Med. Trop. S. Paulo **6:** 17–27.
11. JOHNSON, C. M. 1938. Cardiac changes in dogs experimentally infected with *Trypanosoma cruzi.* Amer. J. Trop. Med. **18:** 197–206.
12. LARANJA, F. S., J. PELLEGRINO & E. DIAS. 1949. Experimental Chagas' heart disease. Amer. Heart J. **37:** 646.
13. GOBLE, F. C. 1952. Observations on experimental Chagas' disease in dogs. Amer. J. Trop. Med. Hyg. **1:** 189–204.
14. ANSELMI, A., F. C. PIFANO, J. A. JUAREZ & O. GURDIEL. 1966. Myocardiopathy in Chagas' disease. I. Comparative study of pathologic findings in chronic human and experimental Chagas' myocarditis. Amer. Heart. J. **72:** 469–481.
15. FEDERICI, E. E., W. H. ABELMANN & F. A. NEVA. 1964. Chronic and progressive myocarditis and myositis in C3H mice infected with *Trypanosoma cruzi.* Amer. J. Trop. Med. Hyg. **13:** 272–280.
16. ELSON, S. H. & W. H. ABELMANN. 1965. Effects of muscular activity upon the acute myocarditis of C3H mice infected with *Trypanosoma cruzi.* Amer. Heart J. **69:** 629–636.
17. LIEBER, C. S., D. P. JONES & L. M. DECARLI. 1965. Effects of prolonged ethanol intake: Production of fatty liver despite adequate diets. J. Clin. Invest. **44:** 1009–1021.
18. YAEGER, R. G. & O. N. MILLER. 1960. Effect of malnutrition on susceptibility of rats to *Trypanosoma cruzi.* III. Pantothenate deficiency. Exp. Parasit. **10:** 232–237.
19. YAEGER, R. G. & O. N. MILLER. 1960. Effect of malnutrition on susceptibility of rats to *Trypanosoma cruzi.* IV. Pyridoxine deficiency. Exp. Parasit. **10:** 238–244.
20. YAEGER, R. G. & O. N. MILLER. 1963. Effect of lysine deficiency on Chagas' disease in laboratory rats. J. Nutr. **81:** 169–174.
21. TILLES, J. G., S. H. ELSON, J. A. SHAKA, W. H. ABELMANN, A. M. LERNER & M. FINLAND. 1964. Effects of exercise on Coxsackie A9 myocarditis in adult mice. Proc. Soc. Exp. Biol. Med. **117:** 777–782.
22. ABELMANN, W. H. 1966. Current Concepts: Myocarditis. New Eng. J. Med. **275:** 832–834 and 944–945.
23. COUDERT, J., J. DESPEIGNES, M. R. BATTESTI & J. MICHEL-BRUN. 1964. Un cas de maladie de Chagas par contamination accidentelle de laboratoire avec *T. cruzi.* Bull. Soc. Path. Exot. **57:** 208–213.

TRYPTOPHAN METABOLISM AND CARDIAC DISEASE

Maria Spatz

Section on Histochemistry, Laboratory of Experimental Pathology
National Institute of Arthritis and Metabolic Diseases
National Institutes of Health, Bethesda, Md.

The pathogenesis of heart lesions in the carcinoid syndrome was the starting point for the investigations reported in this paper. The experiments included a study of tryptophan deficiency as part of the carcinoid syndrome and provided an opportunity to examine the effect of this deficiency on the myocardium. Several aspects of these investigations have been reported previously.[1-3] They will be reviewed here and enlarged upon with more recently obtained information. All studies were done in guinea pigs, which were found to be more suitable than other animals for these investigations on the basis of preliminary studies.

Endocardial lesions that mimicked in many respects those seen in the hearts of patients suffering from the carcinoid syndrome were successfully induced in guinea pigs by experimentally creating a triad of metabolic disorders analogous to the disease in man. The cardinal features of the triad were: (1) hyperserotonemia, (2) relative tryptophan deficiency of various degrees, and (3) alteration of liver function produced by a hepatotoxic agent. The effect of each feature and of various combinations will first be reviewed briefly.

Experimental Results

Hyperserotonemia

Intraperitoneal and subcutaneous injections of 5-hydroxytryptamine produced transient tachycardia and a reddish discoloration of the lips and ear lobes. Flooding of the tissues with this compound was indicated by a two- to threefold increase in the 5-hydroxyindoleacetic acid excretion in urine. Repeating the injections at regular intervals produced a fluctuant state of hyperseroteonemia. Microscopical study of the endocardium and heart valves of guinea pigs thus treated revealed slight edema associated with mononuclear cellular infiltration.

Tryptophan Deficiency

Dietary tryptophan deficiency resulted in: (a) loss in body weight; (b) diarrhea and rectal prolapse noted in one-fourth of the guinea pigs; (c) decreased urinary excretion of 5-hydroxyindoleacetic acid and disappearance of urinary tryptophan; and (d) high mortality. The severity of these effects was directly proportionate to the level of the tryptophan deficiency. The high mortality rate could be reduced by treatment with 5-hydroxytryptamine and its precursor 5-hydroxytryptophan. A similar reduction in the death rate was obtained by carefully alternating the tryptophan-deficient diet with the basal diet. Microscopical study of the endocardium and heart valves of tryptophan-deficient guinea pigs revealed slight subendothelial edema, focal accumulations of mononuclear cells, and evidence of myocardial injury, which is described in greater detail in a subsequent section.

Toxic Liver Injury

In the absence of a transplantable or inducible carcinoid tumor in guinea pigs, the importance of liver injury per se was investigated. Cycad meal, which contains a hepatotoxic principle (cycasin), was added to the basal diet in small concentrations. There was a slight loss in body weight and microscopical evidence of centrilobular liver cell injury. The endocardium and heart valves were essentially normal, except for mild edematous changes.

Combined Effect of Tryptophan Deficiency and 5-Hydroxytryptamine

Injections of 5-hydroxytryptamine reduced the loss in body weight and decreased the death rate of tryptophan-deficient guinea pigs. It increased the excretion of 5-hydroxyindoleacetic acid, but not to the levels obtained in guinea pigs injected with 5-hydroxytryptamine on a complete basal diet. It did not prevent the diarrhea and rectal prolapse, both of which were more severe and often associated with rectal bleeding under this combined regimen; in addition, vaginal bleeding occurred among the female guinea pigs. Microscopical study of the endocardium and heart valves revealed a moderate degree of mononuclear cellular infiltration.

Combined Effect of Tryptophan Deficiency and 5-Hydroxytryptamine in the Presence of Liver Injury

The metabolic effects of the combined regimen were essentially similar to those outlined in the preceding section. Gross and microscopical study of the hearts, however, revealed nodular or diffuse plaques on the mural endocardium and on the valvular surfaces (FIGURES 1 and 2). The plaques were found in various combinations involving one or both surfaces of the atrioventricular valves, the base and cusps of the pulmonary artery, the mural endocardium of the right atrium and ventricle, and occasionally the ventricular surface of the aortic valve. Plaques found on the left side of the heart were usually associated with an open foramen ovale. Nodules and plaques were composed of young fibroblasts and mononuclear cells within a metachromatically staining intercellular substance, and they were covered by endothelial cells. Elastic fibers were absent from the plaques, but were well preserved and continuous at the valvular rings and beneath the plaques covering the mural endocardium.

The Myocardium in Tryptophan Deficiency

As noted previously, evidence of myocardial injury was found in guinea pigs on tryptophan-deficient diets. Foci of myofibrillar necrosis developed, in which necrotic fibers had a central basophilic area surrounded by an eosinophilic zone in sections stained with hematoxylin and eosin (FIGURE 3, top). These fibers, and especially their margins, stained positively with the periodic acid-Schiff method after pretreatment with diastase (FIGURE 3, bottom). Special staining procedures for calcium salts gave negative results. Foci of myocardial necrosis were seen particularly well in guinea pigs receiving a diet that was 80–100% deficient in tryptophan. Less severe deficiency states (60%) produced myofibrillar degeneration characterized by a loss of striation and karyolysis and pycnosis of muscle cell nuclei (FIGURE 4). Animals fed a 40% tryptophan-deficient diet for six months had foci of fibroblastic proliferation

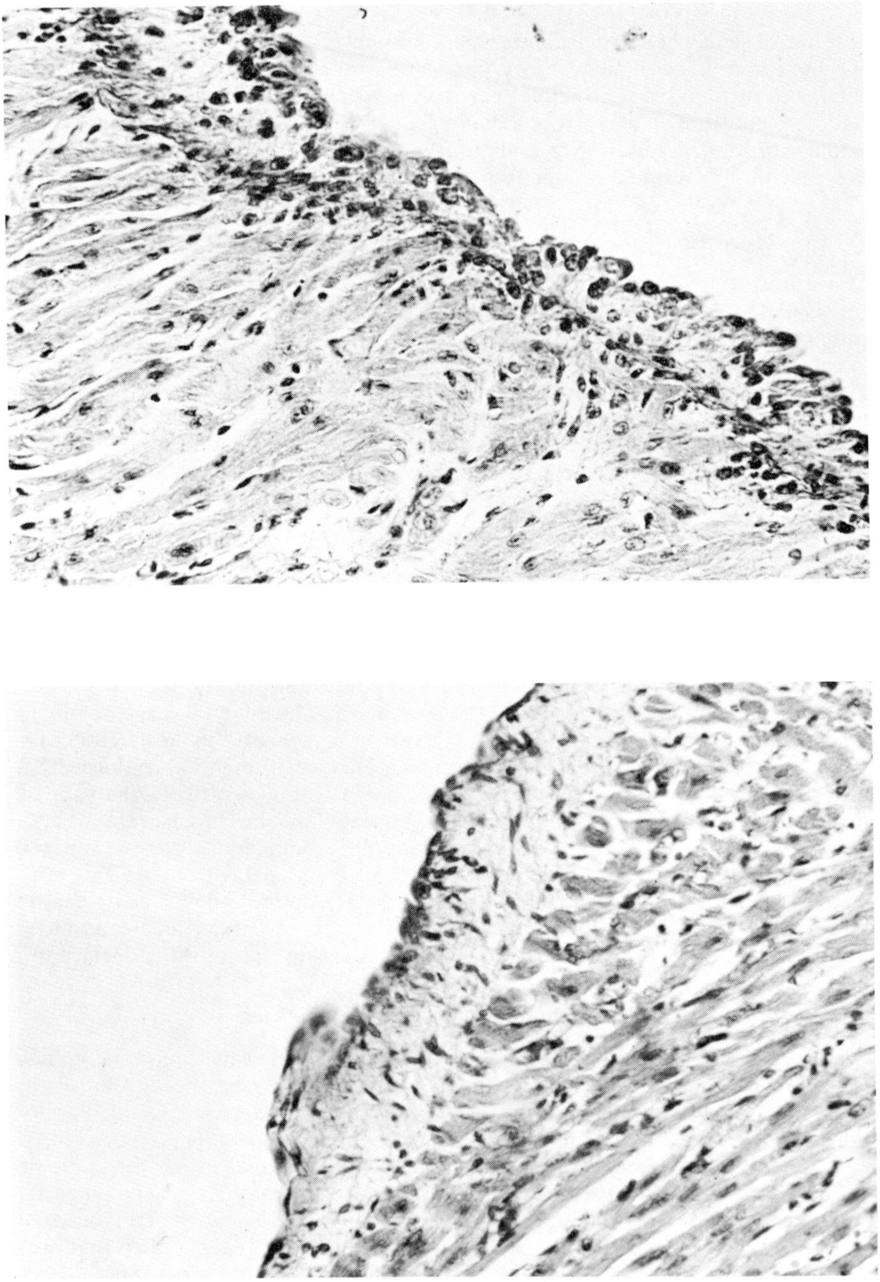

FIGURE 1. Heart sections from guinea pigs treated with hepatotoxin, 5-hydroxytryptamine, and a tryptophan-deficient diet, showing endocardial fibrous proliferation. (*Top*) Right atrium. Note preservation of elastic fibers. Stain: Weigert and Van Giessen. (*Bottom*) Right ventricle. Stain: hematoxylin and eosin. × 238.

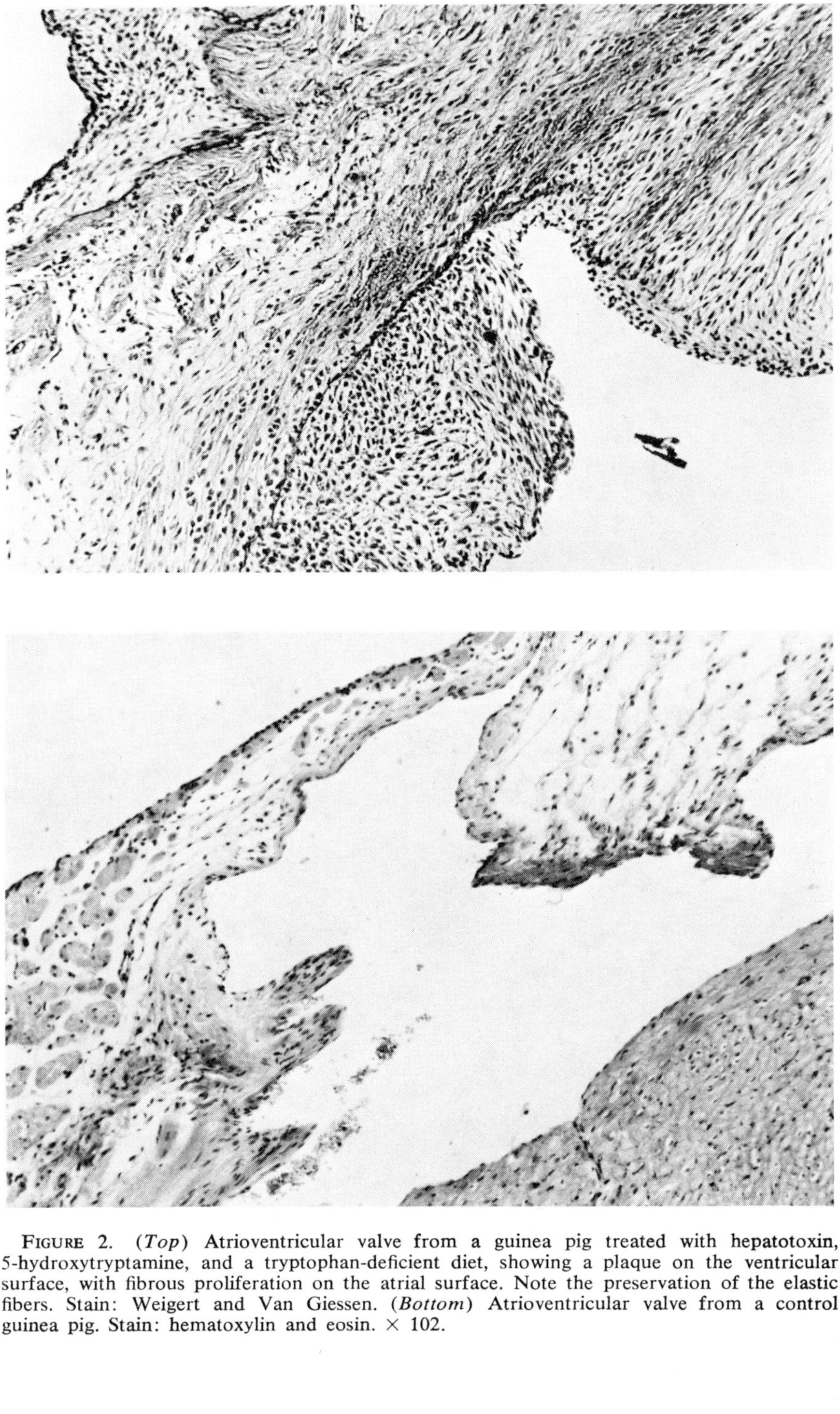

FIGURE 2. (*Top*) Atrioventricular valve from a guinea pig treated with hepatotoxin, 5-hydroxytryptamine, and a tryptophan-deficient diet, showing a plaque on the ventricular surface, with fibrous proliferation on the atrial surface. Note the preservation of the elastic fibers. Stain: Weigert and Van Giessen. (*Bottom*) Atrioventricular valve from a control guinea pig. Stain: hematoxylin and eosin. × 102.

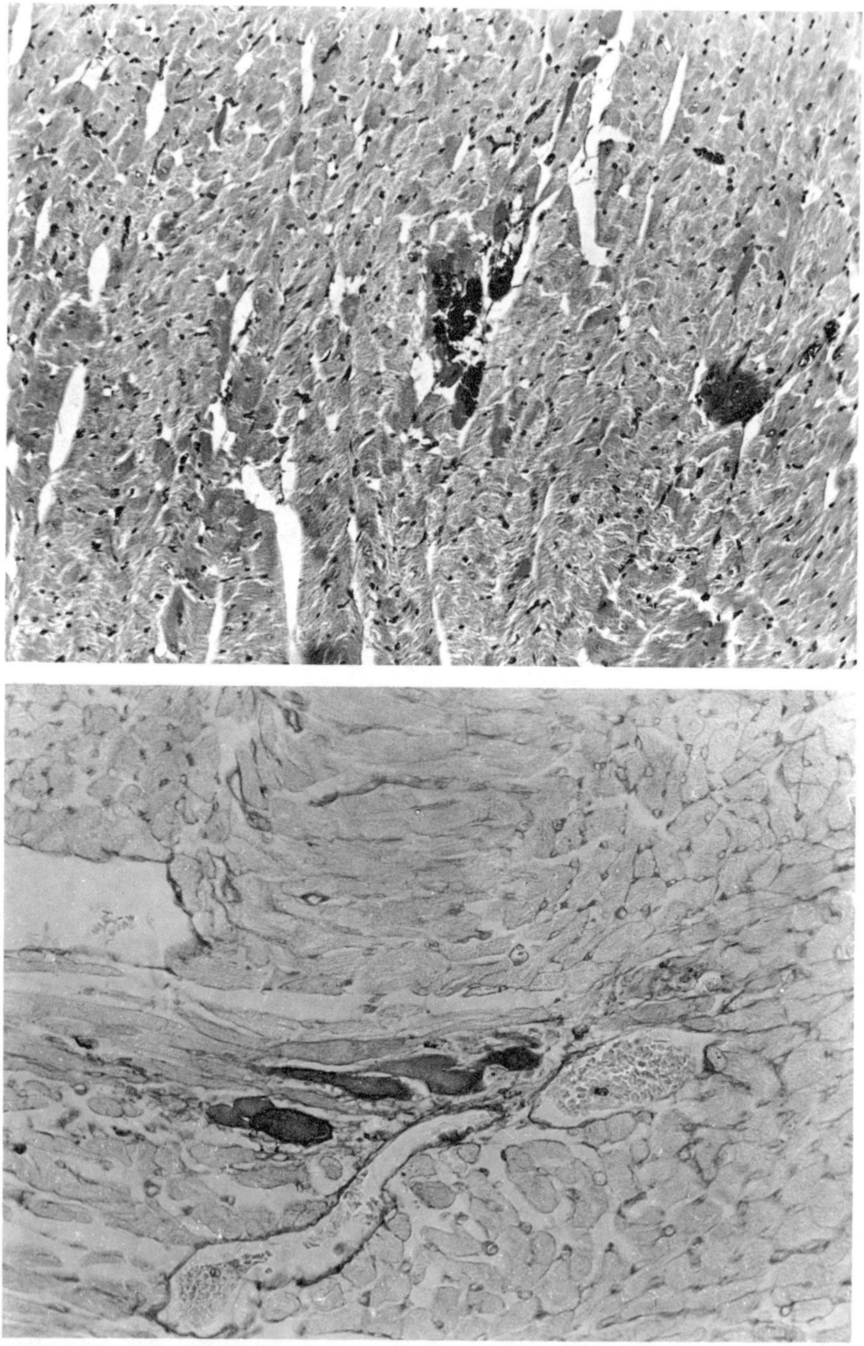

FIGURE 3. Heart sections from guinea pigs fed an 80% tryptophan-deficient diet. (*Top*) Myocardium showing basophilic necrosis. Stain: hematoxylin and eosin. × 143. (*Bottom*) Myocardium showing periodic acid-Schiff-positive fibers. Note the more intense staining of the fibers at the periphery. Stain: pretreated with diastase; periodic acid-Schiff. × 250.

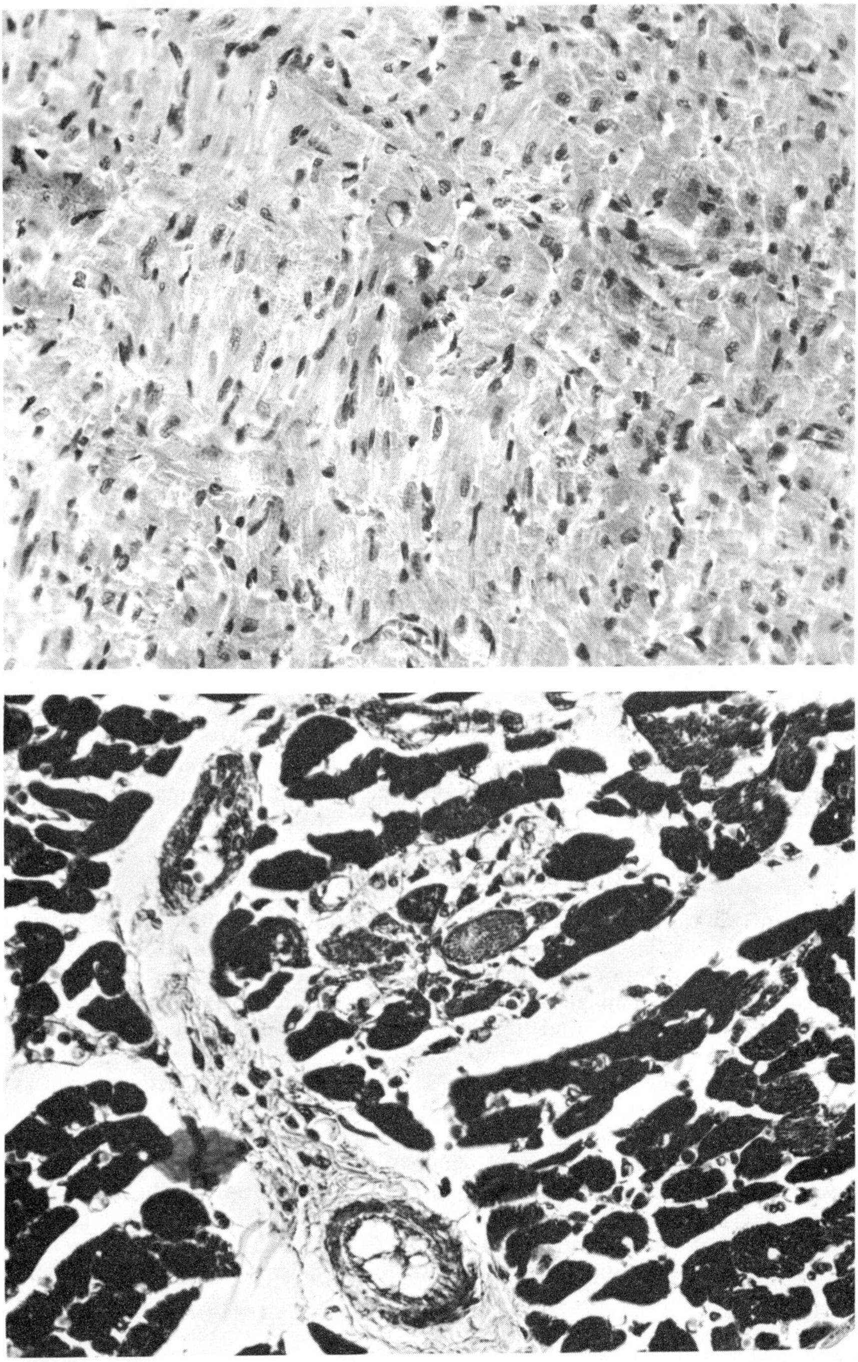

FIGURE 4. Heart sections from guinea pigs fed a 60% tryptophan-deficient diet. (*Top*) Myofibrillar degeneration with nuclear pycnosis and karyolysis. Stain: hematoxylin and eosin. × 250. (*Bottom*) Myofibrillar loss of striation. Note the surrounding mononuclear cellular reaction: Stain: phosphotungstic acid hematoxylin. × 350.

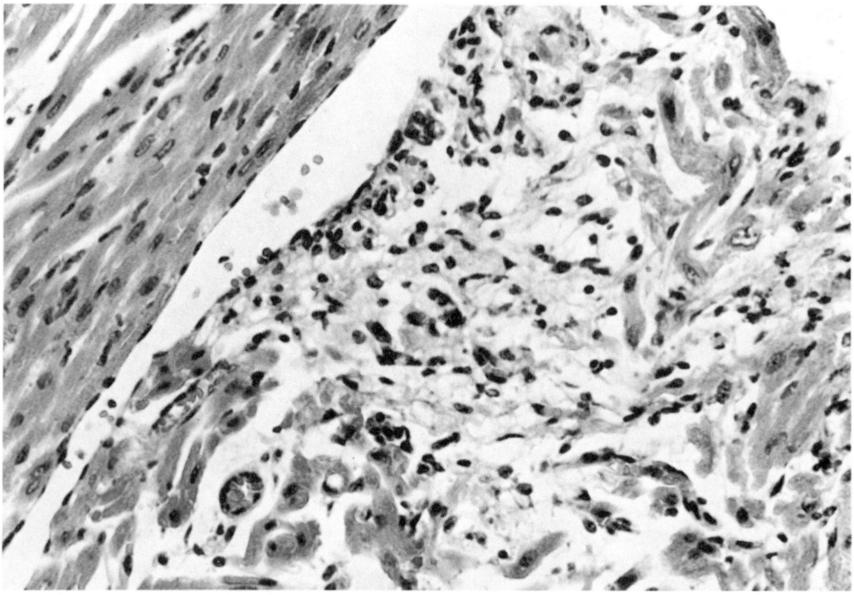

FIGURE 5. Heart section from a guinea pig fed a 40% tryptophan-deficient diet, showing myocardial fibrous proliferation. Stain: hemotoxylin and eosin. × 270.

in the myocardium (FIGURE 5). Similar proliferative myocardial lesions were found in guinea pigs surviving for periods as long as 12 months on a 60% tryptophan-deficient diet, with interposed periods on the complete basal diet (FIGURE 6).

Protective Effect of 5-Hydroxytryptamine on Myocardium

Foci of myocardial necrosis were not found when guinea pigs received one or two daily injections of 5-hydroxytryptophan or 5-hydroxytryptamine. Subsequent investigations of the "protective effect" of 5-hydroxytryptamine against myocardial damage showed a good correlation between levels of total phosphorylase activity* and the presence of myocardial lesions. Whereas normal guinea pigs had an activity of 24.850 ± 1.097 μg, those on a 60% tryptophan-deficient diet for 21 days showed a decrease in activity to 16.60 ± 0.850 μg. Supplementation of the deficient diet with 0.2% DL-tryptophan raised the level to 20.90 ± 1.070 μg, and administration of 5-hydroxytryptamine produced a nearly normal value of 22.40 ± 1.280 μg. If the guinea pigs were maintained on a tryptophan-deficient diet prior to the injection of 5-hydroxytryptamine, phosphorylase activity remained low (16.20 ± 1.190 μg), and myocardial lesions were found.

Although supplementation of the tryptophan-deficient diet with DL-tryptophan

* Total phosphorylase activity is expressed as micrograms of phosphate per milligram × 10^{-1} of protein ($\mu g/mg^{-1}$), with standard error. The percent contribution of phosphorylase a activity in controls was 50.4 ± 1.61%; it increased to 72.5 ± 5.7% in control guinea pigs injected with 5-hydroxytryptamine, since some phosphorylase b was converted to phosphorylase a.

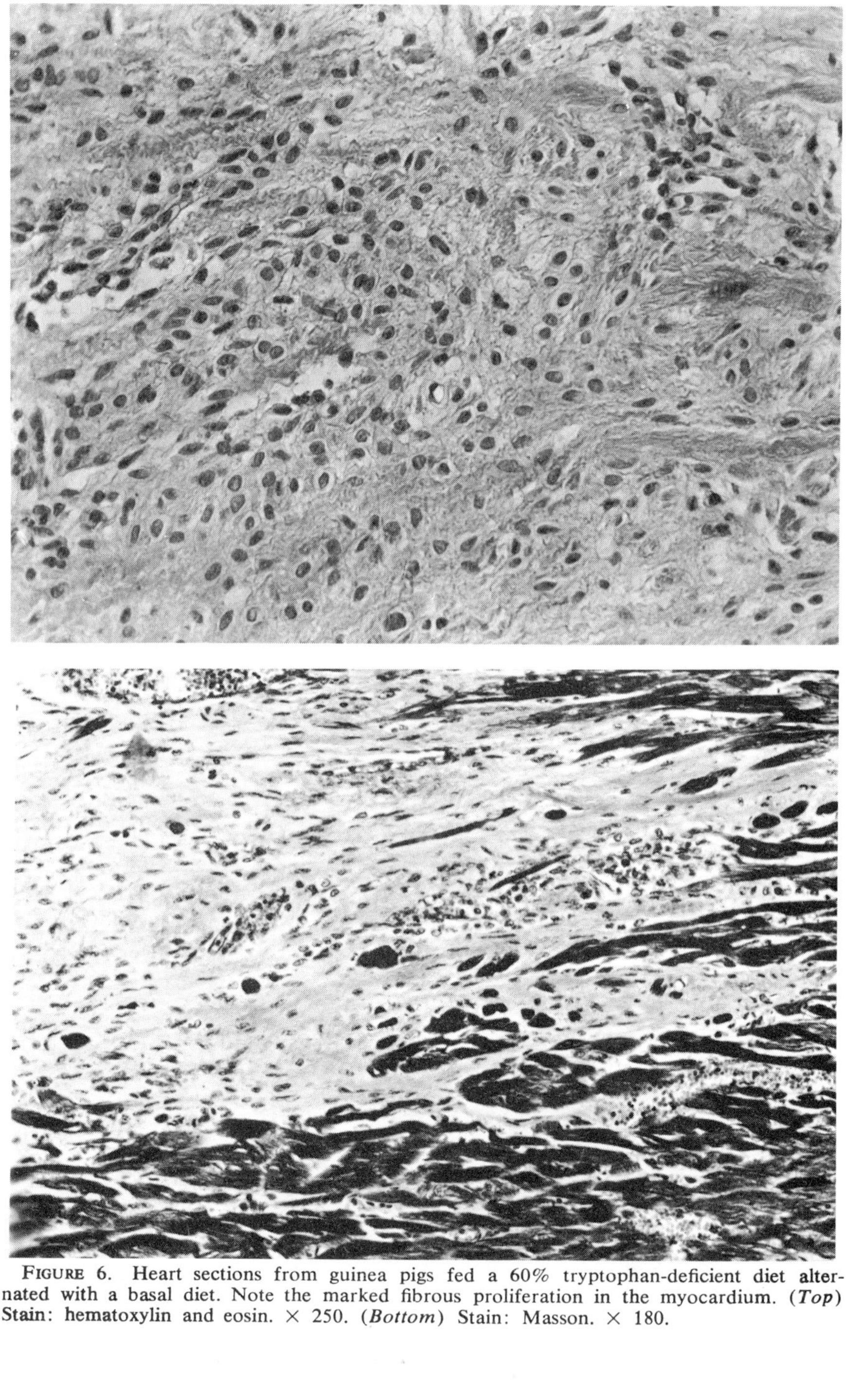

FIGURE 6. Heart sections from guinea pigs fed a 60% tryptophan-deficient diet alternated with a basal diet. Note the marked fibrous proliferation in the myocardium. (*Top*) Stain: hematoxylin and eosin. × 250. (*Bottom*) Stain: Masson. × 180.

TABLE 1

SUPPLEMENTATION OF A TRYPTOPHAN-DEFICIENT DIET AND ITS EFFECT ON THE TOTAL PHOSPHORYLASE ACTIVITY IN THE GUINEA PIG HEART

Group	Diet	Supplement	No. of Assays	Total Phosphorylase*	Correlation between Groups
1	Basal	None	7	22.4 ± 1.24	
2	60% Tryptophan-deficient	0.2% L-Tryptophan	10	20.2 ± 1.56	1 and 3: no significance 4 and 5: $p < 0.001$ 6: $p < 0.05$
3	60% Tryptophan-deficient	0.2% DL-Tryptophan	9	17.3 ± 2.00	1 and 5: $p < 0.05$ 2 and 6: no significance 4: $p < 0.02$
4	60% Tryptophan-deficient	Tryptamine†	11	10.9 ± 1.46	1 and 2: $p < 0.001$ 3: $p < 0.02$
5	60% Tryptophan-deficient	Tyramine†	9	12.13 ± 1.36	1 and 2: $p < 0.001$ 3: $p < 0.05$
6	60% Tryptophan-deficient	5-Hydroxyindoleacetic acid†	7	15.16 ± 2.07	1 and 2: $p < 0.001$ 3: no significance

* Expressed as micrograms of phosphate per milligram $\times 10^{-1}$ of protein, ($\mu g/mg^{-1}$), with standard error.
† By intraperitoneal injection.

only partially restored total phosphorylase activity levels in the heart toward control values, recent experiments with L-tryptophan as the supplement gave values for this enzyme not significantly different from those of the controls assayed concomitantly (see Table 1). The reason is unknown for the generally lower values of total phosphorylase activity in all groups of this experiment when compared with the corresponding values in the earlier experiment. No effect on total phosphorylase activity was seen when guinea pigs on a tryptophan-deficient diet were injected with tyramine, tryptamine, or 5-hydroxyindoleacetic acid (see groups 4–6 in TABLE 1).†

Discussion

Experimental results indicate that dietary tryptophan deficiency is an important factor in the production of endocardial and myocardial diseases in guinea pigs. On occasion, involvement of both endocardium and myocardium produced a picture of endomyocardial disease. It seems reasonable to assume that tryptophan deficiency, in an overt or disguised form, may play an equally important or contributing role in certain diseases in man. It is therefore proper, within the general framework of this monograph, to point out possible similarities between the experimentally induced metabolic disturbances and certain human diseases. Although such comparisons can only be tentative, they may suggest ideas for further studies in man and experimental animals.

Similarities between the experimentally induced endocardial lesions and those seen in patients suffering from the carcinoid syndrome have been described in detail in a previous communication,[2] which also contained a discussion of some of the underlying metabolic disturbances in patients with the carcinoid syndrome. The recognition of these disturbances led to the attempt to reproduce the lesions in the hearts of experimental animals. They are briefly reiterated here.

Hyperserotonemia due to secretion of serotonin by the carcinoid tumor was imitated in the experimental animal by injecting serotonin subcutaneously or intraperitoneally at frequent intervals and over long periods of time. This resulted in an increased excretion of 5-hydroxyindoleacetic acid, which also occurs in patients with the carcinoid syndrome. Since a substantial percentage of dietary tryptophan is diverted into the serotonin pathway in patients with carcinoid disease, relative tryptophan or niacin deficiency may occur. A comparable deficiency state was induced by feeding tryptophan-deficient diets to the guinea pigs over long periods of time. This particular aspect of the experiment was the most difficult to control, and required almost continuous observation of the animals. Frequent periods on the basal diet were required to assure longevity of the animals, which were remarkably sensitive to prolonged states of tryptophan deficiency.

Metastatic disease in the liver is a frequent occurrence in patients with the carcinoid syndrome. Although there was no simple experimental way of reproducing this aspect of the human disease, it seemed worthwhile to examine the effect of hyperserotonemia and of tryptophan deficiency in the presence of an altered liver function per se. This was accomplished by adding to the experimental regimen a hepatotoxin in which there was a general interest in

† Tryptamine and 5-hydroxyindoleacetic acid were administered in a concentration of 6.8 mg/ml/kg of body weight. Tyramine hydrochloride was given in a concentration of 8 mg/ml/kg of body weight. Each compound was dissolved in 0.9% saline and filtered prior to use.

the laboratory when the investigations were performed. The combined experimental procedures resulted in the production of proliferative endocardial lesions that had several features in common with those seen in the hearts of patients with the carcinoid syndrome. These lesions consisted of a nodular or diffuse type of endocardial fibrosis, involvement of the pulmonary valve in this process, absence of elastic fibers in the newly formed tissues but preservation of preexisting elastic fibers, and a metachromasia of the ground substance in the plaques.

It is of interest that recent investigations have demonstrated an elevated level of bradykinin in the serum of patients with the carcinoid syndrome. Several short-term experiments in which bradykinin was administered to animals have not afforded additional information. These negative results do not exclude the possibility that bradykinin may play a contributory role in the development of the carcinoid heart disease. The extremely short half-life of bradykinin (30 seconds) may be responsible for the lack of results obtained to date.

Although tryptophan deficiency was found to be an integral part of the total mechanism that results in endocardial fibroblastic proliferation, it also had an additional and separate effect on the myocardium. The severity of the myocardial lesions depended on the degree and duration of the deficiency state, and the most pronounced myocardial changes were found within a short period of time in animals having the lowest tryptophan concentration in their diets. Mortality among these guinea pigs was high, but it is more likely that death was caused by metabolic events resulting from this deficiency than by myocardial damage alone.

The "protective effect" of 5-hydroxytryptamine against myocardial injury in guinea pigs on tryptophan-deficient diets was striking. It also prevented the decrease in total phosphorylase activity usually produced in guinea pigs on tryptophan-deficient diets. The protective effect was not observed when compounds structurally similar to 5-hydroxytryptamine, such as tyramine, tryptamine, and 5-hydroxyindoleacetic acid, were administered. Feeding of DL-tryptophan only partially prevented the effect of the tryptophan-deficient diet, whereas L-tryptophan was effective in preventing myocardial degeneration and in restoring total phosphorylase activity to control levels.

It has recently been suggested that an elevated level of 5-hydroxytryptamine may be the common denominator for the development of carcinoid heart disease and endomyocardial fibrosis.[4] This suggestion was based on observations made in Central and West Africa, where endomyocardial disease commonly occurs among populations using plantain (cooked bananas) as staple food. This diet is known to have high levels of 5-hydroxytryptamine. Metabolic study in which patients with and without endomyocardial disease were fed a plantain diet showed clearly that the excretion of 5-hydroxyindoleacetic acid was considerably less in the patients with endomyocardial disease than in the control group.[5] If it can be shown in the future that the plantain diet is poor in tryptophan, a fact presently unknown, the findings in patients with endomyocardial disease would be comparable to those obtained in the chronically tryptophan-deficient guinea pigs. Injections of 5-hydroxytryptamine resulted in a much smaller excretion of 5-hydroxyindoleacetic acid in chronically tryptophan-deficient guinea pigs than in guinea pigs on a basal diet.

Another possible explanation for the metabolic changes noted in patients with endomyocardial disease is that the high content of 5-hydroxytryptamine may have affected intestinal motility, resulting in poor absorption of tryptophan by the intestinal tract and, therefore, a relative tryptophan-deficiency state. An elucidation of the operative mechanism may be expected to come from amino acid analyses of the plantain diet.

Another type of endomyocardial disease, which was described in South Africa, has been related to a low-protein maize diet. Experimental studies in rats on a maize diet have produced myocardial lesions. The tryptophan content of the maize diet was found to be low, and the serum of rats fed this diet showed a low tryptophan level.[6]

In view of these observations, relative tryptophan deficiency is suggested as a common denominator responsible for the development of cardiac disease in the carcinoid syndrome and endomyocardial disease reported in Africa.

Acknowledgments

The author wishes to thank Dr. Gert L. Laqueur for helpful discussions, as well as for the preparation of this manuscript. The technical assistance of Mrs. Marilyn T. Beale is gratefully acknowledged.

References

1. Spatz, M. 1963. Protective action of serotonin against induced tryptophan-deficient cardiac necrosis. Amer. J. Path. **123:** 8a.
2. Spatz, M. 1964. Pathogenetic studies of experimentally induced heart lesions and their relation to the carcinoid syndrome. Lab. Invest. **13:** 288.
3. Spatz, M. 1966. Myocardial "protective effect" of 5-OH-tryptamine during tryptophan deficiency. Life Sci. **5** (10): 939.
4. Crawford, M. A. 1963. Endomyocardial fibrosis and carcinoidosis. A common denominator? Amer. Heart J. **662:** 272.
5. Ojo, G. O. & J. R. Parratt. 1966. Urinary excretion of 5-hydroxyindoleacetic acid in Nigerians with endomyocardial fibrosis. Lancet **i:** 854.
6. Reid, J. V. O. & P. Berjak. 1966. Dietary production of myocardial fibrosis in the rat. Amer. Heart J. **71:** 240.

MYOFIBRILLAR DEGENERATION: A COMMON FORM OF CARDIAC MUSCLE INJURY*

Dennis Reichenbach and Earl P. Benditt

Department of Pathology
University of Washington School of Medicine
Seattle, Wash.

Myocardial lesions that differ from ordinary coagulation necrosis of ischemic infarction have been produced experimentally by several chemical, metabolic, and mechanical means.[1-8] One of the striking histological features of these lesions is the segmented or banded appearance of the myocardial cell cytoplasm. Similar changes can be seen in human myocardium at autopsy associated with several clinical conditions. The changes occurring in this lesion do so in a regular and reproducible sequence extending over days to weeks. This indicates that the change is not merely agonal or an artifact. In this communication we shall present the characteristic histological features of cardiac lesions produced experimentally in the dog by electric shock and compare them with those seen in human myocardium after cardiac surgery.

Lesions Induced by Electric Shock

An electric current discharge applied to the surface of canine myocardium with steel electrodes (5 cm in diameter) produces a lesion in which the sequential changes of the injury reaction can be readily studied.[3] The extent of the lesion is related to the voltage of the discharge. A 250-volt alternating current (AC) shock produces an area of damage which regularly extends through the entire thickness of the right ventricle, or, if applied to the left ventricular wall, extends to a depth of 5–8 mm. One group of ten dogs received a single 250-volt AC electric shock, and a second group of 25 dogs received five AC electric shocks to the myocardium at two-minute intervals, with the voltage of the discharge ranging from 100–250 volts.

Animals were sacrificed at 5 minutes, 6, 19, and 24 hours, and 2, 3, 5, 7, 8, 14, 21, and 30 days. TABLE 1 lists the frequency of occurrence of several histological features of this lesion grouped in time intervals following the injury.

Features of the Lesion

Within a few minutes following electric shock, the myocardial cell cytoplasm showed a loss of striations and the appearance of homogeneous eosinophilic transverse bands or clumps, with intervening areas of fine granulation throughout the cell (FIGURE 1). Although this change was evident with hematoxylin and eosin staining, it was more apparent with the Gomori trichrome stain, in which the cytoplasmic bands appeared bright red. This alteration involved individual myocardial cells and in many instances was abruptly limited at the intercalated disc. At the periphery of confluent areas of injury, scattered cells, singly or in small groups showing this change, were surrounded by unaltered myocardial cells. The cytoplasmic segmentation was the most common feature of the lesion and could be seen in some cells through the eighth day following injury.

* The investigation reported in this paper was supported in part by United States Public Health Service grants nos. GM-13543, HE-03174, and GM-100.

TABLE 1

HISTOLOGICAL FEATURES OF MYOFIBRILLAR DEGENERATION IN DOGS FOLLOWING ELECTRIC CURRENT DISCHARGE

	Frequency of Occurrence				
Histological Features	1 day or less	2–3 days	5–8 days	14–21 days	30 days
Prominent nucleoli	2	14	4	2	2
Mineralization	0	14	1	1	1
Polymorphonuclear leukocyte	2	5	0	0	0
Mononuclear proliferation	1	20	4	0	0
Loss of nuclear staining	0	7	2	0	0
Fading of nuclear staining	1	15	0	0	0
Clumping of nuclear chromatin	3	0	0	0	0
Banding of cytoplasm	4	20	2	0	0
Number of cases	4	20	4	3	4

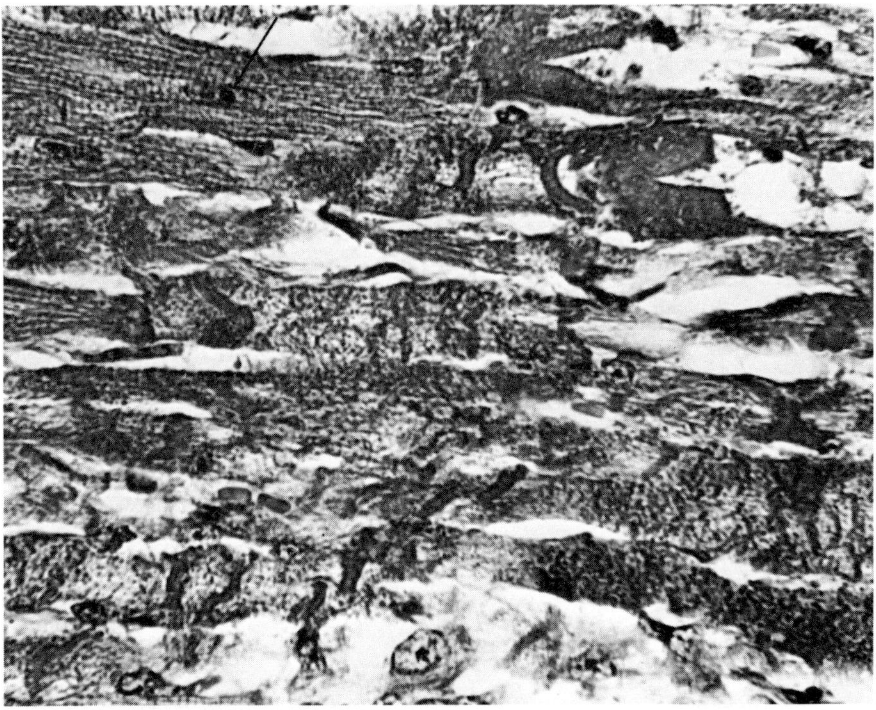

FIGURE 1. Dog myocardium, three days following electric shock to the surface of the myocardium. In the upper left is a cell showing normal striated appearance and a nucleus with a prominent nucleolus (arrow). The other cells shows alteration of cytoplasmic architecture, with transverse bands and intervening granularity. Nuclei of interstitial cells and capillaries are seen, but myocardial nuclei are not evident. Stain: Gomori trichrome. × 640.

Within the first 24 hours, the nucleus exhibited accentuated clumping of the chromatin, followed by a decrease and then a loss of staining within four days. Cells of the interstitial stroma and capillaries appeared unaltered.

Within three days, many myocardial cells showed punctate basophilic granular material aggregated between the cytoplasmic bands (FIGURE 2). This material gave a positive staining reaction for calcium and phosphates, with alizarin red and Von Kóssa stains, respectively, indicating the mineralization. The material was not seen in all cases and did not correlate with the amount of energy applied in the electric shock.

Scattered polymorphonuclear leukocytes were seen between one and three days following the injury but were never a prominent feature. Within three days, a proliferative cellular reaction was evident in the interstitial stroma of the injured myocardial cells (FIGURE 3). The cells were slightly elongated, with round to oval nuclei, moderately prominent nucleoli, and slightly basophilic cytoplasm. Some of these cells could be clearly identified as enlarged and prominent vascular endothelial cells, but the other cells could not be definitely classified; they might have been macrophages, fibroblasts, or monocytes. Mitotic figures were frequently seen in these interstitial cells. None of the cells exhibiting mitotic activity was identified as a myocardial cell. As the

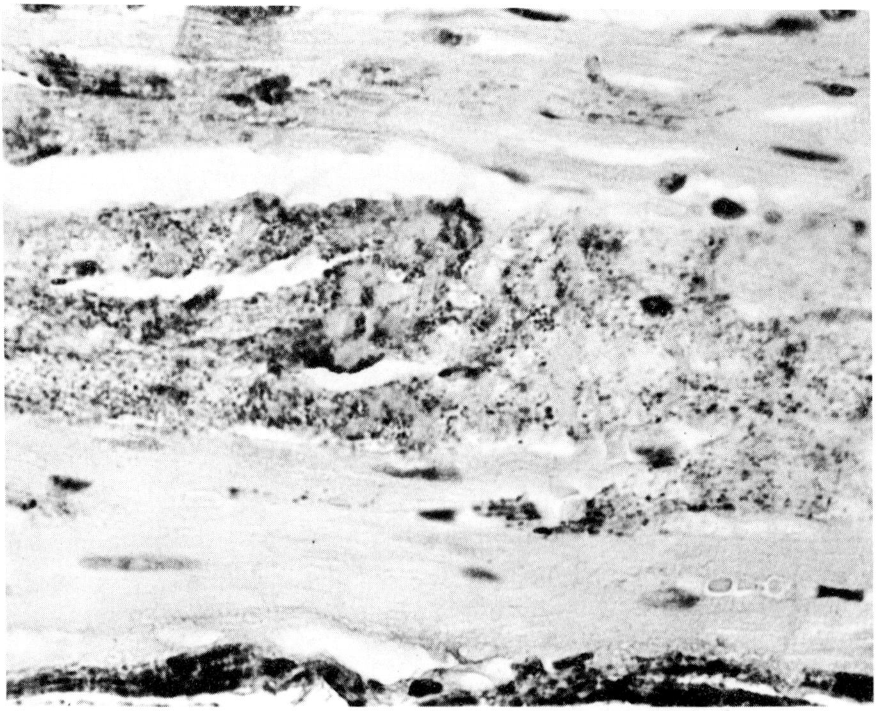

FIGURE 2. Dog myocardium, three days following electric shock. The cytoplasm of the myocardial cells in the center of the picture is altered, with the formation of bands of lighter-staining cytoplasm between punctate basophilic granules of mineralization. Stain: hematoxylin and eosin. × 640.

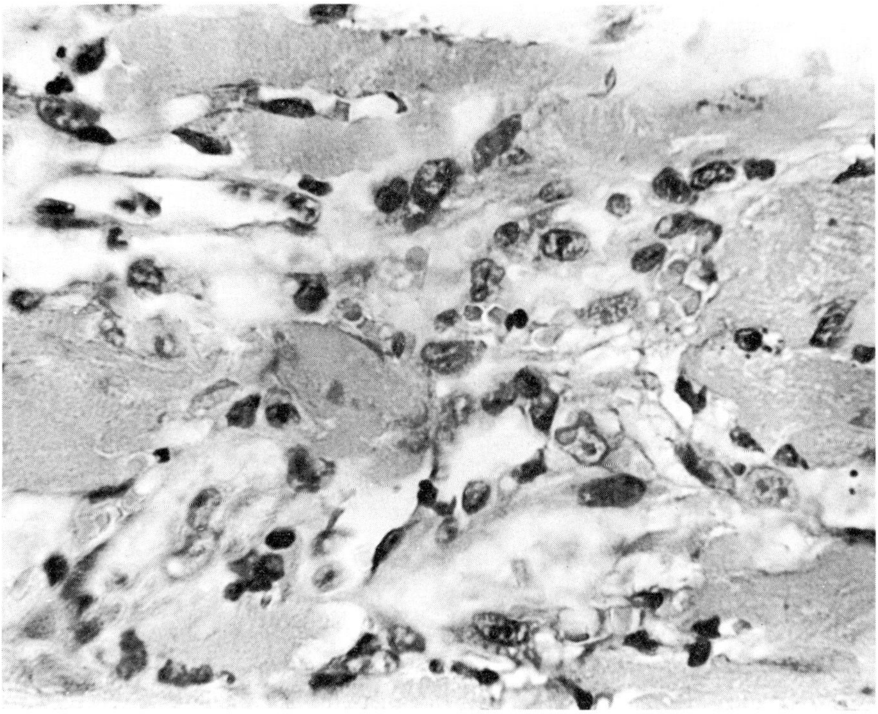

FIGURE 3. Dog myocardium, three days following electric shock. Most myocardial cells have absent nuclear staining and banding of the cytoplasm. Cells of the interstitial area are prominent, and polymorphonuclear leukocytes are not present. Stain: hematoxylin and eosin. × 640.

interstitial cell proliferation became prominent, the number of myocardial cells exhibiting cytoplasmic banding became less prominent, and the reticulum of the stroma surrounding damaged cells appeared to have collapsed (FIGURE 4). Intact myocardial cells along the periphery of the injury showed enlarged vesicular nuclei and prominent nucleoli. These changes were most prominent three to eight days following injury. Myocardial cells with double nuclei were frequently seen during this time.

Within two weeks the cellular interstitial reaction had essentially disappeared. Areas of loose connective tissue showed collapsed reticulum and pigmented macrophages with a variable amount of fibrous tissue (FIGURE 5). Between 21 and 30 days following injury, the residual damage varied from small subepicardial zones of loose connective tissue and occasional foci of loose connective tissue and fibrosis scattered throughout the myocardium to more extensive scars exhibiting focal replacement of the entire thickness of the right ventricular wall by fibrous connective tissue.

In no instance was the amount of residual damage seen after three to four weeks as extensive as that seen after three days. Confluent damage extending through the thickness of the right ventricle was reproducible and consistently seen three days following a 250-volt electric shock, but only occasionally did the residual damage involve the thickness of the right ventricle. Collapse and condensation of the stroma in the injured area account for a portion of the difference noted in the size of the damaged area.

When mineralization occurred in the lesion, it persisted after three to four weeks as basophilic foci with occasional foreign-body giant cells surrounded by collapsed stroma and some fibrous tissue. These foci of mineralization were scattered throughout the thickness of the ventricular chamber, with normal-appearing myocardium between them.

Electron Microscopy of the Myocardial Lesion

Electron microscopical studies of the lesion induced in dogs by electric current discharge showed a change evident within five minutes following injury. This reaction consisted of a loss of cytoplasmic organization manifested by the appearance of transverse bands of granular material, with a loss of definition of thick and thin filaments. Some filament strands frequently extended out from the granular mass. The translocated mitochondria became aggregated between these cytoplasmic bands, and many showed increased density of the matrix, consistent with mineralization. The capillary endothelium adjacent to injured myocardial cells appeared normal. Within 24 hours, macro-

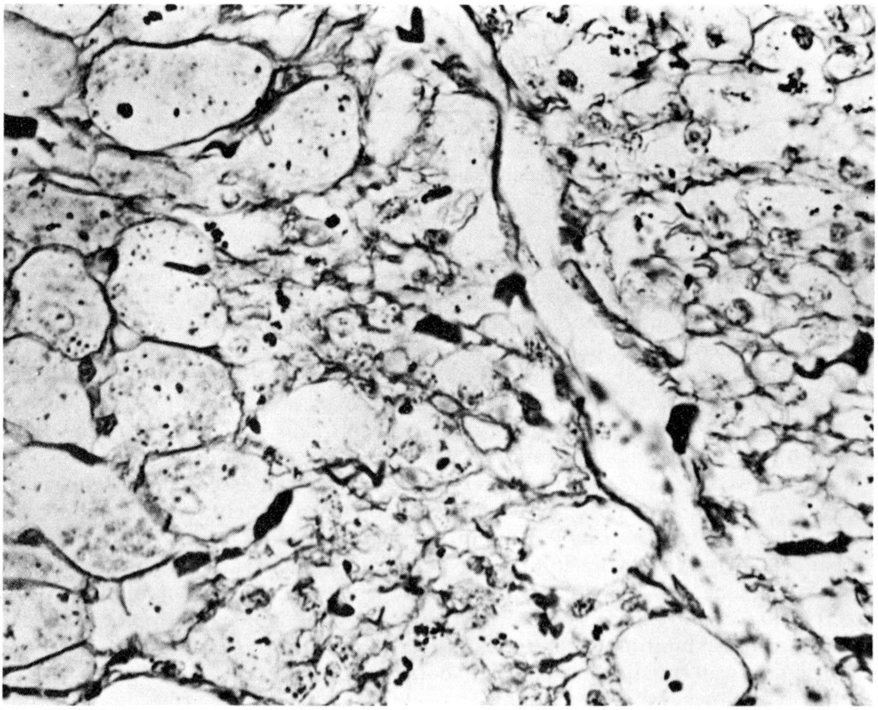

FIGURE 4. Dog myocardium, seven days following electric shock. The reticulum surrounding unaltered myocardial cells is seen on the left. On the right, the reticulum is collapsed and distorted. Stain: reticulum. × 640.

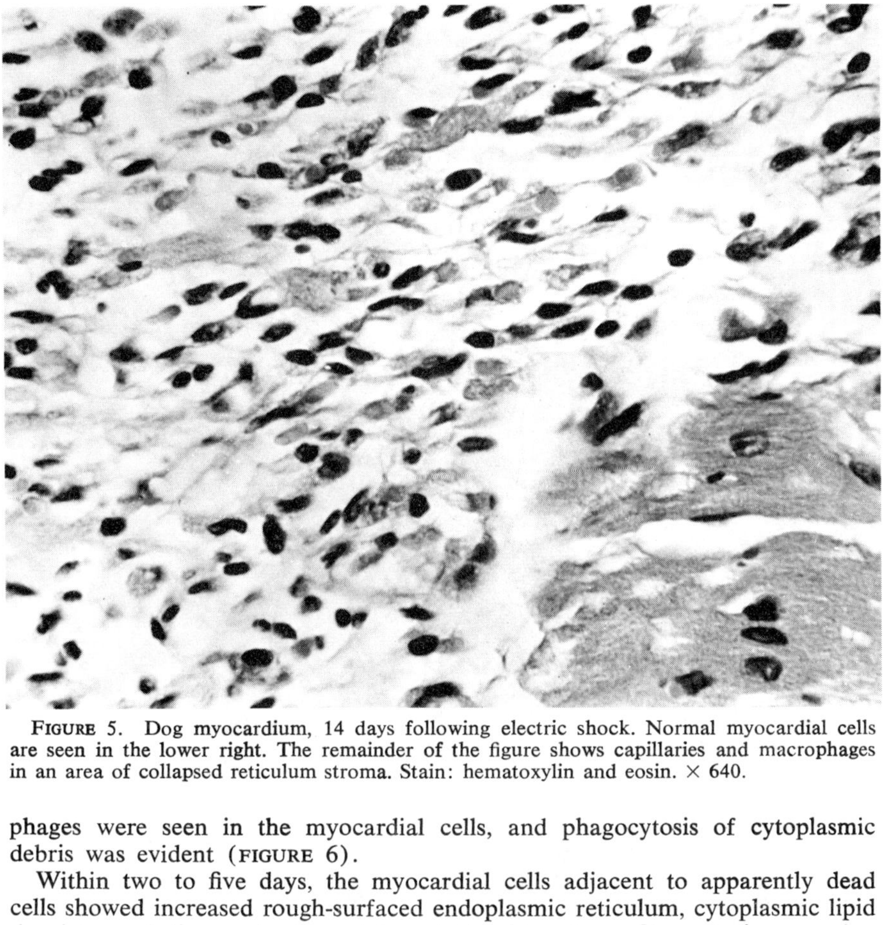

FIGURE 5. Dog myocardium, 14 days following electric shock. Normal myocardial cells are seen in the lower right. The remainder of the figure shows capillaries and macrophages in an area of collapsed reticulum stroma. Stain: hematoxylin and eosin. × 640.

phages were seen in the myocardial cells, and phagocytosis of cytoplasmic debris was evident (FIGURE 6).

Within two to five days, the myocardial cells adjacent to apparently dead cells showed increased rough-surfaced endoplasmic reticulum, cytoplasmic lipid droplets, and disorganization of the relationship of myofilaments in a portion of the cell. The structure of the filaments appeared intact, and there was no formation of amorphous band-like aggregates in these cells.

Some of the interstitial cells that became prominent after three to five days were macrophages, but most of the cells were difficult to identify, and none could be clearly identified as cardiac muscle cells. By the eighth day following injury, however, many cells could be identified as muscle cells, although their morphology was not that of mature cardiac muscle. They had features similar to those seen in embryonic cardiac muscle and, to some extent, in regenerating skeletal muscle.

The cells had sparse contractile elements that formed a peripheral zone near the plasma membrane; glycogen was abundant within the central portion of the cell. Mitochondria were not prominent, and the cristae were not as extensive as in mature myocardial cells. Ribosomes were prominent, and the Golgi apparatus was well developed. Within two weeks, the cells appeared similar to mature cardiac muscle cells except for the increased rough-surfaced endoplasmic reticulum.

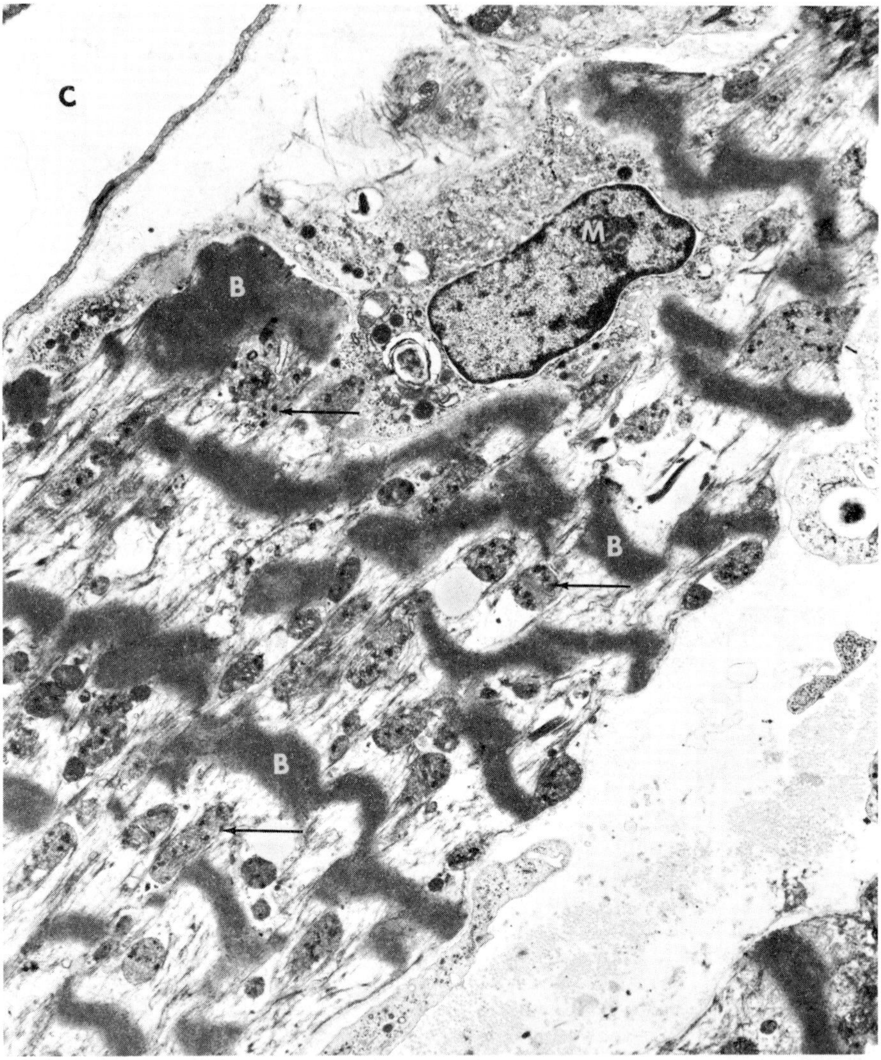

FIGURE 6. Electron micrograph of dog myocardium, 24 hours following electric shock. The myocardial cell cytoplasm appears as band-like aggregates (B) between translocated mitochondria. The mitochondria have increased density, which is consistent with mineralization (arrows). A macrophage (M) is present within the cell debris. The adjacent capillary endothelial cell (C) seen along the upper left appears unremarkable. Fixation: glutaraldehyde and osmium tetroxide; stain: lead and uranyl acetate. × 6,000.

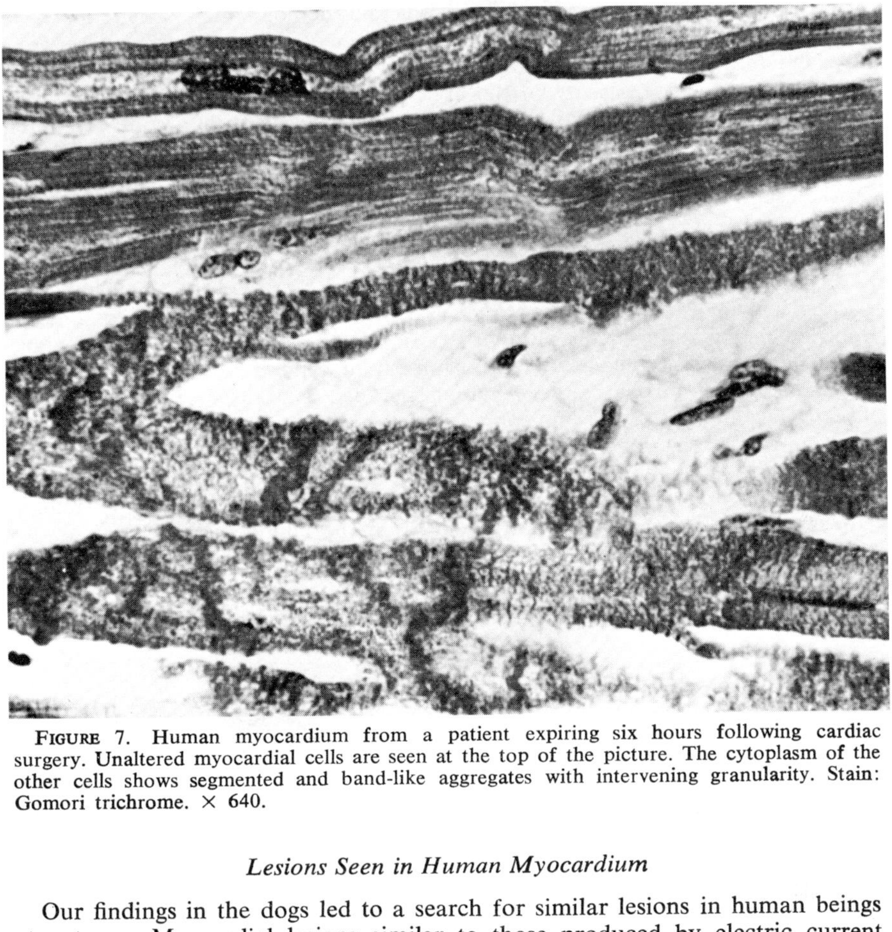

FIGURE 7. Human myocardium from a patient expiring six hours following cardiac surgery. Unaltered myocardial cells are seen at the top of the picture. The cytoplasm of the other cells shows segmented and band-like aggregates with intervening granularity. Stain: Gomori trichrome. × 640.

Lesions Seen in Human Myocardium

Our findings in the dogs led to a search for similar lesions in human beings at autopsy. Myocardial lesions similar to those produced by electric current discharge could be found in the human myocardium associated with a variety of clinical conditions. We have found them regularly associated with cardiovascular surgery postoperatively; they can be found around the periphery of myocardial infarctions, and are frequently seen in relation to foci of myocarditis.

Histological studies of 50 patients who expired at various time intervals following cardiac surgery showed a sequence of changes similar to those seen in experimental animals, suggesting that the myocardial injury occurred in relation to the cardiac surgery (FIGURES 7–11). Cytoplasmic banding was the most prominent feature of the lesion and was seen in 96% of patients expiring within eight days following cardiac surgery. The extent of the interstitial cell reaction was not as marked as it was in the experimental animals, nor did myocardial cells with prominent nucleoli occur around the periphery of the lesion as frequently.

Gross demonstration of dehydrogenase activity[9] in myocardial slices showed substrate deficiency in the area of the lesion in patients expiring four hours after surgery, but enzyme activity could be demonstrated when substrate (succinate) was added to the incubation medium. In patients expiring between two and four days following surgery, however, it was not possible to demonstrate dehydrogenase activity in the area of the lesion.

The extent of involvement of the myocardium varied from a zone of altered epicardial cells to large areas of injury involving more than half the thickness of the left ventricle. Occurrence of the lesion was not affected by variations in the use of cardiopulmonary bypass or procedures for resuscitation or cardiac arrest.

Discussion

The histological changes seen in this distinctive type of myocardial lesion indicate that it differs from ordinary coagulation necrosis of ischemic infarction. Features of this cell injury and interstitial cellular reaction include: (1) segmentation of myocardial cell cytoplasm, seen as transverse bands between areas of granularity; (2) appearance of the alteration within minutes after appropriate stimulation; (3) prominent interstitial mononuclear cell response; (4) paucity of polymorphonuclear leukocytes in the cellular reaction; (5) sparing of the reticulum stroma, vessels, and nerves; and (6) the frequent appearance of punctate mineralization within the altered cells.

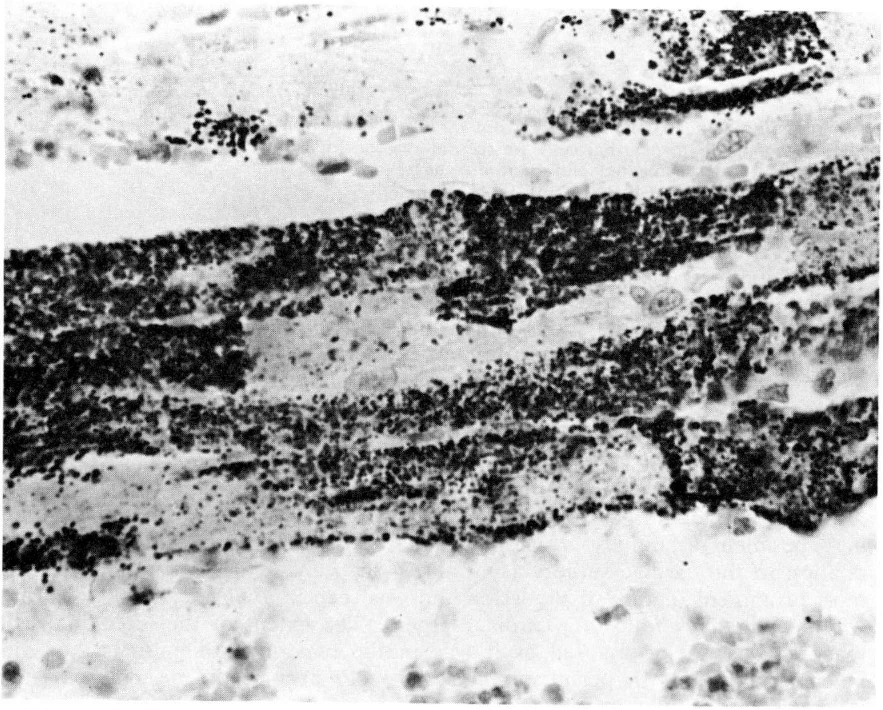

FIGURE 8. Human myocardium from a patient expiring ten days following cardiac surgery. Myocardial cell cytoplasm is segmented, and many punctate granules of mineralized material are seen. Stain: von Kóssa. × 640.

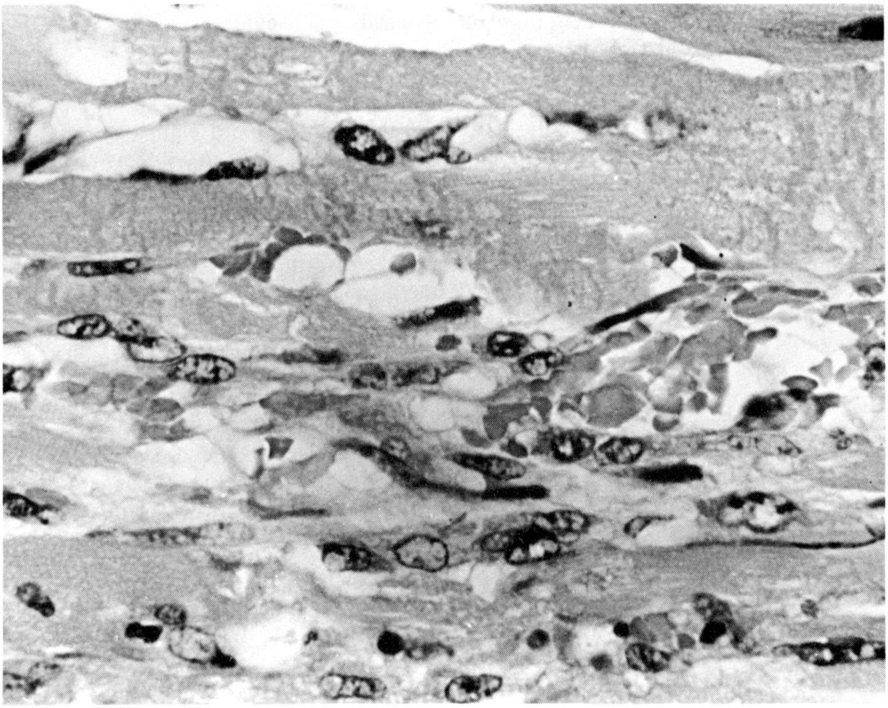

FIGURE 9. Human myocardium from a patient expiring three days following cardiac surgery. Myocardial cells show segmentation and banding of the cytoplasm and loss of nuclear staining. Prominent interstitial cells are present. Polymorphonuclear leukocytes are not present. Stain: hematoxylin and eosin. × 640.

Electric shock may be used to produce this lesion experimentally. However, since only 30 of the 50 human cases had defibrillating electric shock, it appears that other factors may produce an injury with similar morphological features. At present, it is difficult to be certain what these other factors might be in patients subjected to cardiac surgery, inasmuch as these patients usually receive a number of pressor agents and a variety of electrolytes along with the mechanical trauma and stress of the operative procedure.

Mention of some of the experimental conditions associated with this lesion may indicate the types of agents having a possible role in producing the lesion in human beings. An injury reaction of this type may be produced by hypokalemia,[1, 6] temporary occlusion of a coronary artery,[2] large doses of catecholamines,[5] and 9-fluorocortisol plus sodium phosphate.[7] The diversity of these injurious agents suggests that they may affect a common metabolic structural portion of the myocardial cell, resulting in a similar morphological response to injury. Other clinical conditions associated with this lesion include: myocardial infarction, where it is occurs around the periphery of the infarct, myocarditis, and ruptured central nervous system aneurysm.

One of the prominent alterations in the myocardial lesion described here is the structural change seen in the myofibrils in which there is a loss of definition of individual myofilaments, as seen by electron microscopy. This change is readily observed as a segmentation of myocardial cell cytoplasm, seen as transverse bands in the light microscope. The striking appearance of the cytoplasm differs from that seen in ordinary ischemic infarction, in which the usual striated appearance of the muscle cell may persist for several days.

The lesion is at least partially reversible. Between five and eight days following injury, there are nuclear and nucleolar changes that are consistent with increased metabolic activity and protein synthesis, and some cells show changes consistent with the formation of new contractile elements. A reproducible confluent injury is evident after three days, but the residual damage seen after three to four weeks is usually not extensive or confluent. Focal areas of collapsed reticulum or mineralization are not in continuity, but may be separated by normal-appearing myocardial cells. The origin of these cells is uncertain. They may represent severely injured myocardial cells in which degenerated cytoplasmic material has been removed, rendering them temporarily unidentifiable as muscle cells. Nevertheless, they may still be capable of forming new contractile fibrils. At present, it seems less likely that they originate from cells capable of differentiating into myocardial cells. Since there are morphological changes indicating that the injury is partially reversible, we have tended to characterize the lesion as a degenerative process. However, there is no

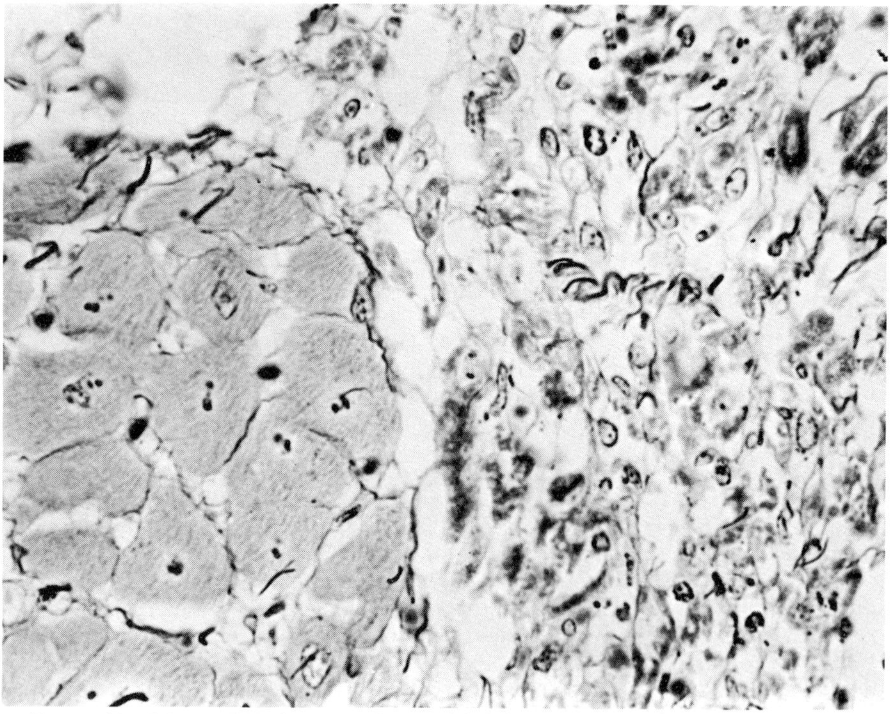

FIGURE 10. Myocardium from a patient expiring three days following cardiac surgery. On the left are normal myocardial cells and reticulum. Collapse and fragmentation of the reticulum stroma are seen on the right. Stain: reticulum. × 640.

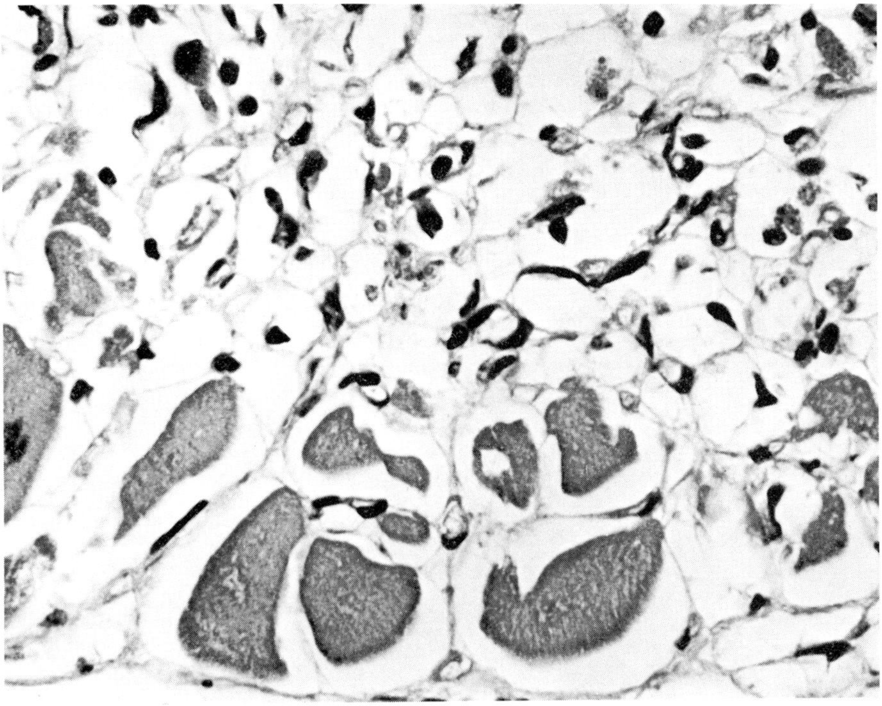

FIGURE 11. Myocardium from a patient expiring three months following cardiac surgery. There is collapse of the reticulum stroma resulting in a loose area of connective tissue which contains pigment-laden macrophages. There is no significant fibrosis. Stain: hematoxylin and eosin. ×·640.

question that myocardial necrosis and cell death occur in this lesion. In such damaged areas, there is collapse of the reticulum stroma, and fibrosis frequently ensues in more severely damaged areas.

The structural alteration of myofilaments of the injured myocardial cells suggests that it must be associated with a loss of contractile function. Altered cellular function is suggested by the loss of dehydrogenase activity in this lesion. The demonstration of the initial loss of substrate in the lesion, followed by a loss of enzyme activity, is additional evidence that the morphological changes are not artifacts. Since a significant portion of the myocardium may be involved in this injury, it is reasonable to suppose that it may contribute to the poor cardiac function seen in many patients following cardiac surgery.

Summary

Histological features are described of a common cardiac lesion that differs from ordinary coagulation necrosis of ischemic infarction. The lesion is seen at autopsy associated with several clinical conditions and may be produced experimentally by several chemical, metabolic, and mechanical means. The injury affects the structural organization of the myofibrils and is at least partially reversible.

References

1. MOLNAR, Z., K. LARSEN & B. SPARGO. 1962. Cardiac changes in the potassium-depleted rat. Arch. Path. (Chicago) **74:** 339.
2. HERDSON, P. B., H. M. SOMMERS & R. B. JENNINGS. 1965. A comparative study of the fine structure of normal and ischemic dog myocardium with special reference to early changes following temporary occlusion of a coronary artery. Amer. J. Path. **46:** 367.
3. ANDERSON, H. N., D. REICHENBACH, G. P. STEINMETZ, JR. & K. A. MERENDINO. 1964. An evaluation and comparison of effects of alternating and direct current electrical discharges on canine hearts. Ann. Surg. **160:** 251.
4. HEGGTVEIT, H. A., L. HERMAN & R. K. MISHRA. 1964. Cardiac necrosis and calcification in experimental magnesium deficiency. A light and electron microscopic study. Amer. J. Path. **45:** 757.
5. RONA, G., C. I. CHAPPEL, T. BALAZS & R. GANDRY. 1959. An infarct-like myocardial lesion and other toxic manifestations produced by isoproterenol in the rat. Arch. Path. (Chicago) **67:** 443.
6. FRENCH, J. E. 1952. A histological study of the heart lesions in potassium-deficient rats. Arch. Path. (Chicago) **53:** 485.
7. D'AGOSTINO, A. N. 1964. An electron microscopic study of cardiac necrosis produced by 9 α-fluorocortisol and sodium phosphate. Amer. Path. **45:** 633.
8. MARTIN, JR., A. M. & D. B. HACKEL. 1966. An electron microscopic study of the progression of myocardial lesions in the dog after hemorrhagic shock. Lab. Invest. **15:** 243.
9. NACHLAS, M. M. & T. S. SHNITKA. 1963. Macroscopic identification of early myocardial infarcts by alterations in dehydrogenase activity. Amer. J. Path. **42:** 379.

EXPERIMENTAL STUDIES ON THE HEALING OF CARDIAC NECROSIS

George Rona and David S. Kahn

Departments of Pathology, The Lakeshore General Hospital and St. Mary's Memorial Hospital and Institute of Pathology McGill University, Montreal, Canada

General Considerations

Experimental studies have contributed to an understanding of some of the factors governing the healing of human myocardial infarction.[1] These studies could also be used to determine the modifying effect of various conditions and drugs on the repair process. Cardiac muscle, irreversibly damaged, cannot regenerate, and its repair takes place primarily by means of fibrous tissue substitution (organization); thus, the same general principles that govern connective tissue proliferation operate in myocardial repair. The healing of myocardial necrosis may be thought of as taking place in three stages: (1) the evolution of necrobiosis, lasting from the original injury to the peak of the regressive changes; (2) the removal of the necrotic debris; and (3) the repair period. There is, however, a considerable overlap among these stages. As has been shown by incorporation of radioactive glycine into protein and nucleic acids, the repair process starts a few hours after infarction.[2] However, persistence or perpetuation of noxious conditions following the initial precipitating insult may lead to repeated regressive myocardial changes at a time when removal of the original necrotic debris is taking place and also during repair. Difficulties in interpretation may result from the equivocal usage of the terms "recuperation," "repair," and "regeneration" by biochemists, experimental cardiologists, and pathologists.

To obtain reliable data on the chronology of the healing process, as well as an accurate assessment of the modifying factors, it is necessary to specify the experimental method and the morphological characteristics of a particular model. Various techniques have been used to produce myocardial necrosis: (1) restriction of the coronary blood supply (temporary and relative myocardial ischemia); (2) metabolic factors (electrolyte imbalance); (3) sympathomimetics; (4) mechanical means; (5) chemical agents; and (6) sundry factors. A simple and standardized method that produces necrosis of sufficient size in the presence of a low mortality rate is preferable for healing studies. Three experimental models fulfill these criteria: myocardial necrosis produced by coronary artery ligation, thermal injury, and catecholamines.[3]

The possibility of myocardial survival or repair depends upon the severity of the actual injury, the duration and extent of oxygen deprivation (restoration of blood flow and collaterals), and the metabolic requirement of the myocardial fibers. Following temporary or relative ischemia, groups of myocardial fibers may survive the acute episode; myocardial recuperation and repair will both be facilitated by the reopening of coronary vessels and the reestablishment of coronary blood flow. These characteristics make isoproterenol-induced myocardial necrosis particularly suited for healing studies.

The Healing of Isoproterenol-Induced Myocardial Necrosis

In 1959, we demonstrated that isoproterenol [1(3,4-dihydroxyphenyl)–2-isopropylaminoethanol], a synthetic depressor (beta-adrenergic receptor stim-

ulator) catecholamine, produces infarct-like myocardial necrosis in experimental **animals.**[4] The acute lesion was of uniform severity and grossly resembled human myocardial infarction. In male or female Wistar rats weighing an average of 250 g, the optimal infarct-producing dose of isoproterenol hydrochloride ranged between 5.25 and 85 mg/kg subcutaneously (s.c.) on two consecutive days.[5] On gross examination, the infarct was well demarcated within 48 hours. It involved almost the entire left ventricle and the apical portion of the right ventricle (FIGURE 1). It had a granular appearance, turned

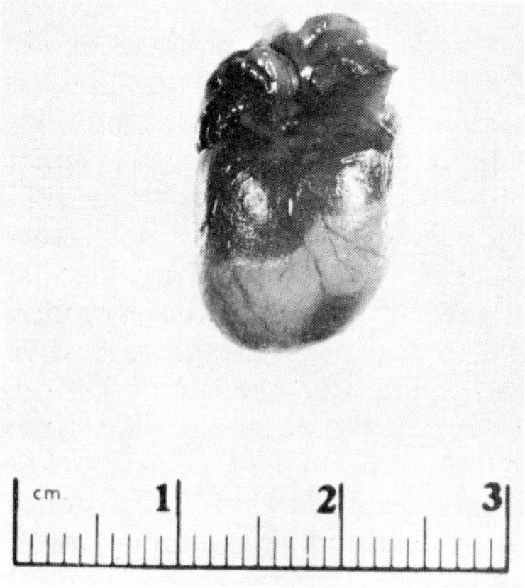

FIGURE 1. Infarct-like necrosis, 48 hours after injections of isoproterenol (85 mg/kg, s.c.) on two consecutive days. The pale area of necrosis is evident at the apical portion of the heart.

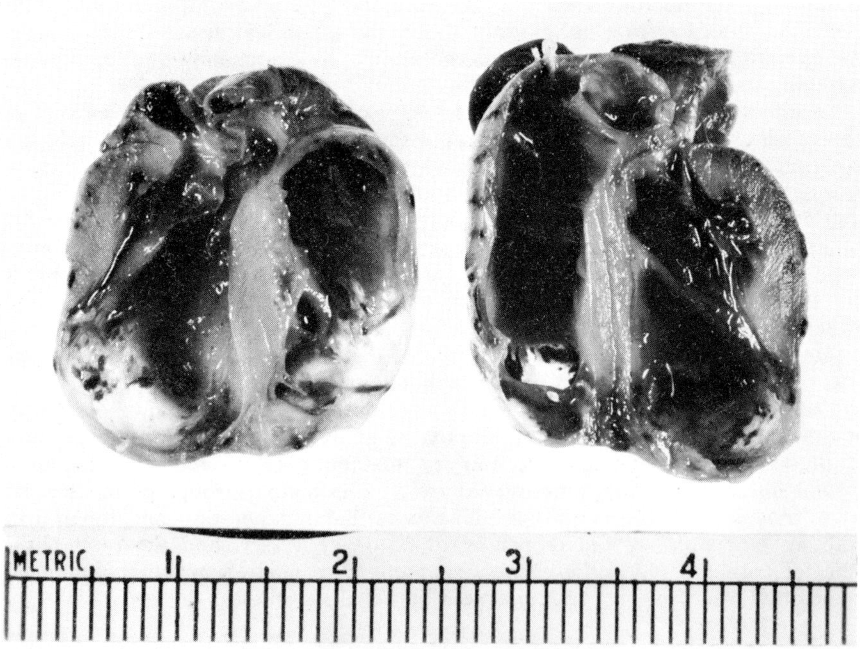

FIGURE 2. Chronic aneurysm and myocardial hypertrophy, shown in a frontal bisection of the heart of a rat, two years following injections of isoproterenol (85 mg/kg) on two consecutive days.

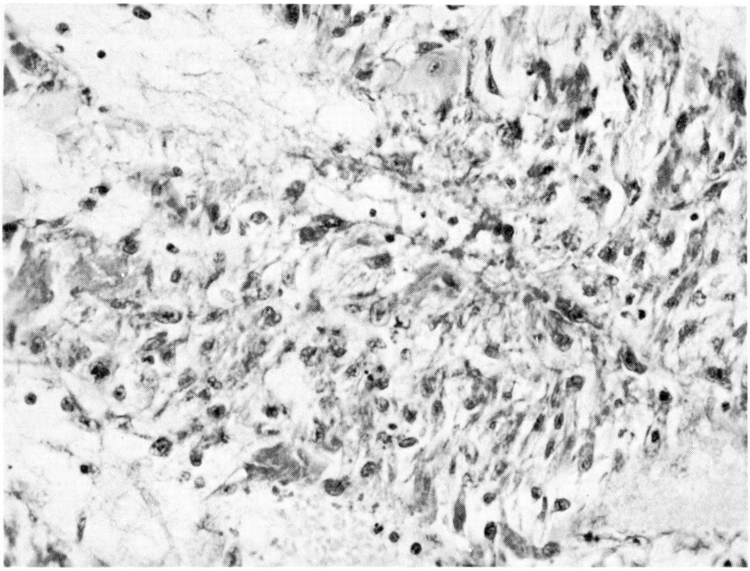

FIGURE 3. Massive necrosis of the myofibers, 48 hours after isoproterenol injection. Stain: periodic acid—Schiff. × 300.

pale greyish-yellow in color, and was friable in consistency. An acute aneurysm with mural thrombi was occasionally observed. Following the acute phase, gradual fibrous replacement of the infarct took place, with transformation of the necrotic friable myocardium into firm elastic tissue. In two to three weeks, some of the infarcts appeared to be diminished in size, and within six weeks became quite indistinct. In roughly one-half of the animals, however, the extent of the infarct increased,[6] and marked cardiac enlargement with chronic apical aneurysm of both ventricles developed within 16 weeks (FIGURE 2).

The early electron microscopical, histochemical, and light microscopical changes of the isoproterenol-induced heart necrosis have been discussed in detail elsewhere.[3] For an analysis of the repair process, knowledge of the histological components of the fully evolved myocardial necrosis (peak at 48 hours) is pertinent.[7] These components have been grouped in two categories: regressive myofiber changes and stromal reaction. Cytoplasmic eosinophilia, fatty change, vacuolar swelling, and hyaline necrosis of the muscle fibers were grouped in the former category; the involved fibers became homogeneous, strongly eosinophilic, and periodic acid-Schiff (PAS) positive. Finally, the striation of the muscle fibers disappeared, and the nuclei were either shrunken or completely absent (FIGURE 3). The reactive changes of the stroma consisted of capillary dilatation, interstitial edema with a mucoid component, infiltration by polymorphonuclear leukocytes, and proliferation of mononuclear cells. Fibroblastic swelling was one of the most consistent reactive changes.

Examination 72 hours after injury showed the necrotic debris being removed by histiocytes that contained fat globules and hemosiderin. Empty sarcolemmal sheaths marked the site of the dissolved necrotic myocardial fibers. Only a few PAS-positive granular fibers remained. The edema regressed, and a proliferation of mononuclear cells and plump fibroblasts dominated the picture (FIGURE 4). These, along with capillaries, penetrated into the necrotic areas. Five days after injury, some muscle fiber nuclei showed a peculiar chromatin alteration suggesting attempted mitosis (FIGURE 5). Histiocytes, fibroblasts, Anitschkow myocytes, and Aschoff giant cells surrounded the residual necrotic foci forming granulomata (FIGURE 6). At seven days, the organization process progressed; reticulin and collagen fibers became prominent. In rats sacrificed at two to five weeks after injury, the fibrous scars contained spindle-shaped fibroblasts, pigment-laden macrophages, and lymphocytes (FIGURE 7). The cellularity of the scars further diminished at eight to 12 weeks. Within 16

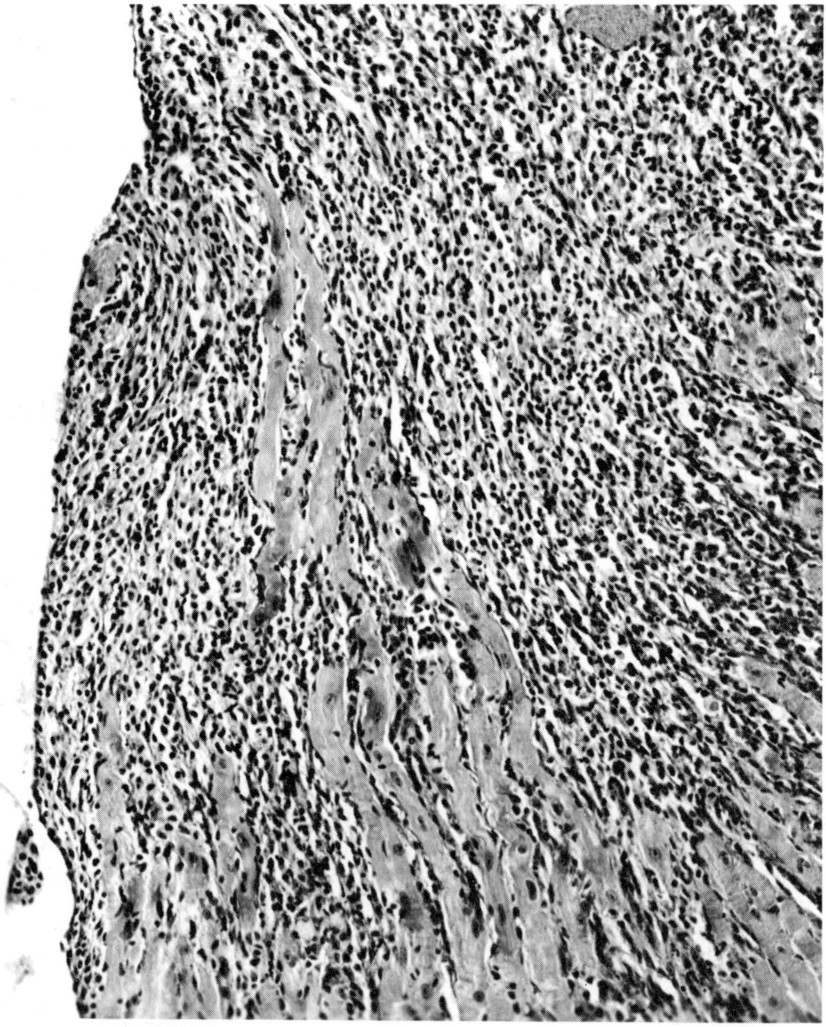

FIGURE 4. Replacement of necrotic myofibers by mononuclear cells and fibroblasts. Stain: hematoxylin and eosin. × 150.

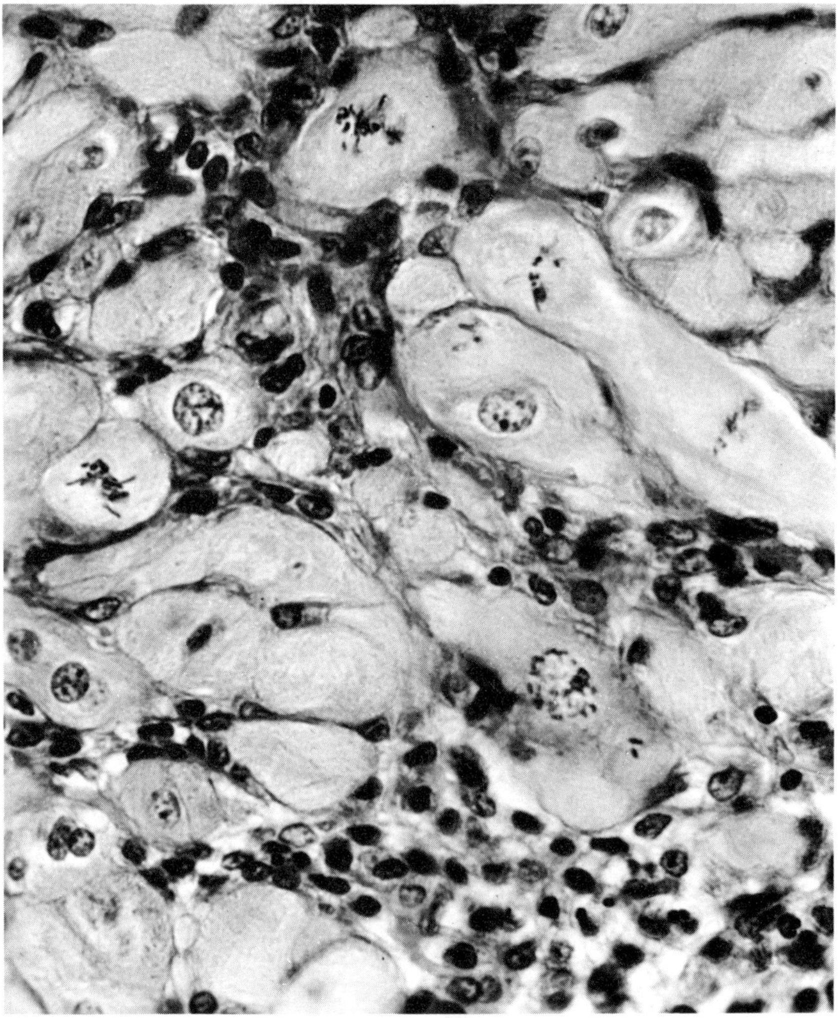

FIGURE 5. Changes of the myofiber nuclei, indicating excessive stimulation and mitoses, five days following isoproterenol injection. Stain: hematoxylin and eosin. × 500.

weeks, unless aneurysm formation took place, the necrosis healed with an indistinct linear scar (FIGURE 8). In rats with chronic aneurysms, the aneurysmal wall was formed by mature fibrous connective tissue revealing focal cartilaginous or bony metaplasia. Although the myofibers generally were enlarged, some close to the aneurysmal wall showed eosinophilia and loss of striation. Some loosely textured cellular foci containing lymphocytes and plump mononuclear cells were also found at the transition zone (FIGURE 9). There was little difference in the findings at 16 weeks and up to 12, 18, and 24 months following the myocardial injury.[8] At the border of the aneurysm, a few eosinophilic or fading myofibers were still recognizable, and proliferation of histiocytes, fibroblasts, Anitschkow myocytes, and multinucleated giant cells formed predominantly perivascular and subendocardial granulomata. Occasional arterioles showed a swollen endothelial lining, a thickened fibrotic wall, and a prominent mantle of adventitial histiocytes.

Discussion

The early stage of isoproterenol-induced myocardial necrosis has a characteristic morphology and corresponding serum enzyme findings that differ from the changes following coronary artery ligation. In the former, the rapid re-

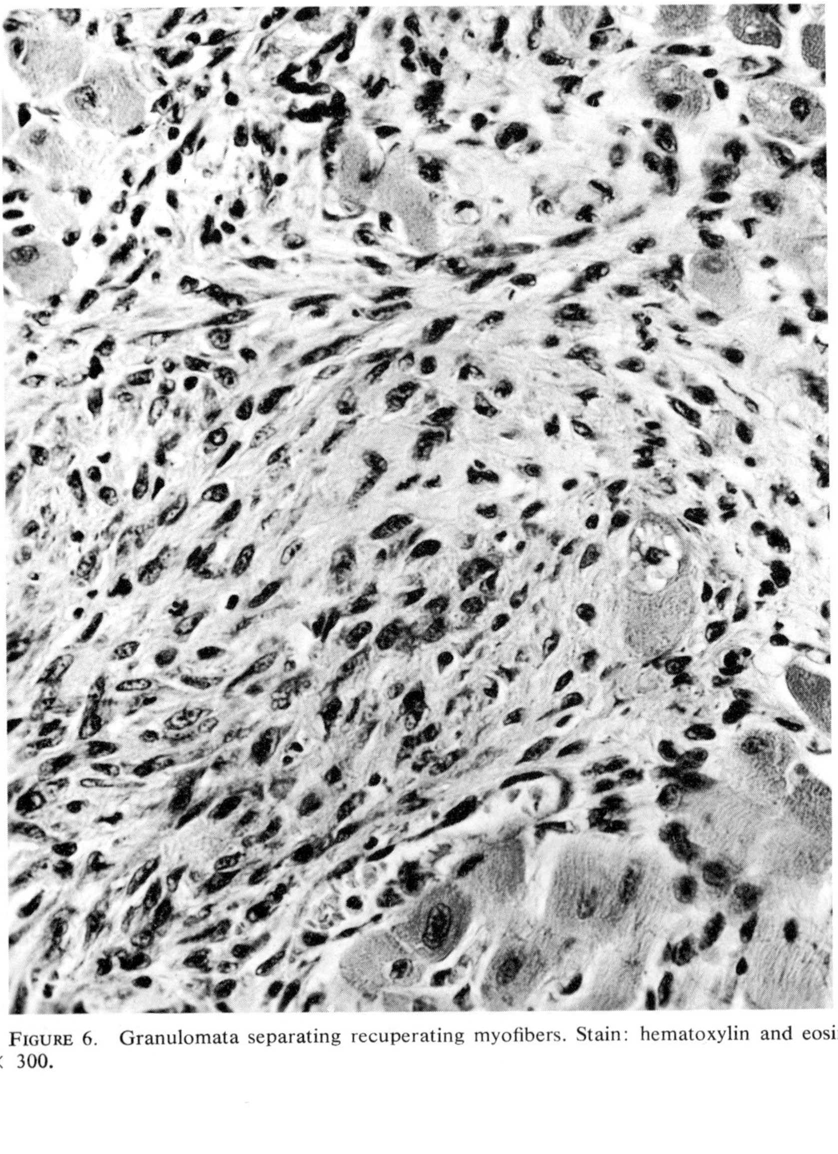

FIGURE 6. Granulomata separating recuperating myofibers. Stain: hematoxylin and eosin. × 300.

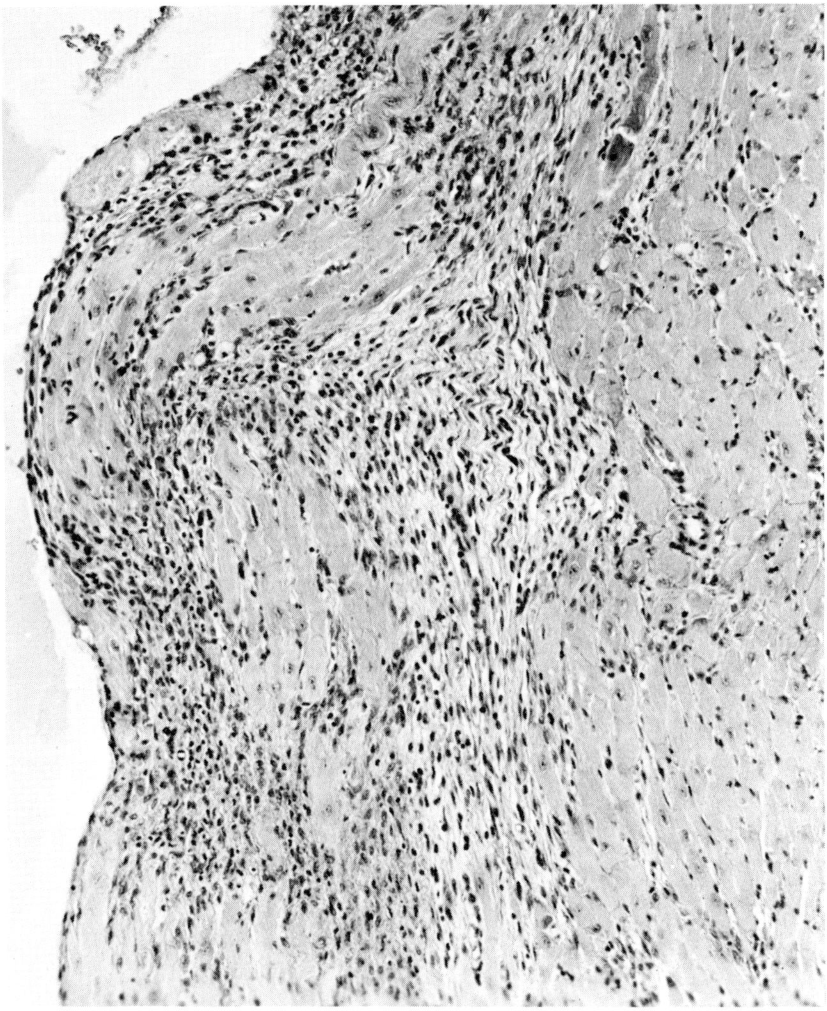

FIGURE 7. Repair after two weeks. The predominant cells are spindle-shaped fibroblasts. Stain: hematoxylin and eosin. × 150.

moval of the necrotic debris and return of serum enzyme levels to normal[9,10] are probably related to the patency of coronary arteries. In isoproterenol experiments, the necrotic fibers are completely removed and replaced by an organization process within three to five days after injury, whereas this process may take weeks in infarcts produced by coronary ligation.[11,12] A sufficient oxygen supply to an excessively stimulated and damaged area of myocardium also leads to a prominent capillary engorgement, cellular reaction, and edema. If the circulation is restored in an animal with a coronary artery ligation, the ensuing hemorrhagic and exudative response differs from the predominantly regressive myocardial lesions produced by permanent coronary occlusion[13,14]

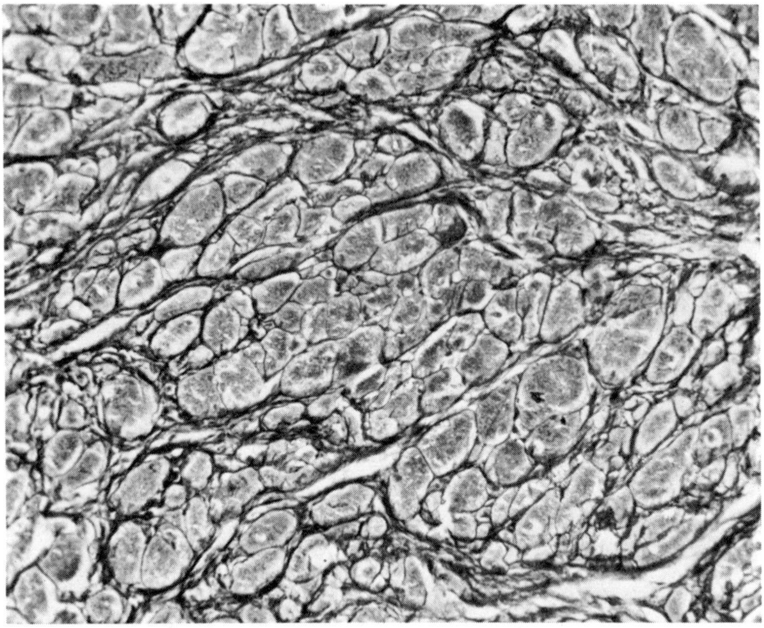

FIGURE 8. Healing by linear scars. Stain: reticulin. × 180. (Courtesy of Dr. G. Korb. Marburg, Germany.)

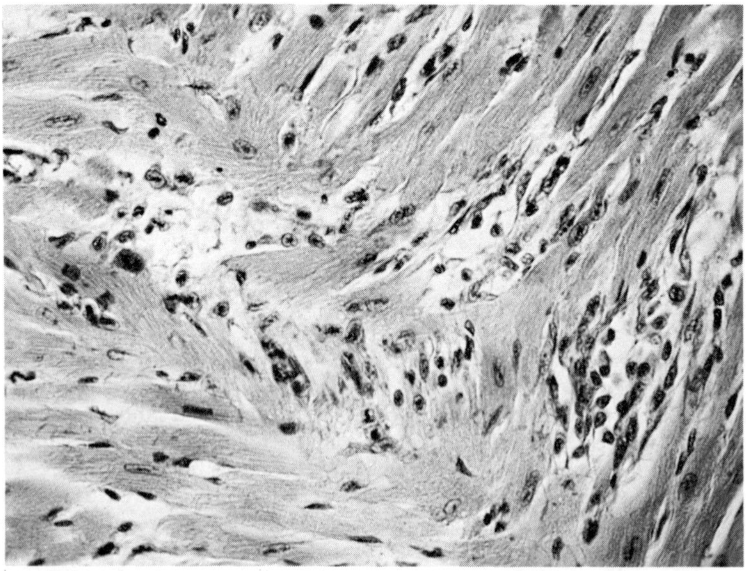

FIGURE 9. Formation of granulomata at the transition zone of a chronic heart aneurysm. Stain: hematoxylin and eosin. × 300.

and resembles closely that seen in the early evolutionary stage of isoproterenol-induced necrosis.[15, 16]

The electron microscopical investigations of Korb[17, 18] and Ferrans and his colleagues,[19] by differentiating reversible and irreversible myofiber changes in acute experiments, supplied significant information regarding the two distinct sequelae in the healing of isoproterenol-induced heart necrosis. Collapse of the endoplasmic reticulum, disappearance of the nuclear and mitochondrial membranes, transformation of the nuclear structure, and extensive disintegration of the myofibers indicated irreversible damage. Loss of glycogen, intracellular edema, swelling of the endoplasmic reticulum, and condensation of the mitochondrial matrix were examples of reversible myofiber alteration. Muscle fibers with slight or moderate fatty change and green fluorescence under electron microscopy possess normal mitochondria and may recover.[20]

Restoration of blood flow subsequent to a relative[6, 7] or temporary[21] ischemia may limit the damage and favorably influence the ensuing healing process. Although the interstitial tissue is destroyed together with the parenchymal cells in regions of permanent absolute anoxia, some of the reticulin framework with capillaries and fibroblasts remain viable in isoproterenol-induced lesions. Thus, proliferation occurs readily from multiple foci and achieves a pattern roughly restoring the original architecture (with some diminution) of the myocardium and prevents the formation of large deforming scars. Remodeling of the newly formed connective tissue reduces the myocardial lesion to small indistinct fibrotic foci; thus, one is unable to estimate the original size of these infarcts from the scar.[6] In other cases, excessive myocardial stimulation apparently produces irreversible damage of the myofibers and, in some way, the stromal components. The repair of the coalescent necrotic fields results in large deforming scars, with formation of chronic heart aneurysms.

Electron microscopical and histochemical studies on isoproterenol-induced heart necrosis revealed prominent and early mitochondrial swelling and an increase of succinic dehydrogenase activity.[19] These changes were regarded as an indication of mitochondrial stimulation leading to a relative ischemia. Whereas in isoproterenol-induced heart necrosis the blood supply through the patent coronary arteries satisfies the oxygen demand during the repair period, in permanent coronary artery ligation, an absolute myocardial ischemia is present during both the evolution and the healing stage; the outcome will be influenced by the availability of a blood supply through collateral channels.[22]

The duration of ischemia effects the severity of the original injury and also modifies the circulatory dynamics in the postinfarction period. Coronary ligation lasting 60 minutes or longer produces a prolonged disturbance of blood flow at the periphery of its region of supply.[23] Intramyocardial capillary thrombosis, intracellular and interstitial edema, and elevated intraventricular pressure have been suggested as possible mechanisms.[24, 25] These postinfarction ischemic alterations must be considered in establishing the revival time of the myocardium (the length of time from the beginning of ischemia to the development of irreversible damage) and for therapeutic management.[26]

The granulomata observed during the first week of repair of isoproterenol-induced heart necrosis resemble the myofiber Aschoff bodies.[27] For granuloma formation, normal blood supply to the injured myocardium appears to be necessary, since no such reaction is reported in the rat myocardium following coronary artery ligation.[28] An additional factor may be related to an indirect stimulation of cellular proliferation by an isoproterenol effect on protein[29] and nucleoprotein[30] synthesis. Murphy suggested that the multinucleated giant cells in granulomas of rheumatic fever are of myogenic origin, as are Anitschkow myocytes.[27] These cells represent a primitive regenerative response to primary myofiber damage.[31] Occasional mitotic divisions observed in the differentiated muscle fibers also indicate excessive stimulation and possible regenerative activity.

We have previously suggested that minor mechanical injuries mediated by altered tension forces at the transition zone of the chronic heart aneurysm may be responsible for the small granulomatous foci found in this region many months after the original insult.[6] The possibility that they are related to heart-specific antibodies[32] seems unlikely in view of their localized nature and the lack of circulating antibodies in isoproterenol-induced heart necrosis.[33] The cardiac enlargement observed in animals with chronic aneurysms may be based on altered intracardiac circulatory dynamics leading to overload and an abnormal stretching of the muscle which is known to produce cardiac dilatation and hypertrophy.[34]

The effects of intrinsic and extrinsic factors that modify anabolic biochemical processes[35] and the incidence and extent of myocardial necrosis[36-39] in acute experiments have not been properly investigated in the late phase of healing. It has been shown that insulin and methandrostenolone protect the heart infarcted by coronary artery ligation against aneurysm formation, whereas a protein-free diet leads to a more frequent development of aneurysm.[35] The present paper demonstrates the modifying role of one of the most important local factors, the patency of coronary arteries (myocardial blood supply), on the morphology of the repair process. There is a need for further studies concerning the effect of other local (heart size, collaterals, the site of necrosis) and systemic factors[40] that might be expected to influence repair processes in the heart. It would be interesting to know the effect of the following on the healing of myocardial necrosis: sex and age of the animals, physical activity and rest, diet (vitamin, salt, lipid, and protein- and sulphur-containing amino acid content), hormones (pituitary growth hormone, insulin, sex, and adrenocortical hormones), and various drugs. These experiments could yield some significant practical information concerning factors that influence the healing of a myocardial infarct and its complications, such as aneurysm formation and rupture.

Summary

Experimental myocardial necrosis has been used for studying factors that may modify its healing process. Since cardiac muscle fibers cannot regenerate, myocardial necrosis heals primarily by connective tissue replacement. Thus, the healing is governed by the same principles that regulate connective tissue proliferation in general. In addition to systemic factors, the extent and rate of healing of myocardial necrosis may be affected by some specific local conditions.

For accurate assessment of the healing process and the modifying factors, it is necessary to specify the exact method of the production and the morphological characteristics of a particular experimental model. Myocardial necrosis can be produced by: (1) restriction of coronary blood supply, (2) metabolic factors, (3) symphatomimetics, (4) mechanical means, (5) chemical means, and (6) sundry factors.

Three well-standardized techniques lend themselves for use in detailed healing studies. These are experimental myocardial infarction produced by coronary artery ligation, thermal myocardial injury, and isoproterenol-induced myocardial necrosis.

The healing of isoproterenol-induced myocardial necrosis has been presented in detail and the data compared with that of experimental myocardial infarct produced by coronary artery ligation. Although the original myocardial injury appeared to be uniform in severity, there were two distinct sequelae of isoproterenol-induced myocardial necrosis: healing with a residual linear scar and formation of a chronic aneurysm. This suggests that the healing process was influenced by factors independent of the extent of the original injury. The difference in the manifestation and healing between cardiac necroses occurring in hearts with patent coronary arteries and those in which the necrosis results from permanent coronary occlusion has been discussed.

Some factors have been shown to modify the severity of the acute lesion. However, the effect of either local or systemic conditions on the healing process beyond the acute stage has not been sufficiently studied. This would be a profitable subject for further investigations.

Acknowledgment

The authors would like to thank Mrs. G. Henderson for her help in preparing the manuscript.

References

1. LODGE-PATCH, I. 1951. The ageing of cardiac infarcts and its influence on cardiac rupture. Brit. Heart J. **13**: 37–42.
2. GUDBJARNASON, S., C. DESCHRYVER, C. CHIBA, J. YAMANAKA & R. J. BING. 1964. Protein and nucleic acid synthesis during the reparative processes following myocardial infarction. Circ. Res. **15**: 320–326.
3. RONA, G. & D. S. KAHN. 1967. The healing of cardiac necrosis as reflected by experimental studies. *In* Methods and Achievements in Experimental Pathology. E. Bajusz & G. Jasmin, Eds. **3**: 200–249. S. Karger. Basel, Switzerland.
4. RONA, G., C. I. CHAPPEL, R. BALAZS & R. GAUDRY. 1959. An infarct-like myocardial lesion and other toxic manifestations produced by isoproterenol in the rat. Arch. Path. Chicago) **67**: 443–455.
5. CHAPPEL, C. I., G. RONA, R. BALAZS & R. GAUDRY. 1959. Severe myocardial necrosis produced by isoproterenol in the rat. Arch. Int. Pharmacodyn. **122**: 123–128.
6. RONA, G., D. S. KAHN & C. I. CHAPPEL. 1961. Study on the healing of cardiac necrosis in the rat. Amer. J. Path. **39**: 473–489.
7. RONA, G., D. S. KAHN & C. I. CHAPPEL. 1963. Studies on infarct-like myocardial necrosis produced by isoproterenol. A Review. Rev. Canad. Biol. **22**: 241–255.
8. RONA, G., C. I. CHAPPEL & D. S. KAHN. 1963. Experimental production of chronic cardiac aneurysm and congestive heart failure in the rat. Exp. Molec. Path. **2**: 40–51.
9. WEXLER, B. C. & G. W. KITTINGER. 1963. Myocardial necrosis in the rats: Serum enzymes, adrenal steroid and histopathological alterations. Circ. Res. **13**: 159–171.
10. ANSHELEVITCH, Y., A. AMELIN & M. MELZOBS. 1961. The production of myocardial necrosis in rabbits by Isadrine (isopropylnoradrenaline). Latvian Acad. Sci. News **173**(12): 91–94.
11. KASNER, H. T. & J. E. DWYER. 1916. Studies in infarction. IV. Experimental bland infarction of the myocardium, myocardial regeneration and cicatrization. J. Med. Res. **34**: 21–39.
12. KAUFMAN, N., T. L. GAVAN & R. W. HILLS. 1959. Experimental myocardial infarction in the rat. Arch. Path. (Chicago) **67**: 482–488.
13. BAJUSZ, E. & G. JASMIN. 1964. Histochemical studies on the myocardium following experimental interference with coronary circulation in the rat. I. Occlusion of coronary artery. Acta. Histochem. **18**: 222–237.
14. BAJUSZ, E. & G. JASMIN. 1963. Comparative morphogenesis and enzyme histogenesis of some occlusive and metabolic cardiac necroses. Rev. Canad. Biol. **22**: 181–199.

15. TENNANT, R., D. M. GRAYZEL, F. A. SUTHERLAND & S. W. STRINGER. 1936. Studies on experimental coronary occlusion. Chemical and anatomical changes in the myocardium after coronary ligation. Amer. Heart J. **12:** 168–173.
16. BRONSON, L. H. 1937–1938. Anatomical and chemical changes in the myocardium following short term coronary artery occlusion in dogs. Yale J. Biol. Med. **10:** 405–410.
17. KORB, G. 1964. Elektronenmikroskopische Befunde am Herzmuskel nach hohen Aludrininjektionen. Verh. Deutsch. Ges. Path. **48:** 245–250.
18. KORB, G. 1965. Elektronenmikroskopische Untersuchungen zur Aludrin (Isoproterenosulfat)-Schädigung des Herzmuskels. Virchow. Arch. Path. Anat. **339:** 136–150.
19. FERRANS, V. J., R. G. HIBBS, W. C. BLACK & D. G. WEILBAECHER. 1964. Isoproterenol-induced myocardial necrosis. A histochemical and electron microscopic study. Amer. Heart J. **68:** 71–90.
20. KORB, G. & V. TOTOVIC. 1963. Licht- und fluoreszenz-mikroskopische Befunde am Herzmuskel nach einer akuten, kurzfristigen Coronarinsuffizienz. Virchow. Arch. Path. Anat. **336:** 475–484.
21. JENNINGS, R. B., J. H. BAUM & P. B. HERDSON. 1965. Fine structural changes in myocardial ischemic injury. Arch. Path. (Chicago) **79:** 135–143.
22. JENNINGS, R. B. & W. B. WARTMAN. 1957. Reactions of the myocardium to obstruction of the coronary arteries. Med. Clin. N. Amer. **41:** 3–15.
23. KRUG, A. & G. KORB. 1966. Durchblutungsstörungen und histologische sowie enzymhistochemische Frühveränderungen am Katzenherzen nach temporärer Unterbindung von Coronargefässen. Beitr. Path. Anat. **134:** 29–51.
24. WEBB, W. R. & H. S. HOWARD. 1957. Extension of limits of cardiac viability with total coronary occlusion. Surgery **42:** 92–100.
25. KRUG, A., W. DU MESNIL DE ROCHEMONT, G. KORB. 1966. Blood supply of the myocardium after temporary coronary occlusion. Circ. Res. **19:** 57–62.
26. KRUG, A. 1965. Untersuchungen am Katzenherzen nach temporärer Unterbindung einer Koronararterie. Z. Kreislaufforsch. **54:** 510–516.
27. MURPHY, G. E. 1952. Evidence that Aschoff bodies of rheumatic myocarditis develop from injured myofibres. J. Exp. Med. **95:** 319–322.
28. JOHNS, T. N. P. & B. J. OLSON. 1954. Experimental myocardial infarction. I. A method of coronary occlusion in small animals. Ann. Surg. **140:** 675–682.
29. ZBINDEN, G. & R. A. MOE. 1968. Pharmacological studies on heart-muscle lesions induced by isoproterenol. This monograph.
30. SELYE, H., R. VEILLEUX & M. CANTIN. 1961. Excessive stimulation of salivary gland growth by isoproterenol. Science **133:** 44–45.
31. MURPHY, G. E. & C. G. BECKER. 1966. Occurrence of caterpillar nuclei within normal immature and normal appearing and altered mature heart muscle cells and the evolution of Anitschkow cells from the latter. Amer. J. Path. **48:** 931–957.
32. HEINE, W. I., H. FRIEDMAN, M. S. MANDELL & H. GOLDBERG. 1966. Antibodies to cardiac tissue in acute ischemic heart disease. Amer. J. Cardiol. **17:** 798–803.
33. ROSENMANN, E., E. GAZENFIELD, A. LAUFER & A. M. DAVIES. 1964. Isoproterenol-induced myocardial lesions in the immunized and non-immunized rat. I. Histopathological lesions in normal rats. Path. Microbiol. (Basel) **27:** 303–309.
34. WARIS, E. K., L. SIITONEN & E. HIMANKA. 1966. Heart size and prognosis in myocardial infarction. Amer. Heart J. **71:** 187–195.
35. GUDBJARNASON, S., J. C. FENTON, P. L. WOLF & R. J. BING. 1966. Stimulation of reparative processes following experimental myocardial infarction. Arch. Intern. Med. (Chicago) **118:** 33–40.
36. RONA, G., C. I. CHAPPEL & D. S. KAHN. 1963. The significance of factors modifying the development of isoproterenol-induced myocardial necrosis. Amer. Heart J.. **66:** 389–395.
37. BAJUSZ, E. & G. JASMIN. 1962. Protective action of serotonin against certain chemically and surgically induced cardiac necroses. Rev. Canad. Biol. **21:** 51–62.
38. ZBINDEN, G. & R. E. BAGDON. 1963. Isoproterenol-induced heart necrosis, an experimental model for the study of angina pectoris and myocardial infarct. Rev. Canad. Biol. **22:** 257–263.
39. BREINING, H. & O. STRUBELT. 1965. Die Bedeutung der adrenergischen beta-Rezeptoren für die cardiotoxische Wirkung sympathicomimetischer Amine. Med. Pharmacol. Exp. (Basel) **13:** 169–176.
40. EDWARDS, L. S. & J. E. DUNPHY. 1958. Wound healing. I. Injury and normal repair. II. Injury and abnormal repair. New Engl. J. Med. **259:** 224–233 and 275–285.

MYOCARDIAL TOXICITY OF COBALT IN THE RAT

H. C. Grice, T. Goodman, I. C. Munro, G. S. Wiberg, and A. B. Morrison
Food and Drug Research Laboratories, Department of National Health and Welfare
Ottawa, Canada

It is a well-established fact that the rat myocardium oxidizes long-chain fatty acids for its energy requirements in preference to either pyruvate or glucose.[1-4] In the absence of long-chain fatty acids, pyruvate becomes the preferred substrate.[2-4] Investigations carried out in this laboratory have shown that heart mitochondria of rats pretreated with cobalt (Co^{++}, at 4 mg/kg intraperitoneally daily for eight days) demonstrated a reduced ability to oxidize octanoate or pyruvate. A preliminary description of these biochemical studies has been presented elsewhere.[5] As part of continuing investigations in our laboratory on cobalt metabolism and toxicity, this report deals with heart lesions observed in rats given high levels of cobalt.

Material and Methods

Young male rats of the Wistar strain, averaging 100 g in body weight, were divided into three comparable groups of 20 rats each and housed in individual cages maintained in an air-conditioned room kept at 74–76° F. The first group received the protein-free diet of Chapman and co-workers,[6] supplemented by 8% wheat gluten and 3.3% casein, with the Jones and Foster[7] salt mixture rather than USP XIV salt mixture. Group 2 received a diet similar to group 1, except that the thiamine content of the diet was reduced to 40 μg/100 g of diet. Group 3 received the same diet as group 2, except that the salt mixture was adjusted in composition to contain twice the normal level of dibasic potassium phosphate and one-half the normal level of calcium carbonate. The diets tested were chosen because it was considered possible that cobalt toxicity could be influenced by concomitant nutritional deficiency or excess. After eight weeks, half of the rats fed each diet were given an initial oral dose of 100 mg/kg of cobalt (as cobalt sulfate) dissolved in 0.5 ml of water, followed by daily oral doses of 26 mg/kg of cobalt for eight weeks. At the end of this time, the surviving rats were sacrificed, and the hearts were removed and examined histologically.

Results

Of the 30 animals given cobalt, 15 (five from each diet) died before the experiment was terminated. Histological changes, involving both myocardial cells and interstitium, were seen in 26 of the 30 rats given cobalt. Changes seen in the thiamine-deficient animals given added cobalt tended to be somewhat more severe than those in the animals given diet 1 plus cobalt. The cobalt-induced changes in animals on all three diets were varied and were observed both in rats dying during the experiment and in those sacrificed at the termination of the study. The initial changes involved edematous separation of cells, some fragmentation and vacuolization of myocardial cells, and minimal inflammatory cellular response.

There was a slight swelling of the myocardial cells and an apparent increase in ground substance, along with a decrease in the number of myofibrils so that only a few myofibrils remained in some cells. This resulted in an "unmasking" of the mitochondria which stood out vividly between myofibrillar elements. In areas where myofibrillar loss was complete, the mitochondria were aggregated within intact sarcolemmal sheaths filled with diluted ground substance (FIGURE 1). With complete disappearance of cellular components, residual empty endomysial sheaths collapsed and were replaced by fibrous tissue.

With special stains,[8] there was little difficulty in recognizing the mitochondria, but in some cells, small globular structures, larger than normal mitochondria, were observed between the myofibrils. These globular structures could represent swollen coalesced mitochondria or fragmented contracted myofibrillar substance. Electron microscopy indicated that mitochondria in areas of greatest damage tended to be slender and smaller than normal, averaging 0.12μ in diameter (FIGURES 2 and 3). Prominent myofibrillar degeneration was evidenced by the focal and segmental occurrence of brightly acidophilic contraction bands in some myocardial cells (FIGURE 1).

In certain cells the thinning, disappearance, and separation of myofibrils was associated with an accumulation of small vacuoles appearing in rows between the myofibrils. The vacuoles were considered to represent spaces formerly occupied by liposomes or fat droplets. The droplets tended to coalesce and form large globules that imparted a "moth-eaten" appearance to a few fibers. Similarly, electron microscopical observations revealed focal areas of degeneration,

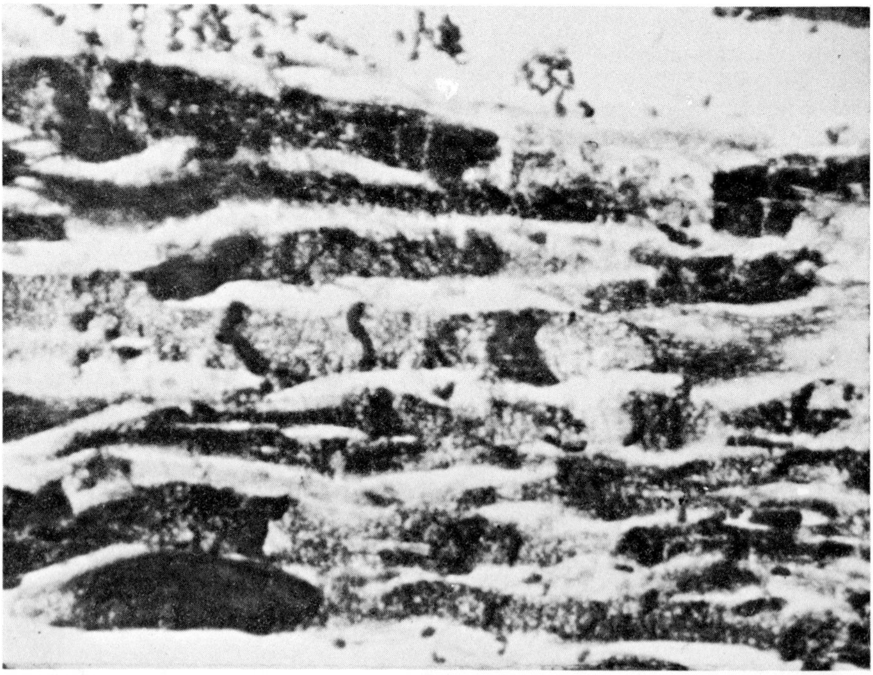

FIGURE 1. Fragmentation, separation, and swelling of myocardial cells in the rat. Mitochondria, vacuolization, and contraction bands are apparent in the cell in the center of the field. Stain: Fuchsin acid-light green. × 400.

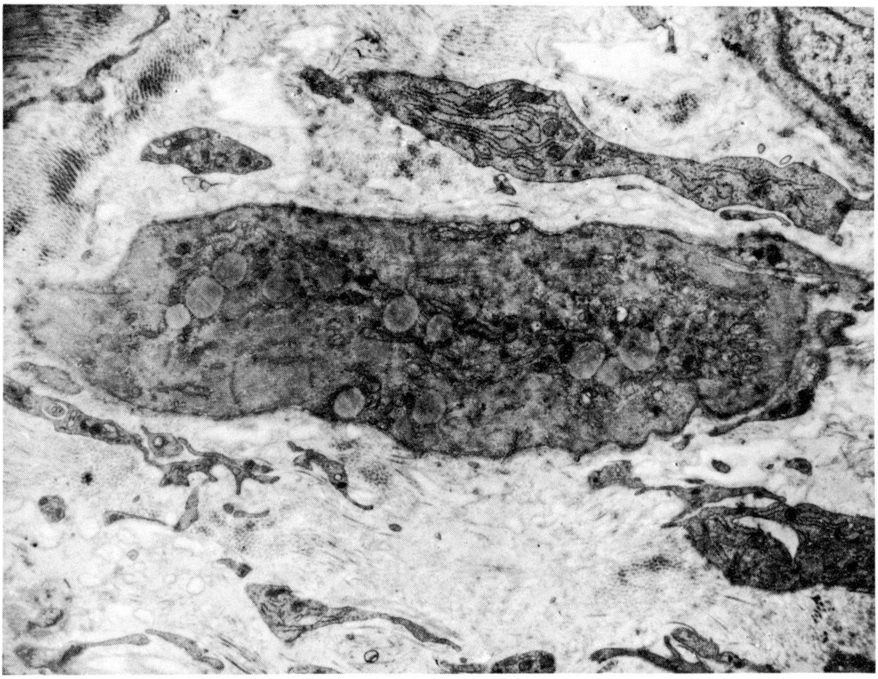

FIGURE 2. Electron micrograph through a focal area of muscle cell degeneration in the left ventricle. In the center is an isolated slightly rounded muscle cell, surrounded by a large interstitial space filled with collagen fibers and connective tissue cells. In the muscle cell are many fat droplets. The heart was perfused with 20 ml of 5% glutaraldehyde at 4° C, prefixed with 5% glutaraldehyde for 90 minutes, postfixed with buffered osmic acid (pH 7.2) for two hours, dehydrated with acetone, and Epon-embedded. Stain: uranyl acetate and lead citrate. × 6,000.

in which some muscle cells contained fat droplets, 0.4–0.8μ in diameter (FIGURES 2 and 3).

The focal fragmentation of muscle fibers was pronounced in some areas, and fragmented fibers became rounded, decreased in number and size, and replaced by loose fibrous tissue. The rounded character of the fibers also was apparent in electron micrographs. Initially, there appeared to be a widening or pulling apart of the muscle cells at the intercalated discs and a "rounding off" of the ends of the cells. These cells became completely isolated and surrounded by interstitial space containing collagen fibers (FIGURE 2). In the isolated muscle cells, there was a sparse and irregular distribution of myofibrils, some of which contained cross-bands. Light microscopy of older lesions revealed small shrunken muscle cells, sometimes consisting of a nucleus with only a few frayed myofibrils, embedded in or surrounded by fairly dense fibrous tissue (FIGURE 4).

In one rat, an aneurysmal dilatation of the apex of the heart was observed. In this animal, an organizing mural thrombus, attached to the endocardium, was seen under light microscopy (FIGURE 5). In the area of the aneurysmal sac, the full thickness of the ventricular wall was replaced by fibrous tissue.

Histological changes involving slight separation of muscle fibers and small focal areas of fibrous tissue replacement of myocardial cells were seen in two rats given diet 2 without added cobalt and in four rats given diet 3 without added cobalt. No abnormalities were seen in the hearts of animals given diet 1 alone.

Discussion

These studies show clearly that high levels of cobalt given daily for eight weeks produced degenerative heart lesions in rats. The lesions were characterized by edematous separation of cells, accumulation of fat droplets, a decrease in the number of myofibrils, and only minimal inflammatory cellular response. In these preliminary studies, the cobalt-induced heart lesions tended to be somewhat more marked in animals given thiamine-deficient diets (diets 2 and 3). Since cardiomyopathies of nutritional or metabolic origin are well known, other studies are underway in our laboratory to investigate more fully the possible role of nutrition in influencing the production of the lesions described in this report.

It is interesting to speculate on the possible relationship between the cobalt-induced lesions produced in this study and the biochemical effects of cobalt on the heart. In previous investigations,[5] we found that pretreatment of the rats with cobalt reduced the ability of the heart mitochondria to oxidize pyru-

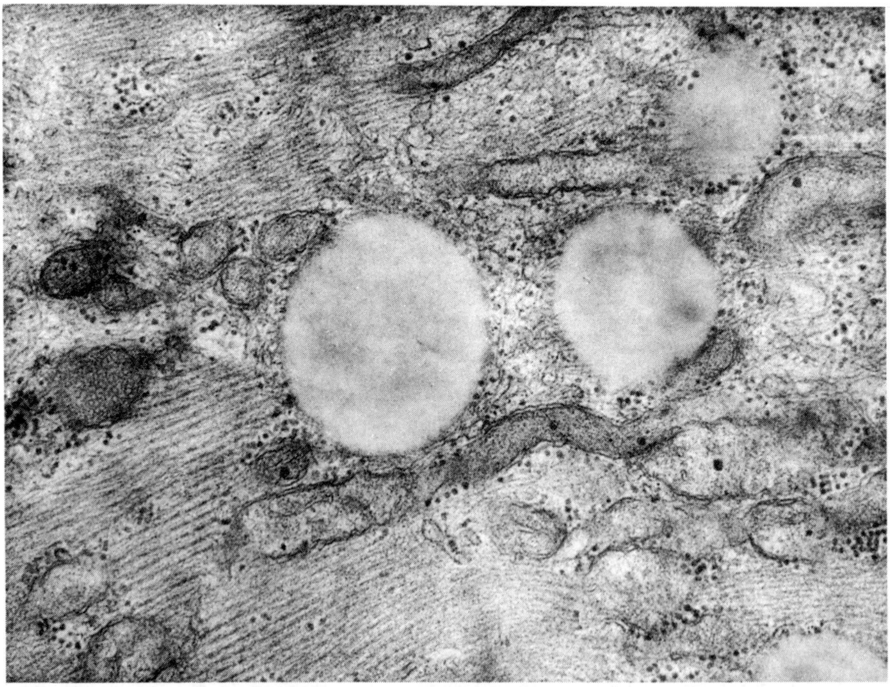

FIGURE 3. An enlarged portion of the muscle cell in FIGURE 2, showing in greater detail the fat droplets, a few remaining myofilaments, and slender mitochondria. × 34,200 (orig. mag. × 36,000).

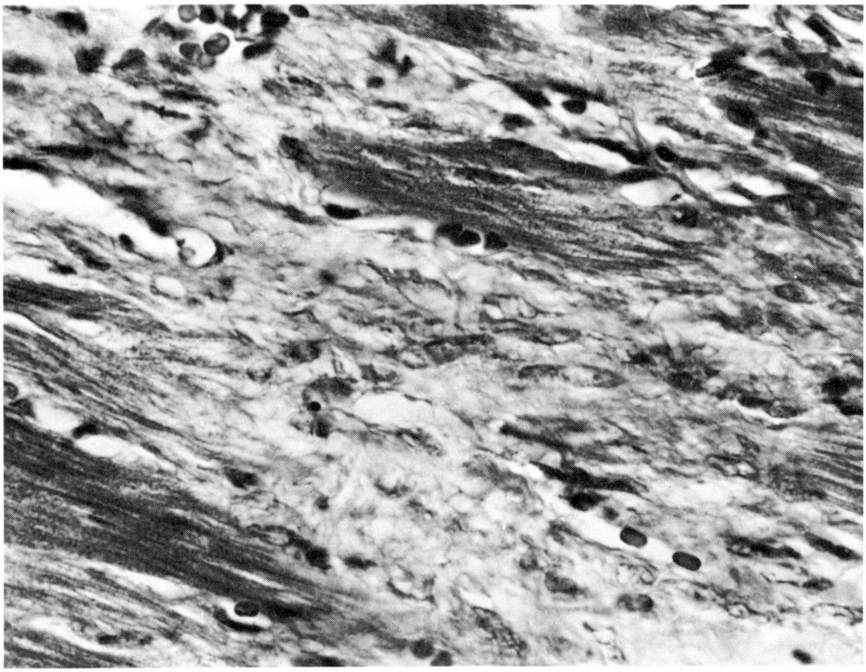

FIGURE 4. A section of left ventricular myocardium of rat with the myocardial cells being replaced by fibrous tissue. The heart was perfused with 20 ml of 5% glutaraldehyde. Stain: hematoxylin-saffron-phloxin. × 140.

vate or octanoate. The addition of α-lipoic acid to the *in vitro* system completely restored the ability of these rat heart mitochondria to metabolize pyruvate, but had no effect on pyruvate metabolism in heart mitochondria from untreated control rats that had not received cobalt. Dingle and his associates[9] have shown previously that cobalt depresses pyruvate metabolism in mitochondria of rat liver and thigh muscle. Our observation that α-lipoic acid restored the ability of heart mitochondria to metabolize pyruvate may be related, in part, to the observation of Webb[10] that cobalt can form a complex with the sulfhydryl groups of lipoic acid and thus render it unavailable for the metabolism of α-ketoglutarate. It would appear, therefore, that cobalt can markedly inhibit cardiac energy metabolism by inactivating lipoic acid, an essential cofactor required for the metabolism of fatty acids, pyruvate, and α-ketoglutarate. Interference with α-ketoglutarate metabolism would be of particular significance in the present studies, since wheat gluten, which made up most of the dietary protein, contains a high level of glutamic acid.[11]

From a consideration of the metabolic pathways involved, it is obvious that interference with normal energy metabolism in the heart could lead to accumulation of cardiac lipid. It is noteworthy, therefore, that the present studies showed an accumulation of fat droplets in myocardial cells of cobalt-treated rats. The cardiac changes noted in the animals given diets 2 and 3, which were partially deficient in thiamine, were similar to those described previously in thiamine-deficient rats.[12]

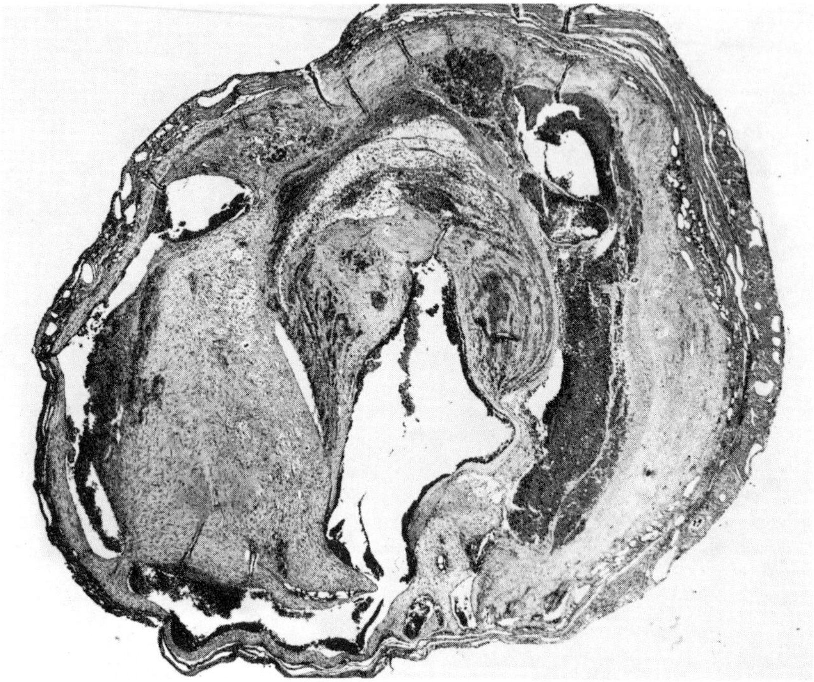

FIGURE 5. Cross-section of the apex of a rat heart, with mural thrombus and replacement of myocardial cells by fibrous tissue. The heart was perfused with 20 ml of 5% glutaraldehyde. Stain: hematoxylin-saffron-phloxin. × 25.

Acknowledgments

The authors are indebted to T. K. MacGregor, Z. Zawidzka, S. Gray, E. Millard, and R. Neugebauer for technical assistance.

References

1. EVANS, J. R., L. H. OPIE & J. C. SHIPP. 1963. Amer. J. Physiol. **203**: 766.
2. WILLIAMSON, J. R. 1965. J. Biol. Chem. **240**: 2308.
3. RANDLE, P. J., E. A. NEWHOLME & P. B. GARLAND. 1964. Biochem. J. **93**: 652.
4. GARLAND, P. B., E. A. NEWHOLME & P. J. RANDLE. 1964. Biochem. J. **93**: 665.
5. WIBERG, G. S., I. C. MUNRO & A. B. MORRISON. 1967. Canad. J. Biochem. **45**: 1219.
6. CHAPMAN, D. G., R. CASTILLO & J. A. CAMPBELL. 1959. Canad. J. Biochem. Physiol. **37**: 679.
7. JONES, J. H. & C. FOSTER. 1942. J. Nutr. **24**: 245.
8. GURR, E. 1962. Staining Animal Tissues. Practical and Theoretical. Leonard Hill Books, Ltd. London, England.
9. DINGLE, J. T., J. C. HEATH, M. WEBB & M. DANIEL. 1962. Biochem. Biophys. Acta **65**: 34.
10. WEBB, M. 1962. Biochem. Biophys. Acta **65**: 47.
11. BLOCK, R. J. & K. W. WEISS. 1956. *In* Amino Acid Handbook. : 312. Charles C Thomas, Publ. Springfield, Ill.
12. ASHBURN, L. L. & J. V. LOWRY. 1944. Arch. Path. (Chicago) **37**: 27.

PART III. GENESIS AND PREVENTION OF CARDIOPATHIES: HORMONAL, NEURAL, NEUROENDOCRINE, AND MISCELLANEOUS MECHANISMS

THE PLURICAUSAL CARDIOPATHIES*

Hans Selye

Institut de Médecine et de Chirurgie Expérimentales
Université de Montréal, Montréal, Canada

The very fact that scientists of so many countries have contributed to this monograph on "metabolic" cardiopathies bears witness to the great change in outlook that has taken place in the interpretation of the pathogenesis of heart disease during the last decade. Barely eight years ago, in September, 1959, at the International Symposium on Arteriosclerosis and Coronary Disease in Mexico City, I tried to prove that infarct-like cardiac necroses can be produced without vascular obstruction, e.g. by combined treatment with corticoids and electrolytes or corticoids and stress; at that time, with the notable exception of Dr. Sodi-Pallares, few of the participants were prepared to believe that such metabolic factors could play a role in the genesis of "true" cardiac infarcts in man. Although the functional effect of many electrolytes upon the heart had long been known, the finding that sodium increases and potassium and magnesium diminish the susceptibility to cardiac necrosis was also received with the greatest reserve. Seemingly even more incongruous were the observations showing that many essentially distinct experimental cardiopathies (characterized by hyalinization, calcification, inflammation, and endomyocardial fibrosis) can be produced merely by varying the types of steroids and electrolytes used, or the length of treatment. It was especially puzzling how potassium and magnesium could offer protection against so many cardiac lesions differing from one another in their morphological structure and the method of their production.

The basic facts have since been confirmed in many laboratories, and, although their interpretation is still very difficult, several contributors to this monograph begin to show the direction that future research must take. It appears that the heart is capable of responding only with a limited number of reactions to the innumerable agents and combinations of agents that can act upon it. There must be a limited number of final common pathways of response. The morphologists look for them in cell membranes, structurally identifiable subcellular particles, or the "transit zone" of Hauss; the biochemist thinks of them primarily in terms of enzyme systems related to the production and utilization of energy. Undoubtedly, it is along some of these lines that a deeper understanding of the metabolic cardiopathies will come. Perhaps the best way to illustrate the limited response of the heart to various stress factors would be to present a brief outline of the concept of "pluricausal diseases," which acted as our guide in this work, and a concise summary of the procedures developed for the production and prevention of various experimental cardiopathies.

* The orignial experiments on which this review is based were supported by United States Public Health Service grant no. HE-06182 from the National Heart Institute, the Canadian Heart Foundation, Ministère de la Santé, Québec, Canada, and Arzneimittelwerk Fischer, Bühl (Baden), Germany.

The Pluricausal Diseases in General

In essence, a pluricausal disease is defined as a derangement produced by combined treatment with two or more agents, none of which is effective in this respect by itself. Most of the pluricausal diseases examined to date were elicited by combined treatment with two agents, one of which (the "conditioner" or "sensitizer") induces a particular type of disease proneness while the other (the "challenger") makes this predisposition manifest and determines the location of the resulting changes.[1] By such a dual treatment, it has been possible to produce calcification,[2] thrombosis with hemorrhage,[3] necrosis,[4, 5] or inflammation and hyalinization,[6] predictably localized in certain organs.

The cardiological implications of this concept have been discussed at length in two monographs;[7, 8] hence, it will suffice to give a mere outline here. For comparison, we shall also mention a few cardiopathies that are apparently monocausal inasmuch as they are elicited by treatment with a single agent; yet, even in some of these, we have reason to suspect that the apparently unique pathogen acts through the combined effect of several of its distinct pharmacological properties.

Experimental Cardiopathies with Vascular Involvement

First, we shall discuss those cardiopathies that are always accompanied by histologically detectable changes in the coronary vessels. These changes range from calcification to lipid deposition or hyalinization, but, whatever their nature, it seems likely that they affect the metabolism of myocardial fibers.

Hyalinizing Cardiopathies

The Electrolyte-Steroid Cardiopathy with Hyalinization

The electrolyte-steroid cardiopathy with hyalinization (ESCH) is normally produced by combined treatment with certain steroids (mineralocorticoids) and electrolytes (sodium salts) in animals pretreated by unilateral nephrectomy.[8] It is characterized by precipitation of hyaline material within the myocardium and in the coronary arteries.

Macroscopically, the heart is hypertrophic; on its surface it exhibits multiple, small, light-brown or grayish patches that correspond to the hyalinized myocardial granulomas. Similar lesions are sometimes visible along the course of the coronary arteries, particularly when periarteritis nodosa is present.

The periodic acid-Schiff (PAS) stain is a good histological technique for the study of all hyalinizing cardiopathies. We also employ a trichrome (alcian blue, phosphotungstic acid, and aldehyde fuchsin) stain, which is especially useful in detecting the earliest lesions.[9, 10]

Histologically, the ESCH is easily recognized by the formation of homogeneous hyaline masses within the myocardium and its arteries. In the myocardium, the hyaline material appears partly in disintegrating muscle fibers ("hyaline or fibrinoid necrosis") and partly in the stroma around the muscles. The homogeneous masses thus deposited soon become surrounded by a granuloma, which consists mainly of young fibroblasts and histiocytes, although it may also contain Anitschkow cells ("caterpillar cells") or even eosinophilic leukocytes.

In the coronary vessels, the lesions begin by the deposition of hyalin underneath the intima and in the media. Eventually, the entire vessel wall may be transformed into a hyaline mass, which is surrounded and infiltrated by a granuloma.

The Isoproterenol Cardiopathy

This subject is discussed at length by various other contributors to this monograph. Under certain experimental conditions, isoproterenol can produce not only the typical necroses revealed by the classical work of Rona and his colleagues,[12, 13] but also intense hyalinization of the coronary arteries,[8] as well as dissecting aneurysms of the aortic arch.[14] The isoproterenol necroses (like those produced by adrenaline or noradrenaline) are apparently monocausal, but catecholamines can also act as ingredients of pluricausal pathogenic situations; for example, their ability to produce cardiac necroses is enormously increased by concurrent treatment with mineralocorticoids.[7]

Calcifying Cardiopathies

The Electrolyte-Steroid Cardiopathy with Calcification

Whereas in the ESCH the main morphological lesion is fibrinoid degeneration, the principal characteristic of the electrolyte-steroid cardiopathy with calcification (ESCC) is a deposition of calcium salts, with essentially the same localization as that of hyalin in the ESCH. The ESCC is induced by treatment with certain steroids and electrolytes; concurrent exposure to acute stress greatly facilitates the production of this cardiopathy.[8]

Histologically, the ESCC is characterized by the appearance of more or less massive calcium deposits in the cardiac muscle fibers, the stroma, and the coronary arteries. Calcification tends to occur in patches rather than diffusely, but the affected areas are quite irregularly distributed throughout the heart. The coronary veins are not affected. The relative severity of calcification in muscles, stroma, and arteries is subject to great variations. The heavily calcified myocardial regions undergo necrosis, but in this cardiopathy it is very unusual to find necrotic regions without any trace of calcification. It is also exceptional to see an advanced ESCC in which the arteries are not calcified; usually, even the periarterial striated muscle fibers are preferential sites for calcification. On the other hand, inflammatory changes are never conspicuous, and even the totally calcified necrotic muscle fibers show little tendency to become absorbed or invaded by inflammatory infiltrates.

The Calciphylactic Cardiopathies

Calciphylaxis is a condition of induced systemic hypersensitivity in which tissues respond to appropriate challenging agents with calcification.[2] The components of this phenomenon are a systemic calcifying agent or sensitizer [e.g. parathyroid hormone, vitamin D compounds, or dihydrotachysterol (DHT)] and an inorganic or organic challenger (e.g. $CrCl_3$ or serotonin) which is administered during a specific interval ("critical period") after the sensitizer. We distinguish between topical calciphylaxis, in which the challenger is applied directly to the target, and systemic calciphylaxis, in which the challenger is injected parenterally and yet acts selectively on certain organs.

The Phosphate Cardiopathy. This type of lesion is induced by oral administration of sodium phosphate to a calciphylactically sensitized animal.[8] Macroscopically, it is characterized by the presence of multiple polymorphic foci that are somewhat irregularly distributed throughout the heart. Histologically, the outstanding feature is an abscess-like nodule in which the myocardial fibers have undergone necrosis and dissolution. Calcification is slight or absent. The predominating structural element is the polymorphonuclear leukocyte. In this case, therefore, we may speak of miliary abscesses or of a focal suppurating myocarditis.

The Adrenaline Cardiopathy. Adrenaline (in a dose which alone does not cause structural changes in the heart) induces a high incidence of macroscopically visible auricular thromboses when administered following pretreatment with either DHT or parathyroid extract.[15] The thrombi are invariably localized in the left auricular appendage or the left atrium and take the shape of yellowish or reddish nodules, usually adherent to the arterial wall. A similar lesion may be produced by adrenaline or methoxamine in animals pretreated with an intravenous (i.v.) injection of lead acetate.[16]

The Histamine-Liberator Cardiopathy. The treatment of sensitized animals with dextran, dextrin, polymyxin, or compound 48/80, especially on the third day after DHT, induces an intense aggravation of muscular and vascular calcification in the heart, accompanied by a selective, macroscopically visible apical lesion.[17] Histologically, there is intense calcification of muscle fibers, with giant-cell formation and connective tissue proliferation in the apex.

The Ferric Oxide Saccharate Cardiopathies. Administration of ferric oxide saccharate (Fe-OS) can induce two types of lesions in rats pretreated with DHT, depending upon the "critical period."[18] One type appears when Fe-OS is injected a short time (one to two days) after sensitization; it is characterized by calcification of the left cardiac auricle. Histochemically, it is possible to demonstrate the selective deposition of iron in the extracellular tissue of the region, which subsequently undergoes calcification.[19]

The picture is entirely different in rats treated with Fe-OS ten days after sensitization. Auricular calcification is absent, but myocardial necroses are much more extensive and rather irregularly distributed throughout the myocardium. In these animals, calcium salts are also present in all branches of the coronary arterial system. The calcium deposits form plaques surrounded by proliferating fibrous tissue and often conducive to thrombosis.[2]

The Aorta Ligature Cardiopathy. In rats conditioned with DHT, a constricting but incomplete ligature placed above the renal arteries greatly raises the blood pressure and produces intense calcification of the coronary arteries and of the aorta above the ligature. Below the ligature, calcification is minimal. Apparently, the high blood pressure can act as a calciphylactic challenger. It is interesting to speculate whether calcification at the bifurcation of blood vessels, where the arterial wall is exposed to great pressure, might not also depend on a similar mechanism.[20]

Other Calcifying Cardiopathies

There is a group of lesions in which it is always possible to detect calcium salts histologically in the coronary arteries and in myocardial fibers. The methods of eliciting these lesions vary in each case, so they will be described separately.

The Antibiotic Cardiopathy. This lesion, which is structurally similar to the one seen in the ESCC, is induced by treatment with polymyxin plus stress, or polymyxin plus gluco- or mineralocorticoids.[21]

The Uremic Cardiopathy. Following bilateral nephrectomy, the adult rat usually survives for three to four days and then shows at least microscopical evidence of typical lesions consisting primarily of calcium deposition in the myocardium coronary arteries and aorta.[22-24] This uremic effect greatly resembles that of parathyroid hormone or acute vitamin D overdosage.

The Parathyroid Hormone Cardiopathy. Lesions can be produced simply by the injection of parathyroid extract in toxic amounts. They consist almost exclusively of calcifying necroses in the myocardium, with a Mönckeberg sclerosis type of calcification in the coronary arteries.[8]

Vitamin D Group Steroid Cardiopathies. Two distinct types of lesions can be produced by overdosage with the steroids of the vitamin D group (vitamin D_2, vitamin D_3, and DHT). One is due to acute[8] and the other to chronic[25, 26] overdosage with these compounds. In the former, the lesions are similar to those produced by acute intoxication with parathyroid extract, but they are accompanied by a more intense involvement of the coronary and other arteries, especially the arch of the aorta, which exhibit an intense calcification. The deposition of calcium salts appears to start in connection with elastic fibers of the media.[27, 28]

The second type of vitamin D cardiopathy occurs when the dose is diminished and the treatment more chronic. In this way, it is possible to induce lesions localized almost completely in the arterial walls. Macroscopically, the coronary arteries show interrupted rings of calcification along their course; these rings correspond histologically to a Mönckeberg type of sclerosis. The extracardiac manifestations of this cardiopathy constitute a syndrome resembling premature aging.[25, 26]

Occlusive Cardiopathies

Cardiac Infarcts Induced by Ligature of Coronary Arteries

Using various surgical techniques, it is possible to produce complete occlusion of coronary arteries in the rat.[8, 29] Comparative observations have shown that, even after ligation of the main coronary arteries, the resulting infarcts always leave the subendocardial and subepicardial muscle layers intact; usually, the myocardial fibers surrounding the cardiac veins within the necrotic area are also spared.

Cardiac Lesions Induced by Coronary Vein Ligature

The morphological consequences of coronary vein ligature are entirely different from those of coronary artery occlusion.[29] In the rat, the obstruction of even major coronary veins leaves the myocardium unaffected.

The Atherosclerotic Cardiopathy Produced by Thrombogenic Diets

The cardiopathy produced in rats by the so-called "thrombogenic diets" is characterized by coronary atheromatosis, sometimes in association with thrombosis and myocardial infarction.[30-32] Important ingredients of the thrombogenic diets appear to be saturated fats, cholesterol, propylthiouracil, and bile salts.

Thrombohemorrhagic Cardiopathies

The main feature of these cardiopathies is the concurrent presence of multiple hemorrhages and microthromboses located mainly in heart, kidneys, and lungs. Thrombohemorrhagic lesions may be obtained by the i.v. injection of reticuoendothelial system-blocking agents, various metal combinations, and certain agar preparations, especially if these substances are given in conjunction with corticoid hormones, severe systemic stressors, or catecholamines (adrenaline or noradrenaline).[33-35] Macroscopically, there is intense hemorrhagic infiltration of the myocardium, sometimes with massive hemorrhages around the pulmonary cone and root of the aorta. Histologically, areas of necrosis are seen, with thrombus formation in the small vessels and often hemorrhages around the necrotic areas. The thrombi are composed primarily of fibrin and platelets. In animals properly sensitized (e.g. by $ScCl_3$, i.v.) injection of catecholamines in the vicinity of large veins causes a topical thrombosis that may result in pulmonary embolism.[3]

Experimental Cardiopathies without Vascular Involvement

The lesions described in this section are not necessarily associated with blood vessel damage. As judged by microscopical examination, the primary lesion is apparently situated in the myocardial fibers. The concept of cardiac necrosis without vascular involvement is now beginning to receive increasing attention in clinical medicine.[36,37]

The Electrolyte-Steroid Cardiopathy with Necrosis

The electrolyte-steroid cardiopathy with necrosis (ESCN) is characterized by large infarctoid necroses that develop in the absence of coronary occlusion as a result of the combined action of certain steroids and sodium salts.[8] The techniques used for the production of the ESCN are based upon the administration of sensitizing electrolytes and corticoids, with or without subsequent exposure to stress.

The appearance of the ESCN is very distinctive: Inspection of the surface of the heart reveals multiple large infarctoid areas of necrosis, which are recognizable because of their light-yellowish color. The margins of these regions are usually quite sharply drawn and sometimes accentuated by a reddish line of demarcation separating them from the normal myocardium. The surface veins that course over the necrotic territories are well filled with blood and retain their normal coloration.

Histologically, the appearance of the infarctoid necroses varies during the course of their evolution. The first change detectable by the light microscope is necrosis of the muscle fibers, which manifests itself by pycnosis of the nucleus and disintegration of the myofibrils, which become granular. This change is not accompanied by the appearance of any significant amount of PAS-positive material and, thus, differs sharply from the hyaline necrosis characteristic of the ESCH.

A particularly useful technique for detecting the early myocardial changes during the ESCN is the staining by acid fuchsin of formalin-fixed myocardium.[38] This "fuchsinophilia" also occurs in recent myocardial infarcts in man.[39] The myocardial fiber segments that undergo early necrosis are selectively fuchsinophilic, and the first lesions appear to be along the Z band. With increasing damage, the fuchsinophilia is extended to the entire sarcoplasm of the fiber and stains the muscle dark red.

Electron microscopical investigation of the cardiac necrosis produced by the combined administration of corticoids and Na_2HPO_4 showed the early presence in the myocardial cells of electron-dense particulate inclusions located in the mitochondria. Macrophages present in such fibers contain similar inclusion-bearing mitochondria within cytoplasmic compartments. The intramitochondrial inclusions are presumed to represent deposits of calcium.[40]

In the necrotic muscle fibers, more or less heavy precipitates of calcium salts can be demonstrated with the von Kóssa stain. However, in the typical

ESCN, calcification does not affect the coronary arteries; this helps to distinguish even heavily calcified ESCN lesions from those of the ESCC.

In a second stage, the necrotic muscle is gradually absorbed, and the area is invaded mainly by histiocytes and fibroblasts, although occasional lymphocytes, neutrophils, and eosinophils may also appear. Finally, the entire necrotic area is replaced by a connective tissue scar, which often contains large numbers of elastic fibers.

The endocardium, pericardium, and valvular system are not selectively affected in this cardiopathy. It is especially noteworthy, however, that the necrotic areas are frequently situated in the subendocardial muscle layer. By contrast, as previously mentioned, this innermost region is invariably spared in true infarcts produced by ligature of coronary arteries, presumably owing to direct nutrition from the ventricular cavities. The necroses of the ESCN are evidently not due to thrombosis or embolism; it is also unlikely that they arise as a result of a sudden functional occlusion of coronary branches, since this could be expected to produce a picture similar to that obtained by coronary ligature. It is more probable that metabolic derangements are responsible for these necroses.[7]

Endomyocardial Fibrosis

A syndrome reminiscent of clinical endomyocardial fibrosis develops in the rat, under certain circumstances, after the interruption of a transient treatment with methylchlorocortisol and NaH_2PO_4, while time is allowed for abundant scar formation.[7] Whether there is any close relationship between this model and the clinical disease is debatable. However, allegedly, the spontaneous malady in man depends upon metabolic derangements in which potassium, magnesium, and stress play important roles; therefore, potassium and magnesium treatment has been recommended.[11]

Cardiopathies Caused by Dietary Potassium, Magnesium, or Chloride Deficiency

Deficiency in potassium, magnesium, or chloride predisposes to cardiac necroses that closely resemble those of the ESCN in both their morphological characteristics and their response to various agents. Like the ESCN, the cardiopathies elicited by deficiency in potassium, magnesium, or chloride consist primarily of more or less extensive and often multiple foci of myocardial necrosis, with little or no hyalinization. Usually, there is considerable calcium deposition in the coronary arteries (for literature see References 7 and 8).

Cardiopathies Caused by Antibiotics

Several antibiotics can induce necrotizing cardiopathies, both in experimental animals and in man. It has been shown that most experimental cardiopathies of this group are considerably aggravated by stress, if not wholly dependent upon concurrent conditioning with some strong stressor agent. A prototype of the antibiotic-induced necrotizing cardiopathy is that produced by neomycin plus stress, which has been the subject of particularly extensive studies in our Institute.[41, 42]

Cardiopathy Induced by Cardiac Glycosides

The fact that myocardial necroses can be produced with cardiac glycosides has long been known. The possible interrelations between corticoids, electrolytes, and cardiac glycosides have been discussed at some length in connection with the pathogenesis of the ESCN.[7]

The literature on the effect of digitoxin and deoxycorticosterone upon the structure and chemical composition of the heart has also been reviewed. It appears that the effect of these compounds upon the potassium content of the myocardium represents the principal connecting link between them.[43]

The Plasmocid Cardiopathy

Plasmocid (a rather toxic antimalarial agent no longer in clinical use) has been shown to induce large infarctoid myocardial necroses that are unaccompanied by any characteristic extracardiac manifestations such as nephrocalcinosis or hepatic necrosis.[7]

The Stress Cardiopathy

The stress cardiopathy consists of disseminated micronecroses induced by exposure to sudden intense stress, without any special conditioning.[8]

Ossification of the Heart Induced by Cardiac Ligature

Ossification can occur in inflamed connective tissue exposed to pressure. It was therefore thought that ossification might also be induced in the heart, if pressure were increased simultaneously with the induction of a large inflamed surface. To test this possibility, the lower third of both cardiac ventricles was tied off by a complete ligature in the rat. This operation regularly transforms the resulting apical scar into a cup-shaped bone having two laminae separated by diploë-like bone marrow. This is apparently a monocausal lesion, since only a single intervention was used to produce it, but it may well be pluricausal in that both scar formation and increased pressure are essential for its production.[44, 45]

Prevention of the Various Cardiopathies by Stress

Stress not only induces various cardiac lesions, but, when applied prophylactically, it can also protect the heart against diverse forms of injury.

Cardiopathies with Vascular Involvement

Stress neither elicits nor prevents the ESCH and the other forms of hyalinizing cardiopathies.[8] It also offers very little protection against the ESCC, although it can facilitate the induction of the characteristic lesions.[8]

The cardiovascular and renal calcification induced by acute or chronic overdosage of vitamin D compounds are only slightly influenced by pretreatment with various stressors,[46] whereas the stress of forced restraint is most effective in inhibiting the lesions induced by intoxication with parathyroid extract.[47, 48] This action seems to be independent of the adrenals, since it also occurs in adrenalectomized animals maintained with small doses of corticoids. Furthermore, pretreatment with various stressors on the day of sensitization inhibits the selective calcifications induced by local and systemic calciphylaxis.[2, 16]

Cardiopathies without Vascular Involvement

As previously noted, after conditioning with corticoids and sodium salts, sudden exposure to the stress of intense muscular exercise induces severe cardiac necroses (ESCN) and high mortality in the rat. If the animals are previously exposed to repeated short periods of stress, this same stressor subsequently fails to elicit the usual ESCN. Under identical conditions, the ESCN-producing effect of muscular exercise can be prevented by pretreatment with cold, that of cold by muscular exercise, that of noradrenaline by restraint, that of restraint by noradrenaline, and that of bone fracture by muscular exercise.[49] Pretreatment with stressor agents also inhibits the cardiopathies induced by plasmocid and proteolytic enzymes, such as papain.[50]

Prevention of Various Cardiopathies by Electrolytes

The concept that changes in ionic equilibrium play a decisive role in the pathogenesis of pluricausal experimental cardiopathies suggested that these lesions may be prevented by the administration of electrolytes which correct the changes induced by the various treatments.

Cardiopathies with Vascular Involvement

One of the most effective means of preventing the ESCH is treatment with the so-called "acidifying salts," particularly NH_4Cl and $CaCl_2$.[24] The ESCC, produced in the rat by corticoids plus calcium acetate plus stress, can be at least partially inhibited by oral administration of KCl or NH_4Cl, but the accompanying mortality remains uninfluenced and may even be increased.[7,8]

Among the other calcifying cardiopathies, those induced by overdosage of vitamin D compounds seem to be dependent upon uptake of calcium and phosphate from the diet.[51,52] Calciphylactic lesions are also highly dependent upon the oral uptake of calcium and phosphate.[53,54] The inhibition by potassium salts of the cardiac lesions induced by acute DHT or vitamin D_3 overdosage has recently been demonstrated.[55]

Certain preliminary experiments have suggested that KCl and $MgCl_2$ may protect the rat against necroses resulting from occlusion of coronary vessels, but this has not been confirmed in successive experiments.[56] Nevertheless, in the dog it was possible to prevent the same type of lesion by administration of glucose, potassium, and insulin.[57]

Cardiopathies without Vascular Involvement

During the course of the ESCN, the modification of electrolyte equilibrium seems to play a decisive role, as previously stated. This interpretation receives further confirmation from the fact that treatment with certain electrolytes can completely inhibit the development of the necrotic lesions.[7,8]

The ESCN (as well as accompanying nephrocalcinosis) can be inhibited not only by potassium-sparing agents (spironolactone, amiloride) and KCl but also by a variety of other potassium salts, although the chloride and nitrate appear to be the most effective. The ESCN can also be inhibited by a variety of chlorides, irrespective of the cation to which the chloride ion is attached. We can therefore conclude that potassium salts and, to a lesser extent, $MgCl_2$, are effective in protecting the myocardial cells against various forms of experimental cardiopathies.

Summary

After a brief outline of the pluricausal disease concept in general, its implications in experimental cardiology have received special consideration. Many examples are given to show that certain cardiopathies can be experimentally produced only by the simultaneous or appropriately spaced application of several agents; even at fatal dose levels, none of these factors exerts a similar effect by itself. It is assumed that the cardiac muscle possesses several alternative protective mechanisms, and, hence, certain morbid lesions develop only when all metabolic pathways of homeostasis are blocked.

Various qualitatively distinct forms of experimental pluricausal cardiopathies can be produced or prevented by appropriate combinations of stress, corticoids, and electrolytes. Special attention is given to the most recent observations on the production of cardiovascular lesions through calciphylaxis and the thrombohemorrhagic phenomenon, as well as the experimental induction of true bone formation in the heart.

It appears that essentially different cardiac lesions can be compounded at will by appropriate combinations of comparatively simple agents. Through this process of "pathosynthesis," we hope to gain insight into the elementary factors that constitute pathogenic situations for the heart.

References

1. Selye, H. 1966. Pluricausal diseases. Exp. Med. Surg. **24:** 191.
2. Selye, H. 1962. Calciphylaxis. University of Chicago Press. Chicago, Ill.
3. Selye, H. 1966. Thrombohemorrhagic Phenomena. Charles C Thomas, Publ. Springfield, Ill.
4. Selye, H., P. Rohan & U. S. Pahk. 1966. Humoral conditioning for necrosis. Part I. The conditioning factors. Naunyn. Schmiedeberg. Arch. Exp. Path. **255:** 133.
5. Selye, H. & P. Rohan. 1966. Humoral conditioning for necrosis. Part. II. The challenges. Naunyn. Schmiedeberg. Arch. Exp. Path. **255:** 142.
6. Selye, H. 1950. Stress. Acta Inc. Montreal, Canada.
7. Selye, H. 1958. The Chemical Prevention of Cardiac Necroses. The Ronald Press Co. New York, N. Y.
8. Selye, H. 1961. The Pluricausal Cardiopathies. Charles C Thomas, Publ. Springfield, Ill.
9. Selye, H. & G. Gabbiani. 1966. Fragen der Elektrolyte, des Stress und der Herznekrose. *In* Lehrbuch der speziellen pathologischen Anatomie. Kaufmann & Staemmler, Eds. 11th–12th edit. **1** (Suppl.): part 1, 1–57.
10. Selye, H., K. Nielsen & B. Tuchweber. 1965. An experimental obliterating thromboangiitis limited to the posterior part of the body. Thromb. Diath. Haemorrh. **14:** 184.
11. Michon, P., G. Rauber, A. Larcan & P. Vert. 1959. Endomyofibrose de myocardique. Sem. Hop. Paris **35:** 3301.
12. Rona, G., C. I. Chappel, T. Balazs & R. Gaudry. 1959. The effect of breed, age, and sex on myocardial necrosis produced by isoproterenol in the rat. J. Geront. **14:** 169.
13. Rona, G., C. I. Chappel & R. Gaudry. 1959. Relationship between thyroid function and cardiotoxic properties of isoproterenol. Montreal Physiol. Soc. Meet., March 6. : 17.
14. Selye, H., E. Bajusz & R. Veilleux. 1960. Production of dissecting aneurysms by chronic isoproterenol treatment. Cor Vasa **2:** 273.
15. Tuchweber, B., G. Gabbiani & H. Selye. 1964. Humoral production of mural and ball thrombi in the cardiac cavities. Angiologica (Basel) **1:** 49.
16. Gabbiani, G. & J. M. Rojo Ortega. 1964. Stress et calciphylaxie. Path. Biol. (Paris) **12:** 192.
17. Gabbiani, G., B. Tuchweber & H. Selye. 1964. A calciphylactic dermatosis produced by histamine liberators. J. Invest. Derm. **42:** 49.
18. Grasso, S. & H. Selye. 1962. Calciphylaxis in relation to the humoral production of occlusive coronary lesions with infarction. J. Path. Bact. **83:** 495.
19. Gabbiani, G. & B. Tuchweber. 1963. The role of iron in the mechanism of experimental calcification. J. Histochem. Cytochem. **11:** 799.
20. Selye, H. & L. Savoie. 1967. Calciphylaxie der Gefässe. Zbl. Chir. **92:** 1493.
21. Selye, H., P. Prioreschi & M. Cantin. 1961. Factors that determine the production of cardiovascular and renal lesions by polymyxin. Antibiot. Chemother. (Basel) **11:** 12.
22. Jasmin, G. & P. Bois. 1958. Histogenesis and prevention of gastric ulcers induced by a histamine releaser 48/80. Montreal Physiol. Soc. Meet., March 7. : 4.
23. Lehr, D., I. Wajda & M. Krukowski. 1957. Pathogenesis of cardiovascular necrosis induced by nephrectomy. Fed. Proc. **16:** 316.

24. Toussaint, C. 1952. Les modifications pathologiques provoquées par l'ischemie partielle du rein, l'hydronephrose bilatérale et la néphrectomie totale chez la rat intact et chez le rat surrénalectomisé. Rev. Belg. Path. **21**: 465.
25. Selye, H. & R. Strebel. 1962. Prevention by calciphylaxis of the progeria-like syndrome induced by chronic dihydrotachysterol overdosage. Proc. Soc. Exp. Biol. Med. **110**: 673.
26. Selye, H., R. Strebel & L. Mikulaj. 1963. A progeria-like syndrome produced by dihydrotachysterol and its prevention by methyltestosterone and ferric dextran. J. Amer. Geriat. Soc. **11**: 1.
27. Eisenstein, R. & L. Zeruolis. 1964. Vitamin D-induced aortic calcification. Arch. Path. (Chicago) **77**: 27.
28. Hass, G. M., R. E. Trueheart, C. B. Taylor & M. Stumpe. 1958. An experimental histologic study of hypervitaminosis D. Amer. J. Path. **34**: 395.
29. Selye, H., E. Bajusz, S. Grasso & P. Mendell. 1960. Simple techniques for the surgical occlusion of coronary vessels in the rat. Angiology **11**: 398.
30. Renaud, S. & C. Allard. 1962. Thrombosis in connection with serum lipidic changes in the rat. Circ. Res. **11**: 388.
31. Thomas, W. A., W. S. Hartroft & R. M. O'Neal. 1959. Modification of diets responsible for induction of coronary thromboses and myocardial infarcts in rats. J. Nutr. **69**: 325.
32. Thomas, W. A., W. S. Hartroft & R. M. O'Neal. 1960. Myocardial infarction in man and experimental animals. A.M.A. Arch. Path. **69**: 104.
33. Gabbiani, G. 1964. Sensitization by stress for renal lesions resembling those of generalized Shwartzman phenomenon. Med. Exp. (Basel) **11**: 209.
34. Selye, H. & S. Grasso. 1961. Chemical production of myocardial necrosis with vascular occlusion. Brit. J. Exp. Path. **42**: 564.
35. Selye, H. & B. Tuchweber. 1964. Ein durch verschiedene Agenzien erzeugbares thrombohämorrhagisches Phänomen. Allerg. Asthma (Leipzig) **10**: 335.
36. Myasnikov, A. L. 1964. Myocardial necroses of coronary and noncoronary genesis. Amer. J. Cardiol. **13**: 435.
37. Spain, D. M. & V. A. Bradess. 1960. Frequency of coronary thrombi as related to duration of survival from onset of acute fatal episodes of myocardial ischemia. Circulation **22**: 816.
38. Nielsen, K., S. Renaud, Y. Lemire & H. Selye. 1958. "Fuchsinophilic degeneration" of myocardial fibers. Proc. Canad. Fed. Biol. Soc., Kingston, June 9–11. : 37.
39. Poley, R. W., C. D. Fobes & M. J. Hall. 1964. Fuchsinophilia in early myocardial infarction. Arch. Path. (Chicago) **77**: 325.
40. D'Agostino, A. N. 1964. An electron microscopic study of cardiac necrosis produced by 9α-fluorocortisol and sodium phosphate. Amer. J. Path. **45**: 633.
41. Renaud, S. 1960. The potentiating effect of tumors on neomycin toxicity. Arzneimittelforschung **10**: 566.
42. Selye, H., E. Bajusz, S. Renaud & M. Nadasi. 1960. Progrès récents dans l'étude de la pathogénie et de la prophylaxie des nécroses cardiaques. Ars Med. (Gand) **15**: 831.
43. Kyser, F. A., H. Teloh & G. C. Sutton. 1959. The effect of digitalis and desoxycorticosterone acetate administration upon intracellular potassium ion concentration. A chemical and morphologic study. J. Lab. Clin. Med. **53**: 216.
44. Selye, H., S. Grasso & G. Gentile. 1961. Surgically induced ossification of the heart. Eksp. Khir. No. **6**: 22.
45. Selye, H., R. Mahajan & S. Mahajan. 1967. Histogenesis of experimentally induced myositis ossificans in the heart. Amer. Heart J. **73**: 195.
46. Selye, H., P. Jean & E. Bajusz. 1961. Résistance croisée et prévention des cardiopathies expérimentales produites par un dérivé de la vitamine D. Path. Biol (Paris) **9**: 331.
47. Selye, H., G. Gabbiani & B. Tuchweber. 1964. Protection by restraint against parathyroid extract intoxication in absence of the adrenals. Amer. J. Physiol. **207**: 573.
48. Selye, H., B. Tuchweber & G. Gabbiani. 1964. Protection by restraint against parathyroid hormone intoxication. Acta Endocr. (Kobenhavn) **43** (Suppl. 90): 203.
49. Bajusz, E. & H. Selye. 1960. Adaptation to the cardiac necrosis-eliciting effect of stress. Amer. J. Physiol. **199**: 453.
50. Selye, H. & E. Bajusz. 1961. Protection afforded by stress against humorally induced cardiac necroses. *In* D. Sodi-Pallares' Memorial Vol., Cardiologia. : 359. Editorial Interamericana. Mexico City, Mexico.

51. HARRIS, L. J. & J. R. M. INNES. 1931. The mode of action of Vitamin D. Studies on the hypervitaminosis D. The influence of the calcium-phosphate intake. J. Biochem. **25:** 367.
52. TUCHWEBER, B. 1965. Studies on a Progeria-like Syndrome. Thesis. University of Montreal. Montreal, Canada.
53. GABBIANI, G. & B. TUCHWEBER. 1965. Influence of exogenous calcium on calciphylaxis and calcergy. Proc. Soc. Exp. Biol. Med. **119:** 24.
54. JEAN, P. & D. DESAULNIERS. 1965. Prevention of cutaneous calciphylaxis in calcium-deficient rats. Canad. J. Physiol. Pharmacol. **43:** 235.
55. PRIORESCHI, P. 1964. Protection of the myocardium by potassium. Exp. Med. Surg. **22:** 60.
56. BAJUSZ, E. & H. SELYE. 1960. The chemical prevention of cardiac necroses following occlusion of coronary vessels. Canad. Med. Ass. J. **82:** 212.
57. SODI-PALLARES, D., A. BISTENI, G. A. MEDRANO, M. R. TESTELLI & A. DEMICHELI. 1963. The polarizing treatment of acute myocardial infarction. Possibility of its use in other cardiovascular conditions. Dis. Chest. **43:** 424.

STUDIES ON THE "NONSPECIFIC MESENCHYMAL REACTION" AND THE "TRANSIT ZONE" IN MYOCARDIAL LESIONS AND ATHEROSCLEROSIS

W. H. Hauss, U. Gerlach, G. Junge-Hülsing, H. Themann, and W. Wirth

Medical Clinic of the Westfalian Wilhelm University
Münster, Germany

Nonspecific Mesenchymal Reaction

For the past few years, we in Münster have studied the effect of external stimulation on mesenchymal metabolism by clinical observations and animal experiments. We use the term "mesenchyme" to denote the system of cells which produce ground substance and fibers and which are present in all organs. In addition to its structural and supporting function, the mesenchyme has other important tasks, particularly in the metabolic exchange between the capillary lumen and the parenchymal cells and in the defense reaction against irritating factors.

We have studied changes in mesenchymal metabolism primarily by the determination of ^{35}S-sulfate incorporation into the sulfomucopolysaccharides (SMPS) of the mesenchymal ground substance.[1-10] It should be noted that sulfate incorporation into SMPS is not the only metabolic function affected by alterations in mesenchymal metabolism; tests with ^{14}C-proline, ^{14}C-leucine, ^{3}H-leucine, ^{3}H-cytidine, and ^{14}C-acetate have demonstrated that the synthesis of collagen, cell protein, ribonucleic acid (RNA), fatty acids, and cholesterol are also affected.

It is of fundamental significance in the pathogenesis of myocardial necrosis and atherosclerosis that the mesenchymal metabolism is extremely sensitive to external stimulation.[7, 8, 11-19] Figure 1 shows the effect of an intraperitoneal (i.p.) injection of endotoxin (pyrexal) on the mesenchymal metabolism of the heart, as reflected by the rate of ^{35}S-sulfate incorporation into the SMPS of the ground substance. There is a distinct acceleration in the metabolism, which returns toward normal after a short period of time. This acceleration of metabolism has been observed in thousands of tests as the regular response of the mesenchyme to miscellaneous nonspecific stimuli; we have therefore termed it the "nonspecific mesenchymal reaction."[16, 17, 20] Table 1 lists various irritating factors capable of stimulating this reaction. The role of the nonspecific mesenchymal reaction in producing reactive diseases is discussed elsewhere.[20a]

An i.p. injection of a small dose of pyrexal stimulates a nonspecific mesenchymal reaction of minor degree, without functional or structural damage to the tissues. However, when a large dose is administered, or when several stimuli are applied, the mesenchymal metabolism is disturbed to an excessive degree, and morphological changes take place in the tissues. For example, an intracutaneous (i.c.) injection of pyrexal results in a moderate mesenchymal reaction in the injection area. If, at the time of maximum metabolic acceleration after the first injection, a second dose of pyrexal is given i.p., an extraordinary rise in the metabolism of the injection area is produced (Figure 2), and tissue necrosis results. This effect is known as the "addition phenomenon."[17, 21]

The addition phenomenon appears to play an important role in the production of structural changes, especially those found in heart muscle necrosis and atherosclerosis. (Figure 3 shows the severe mesenchymal reaction produced by a combination of fatty diet and shock. FIGURE 4 shows the effect of combined stress and fatty diet.[22, 23] The significance of the nonspecific mesenchymal reaction within heart muscle and vascular wall in the pathogenesis of myocardial necrosis and atherosclerosis[8, 11, 14, 18-20, 22, 24-28] will be discussed in the following sections.

MYOCARDIAL NECROSES

It is well known that myocardial necroses can be produced in rats by the application of various stress factors.[29-34] TABLE 2 lists the stress methods by which necroses were produced in our laboratory in order to study their patho-

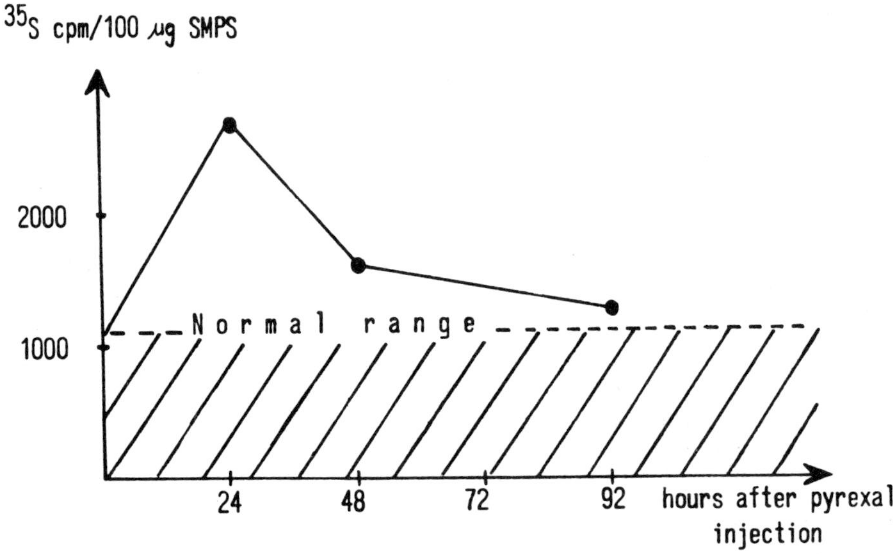

FIGURE 1. Time course of the nonspecific mesenchymal reaction after i.p. injection of pyrexal in a guinea pig heart, as reflected by the ^{35}S-sulfate incorporation into the SMPS of the ground substance.

TABLE 1

IRRITATING FACTORS CAPABLE OF STIMULATING A NONSPECIFIC MESENCHYMAL REACTION AS REFLECTED BY INCREASED INCORPORATION OF ^{35}S-SULFATE INTO SMPS OF CONNECTIVE TISSUE GROUND SUBSTANCE IN ANIMAL EXPERIMENTS

Type of Stimulus	Example
Infection	*Pasteurella multocidum,* staphylococci
Toxins	Pyrexal, staphylococcus or diphtheria toxin
Lack of oxygen	Hypobaric chamber (7,000 m altitude = 20,000 ft)
Foreign proteins	Bovine serum albumin injections
Mechanical irritation	Muscle trauma
Elevated blood pressure	Decreased blood supply to kidneys
Fat overfeeding	Force feeding by stomach tube
Climatic influences	Abrupt changes in atmospheric pressure
Overstrain	Exhaustive running in a running cage
Allergic reactions	Serum injections, Arthus phenomenon
Heterologous materials	Croton oil, plastics
Cerebral alterations	Electrical irritation of thalamus

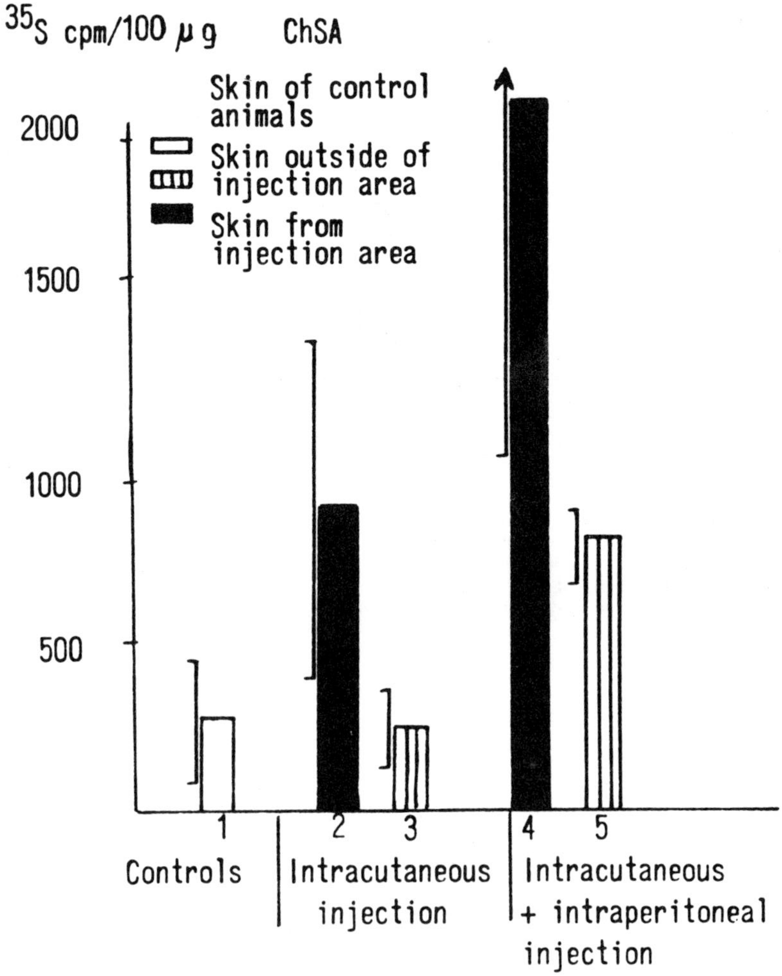

FIGURE 2. Production of the addition phenomenon in rabbit skin by two subsequent injections of pyrexal.

genesis.[14, 24, 26] We wanted to find out how these necroses occur and at what point the injurious agents that were applied produce this effect. There appear to be three possibilities, as shown in FIGURE 5.

Myocardial Necrosis due to Obstruction in the Blood Vessels

If substrates and/or oxygen are transported inadequately by the blood vessels, extreme coronary insufficiency can cause the metabolism of the myocardial fibers to succumb. This phenomenon is frequently observed after coronary artery occlusion in man.

Myocardial Necrosis due to Malfunction of the Intracellular Metabolism

The metabolism of the heart cells may be impaired by the injurious agents to such a great extent[29] that necrosis of the heart muscle results.

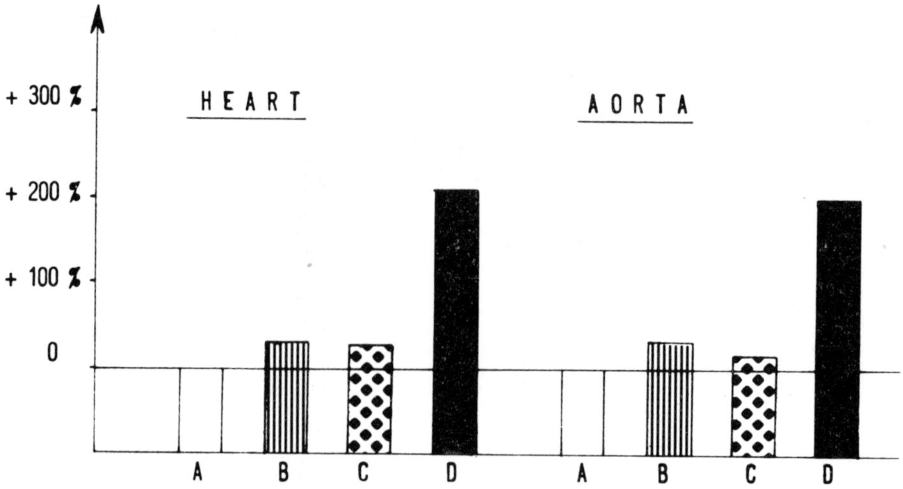

FIGURE 3. The addition phenomenon in the mesenchymal metabolism of guinea pig heart and aorta, as reflected by ^{35}S-sulfate incorporation into the SMPS of the connective tissue ground substance. A = control animals; B = protracted serum shock; C = feeding by stomach tube twice daily of 0.14 g of cholesterol in 2 ml of olive oil; D = combination of protracted serum shock and feeding by stomach tube of the fat mixture.

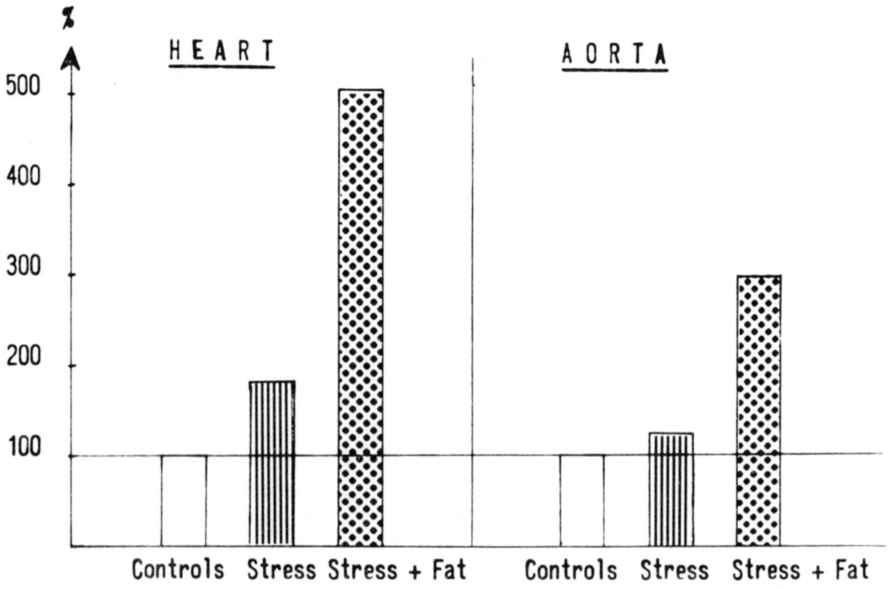

FIGURE 4. Effect of stress plus normal feeding and stress plus fat overfeeding for seven months on the addition phenomenon in the mesenchymal metabolism of the aorta and heart in a rat, as reflected by ^{35}S-sulfate incorporation into the SMPS of connective tissue.

TABLE 2

METHODS OF PRODUCING MYOCARDIAL NECROSIS IN RATS BY STRESS

Type of Stress	Example*
Overstrain	Exhaustive running in a running cage, for five hours at 5 m per minute
Restraining of activity	Complete motor restriction in narrow wire cages over a 5 m per minute
Toxin injection	0.1 ml of staphylococcus toxin i.p., once every three weeks
Electrical irritation	Treatment with low-voltage twitches in cages with metal bars on the ground, for 90 minutes with 25 impulses per minute at 12 volts
Fat overfeeding	Force feeding of an olive oil-cholesterol mixture by stomach tube

* Each method used once a week, unless otherwise noted.

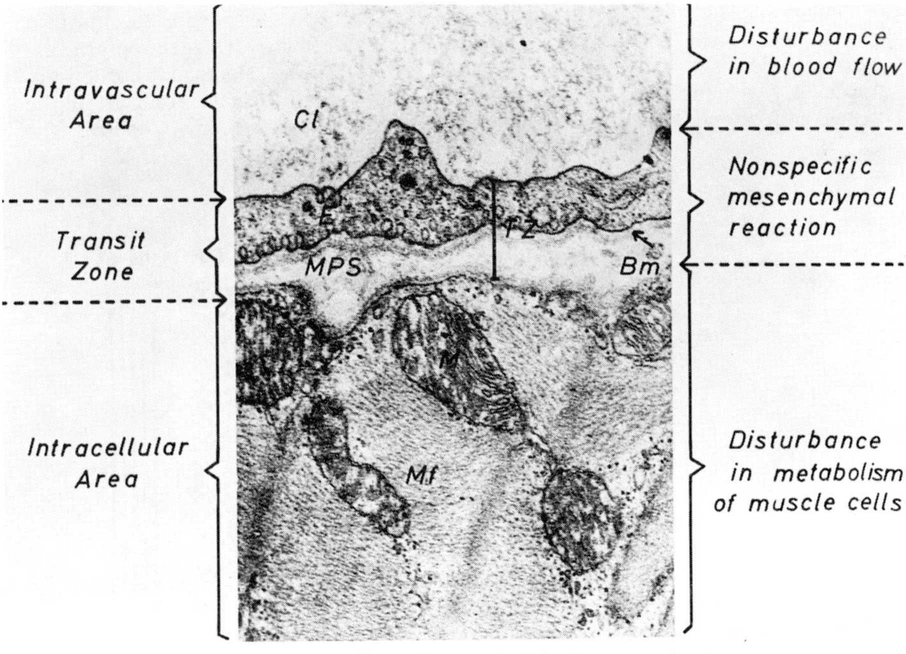

FIGURE 5. Electron photomicrograph of the heart muscle of a rat.

Myocardial Necrosis due to a Block in the Transit Zone

It is possible that damage may occur in the zone between the capillary lumen and the heart muscle fiber; we have named this area the "transit zone."[11, 14, 17, 20, 24, 26] The transit zone consists of the endothelium seam (produced by mesenchymal cells) and the ground substance, in which isolated fibers are interspersed throughout. As noted previously, the metabolism of the ground substance, measured by the rate of incorporation of ^{35}S-sulfate into SMPS, is extremely sensitive to external stimulation.

It is our opinion that irritating factors act on the transit zone: (1) by changing its SMPS metabolism, (2) by damaging its function, and (3) by destroying its structure.

Changing the Metabolism of the Transit Zone. When rats are exposed to stress factors (TABLE 2), the mesenchymal metabolism changes rapidly, even before signs of muscle necrosis appear. This was shown by a measurement of ^{35}S-sulfate incorporation into SMPS of the ground substance (FIGURE 6). During the period of distinct metabolic acceleration, there was no evidence of alterations in the muscle cells.

Damaging the Function of the Transit Zone. The application of stress factors alters the permeability of the transit zone. If normal rats are given intravenous (i.v.) injections of ferritin, it takes 30 minutes for the large ferritin molecules to enter the heart muscle from the capillary. Prior to that time, the ferritin can be found only in the plasma. However, when rats under stress are injected with ferritin, the ferritin can be found in the heart muscle after two minutes; this is a sign that the membrane function has suffered considerable damage, allowing large molecules to pass rapidly through the transit zone.

Destroying the Structure of the Transit Zone. After exposure to injurious agents, the transit zone shows considerable change in structure before the heart muscle cells show any signs of degeneration on electron photomicrographs, e.g. swelling of the mitochondria, loss of the double contour in the cristae mitochondriales, or degeneration of the fibers. FIGURE 7 shows the

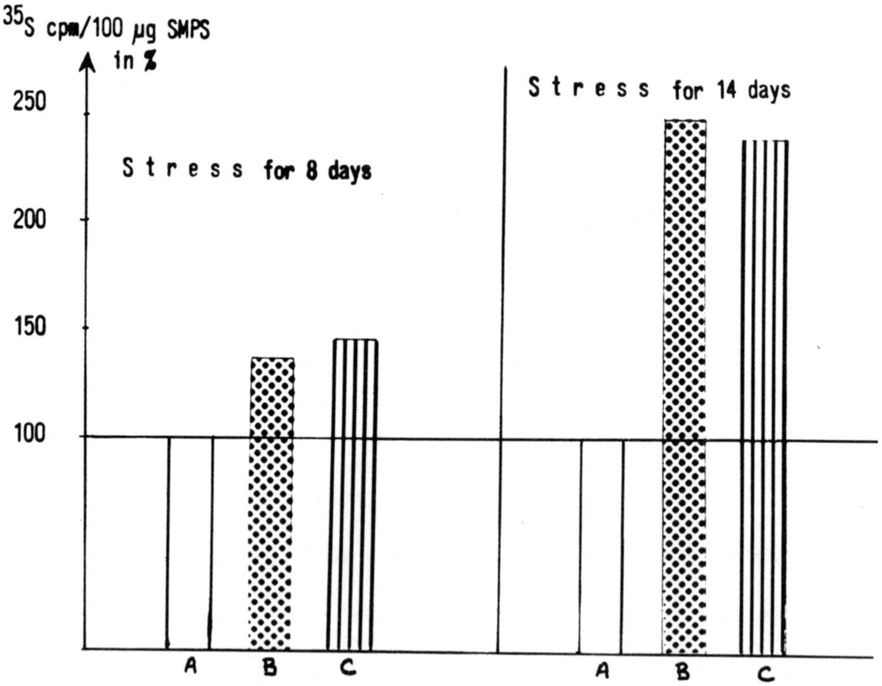

FIGURE 6. Acceleration of the mesenchymal metabolism by stress, as reflected by ^{35}S-sulfate incorporation into the SMPS of the connective tissue of heart and aorta. A = control animals; B = heart; C = aorta (after stress).

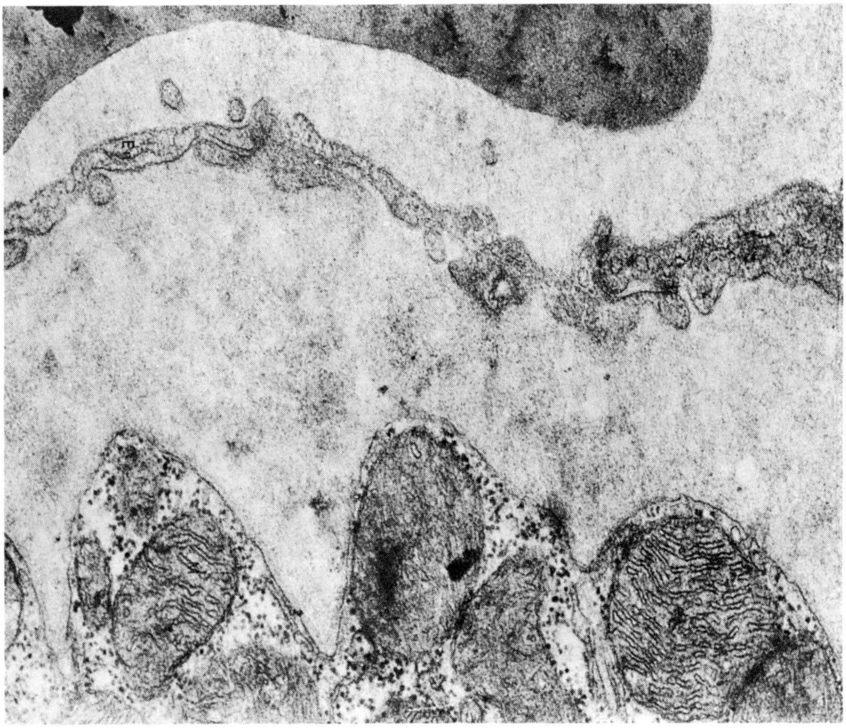

FIGURE 7. Enlargement and condensation of the SMPS in the transit zone.

enlargement and condensation of the SMPS in the transit zone after exposure to stress. FIGURE 8 shows enlargement of the transit zone after injection of toxin by a special technique. FIGURE 9 shows severe deformation of the transit zone, with formation of many endothelial evaginations. FIGURE 10 shows complete destruction of the transit zone, with extravasation of blood plasma into the transit zone and the cell compartments.

On the basis of our experiments, we believe that heart muscle necroses produced by various injurious agents are caused by the nonspecific mesenchymal reaction, which damages the transit zones of the heart muscle capillaries. Thus, the transport of substrates and oxygen is disturbed to the extent that secondary necrosis develops.

ATHEROSCLEROSIS

The effect of irritating factors on the transit zone of the heart muscle is also apparent on the transit zone of the blood vessels. The histology of the arterial wall is such that seepage can occur from the arterial lumen *and* from the lumen of the arterial wall capillaries, with a transit zone in each case. Any severe change in the mesenchymal metabolism will result in a disturbance of the transport of substrates through these transit zones. It is our opinion that mesenchymal metabolic disturbance in the transit zone is the initial step necessary in the development of atherosclerosis.

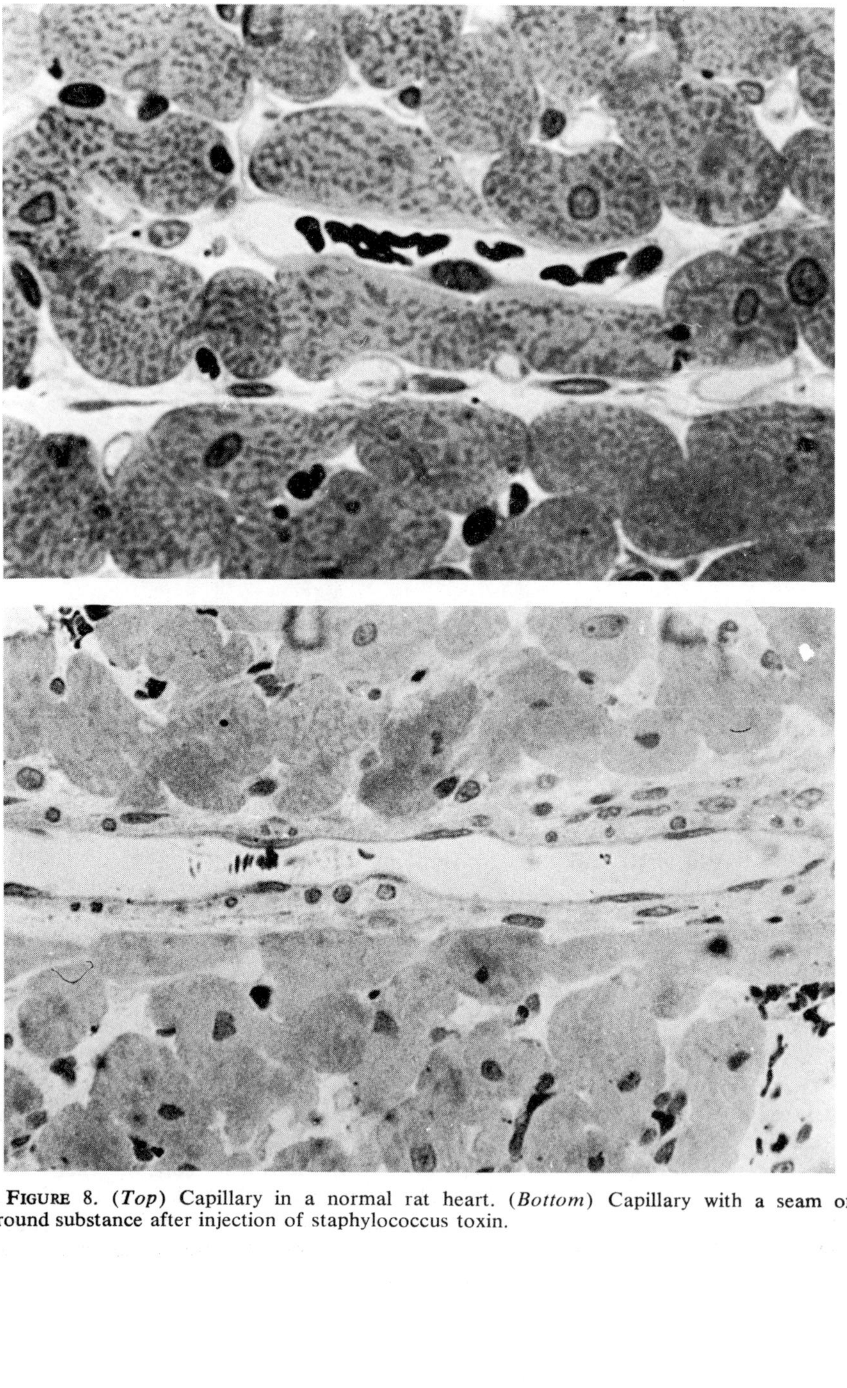

Figure 8. (*Top*) Capillary in a normal rat heart. (*Bottom*) Capillary with a seam of ground substance after injection of staphylococcus toxin.

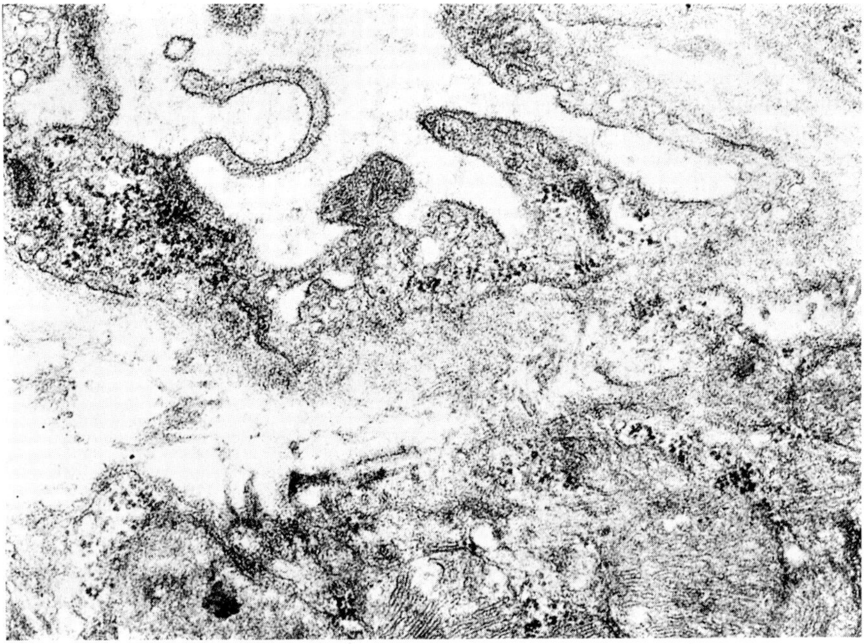

FIGURE 9. Deformation of the transit zone, with marked endothelial evaginations.

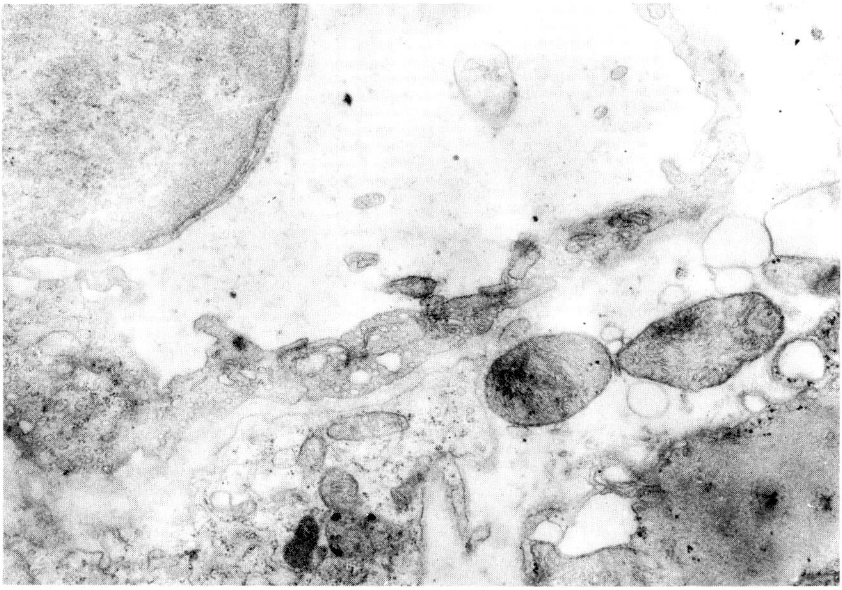

FIGURE 10. Complete destruction of the transit zone, with extravasation of blood plasma into the transit zone and the cell compartments.

It is well known that atherosclerosis may be induced in the blood vessel walls of animals by various experimental procedures. The measurement of ^{35}S-sulfate turnover in the atherosclerotic aorta shows an acceleration of the SMPS metabolism.[11, 15, 18-20, 22, 28] This acceleration of the ^{35}S-sulfate incorporation is noticeable before the histology of the vessel wall shows any sign of pathological change (FIGURE 11). In fact, changes appear only after about two weeks, at which point the ^{35}S-sulfate incorporation into SMPS is still accelerated, although to a lesser degree. As shown in FIGURE 11, the half-life time of ^{35}S-SMPS is also shortened in the atherosclerotic aorta. The result of the nonspecific mesenchymal reaction, which is produced by irritation of the vessel wall, is demonstrable with autoradiographic methods. FIGURE 11

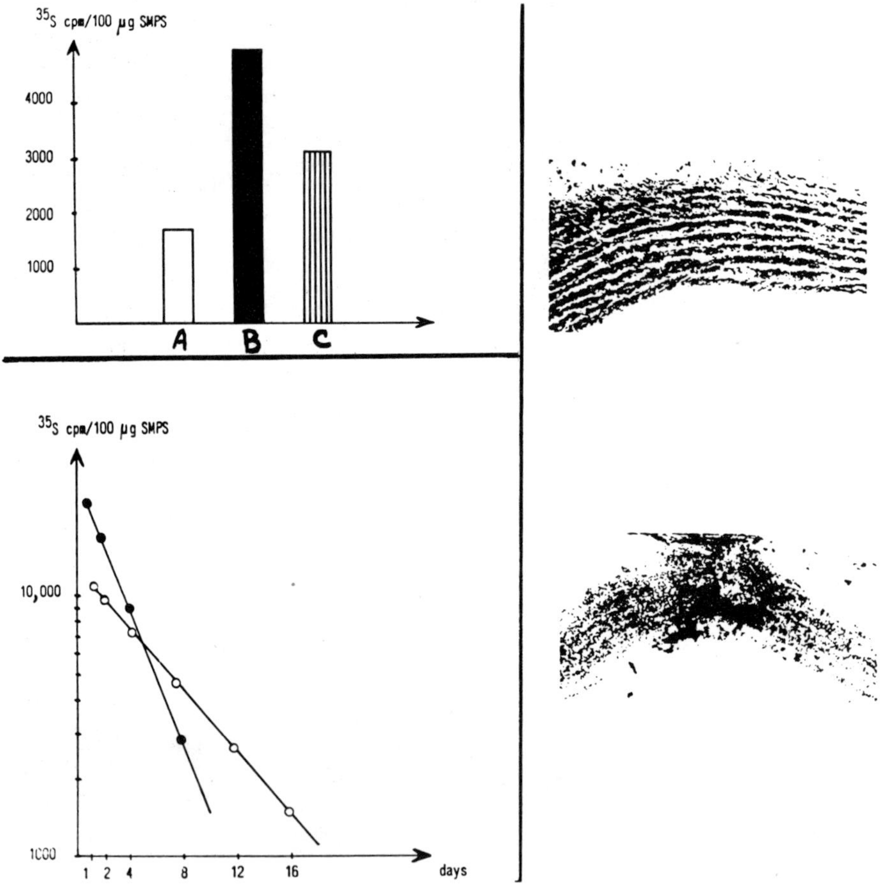

FIGURE 11. Changes in mesenchymal metabolism in experimental atherosclerosis of rats. (*Top left*) Incorporation of ^{35}S-sulfate into SMPS of aortic connective tissue. A = control animals; B = experimental atherosclerosis, early stage with no histological changes; C = experimental atherosclerosis, late stage with remarkable histological changes. (*Bottom left*) Turnover rate of ^{35}S-labeled SMPS in the aorta. ○ = normal aorta, half-life time of seven to eight days; ● = atherosclerotic aorta, half-life time of three to four days. (*Right*) Autoradiographs of ^{35}S-labeled SMPS in the normal (top) and atherosclerotic (bottom) aorta.

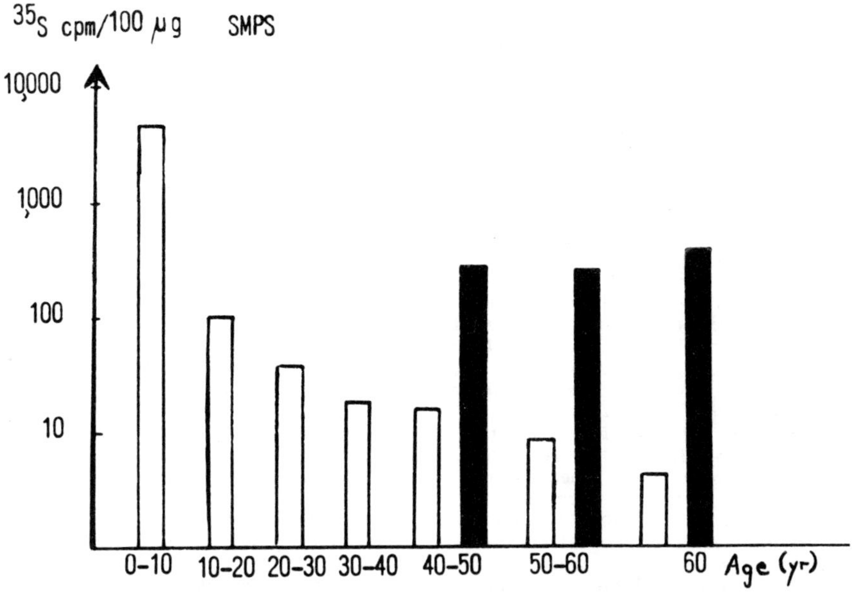

FIGURE 12. Changes in mesenchymal metabolism of the human aorta in atherosclerosis, as reflected by ^{35}S-sulfate incorporation into the SMPS of the connective tissue (incubation assays). □ = normal aorta (n = 68); ■ = atherosclerotic aorta (n = 52).

(right side) shows the fine septal structure of the wall of a normal aorta in an autoradiograph with ^{35}S-sulfate. The disturbance of the mesenchymal metabolism in an atherosclerotic aorta is shown by the disappearance of the normal structure.

It should be noted that human atherosclerosis is also accompanied by an acceleration of the mesenchymal metabolism. We have measured the ^{35}S-sulfate turnover in human aortic strips and confirmed that mesenchymal metabolism in the atherosclerotic aorta was invariably higher than in histologically normal aorta (FIGURE 12).

SUMMARY

On the basis of clinical observations and statistical surveys, it seems probable that the development of coronary sclerosis and myocardial infarction is influenced by many factors,[35] especially the so-called risk factors.[36] We believe that the nonspecific mesenchymal reaction to injurious factors causes a block in the transit zones of the myocardium and the coronary artery wall which results in coronary sclerosis, myocardial necroses, and myocardial infarctions.

REFERENCES

1. BOSTRÖM, H. 1952. J. Biol. Chem. **196:** 477.
2. BOSTRÖM, H. 1960. *In* 2nd Symp. Med. Klin. Münster. Struktur und Stoffwechsel des Bindegewebes. : 20. Georg Thieme. Stuttgart, Germany.
3. DZIEWIATKOWSKI, D. D. 1956. J. Biol. Chem. **223:** 239.
4. DZIEWIATKOWSKI, D. D. 1953. J. Exp. Med. **98:** 119.
5. DZIEWIATKOWSKI, D. D., R. E. BENESCH & R. BENESCH. 1949. J. Biol. Chem. **178:** 931.

6. Dziewiatkowski, D. D. 1945. J. Biol. Chem. **161:** 723.
7. Junge-Hulsing, G. 1959. Z. Rheumaforsch. **18:** 355.
8. Junge-Hulsing, G. 1965. Untersuchungen zur Pathophysiologie des Bindegewebes. A. Hüthig, Ed. Heidelberg, Germany.
9. Lipmann, F. 1945. J. Biol. Chem. **160:** 173.
10. Schiller, S., M. B. Mathews, H. Jefferson, J. Ludowieg & A. Dorfman. 1954. J. Biol. Chem. **211:** 717.
11. Hauss, W. H. 1965. Uber Arteriosklerose und Herzinfarkt. Jahrbuch 1965 des Landesamtes für Forschung des Landes Nordrhein Westfalen.
12. Hauss, W. H. 1964. Her-Kreislauf und Emotion. Muskel und Psyche, Symp., Wien, 1963. : 155–166. S. Karger. Basel, Switzerland.
13. Hauss, W. H., U. Gerlach & G. Junge-Hulsing. 1965. Med. et Hygiene. No. 677. **23:** 208–209.
14. Hauss, W. H. & G. Junge-Hulsing. 1964. In Hochdruckforschung-, Fortschritte auf dem Gebiet der Inneren Medizin. II. Symp. Freiburg, July, 1964. : 125. J. Heilmeyer & H. J. Holtmeier, Eds. Georg Thieme. Stuttgart, Germany.
15. Hauss, W. H. & G. Junge-Hulsing. 1963. Modifications du métabolismé de l'acide chondroitine sulfurique observées dans différentes conditions. Exp. Ann. Biochim. Med. **25**.
16. Hauss, W. H. & G. Junge-Hulsing. 1961. Deutsch. Med. Wschr. **86:** 763.
17. Hauss, W. H., G. Junge-Hulsing, U. Gerlach & W. Wirth. 1965. *In* Stoffwechsel und degenerativer Rheumatismus. V. R. Ott, Ed. (Der Rheumatismus Bd. 36) Verlag. Darmstadt, Germany.
18. Hauss, W. H., G. Junge-Hulsing & F. Konig. 1962. Med. Welt No. **45:** 2371.
19. Hauss, W. H., G. Junge-Hulsing & F. Konig. 1963. Med. Welt No. **3:** 125.
20. Hauss, W. H. 1963. Verh. Deutsch. Ges. Inn. Med. **69:** 554.
20a. Hauss, W. H., U. Junge-Hulsing & G. Gerlich. 1968. Die Unoperifische Mesenchymreaktion. Georg Thieme. Stuttgart, Germany.
21. Hauss, W. H., G. Junge-Hulsing, W. Wirth & H. J. Albrecht. 1962. Z. ges. exp. Med. **135:** 384.
22. Hauss, W. H., G. Junge-Hulsing & H. J. Hollander. 1962. J. Atheroscler. Res. **2:** 50.
23. Hauss, W. H., G. Junge-Hulsing, K. J. Matthes & W. Wirth. 1965. J. Atheroscler. Res. **5:** 451–465.
24. Hauss, W. H. 1964. Verh. Deutsch. Ges. Kreislaufforsch. **30:** 153–168.
25. Hauss, W. H. 1963. Nauheimer Fortbildungslehrgange **28:** 141–153.
26. Hauss, W. H., G. Junge-Hulsing, H. Thermann & J. Unruh. 1965. Z. Alternsforsch. **18:** 218.
27. Hauss, W. H., G. Junge-Hulsing, H. Wehmeyer, H. Zumkley, F. Konig & H. Losse. 1964. Med. Welt No. **12:** 587.
28. Junge-Hulsing, G. 1966. Deutsche Therapiewoche (Karlsruhe, 1965) **16:** 485.
29. Bajusz, E. 1963. Conditioning Factors for Cardiac Necroses. S. Karger. Basel, Switzerland.
30. Raab, W., J. P. Chaplin & E. Bajusz. 1964. Proc. Soc. Exp. Biol. Med. **116:** 665–669.
31. Raab, W. 1963. Amer. Heart J. **66:** 685–706.
32. Selye, H. 1950. Stress. Acta, Inc. Montreal, Canada.
33. Selye, H. & E. Bajusz. 1958. Schweiz. Med. Wschr. **88:** 1147.
34. Selye, H. 1966. Thrombohemorrhagic Phenomena. Charles C Thomas, Publ. Springfield, Ill.
35. Hauss, W. H. 1954. Angina Pectoris. Georg Thieme, Stuttgart, Germany.
36. Kannes, W. B., T. R. Dawber, A. Kagan, N. Revotskie & J. Stokes. 1961. Ann. Intern. Med. **55:** 33–50.

REGIONAL DISTRIBUTION OF CATECHOLAMINES IN THE HEARTS OF VARIOUS SPECIES*

E. T. Angelakos, M. P. King, and R. W. Millard
Department of Physiology, Boston University School of Medicine, Boston, Mass.

It is well known that the heart has extensive afferent and efferent innervation. In fact, the density of nerve elements is so extensive that it is more appropriate to consider the heart a neuromuscular organ. Cardiac innervation has been studied in the past with silver impregnation and other nonspecific nerve-staining techniques (Nonidez, 1943; Tcheng, 1951; Mitchell, 1956; Hirsch, 1963; Hirsch *et al.*, 1963), and more recently with electron microscopical methods (Torri, 1962; Rossi, 1963; Napolitano *et al.*, 1964). Unfortunately, none of these techniques provided a reliable differentiation between the various nerve elements. Thus, in the past, the distinction between sensory, sympathetic, and parasympathetic elements was dependent on rather cumbersome studies involving observations following selective denervation.

Recently, it became possible to study with considerable percision the distribution of one of the neural elements, the sympathetic adrenergic fibers, with specific biochemical and histochemical techniques. Using this approach, the regional distribution of adrenergic innervation of the heart has been studied in a variety of species. A brief review of the key observations made at our laboratory to date appears pertinent at this time.

Basic Questions

Using a combination of the chemical and histochemical approaches, it should be possible to provide answers to some of the basic questions that have been raised in connection with the regional distribution of catecholamines in the heart. Pertinent questions are: (1) What is the distribution of the naturally occurring catecholamines in each part of the heart, and which catecholamine is predominant? (2) What is the relative density of the adrenergic nerve terminals in various parts of the heart, especially in such areas as the sino-auricular node (SAN) and atrioventricular node (AVN)? (3) Are there any catecholamine-containing structures in the heart other than the adrenergic nerve terminals? (4) What is the relationship between cardiac muscle fibers and adrenergic terminals, and what is the mean diffusion distance for the released neurohumor? (5) What is the estimated intraneuronal concentration of catecholamines?

Analytical and Histochemical Methods

The methods used include spectrofluorometric analyses and fluorescence histochemistry. Each of the naturally occurring catecholamines (dopamine, noradrenaline, and adrenaline) was determined spectrofluorometrically in each specific region of the heart. For noradrenaline and adrenaline, the procedure outlined by von Euler and Lishajko (1961) was used. This involves adsorption on alumina followed by oxidation with FeSCN. In general, available methodology permits the specific and accurate determination of noradrenaline and

* The work reviewed here was supported by United States National Science Foundation grants nos. BG-1754 and BG-4386, and National Heart Institute, United States Public Health Service grants nos. HE-05680, HE-09616, and career development award no. K3-HE-15457.

adrenaline in quantities as low as 0.01 μg, and the separation of these two amines when present in ratios as high as 10:1. Dopamine was determined according to the procedure outlined by Carlsson and Weldek (1958). As little as 0.1 μg. of dopamine may be detected with this method.

Histochemically, the Falck-Hillarp technique (Falck, 1962; Falck *et al.*, 1962) has been used for microscopical studies of the distribution of catecholamine-containing structures in the heart (Angelakos *et al.*, 1963; Dahlstrom *et al.*, 1965). This technique is based on the condensation of formaldehyde with monoamines to produce fluorescent products that can be studied under the ultraviolet microscope. Considerable care must be exercised in the interpretation of the observations of fluorescence microscopy, since the specific monoamine fluorescence must be distinguished from a variety of other fluorescent structures. A number of specificity tests have been developed to aid in this differentiation (Falck *et al.*, 1962; Corrodi *et al.*, 1965; Norberg & Hamberger, 1964; Falck and Owman, 1965). Catecholamines can be distinguished from indolamines (such as serotonin) by a distinct difference in the excitation and fluorescence spectra (Corrodi & Hillarp, 1963; Caspersson *et. al.*, 1966). In practice, this is manifested as a distinct difference in the fluorescence color between catecholamines and indolamines (Angelakos, 1964b). Details of the reactions involved and the overall specificity of the method have been published (Corrodi & Hillarp, 1963, 1964). In general, it is not possible to distinguish readily among each of the naturally occurring catecholamines with this histochemical method. Secondary amines, such as adrenaline, require a somewhat longer time to condense with formaldehyde than do primary amines, such as noradrenaline and dopamine (Falck, 1962; Falck *et al.*, 1963; Angelakos *et al.*, 1965b), but this distinction is not very reliable, inasmuch as the condensation time is affected by a number of environmental and other experimental conditions and varies greatly among different laboratories (Falck, 1962; Csillik, 1964; Jacobowitz & Koelle, 1965; Angelakos & King, 1965b).

Recently, a new histochemical method for catecholamines was developed by Angelakos and King (1965a). This is based on oxidation of catecholamines in tissues to form the specific fluorescent lutins according to the well-known trihydroxyindole (THI) reaction employed in the spectrofluorometric analyses for catecholamines (von Euler, 1956; Udenfriend, 1962). This new method permits the differentiation of noradrenaline and adrenaline by the difference in their fluorescence colors (excitation and fluorescence spectra) and gives no detectable fluorescent products with dopamine or indolamines. Thus, far, it has been difficult to utilize this method in the heart, since the demonstration of intraneuronal noradrenaline with this technique requires extensive and/or drastic treatments (such as fixing in boiling solution). Recent studies indicate that this is due to the presence of noradrenaline in a "bound" form within the neuron (Angelakos & King, 1966). Because of this, the method has been adapted for the histochemical demonstration of "free" vs. "bound" neuronal noradrenaline (King & Angelakos, 1966). By contrast, in most cases intraneuronal adrenaline is apparently present in a relatively free form, since it gives the THI reaction according to the Angelakos-King method without the necessity of drastic pretreatment of the tissue (Angelakos & King, 1967). Thus, this method has been employed for the demonstration of intraneuronal adrenaline in the heart (Angelakos *et al.*, 1965a). In this method, adrenaline is readily identified by its characteristic fluorescence color. Intraneuronal noradrenaline, when in the "free" form (as after reserpine), can also be demonstrated with this technique without previous drastic treatment of the tissue and has a different fluorescence color than adrenaline (King & Angelakos, 1966).

FIGURE 1 shows the characteristic pattern of the catecholamine-containing fibers in the guinea pig atrium by means of the Falck-Hillarp histochemical method. This is a whole-mount preparation of the atrium stretched on a microscopical slide. Characteristically, the catecholamine-containing structures form a network of tortuous fibers with distinct varicosities along their length. The same histological picture has been described following nonspecific methylene blue staining, as well as with the highly specific Angelakos-King THI histochemical method. When tissues are examined in histological sections, only short segments of the fibers appear in any given plane because of their tortuous structure.

EXPERIMENTAL RESULTS

Rabbit and Dog Hearts

The regional distribution of catecholamines was evaluated in extensive studies in rabbit and dog hearts with both the chemical and histochemical approaches (Angelakos *et al.*, 1963; Angelakos, 1965). The results of the spectrofluorometric analyses are summarized in FIGURES 2 and 3. Note that in both species

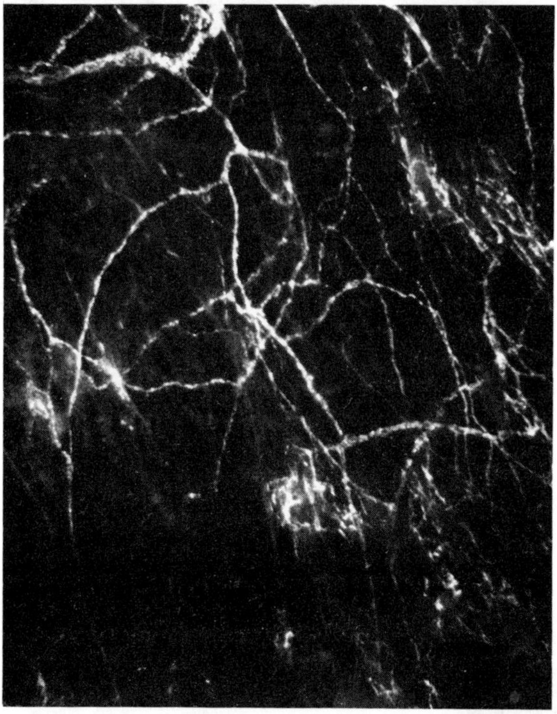

FIGURE 1. Microphotograph of the fluorescent catecholamine-containing nerve fibers in a whole-mount stretch preparation of the guinea pig atrium treated according to the Falck-Hillarp formaldehyde-condensation method. The characteristic fluorescence is blue when appropriate excitation and fluorescence filters are used (see Angelakos, 1964b). × ca. 100.

the predominant catecholamine was noradrenaline in most areas of the heart. This is consistent with the now generally accepted view that noradrenaline is the normal neurohumor in the mammalian sympathetic nervous system (von Euler, 1956). In general, noradrenaline concentration is higher in the right side of the heart than left in both atria and ventricles, although this is more striking in the rabbit than in the dog. In fact, in the dog, no differences were observed in the catecholamine concentration between the right and left auricular appen-

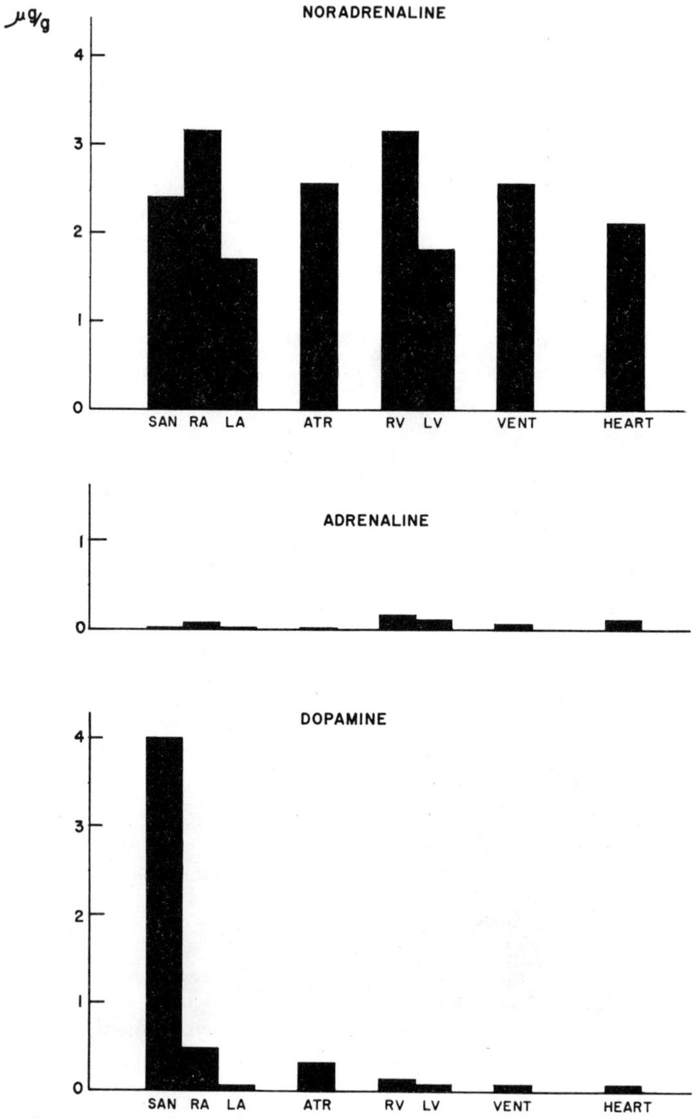

FIGURE 2. Regional distribution of catecholamines in the rabbit heart, determined from spectrofluorometric analyses.

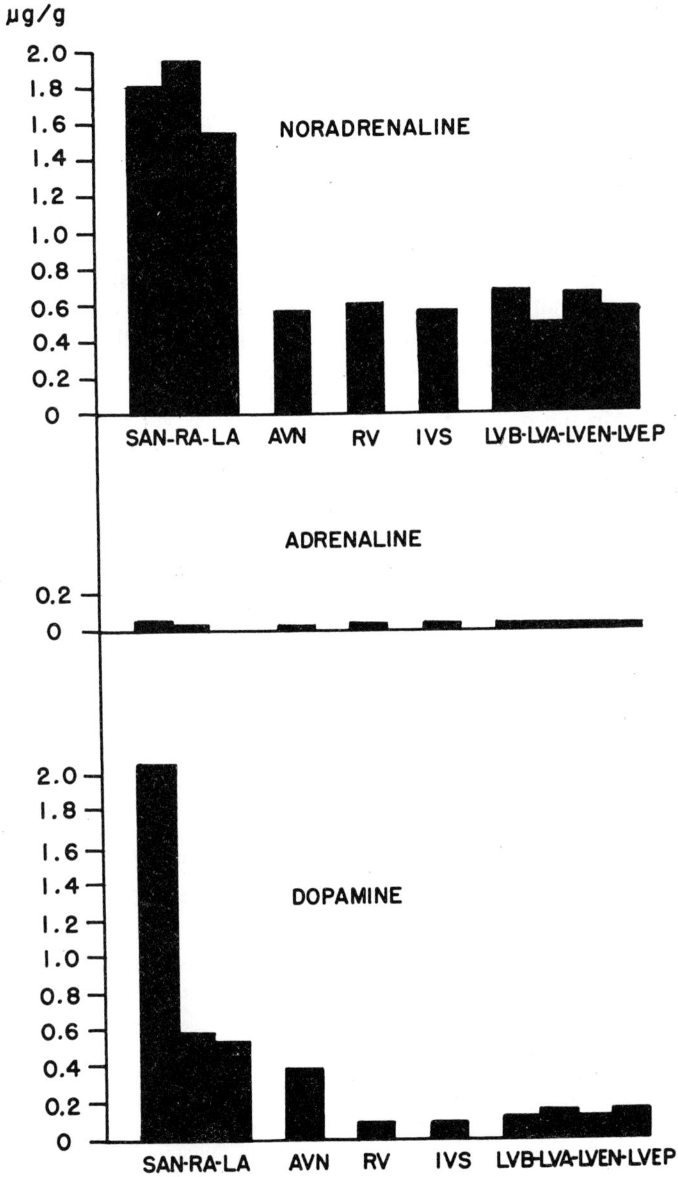

FIGURE 3. Regional distribution of catecholamines in the dog heart, determined from spectrofluorometric analyses.

dages or between certain areas of the right and left ventricle (Angelakos, 1965). In the dog, where the distribution of noradrenaline in various regions of the left ventricle was studied, no definite pattern could be demonstrated, although considerable differences were observed among different regions (e.g. apical vs. basal portions). It is noteworthy that in both species the concentration of noradrenaline in the SAN and AVN regions was not higher than in the surrounding tissues. Essentially similar observations in these species have been reported by others (Goodall & Kirshner, 1956; Shore *et al.*, 1958; Muscholl, 1959; Serrano *et al.*, 1960; Wegman *et al.*, 1961; Klouda, 1963; Jellinek *et al.*, 1964; Li *et al.*, Napolitano *et al.*, 1965; Ueda *et al.*, 1966). Differences in the analytical methodology probably account for some of the discrepancies noted by others (Raab and Gigee, 1955; Kimata, 1965).

The regional distribution of adrenaline was unremarkable, and no significant differences could be detected in either species. In general the concentration of adrenaline was small and variable, which is consistent with the view that adrenaline present in the heart of mammals originates in the adrenal medulla, where the noradrenaline-methylating enzyme is found (Axelrod, 1966).

Small amounts of dopamine were present in all parts of the heart except for the SAN and, in the dog, the AVN regions. Relatively high concentrations of dopamine were found in these nodal areas. In general, there was no correlation between the dopamine and noradrenaline concentrations in various parts of the heart examined. This is not consistent with the view that the amount of dopamine present in the heart is a direct consequence of its role as a metabolic precursor of noradrenaline, unless the turnover rates of noradrenaline are considerably different in various parts of the heart.

Histochemically, the density of the catecholamine-containing fibers was in rough agreement with the catecholamine concentrations determined chemically in most areas of the heart (FIGURES 4 and 5). For instance, a distinctly higher density of fibers was observed in the right atrium of the rabbit than in the left (FIGURE 4), which is consistent with the differences in the analytical results (FIGURE 2). The nodal areas, however, were striking exceptions (Angelakos *et al.*, 1963). Here a dense network of fluorescent fibers was observed in both species (FIGURES 4 and 5), which was in sharp contrast to the noradrenaline conceptions obtained in tissue analyses (FIGURES 2 and 3). Similar histochemical observations in the dog have been reported (Dahlstrom *et al.*, 1965).

Other less striking differences were also observed. In the dog, for instance, no detectable difference in the density of the nerve fibers could be established between most areas of the ventricles when compared to the atria even though there was roughly a twofold difference in noradrenaline content between these tissues (FIGURE 5). Nevertheless, the fluorescence intensity of the nerve fibers found in the dog ventricle was distinctly lower than that found in the atria, suggesting a lower intraneuronal concentration of noradrenaline in the ventricles, which might account for the differences in the results of the analyses. However, no difference in fluorescence intensity was observed between nerve fibers present in the SAN and AVN rgions in either species to account for the discrepancy with the analytical results. In fact, nerve fibers present in these areas were generally intensely fluorescent. Nevertheless, this possibility cannot be excluded, since the fiber fluorescence intensity observed histochemically is affected by a variety of factors and cannot be considered a reliable criterion of intraneuronal amine concentration.

In general, a discrepancy between the concentrations of noradrenaline found

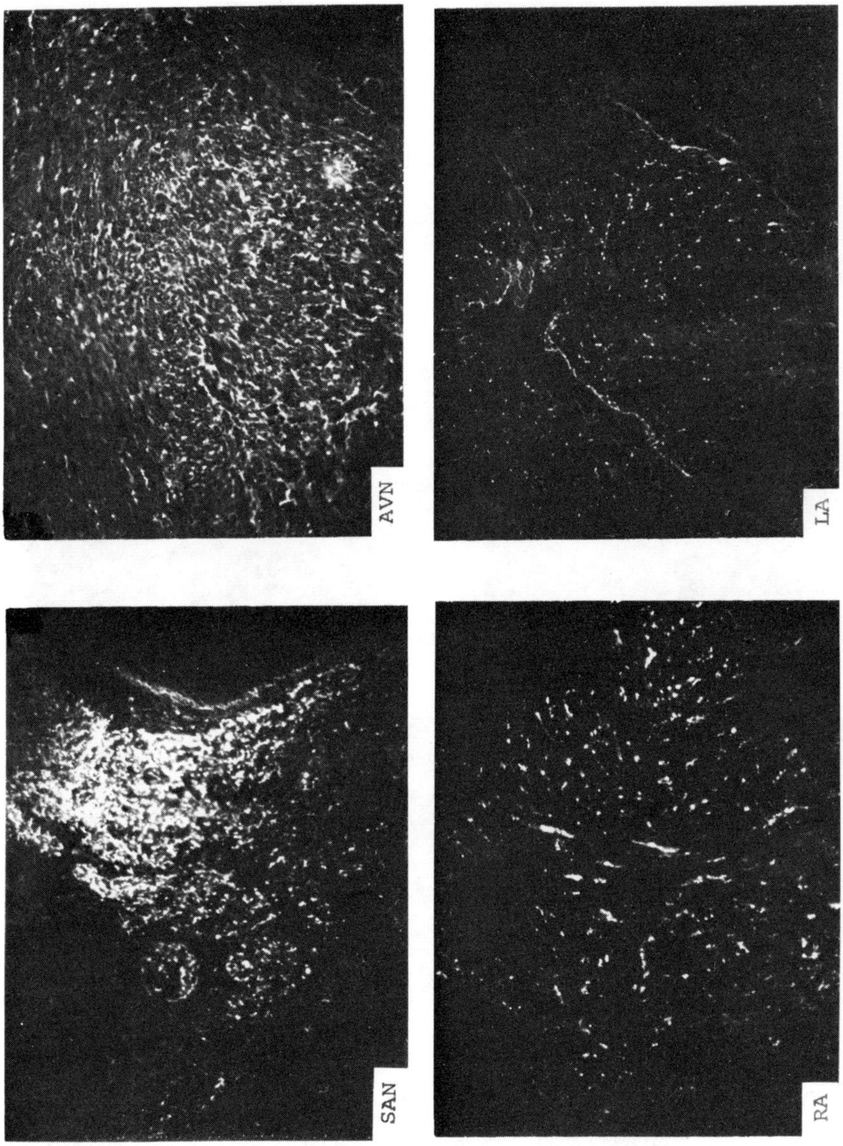

FIGURE 4. Fluorescence microphotographs showing the density of adrenergic fibers in sections from various parts of the rabbit heart: sinoauricular node (SAN), atrioventricular node (AVN), right and left atria (RA and LA). × ca. 100.

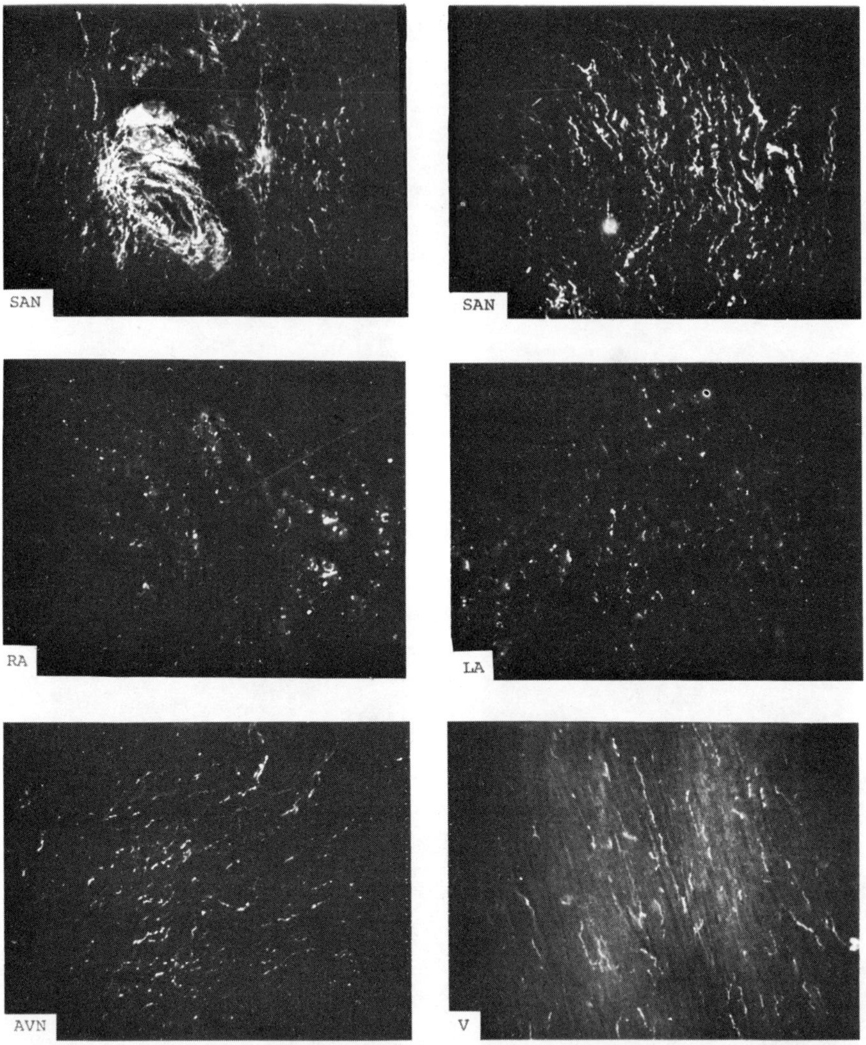

Figure 5. Fluorescence microphotograph showing the density of adrenergic fibers in various parts of the dog heart; two regions of the sinoauricular node (SAN), right and left atria (RA and LA), atrioventricular node (AVN), and right ventricle (V), which is the same as in the left ventricle (not shown). The photographic exposure time was increased by a factor of $\times$ 2.5 for reproducing the ventricular section because of the low fluorescence intensity of the fibers present in this tissue. $\times$ ca. 100.

by tissue analyses and the density of adrenergic fibers suggests different intraneuronal concentrations of noradrenaline, which could be the result of differences in sympathetic activity and, hence, noradrenaline turnover rates.

Hearts of Other Laboratory Species

Spectrofluorometric analyses and histochemical studies were made in the hearts of a number of laboratory species. Although these studies were not as extensive as those performed in the rabbit and dog, the results were quite similar. In all cases, with the exception of frogs and toads (see following sections), the predominant catecholamine found in the heart was noradrenaline. A summary of the results of the distribution of noradrenaline in various parts of the heart is shown in FIGURE 6. In general, the concentration of noradrenaline was higher in the right side of the heart than in the left and, in most cases, higher in the atria than in the ventricles. These results are in agreement, in all essential aspects, with reports from other laboratories.

Preliminary studies in species not previously noted gave similar results. Thus, the cardiac noradrenaline concentration in the desert rat (*Gerbillus gerbillus*) was of the same order as that in the albino rat, while that of the atrium of the thirteen-lined ground squirrel *(Citellus tridecimlineatus)* and of the newborn domestic pig was similar to that found in the atria of hamsters and albino rabbits, respectively (Angelakos *et al.*, 1968).

Reports on cardiac catecholamines in other species indicate a similar range. For instance, mouse hearts are reported to contain roughly 0.4–0.8 $\mu g/g$ of noradrenaline (Lippman *et al.*, 1965; Porter *et al.*, 1965), sheep hearts roughly 0.8 $\mu g/g$, and cattle hearts 0.2–0.4 $\mu g/g$ (Goodall, 1951). The heart of the domestic chicken apparently contains the lowest noradrenaline concentration reported, in the range of 0.12–0.57 $\mu g/g$, distinctly higher in the male than in the female (Jellinek *et al.*, 1963).

In primates, values of cardiac noradrenaline in concentrations of 0.5–1.5 $\mu g/g$ have been reported (Kulinsky, 1964; Ordy *et al.*, 1965). For human cardiac tissue, values of 0.5–2.5 $\mu g/g$ (mean, 1.8 $\mu g/g$) were reported for the noradrenaline concentration of atrial tissue obtained by biopsy during cardiac surgery (Chidsey *et al.*, 1964).

In general, the noradrenaline concentrations in the hearts of all the species that have been studied (except for frogs and toads; see following sections) are in the range of 0.15–4.5 $\mu g/g$ with most species falling in the range of 0.5–2.5 $\mu g/g$. Limited histochemical studies made in other species gave results similar to those obtained in the dog and rabbit. A dense network of intensely fluorescent fibers was always found in the SAN region. In other areas, the tissue concentrations of noradrenaline corresponded roughly to the density of the adrenergic fibers, although a close correlation was not always present.

Catecholamine-Containing Structures

In all the species studied, only nerve fibers could be identified histochemically as the catecholamine-containing structures. No catecholamine-containing cells were found. Reports describing such cells (Jacobowitz *et al.*, 1966) could not be confirmed in these and previous studies (Angelakos *et al.*, 1963; Falck, 1964; Dahlstrom *et al.*, 1965). Fluorescent cells were occasionally seen in the hearts of some species. However, the fluorescence color and excitation and fluorescence spectra obtained from these structures were distinctly different

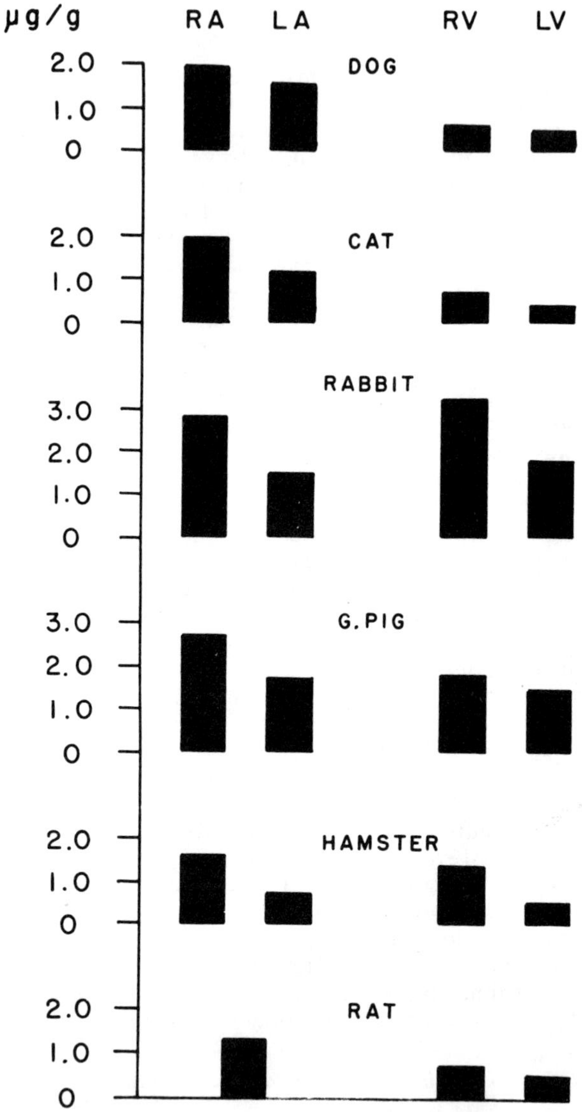

FIGURE 6. Noradrenaline concentrations in atria and ventricles of various laboratory species. The results are based on no less than five determinations. In the smaller species, tissues from three to five animals were pooled. The right and left atria were pooled in the rat.

than those for catecholamines: the contents of the cells exhibited a yellow fluorescence when excited with monochromatic 405 mμ light, whereas under the same conditions, catecholamines exhibited a distinctly blue fluorescence (Angelakos, 1964b). Furthermore, these structures did not give the specificity reactions for catecholamines which have been proposed in connection with this histochemical method (Falck & Owman, 1965). Thus, it appears likely that such cells may contain serotonin or a similar indolamine, or some other compound such as histamine. Serotonin and related compounds are known to give yellow fluorescent products when condensed with formaldehyde (Falck *et al.*, 1962; Corrodi & Hillarp, 1963). Another yellow fluorescent product has been described after condensation of formaldehyde with histamine (Lagunoff *et al.*, 1961). Similar yellow fluorescent cells have been found at an early stage in development in the heart of the chick embryo and in the frog heart, confirming previous reports (Enemar *et al.*, 1965; Falck *et al.*, 1963). In all cases, these cells have been shown to contain tryptamine derivatives rather than catecholamines.

Frog and Toad Hearts

Of all the common laboratory species, only frog and toad hearts were found to contain adrenaline rather than noradrenaline as a predominant catecholamine. The regional distribution of each of the naturally occurring catecholamines in the various parts of the heart of the common frog *(Rana pipiens)* is shown in FIGURE 7. Similar results were obtained in other species of frogs and toads (Angelakos *et al.*, 1965b). This is in agreement with previous reports (von Euler, 1946; Ostlund, 1954; Falck *et al.*, 1963). Again the presence of high concentrations of dopamine in the pacemaker region (sinus venosus) of this species is noteworthy.

Histochemically fluorescent fibers similar to those seen in other species were

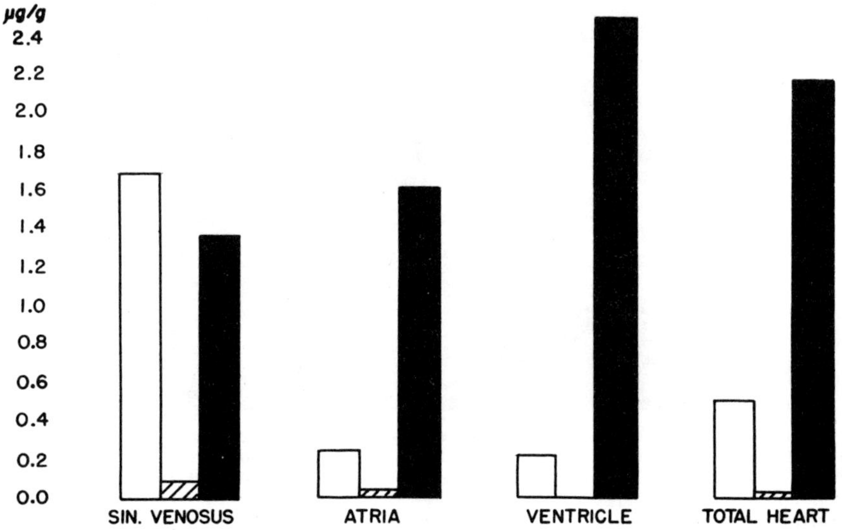

FIGURE 7. Regional distribution of catecholamines in various parts of the heart of the common frog *(Rana pipiens)*. Values are means from 40 animals: white bars = dopamine; cross-hatched bars = norepinephrine; solid bars = epinephrine.

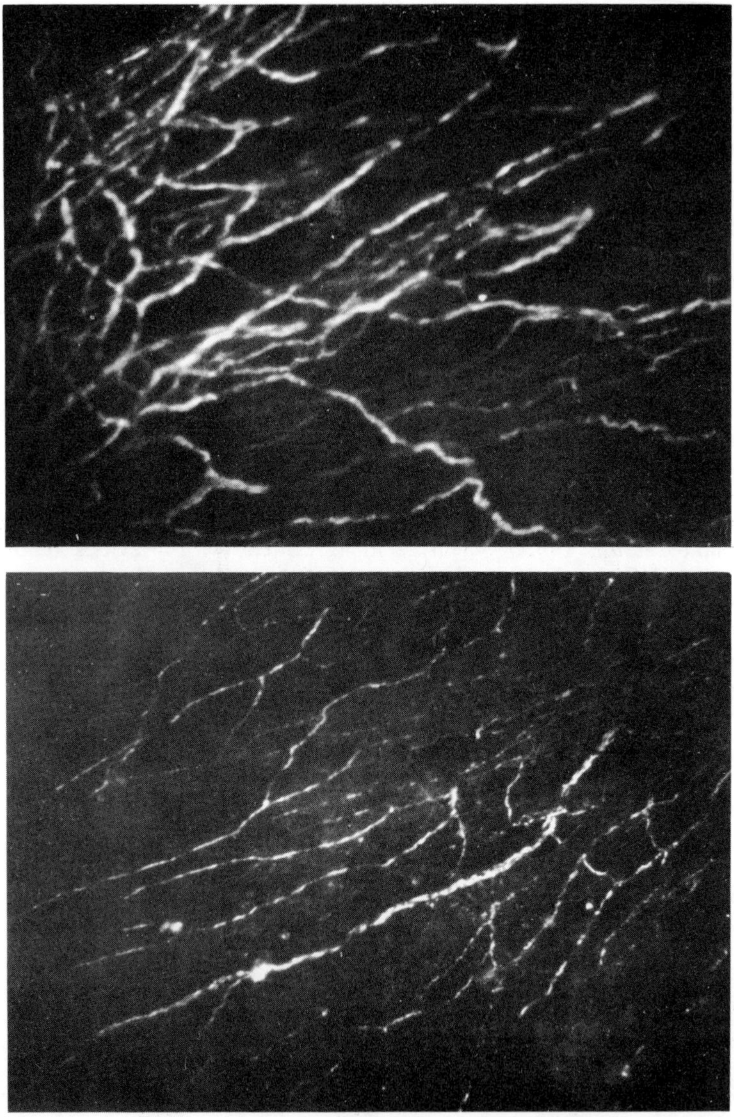

FIGURE 8. Microphotograph of the adrenaline-containing fibers in the frog heart. Whole-mount stretch preparations of sinus venosus (top) and left atrium (bottom) treated according to the Angelakos-King trihydroxyindole (THI) procedure. With this method, adrenaline-containing structures have a characteristic green to green-yellow fluorescence and give the reaction without any pretreatment. By contrast, noradrenaline gives a blue to blue-green color and generally requires some pretreatment of the tissue. × ca. 100.

demonstrated with the Falck-Hillarp method. However, studies based on the time required for condensation suggested that the amine present in these fibers was adrenaline rather than noradrenaline (Falck *et al.*, 1963; Angelakos *et al.*, 1965b; Banister & Mann, 1965). More recent histochemical studies using the Angelakos-King THI method (Angelakos & King, 1967) confirmed the previous findings and indicated clearly the presence of adrenaline in frog fibers (FIGURE 8). Available evidence indicates that the predominance of adrenaline in these species is not limited to the heart but extends to all sympathetically innervated organs (Ostlund, 1954; Falck *et al.*, 1963). Furthermore, Axelrod and associates have recently demonstrated the presence of an *N*-methylating variant enzyme (isozyme?) responsible for the extraadrenal synthesis of adrenaline in frogs (Wurtman *et al.*, 1967). Thus, adrenaline is apparently the sympathetic neurohumor in frogs and toads, and the sympathetic fibers of these species can be properly classified as *adrenergic* in contrast to the *noradrenergic* fibers present in all mammalian species studied.

Fiber Density and Mean Diffusion Distance

All histochemical observations show clearly (FIGURES 1, 4, and 5) that the distribution of the catecholamine-containing fibers within the heart is rather sparse. There is definitely no direct innervation of each cardiac-muscle fiber. Thus, the neurohumor released during sympathetic activation must diffuse over considerable distance before reaching all the cardiac cells. Simple preliminary measurements suggest that the average diffusing distance is on the order of 30 μ. The nodal areas are notable exceptions, in which the dense network of fibers reduces the mean diffusion distance to a few micra. In general, the widely held view (Hirsch, 1963) that every cardiac cell is innervated apparently does not apply to the sympathetic innervation. It may be proposed, of course, that the histochemical methods do not show the finer ramifications of the adrenergic nerve fibers in the heart. Although this possibility cannot be entirely excluded, all the available evidence on the sensitivity of the histochemical reactions employed suggest that, under optimal conditions, all the adrenergic nerve fibers are demonstrable. Further clarification of this problem must await the development of specific histochemical techniques for adrenergic fibers applicable to electron microscopy.

Intraneuronal Concentration of Amines

The density of the adrenergic fibers observed histochemically can be utilized in conjunction with the results of tissue analyses to arrivė at very rough estimates of the mean intraneuronal concentrations of the amines. Rough estimates suggest that the adrenergic nerve plexus accounts for approximately 2–5% of the myocardial mass volume in tissues containing 2–4 μg/g of noradrenaline. Thus the calculated intraneuronal concentration of noradrenaline is 40–200 μg/cc. These values are much smaller than the estimate given by Dahlstrom and her associates (1966) for the intraneuronal concentration of noradrenaline in the varicosities of adrenergic fibers in the iris and vas deferens of the rat. These authors calculated values in the range of 1000–3000 μg/cc. Similar considerations indicate that the intraneuronal concentration of noradrenaline in the terminals innervating the nodal areas must be three to ten times *less* than in other terminals in order to correspond with the high fiber density observed with the same tissue content of noradrenaline. Considering the fiber density, the calculated intraneuronal concentration of dopamine is also relatively low in the nodal areas and may not be higher than in terminals present in other parts of the heart. Thus, on the basis of the fiber density alone, three to ten times as much dopamine may be expected in the nodal regions than in the surrounding areas. This is in close agreement with values of dopamine obtained by tissue analyses. Thus, if these considerations are correct, the high concentrations of dopamine in the nodal regions may only reflect the high density of adrenergic neurons.

The low concentration of noradrenaline in the fibers innervating the nodal regions may suggest a higher turnover rate of noradrenaline in these fibers. Similar considerations would apply to other areas. Thus, observations on the density of adrenergic neurons combined with the results on the tissue noradrenaline analyses suggest that the interaneuronal concentration of this amine is lower in fibers innervating the ventricles than those innervating the atria. This, in turn, might suggest a higher turnover of noradrenaline in the atrial adrenergic fibers than in the ventricular. Actually, in studies made in the isolated dog heart, Chidsey and his colleagues (1963b) have actually found a higher turnover rate for noradrenaline in the ventricles than in the atria.

In any event, it is evident that the noradrenaline concentration in cardiac adrenergic nerves is far in excess of local needs under ordinary conditions. This indicates a high functional reserve for the adrenergic control of cardiac activity and suggests the possibility that the noradrenaline stores of the heart may serve as a general systemic storage site for the neurohumor for release into the general circulation. This suggests a possible endocrine function of the heart in relation to noradrenaline, as has been previously proposed (Braunwald *et al.,* 1964). Evidence of significant concentration of noradrenaline found in the blood leaving the heart during adrenergic stimulation of the organ lends further support to this view (Lammerant *et al.,* 1965).

"Free" and "Bound" Amines

Considerations of the intraneuronal concentration of amines are complicated by the evidence indicating that noradrenaline exists in more than one state within the neurons. Extensive pharmacological observations suggest that there is more than one noradrenaline pool (Carlsson, 1966). Furthermore, more direct evidence from ultracentrifugation of tissue homogenates combined with electron microscope studies indicates that at least a major fraction of the amine is bound within specific microparticles 20–100 mμ in size (Michaelson *et al.,* 1964; Glassman *et al.,* 1965; von Euler & Lishajko, 1965). As much as 60–80% of noradrenaline has been isolated in a particle fraction of heart homogenates (Glassman *et al.,* 1965). Free amine is also found in tissue homogenates. Whether this indicates the presence of significant concentrations of "free" amine within the neuron or is an artifact of the homogenization procedure is open to question. Histochemical studies suggest that no significant concentrations of "free" noradrenaline are present within adrenergic neurons under normal conditions (Angelakos & King, 1966), but this may be altered in stress or under the influence of drugs. In any event, since no extraneuronal pool of noradrenaline has been demonstrated histochemically, it appears likely that all the observed effects of drugs on cardiac catecholamines must be attributed to their effects on different mechanisms of amine synthesis, uptake, binding, or catabolism within the neuron. Interestingly, histochemical studies suggest that the intraneuronal binding of adrenaline may be different than that of noradrenaline (Angelakos *et al.*, 1965a; Angelakos & King, 1967).

Are There Dopaminergic Fibers in the Heart?

Dopamine-containing and presumably *dopaminergic* fibers have been found in the corpus striatum of the brain in extensive analytical and histochemical studies (Carlsson *et al.*, 1960; Falck, 1964; Hillarp *et al.*, 1966). However, no such fibers have been demonstrated in the peripheral nervous system. The presence of a high density of histochemically fluorescent fibers in the SAN and AVN, coupled with the lack of high noradrenaline concentrations in these areas, suggested that these fibers may contain considerable amounts of dopamine (Angelakos *et al.*, 1963; Angelakos, 1965). It is possible that a high turnover of noradrenaline in these regions results in an accumulation of dopamine if the conversion of dopamine to noradrenaline becomes a rate-limiting step. Even though the conversion of dopamine to noradrenaline has not been found to be a limiting step in the tissues that have been studied (Levitt *et al.*, 1965), the possibility cannot be excluded that the turnover rates and limiting steps may be different in various areas of the heart. Clearly, studies on the turnover rate of noradrenaline in the nodal regions of the heart are needed. Alternatively, it is possible that dopamine acts in the nodal areas as a direct neurohumor, and, hence, the fibers in those regions are in fact *dopaminergic*. However, as noted previously, it is quite likely that the high concentration of dopamine in the nodal regions does not indicate a high *intraneuronal* concentration of this amine but is rather a direct consequence of the high density of adrenergic fibers. In this case, the low noradrenaline:dopamine ratio found in the nodal areas may be a reflection of a low intraneuronal concentration of noradrenaline rather than a high intraneuronal concentration of dopamine. At present, no definite answer can be given to this question without further information on the intraneuronal concentration of dopamine, its possible release during nerve stimulation, and the physiological actions of this amine on the nodal fibers. It is noteworthy, however, that the tissue concentration of dopamine bears a closer correlation to the density of adrenergic fibers observed histochemically than does the tissue concentration of noradrenaline. This again suggests different turnover rates of noradrenaline in different parts of the heart.

Development and Aging

Little is known at present regarding the cardiac catecholamines during normal development, growth, and aging. This information is needed particularly for the interpretation of long-term studies and the effects of chronic disease. Preliminary studies have been made in this laboratory in the chick embryo and in the aging rat. It is generally believed that extrinsic innervation reaches the heart of the chick embryo between the fourth and seventh day of incubation (Romanoff, 1960). However, spectrofluorometric analyses and histochemical observations revealed no detectable catecholamines or adrenergic fibers before the 12th to 14th day of incubation.

Yellow fluorescent cells identified as containing a tryptamine derivative were seen in the hearts of four-day-old embryos, but the typical catecholamine-containing fluorescent fibers were not observed before the 16th day of incubation, corresponding with the detection of significant amounts of noradrenaline in the tissue analyses. Essentially similar results have been reported by Enemar and his colleagues (1965). Assuming that the original observations with silver stains were correct and that these histochemical observations do not reflect limitations in methodology, the overall results may suggest either that the sympathetic nerve fibers reach the heart at a later stage than other neural elements or that the appearance of the neurotransmitter and, hence, functional innervation occurs distinctly after the establishment of the anatomical connections.

Preliminary studies were also made in a cohort of growing rats between three and 18 months of age. FIGURE 9 shows some of the results. Note a con-

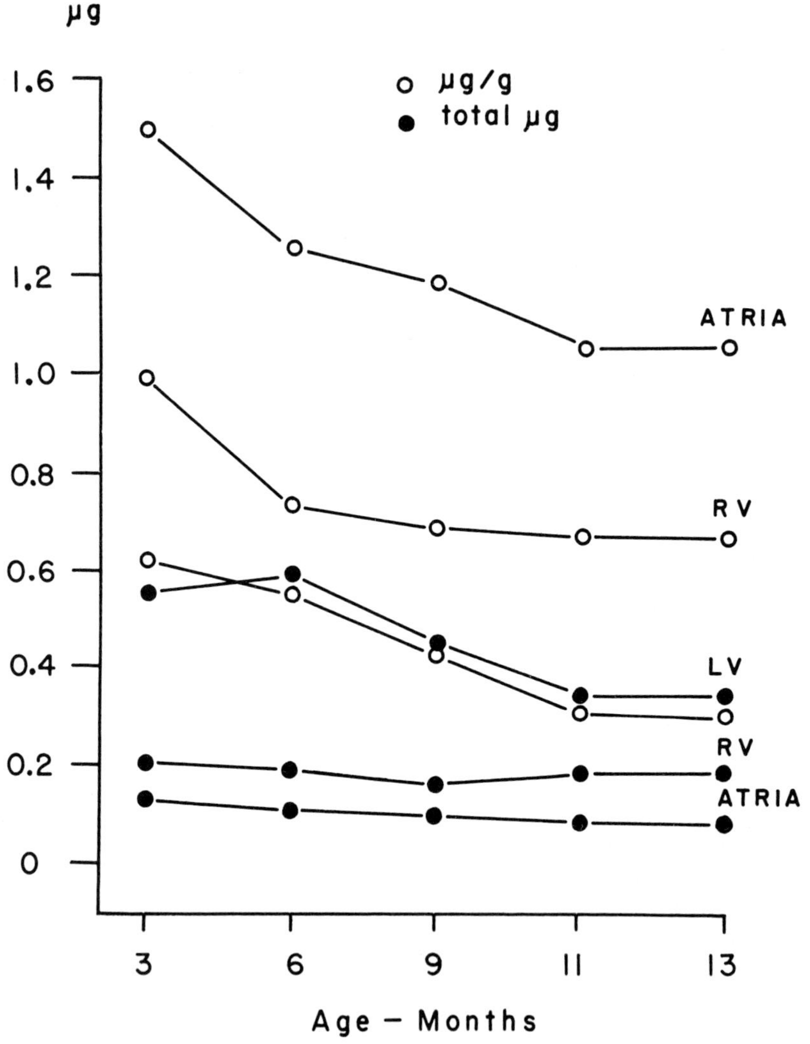

FIGURE 9. Noradrenaline in the heart of rats of different ages. Open circles show the concentration µg/g in heart tissue; solid circles show the total amine per tissue. Values from five animals per age group, obtained from the same original population (cohort).

sistent decrease in left ventricular noradrenaline with age, which is evident whether the results are expressed on a per unit weight or on a per ventricle basis. Atrial and right ventricular noradrenaline concentrations, on the other hand, show only a weight-dependent decrease over this period. In connection with these changes in catecholamines, it is perhaps of some interest that the myocardial cell monoamine oxidase activity apparently increases with age, since it was found to be greater in the 14-month-old rat than in the weaned rat (Studer *et al.*, 1964).

Heart Failure

The decrease in cardiac catecholamine stores in experimentally induced and clinically observed heart failure has been fully documented in a number of studies (Chidsey *et al.*, 1963a; Meerson *et al.*, 1963; Tomomatsu *et al.*, 1963; Chidsey *et al.*, 1964a & b; Torsti *et al.*, 1964; Fischer *et al.*, 1965; Spann *et al.*, 1965; Chidsey *et al.*, 1966).

In collaboration with Dr. Bajusz and his associates of the Bio-Research Institute, preliminary studies were made in this laboratory on the cardiac catecholamine content of a hamster strain in which muscle dystrophy and heart failure develop spontaneously. The characteristics of this dystrophic strain and the cardiac pathology observed are described elsewhere in this monograph (Bajusz *et al.*, 1968a & b). The cardiac catecholamine content of these animals was the same as that of the controls at 35 days of age, when no signs of heart failure has developed (1.18 ± 0.09 μg/g of noradrenaline vs. 0.99 ± 0.12 μg/g). By contrast, at 120 days the cardiac noradrenaline content of the control strain had risen to 1.68 ± 0.28 μg/g, whereas in the dystrophic strain, now exhibiting overt signs of heart failure, cardiac noradrenaline decreased to 0.47 ± 0.11 μg/g. Only part of this decrease could be ascribed to an increase of the weight of the heart of the dystrophic animals. Thus, if the total noradrenaline content of the heart was considered, the dystrophic animals had 1.29 ± 0.30 μg as compared with 2.12 ± 0.30 μg in the controls. All these differences, between the dystrophic and control animals and between the dystrophic animals before and after the development of heart failure, are statistically significant at $p < 0.01$. Thus, depletion of cardiac catecholamines is also evident in this form of heart failure. A similarly low cardiac nonadrenaline concentration has been recently reported in a strain of dystrophic mice (Gordon & Dowben, 1966).

In general, the mechanism responsible for cardiac catecholamine depletion in heart failure has not been established. Furthermore, it is not clear whether this depletion is associated with a partial destruction of neural elements or a decrease in the intraneuronal concentration of neurohumor. Histochemical studies now in progress in this laboratory may help to elucidate this point. It is possible that a defect in the neural uptake and/or retention of noradrenaline, as suggested by Spann *et al.*, (1964), may be the responsible mechanism for the noradrenaline depletion in heart failure. The finding that adenosine triphosphate (ATP) is required for the uptake and binding of noradrenaline by adrenergic neurons (von Euler and Lishajko, 1963; von Euler *et al.*, 1963; Angelakos, 1964a; Stjarne, 1964; Angelakos and King, 1965b; Colburn & Maas, 1965), may be pertinent in this connection. Thus, if heart failure is associated with a decrease in the local concentration of high-energy phosphate compounds, a decreased neuronal uptake and binding of noradrenaline could result. Further studies are needed to test this hypothesis.

Summary and Conclusions

The predominant catecholamine present in the heart of laboratory mammals is noradrenaline. In most species the concentration of noradrenaline is higher in the atria than in the ventricles and generally higher in the right side of the heart than in the left. The SAN and AVN regions have no higher concentrations of noradrenaline than surrounding areas but contain considerably higher amounts of dopamine.

Histochemically, the density of the catecholamine-containing nerve fibers corresponds roughly to the tissue noradrenaline concentrations in most regions of the heart. Thus, differences in the noradrenaline concentrations between the right and left atria reflect, by and large, differences in the density of adrenergic fibers. However, at least some of the differences between atria and ventricles may reflect differences in the intraneuronal concentration of noradrenaline.

In general, no extraneuronal pool of noradrenaline could be demonstrated histochemically, and nerve fibers were the only structures found to contain catecholamines in the hearts of the species studied. Similarly, no catecholamine-containing cells could be identified. Nevertheless, the concentration of noradrenaline and its precursor dopamine may vary in fibers present in different parts of the heart. Thus, the tissue concentration of noradrenaline determined by chemical analyses is not a fully reliable criterion of the extent of adrenergic innervation. Notably the SAN and AVN areas have been shown histochemically to have an extensive adrenergic innervation, many times more dense than the surrounding areas, notwithstanding the unremarkable noradrenaline concentrations found in these regions.

Among the species studied, only frog and toads were shown to have adrenaline-containing nerve fibers. Adrenaline is apparently the normal sympathetic neurohumor in these species. By contrast, only traces of adrenaline were found in the hearts of all other species studied.

With the exception of the nodal areas, the density of adrenergic fibers in the heart muscle is such that diffusion over a roughly estimated mean distance of 30 μ is required for the neurohumor to reach all cardiac cells. In the nodal areas, this distance is reduced to a few micra.

Rough estimates, based on tissue noradrenaline concentrations and on the proportion of nerve fiber volume to the total cardiac mass as indicated by the density of nerve fibers, suggest that the intraneuronal concentration of noradrenaline is 40–200 μg/cc. Similar considerations suggest that the nerve fibers present in nodal areas may contain three to ten times lower concentrations of noradrenaline. By contrast, similar calculations suggest no striking differences in the intraneuronal concentrations of dopamine in various parts of the heart.

The significance of the high concentration of dopamine found in nodal regions has not been established. It is possible that this reflects differences in turnover rates in the metabolism of noradrenaline in these regions, or perhaps the presence of functionally active dopaminergic fibers. However, it is more likely that the high concentration of dopamine is a direct consequence of the high density of adrenergic fibers in these regions, the intraneuronal concentration of dopamine being the same in the nodal regions as in fibers innervating other parts of the heart.

In general, the available evidence suggests that the turnover rates of noradrenaline may be different in adrenergic neurons present in different parts of the heart. Furthermore, it appears that the cardiac concentrations of noradrenaline are far in excess of ordinary local needs but may serve as "endocrine" stores for possible release into the general circulation during adrenergic activation.

Preliminary studies in chick embryos and aging rats suggest that functional sympathetic innervation occurs somewhat later in development than anatomical innervation and that aging may affect the noradrenaline concentrations differerently in different parts of the heart. Other preliminary studies show a striking decrease in cardiac noradrenaline concentration in a dystrophic strain of hamsters during the development of heart failure as compared with normal controls of the same age.

It is concluded that both chemical and histochemical studies, on each of the functionally specific regions of the heart, are needed for any complete evaluation of cardiac catecholamine stores and their possible role under normal or pathological conditions.

References

Angelakos, E. T. 1964a. Histochemical demonstration of uptake of exogenous norepinephrine by adrenergic fibers in vitro. Science **145:** 503–504.

Angelakos, E. T. 1964b. The formaldehyde condensation method for the histochemical demonstration on tissue monoamines. J. Histochem. Cytochem. **12:** 929–931.

Angelakos, E. T. 1965. Regional distribution of catecholamines in the dog heart. Circ. Res. **16:** 39–44.

Angelakos, E. T., E. I. Bloomquist & M. P. King. 1965a. Depletion of norepinephrine from atria by epinephrine. Life Sci. **4:** 1515–1520.

Angelakos, E. T., K. Fuxe & M. L. Torchiana. 1963. Chemical and histochemical evaluation of the distribution of catecholamines in the rabbit and guniea pig hearts. Acta Physiol. Scand. **59:** 184–191.

Angelakos, E. T., P. M. Glassman, R. W. Millard & M. P. King. 1965b. Regional distribution and subcellular localization of catecholamines in the frog heart. Comp. Biochem. Physiol. **15:** 313–325.

Angelakos, E. T. & M. King. 1965a. A new histochemical method for the specific demonstration of CA-containing strucutres. Fed. Proc. **24:** 389.

Angelakos, E. T. & M. King. 1965b. Histochemical demonstration of catecholamine uptake by adrenergic fibers. J. Histochem. Cytochem. **12:** 282–285.

Angelakos, E. T. & M. P. King. 1966. Histochemical evaluation of "free" and "bound" catecholamines in nerve fibers. Fed. Proc. **25:** 383.

Angelakos, E. T. & M. P. King. 1967. Demonstration of adrenaline-containing nerve terminals with a new histochemical technique. Nature. **213:** 391–393.

Angelakos, E. T., M. P. King, J. T. Maher & R. F. Burlington. 1968. Adrenergic innervation and catecholamines in the heart of hibernators. To be published.

Axelrod, J. 1966. Methylation reactions in the formation and metabolism of catecholamines and other biogenic amines. Pharmacol. Rev. **18:** 95–113.

Bajusz, E., J. R. Baker, C. W. Nixon & F. Homburger. 1968a. Spontaneous hereditary myocardial degeneration and congestive heart failure in a strain of Syrian hamsters. This monograph.

Bajusz, E., F. Homburger, J. R. Baker & P. Bogdonoff. 1968b. Dissociation of factors influencing myocardial degeneration and generalized cardiocirculatory failure. This monograph.

Bannister, J. & S. P. Mann. 1965. An investigation of the adrenergic innervation of the heart and major blood vessels of the frog by Falck's methods of fluoresence microscopy. J. Physiol. (London) **181:** 13–15P.

Braunwald, E., D. C. Harrison & C. A. Chidsey. 1964. The heart as an endocrine organ. Amer. J. Med. **36:** 1–4.

Carlsson, A. 1966. Pharmacological depletion of catecholamine stores. Pharmacol. Rev. **18:** 541–549.

Carlsson, A., M. Lindqvist & T. Magnusson. 1960. On the biochemistry and possible functions of dopamine and noradrenaline in brain. *In* Adrenergic Mechanisms. J. R. Vane, Ed. Ciba Found. Symp. : 432–439. Churchill Ltd. Publ. London, England.

Carlsson, A. & B. Waldek. 1958. A fluorometric method for the determination of dopamine (3-OH-tyramine). Acta Physiol. Scand. **44:** 293–298.

Caspersson, T., N.-A. Hillarp & M. Ritzen. 1966. Fluorescence microspectrophotometry of cellular catecholamines and 5HT. Exp. Cell Res. **42**: 415–428.

Chidsey, C. A., E. Braunwald & A. G. Morrow. 1964a. Catecholamine excretion and cardiac stores of norepinephrine in congestive heart failure. Amer. J. Med. **39**: 442–451.

Chidsey, C. A., E. Braunwald, A. G. Morrow & D. T. Mason. 1963a. Myocardial norepinephrine concentration in man. Effects of congestive heart failure. New Eng. J. Med. **269**: 653-658.

Chidsey, C. A., G. A. Kaiser & E. Braunwald. 1963b. Biosynthesis of norepinephrine in isolated canine heart. Science **139**: 828–829.

Chidsey, C. A., G. A. Kaiser, E. H. Sonnenblick, J. F. Spann & E. Braunwald. 1964b. Cardiac norepinephrine stores in experimental heart failure in the dog. J. Clin. Invest. **43**: 2386–2393.

Chidsey, C. A., E. H. Sonnenblick, A. G. Morrow & E. Braunwald. 1966. Norepinephrine stores and contractile force of papillary muscle from the failing human heart. Circulation **33**: 43–51.

Colburn, R. W. & J. W. Maas. 1965. Adenosine triphosphate-metal-norepinephrine ternary complexes and catecholamine binding. Nature **208**: 37–41.

Corrodi, H. & N.-A. Hillarp. 1963. Fluoreszenzmethoden zur histochemischen Sichtbarmachung von Monoaminen. 1. Identifizierung der fluoreszierenden Produkte aus Modellversuchen mit 6, 7-Dimethoxyisochinolinderivaten und Formaldehyd. Helv. Chim. Acta **46**: 2425–2430.

Corrodi, H. & N.-A. Hillarp. 1964. Fluoreszenzmethoden zur histochemischen Sichtbarmachung von Monoaminen. 2. Identifizierung des fluoreszierenden Produktes aus Dopamin und Formaldehyd. Helv. Chim. Acta **47**: 911–918.

Corrodi, H., N.-A. Hillarp & G. Jonsson. 1965. Fluorescence method for the histochemical demonstration of monoamines. 3. Sodium borohydride reduction of the fluorescent compounds as a specificity test. J. Histochem. Cytochem. **13**: 484–487.

Csillik, B. 1964. Histochemcial model experiments on the effect of various drugs on the catecholamine content of adrenergic nerve terminals. J. Neurochem. **11**: 351–355.

Dahlstrom, A., K. Fuxe, M. Mya-Tu & B. E. M. Zetterstrom. 1965. Observations on adrenergic innervation of dog heart. Amer. J. Physiol. **209**: 689–692.

Dahlstrom, A., J. Haggendal & T. Hokfelt. 1966. The noradrenaline content of the nerve terminals varicosities of sympathetic adrenergic neurons in the rat. Acta Physiol. Scand. **67**: 289–294.

Enemar, A., B. Falck & R. Hakanson. 1965. Observations on the appearance of norepinephrine in the sympathetic nervous system of the chick embryo. Develop. Biol. **11**: 268–283.

Falck, B. 1962. Observations on the possibilities of the cellular localization of monoamines by fluorescence method. Acta Physiol. Scand. **56**: (Suppl. 197).

Falck, B. 1964. Cellular localization of monoamines. Progr. Brain Res. **8**: 28–44.

Falck, B., J. Haggendal & C. Owman. 1963. The localization of adrenaline in adrenergic nerves in the frog. Quart. J. Exp. Physiol. **48**: 253–257.

Falck, B., N.-A. Hillarp, G. Thieme & A. Torp. 1962. Fluorescence of catecholamines and related compounds condensed with formaldehyde. J. Histochem. Cytochem. **10**: 348–354.

Falck, B. & C. Owman. 1965. Detailed methodological description of the fluorescence method for the cellular demonstration of biogenic monoamines. Acta Univ. Lund (Sect. II) No. 7.

Fischer, J. E., W. D. Horst & I. J. Kopin. 1965. Norepinephrine metabolism in hypertrophied rat hearts. Nature **207**: 951–953.

Glassman, P. M., E. T. Angelakos & W. F. McNary. 1965. Catecholamine-containing fractions of dog heart homogenates. Life Sci. **4**: 1727–1734.

Goodall, M. 1951. Studies of adrenaline and noradrenaline in mammalian heart and suprarenals. Acta Physiol. Scand. **24**: (Suppl. 85).

Goodall, M. & N. Kirshner. 1956. Effect of cervicothoracic ganglionectomy of the adrenaline content of the mammalian heart. J. Clin. Invest. **35**: 649–656.

Gordan, P. & R. M. Dowben. 1966. Catecholamine distribution in mice afflicted with muscular dystrophy. Amer. J. Physiol. **210**: 728–732.

Hillarp, N.-A., K. Fuxe & A. Dahlstrom. 1966. Demonstration and mapping of central neurons containing dopamine, noradrenaline and 5-hydroxytryptamine and their reactions to psychopharmaca. Pharmacol. Rev. **18**: 727–742.

Hirsch, E. F. 1963. The innervation of the human heart. V. A comparative study of the intrinsic innervation of the heart in vertebrates. Exp. Molec. Path. **2**: 348–401.

Hirsch, E. F., V. L. Willman, M. Jellinek & T. Cooper. 1963. The terminal innervation of the heart. Arch. Path. (Chicago) **76**: 677–692.

JACOBOWITZ, D., T. COOPER & H. B. BARNER. 1966. Histochemical and chemical studies on the localization of adrenergic and cholinergic nerves in normal and denervated rat hearts. Fed. Proc. **25:** 383.

JACOBOWITZ, D. & G. B. KOELLE. 1965. Histochemical correlations of acetylcholinesterase and catecholamines in postganglionic autonomic nerves of the cat, rabbit, and guinea pig. J. Pharmacol. Exp. Ther. **148:** 225–237.

JELLINEK, M., M. P. KAYE, C. A. NIGH & T. COOPER. 1964. Alterations in chemical composition of canine heart after sympathetic denervation. Amer. J. Physiol. **206:** 971–974.

JELLINEK, M., L. L. TUREEN & T. COOPER. 1963. Myocardial catecholamine contents in vitamin E and sulfur-deficient chickens. Proc. Soc. Exp. Biol. Med. **113:** 524–526.

KIMATA, S. 1965. Chemical evaluation of the distribution of catecholamines in the heart. Jap. Circ. J. **29:** 7–10.

KING, M. P. & E. T. ANGELAKOS. 1966. Histochemical demonstration of "free" norepinephrine in reserpinized adrenergic nerve terminals. Pharmacologist **8:** 177.

KLOUDA, M. A. 1963. Distribution of catecholamine in the dog heart. Proc. Soc. Exp. Biol. Med. **112:** 728–729.

KULINSKY, V. I. 1964. Content of catecholamines in tissues of normal macaque monkeys (in Russian). Ukr. Biokhim Zh. **36:** 388–399.

LAGUNOFF, D., M. PHILLIPS & E. P. BENDITT. 1961. The histochemical demonstration of histamine in mast cells. J. Histochem. Cytochem. **9:** 534–541.

LAMMERANT, J., P. DEHERDT & C. DE SCHRYVER. 1965. Direct release of myocardial catecholamines into the left heart chambers. Arch. Int. Physiol. Biochim. **73:** 443–452.

LEVITT, M., S. SPECTOR, A. SJOERDSMA & S. UNDENFRIEND. 1965. Elucidation of the rate-limiting step in norepinephrine biosynthesis in the perfused guinea pig heart. J. Pharmacol. Exp. Ther. **148:** 1–8.

LI, T-H., L. H. LAASBERG & B. ETSTEN. 1964. Effects of anesthesia on myocardial catecholamines. Anesthesiology **25:** 641–649.

LIPPMANN, W., M. WISHNICK & D. A. BUYSKE. 1965. The depletion of noradrenaline from the heart by epsilon amino caproic acid. Life Sci. **4:** 281–286.

MEERSON, F. Z., B. N. MANUKHIN, M. G. PSHENICHNIKOVA & L. S. ROZANOVA. 1963. Mediator metabolism in myocardium in compensatory hyperfunction and hypertrophy of heart. Pat. Fiziol. Eksp. Ter. **7:** 32. Cited in Fed. Proc. (Transl. Suppl.) **23:** T593–T595 (1964).

MICHAELSON, I. A., K. C. RICHARDSON, S. N. SNYDER & E. O. TITUS. 1964. The separation of catecholamine storage vescicles from rat heart. Life Sci. **3:** 971–978.

MITCHELL, G. A. G. 1956. Cardiovascular Innervation. E. & S. Livingstone. Edinburgh, Scotland.

MUSCHOLL, E. 1959. Die Konzentration von Noradrenalin und Adrenalin in den einzelnen Abschnitten des Herzens. Arch. Exp. Path. Pharmacol. **237:** 350–364.

NAPOLITANO, L. M., T. COOPER, V. L. WILLMAN & C. R. HANLON. 1964. Fine structure of the heart after transplantation. Circulation (Suppl. 29) : 81–85.

NAPOLITANO, L. M., V. L. WILLMAN, C. R. HANLON & T. COOPER. 1965. Intrinsic innervation of the heart. Amer. J. Physiol. **208:** 455–457.

NONIDEZ, J. F. 1943. The structure and innervation of the conducting system of the heart of the dog and rhesus monkey as seen with a silver impregnation technique. Amer. J. **26:** 577–597.

NORBERG, K.-A. & B. HAMBERGER. 1964. The sympathetic adrenergic neuron. Acta Physiol. Scand. **63** (Suppl. 238).

ORDY, J. M., T. SAMORAJSKI & D. SCHROEDER. 1966. Concurrent changes in hypothalamic and cardiac catecholamine levels after anesthetics, tranquilizers and stress in a subhuman primate. J. Pharmacol. Exp. Ther. **152:** 445–457.

OSTLUND, E. 1954. The distribution of catecholamines in lower animals and their effect on the heart. Acta Physiol. Scand. **31** (Suppl. 112).

PORTER, C. C., J. A. TOTARO & A. BURCIN. 1965. The relationship between radioactivity and norepinephrine concentration in the brains and hearts of mice following administration of labeled methyldopa or 6-hydroxydopamine. J. Pharmacol. Exp. Ther. **150:** 17–22.

RAAB, W. & W. GIGEE. 1955. Specific avidity of the heart muscle to adsorb and store epinephrine and norepinephrine. Circ. Res. **3:** 553–558.

ROMANOFF, L. 1960. The Avian Embryo. The Macmillan Co., New York, N. Y.

ROSSI, L. 1963. Problems in histology and pathology of the intrinsic nerves of the heart. Amre. J. **66:** 838–840.

SERRANO, M. P. A., A. LERDO DE TEJADA HAY, S. A. VILLANUEVA Y L., B. CHAVEZ LARA & R. COSTERAS. 1960. Contenido y distribution de catecholamines en el corazon del perro. Arch. Inst. Cardiol. Mex. **30:** 777–787.

SHORE, P., V. H. COHN, B. HIGHMAN & H. M. MALING. 1958. Distribution of norepinephrine in the heart. Nature **181**: 848–849.

SPANN, J. F., C. A. CHIDSEY & E. BRAUNWALD. 1964. Reduction of cardiac stores of norepinephrine in experimental heart failure. Science **145**: 1439–1441.

SPANN, J. F., C. A. CHIDSEY, P. E. POOL & E. BRAUNWALD. 1965. Mechanism of norepinephrine depletion in experimental heart failure produced by aortic constriction in the guinea pig. Circ. Res. **17**: 312–321.

STJARNE, L. 1964. Studies of catecholamine uptake storage and release mechanisms. Acta Physiol. Scand. **62** (Suppl. 228).

STUDER, A., H. R. BAUMGARTNER & K. REBER. 1964. Histochemical evidence of monoamine oxidase activity in rats of different ages. Histochemie **4**: 43–47.

TCHENG, K. 1951. Innervation of the dog heart. Amer. Heart J. **41**: 512–524.

TOMOMATSU, T., Y. UEDA, T. MATSUMOTO, T. IKOMA, Y. KONDO. 1963. Catecholamine in congestive heart failure. Jap. Heart J. **4**: 13–24.

TORII, H. 1962. Electron microscope observations of the SA and AV nodes and Purkinje fibers of the rabbit. Jap. Circ. J. **26**: 39–77.

TORSTI, P., O. PENTTILA & E. TORSTI. 1964. The catecholamine content of the failing rabbit heart. Ann. Med. Exp. Fenn. **42**: 33–36.

UDENFRIEND, S. 1962. Fluorescence Assay in Biology and Medicine. Academic Press Inc. New York, N. Y.

UEDA, H., T. IIZUKA, H. YASUDA, Y. TAKABATANE, M. IIZUKA, M. IHORI & M. YAMAMOTO. 1966. Effects of electrical stimulation of the central gray stratum of the mid-brain on the blood and myocardial catecholamine. Jap. Heart. J. **7**: 277–288.

VON EULER, U. S. 1946. A specific sympathomimetic ergone in adrenergic nerve fibers (sympathin) and its relation to adrenaline and noradrenaline. Acta Physiol. Scand. **12**: 73–97.

VON EULER, U. S. 1956. Noradrenaline. Charles C Thomas, Publ. Springfield, Ill.

VON EULER, U. S. & F. LISHAJKO. 1961. Improved technique for the fluoremetric determination of catecholamines. Acta. Physiol. Scand. **51**: 348–355.

VON EULER, U. S. & F. LISHAJKO. 1963. Effect of adenine nucleotides on catecholamine release and uptake in isolated adrenergic nerve granules. Acta. Physiol. Scand. **59**: 454–461.

VON EULER, U. S. & F. LISHAJKO. 1965. Free and bound noradrenaline in the rabbit heart. Nature **205**: 179–180.

VON EULER, U. S., F. LISHAJKO & L. STJARNE. 1963. Catecholamines and adenosine triphosphate in isolated adrenergic nerve granules. Acta Physiol. Scand. **59**: 495–496.

WEGMANN, A., K. KAKO & A. CHRYSOHOU. 1961. Dopa uptake and catecholamine content in heart and spleen. Amer. J. Physiol. **201**: 673–676.

WURTMAN. R. J., J. AXELROD, G. T. ROSS & E. VESSELL. 1967. Fed. Proc. In press.

CENTRAL NERVOUS SYSTEM STIMULATION AND CARDIAC ISCHEMIC CHANGES IN MONKEYS*

K. I. Melville, H. L. Garvey, H. E. Shister, and J. Knaack
Departments of Pharmacology and Pathology, McGill University, Montreal, Canada

Introduction

The role of the cardiovascular changes induced by central nervous system stimulation in the development of ischemic heart disease is still highly speculative. In all types of ischemic heart disease (angina pectoris, coronary atherosclerosis, coronary insufficiency, and myocardial infarction), the primary problem is impairment of coronary function, i.e., myocardial oxygen supply is inadequate to meet myocardial oxygen requirements, to varying degrees. Sudden experimental occlusion of a major coronary blood vessel leads rapidly to fatal ventricular fibrillation, and it is generally believed that acute deaths in ischemic heart disease are of similar origin. Evidence exists that both attacks of anginal pain and electrocardiogram (ECG) ischemic changes (ST alterations) can be precipitated in patients with angina pectoris by excessive physical exertion (effort), exposure to cold, hypoxia or hypoxemia, emotional tension, or injection of epinephrine (Drill, 1965; Hurst & Logue, 1966).

In earlier studies (Melville *et al.*, 1963), it was shown that electrical stimulation of discrete hypothalamic (anterior, posterior, or lateral) areas in cats can lead to pronounced cardiovascular adrenergic (sympathetic) responses: rise in blood pressure and tachycardia associated with varying degrees of ischemic-like changes in the ECG. These effects were also accentuated by vagotomy but completely abolished by spinal cord (C2) section. In some experiments, however, bradycardia and ectopic beats ensued, but these were abolished by vagotomy and appeared to be of parasympathetic or vagal origin.

Varma and co-workers (1961), Melville and Share (1963), and Share and Melville (1963, 1965) have shown that central nervous system pharmacological stimulation, induced by injections of picrotoxin into the lateral cerebral ventricle of rabbits and cats, evoked intense peripheral sympathetic cardiovascular effects (rise in blood pressure, tachycardia, and even ventricular fibrillation in some animals). Smookler and co-workers (1966) and Severs and his associates (1966) have reported that angiotensin II, administered into the perfused lateral ventricle of cats, also induced marked tachycardia and pressor effects of a sympathetic nature. Kisin and Sinitsin (1963) have reported that electrical stimulation of the left frontal lobe of the brain cortex in the regions of the coronal gyrus and orbital gyrus in cats leads to constriction of the coronary blood vessels associated with ischemic changes in the ECG. Carrol and co-workers (1966) showed that unipolar stimulations of various brain areas in dogs (H fields of Forel, ventromedial hypothalamic nucleus, lateral hypothalamic nucleus, and dorsomedial hypothalamic nucleus) evoked marked elevations of blood pressure, coronary hyperemia, and ventricular tachycardia with chaotic heart activity; stimulation of the ventral anterior thalamic or central amygdaloid nuclei did not alter the ECG, and excitation of other points in the amygdaloid complex, hippocampus, or lenticular nucleus did not change coronary flow and/or aortic blood flow.

It is evident from the foregoing that adrenergic mechanisms originating in

* This work was supported by grants from the Medical Research Council of Canada.

the central nervous system may play an important role in coronary function. However, stimulation of cardiac sympathetic nerves and administration of epinephrine or norepinephrine (see Drill, 1965) lead to conflicting coronary responses, i.e., either coronary vasodilatation or coronary vasoconstriction or both, depending presumably upon the species or experimental conditions employed. Barbour (1912) and Barbour and Prince (1915) concluded that epinephrine leads to relaxation of coronary vessels of rabbits, cats, dogs, oxen, sheep, and pigs, but to constriction in isolated human coronary strips or in isolated perfused hearts of rhesus monkeys. The implication from these findings was that adrenergic physiological or drug responses in the human coronary circulation might be more like those observed in rhesus monkeys than in other experimental animals. It was therefore of interest to investigate (1) adrenergic responses (coronary flow and heart contraction changes) in isolated perfused monkey hearts (Melville & Garvey, 1966) and (2) adrenergic responses (blood pressure and cardiac ischemic changes) following hypothalamic stimulation in intact rhesus monkeys. The object of this paper is to present the results obtained in these studies.

Physiological and Pathological Factors Affecting Coronary Blood Flow

Figure 1 shows schematically the multiplicity of factors that have been thought to influence or to regulate coronary blood flow. As is evident, coronary

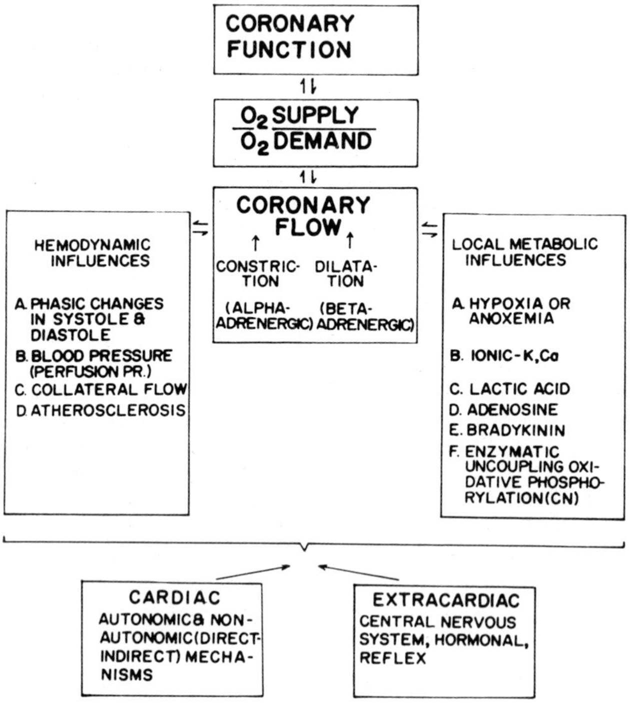

Figure 1. Factors affecting coronary blood flow.

function depends fundamentally upon the balance between oxygen supplied to the myocardium (oxygen supply) and the oxygen required to meet the work demands of the heart (oxygen demand). Considerable evidence exists that the oxygen supply of the heart is in itself an important factor in the regulation of the rate of coronary flow, although the exact mechanism involved is still unknown. In a general way, the various factors indicated may conveniently be subdivided into (1) those of cardiac origin, i.e., autonomic (sympathetic or parasympathetic) or nonautonomic (myogenic or metabolic) effects triggered by direct or indirect mechanisms; and (2) those of extracardiac origin, i.e., changes arising from central nervous system excitation or inhibition, from hormonal release (vasopressin or other substances), or from reflex nervous influences involving, for example, efferent or afferent vagal pathways.

It is also well established that both the so-called "hemodynamic" and "local metabolic" influences, as indicated in FIGURE 1, exert a significant effect upon coronary flow. The rate of coronary flow is not uniform, and increases or decreases might be due to either of these influences. During systole, coronary flow is decreased, presumably due to mechanical compression of the coronary vessels resulting from the heart contractions; conversely, coronary flow increases during diastole. Coronary perfusion pressure is an important determinant of coronary flow; theoretically, increasing aortic blood pressure increases flow, whereas decreasing aortic blood pressure decreases flow. However, as already pointed out, the oxygen supplied to the myocardium is clearly an important factor in regulating coronary flow. Hence, reducing perfusion pressure may also lead to reduction in oxygen supply and, hence, a compensatory increased flow. Acute experimental reduction of coronary blood leads rapidly to "reactive hyperemia," again presumably due to local hypoxia.

Another important hemodynamic factor is collateral blood flow, i.e., opening up of alternate or new vascular pathways to supply the myocardium. The state of the vessel walls i.e., normal or atherosclerotic, may also be important in flow. McGregor and Fam (1966) have emphasized the possible role of collateral flow in diseased states and drug responses. Several workers have observed that coronary dilator responses to nitroglycerin might be rather different in normal and atherosclerotic human coronary vessels (Brachfeld *et al.,* 1959; Gorlin *et al.,* 1959; Luebs *et al.,* 1966), and Melville and Gillis (1965) have found that the coronary constriction induced by sympathetic nerve stimulation is markedly decreased in atherosclerotic rabbit hearts. Whether these differences are due to lack of contractility in atherosclerotic blood vessels or to some unknown metabolic factor is still uncertain.

Among so-called "local metabolites," which may be of importance in regulating coronary flow, are: (1) increase or decrease in oxygen supply; hypoxia or anoxemia is known to lead to increased coronary flow (coronary vasodilatation), whereas excessive oxygen has been reported to decrease flow (coronary vasoconstriction). (2) Increase or decrease in ionic concentrations (potassium or calcium) in perfusing fluids can significantly influence coronary flow and coronary drug responses. (3) Excessive lactic acid production, such as that associated with excessive myocardial stimulation, may increase coronary flow. (4) Release of adenine nucleotides (especially adenosine), polypeptides (such as bradykinin and angiotensin), and histamine have also been considered important in coronary flow regulation (see Berne, 1964). (5) In cyanide poisoning, enzyme inactivation leading to uncoupling of oxidative phosphorylation increases coronary flow. Despite a great deal of interest in these metabolic factors, the exact significance of any of these as physiological or pathological mediators or regulators of coronary blood flow has not been established. However, any complete physiological assessment of coronary function or of the mechanisms of action of so-called "coronary drugs" would require detailed consideration of each of these various factors before final conclusions can be drawn.

In special reference to coronary adrenergic drug responses, Katz and coworkers (1938) observed that, in isolated perfused fibrillating hearts of cats and dogs, epinephrine leads to coronary vasoconstriction in the cat but vasodilatation in the dog. However, varying degrees of coronary vasodilatation and coronary vasoconstriction have been shown to occur in numerous studies in the same species of animals. Melville and Lu (1950) and Lu and Melville (1951) showed that epinephrine and norepinephrine induce both increase and decrease in coronary flow in isolated perfused rabbit hearts. From these and other early studies from this laboratory (Melville and Lu, 1952), using other adrenergic drugs (ephedrine, phenylephrine, isoproterenol, and methoxamine), it was concluded that these differences in adrenergic coronary flow responses might be due to the associated local hemodynamic and metabolic actions of these agents, rather than to any specific effect on adrenergic receptor mechanisms. Berne (1958) has reported that intracoronary injection of epinephrine or norepinephrine in fibrillating dog hearts leads to a brief initial decrease in coronary flow, followed by a more prolonged increase, which was associated with a reduction in coronary sinus blood oxygen tension. In potassium-arrested hearts, however, only reduction in coronary flow was observed. Hashimoto and his colleagues (1960), using the isolated dog heart preparation, concluded that epinephrine and levarterenol produced coronary vasodilation by increasing myocardial oxygen consumption, after initially producing a vasoconstriction. These authors also considered that coronary vasodilatation following isoproterenol administration was due only *secondarily* to cardiac stimulation, since it was found that phenoxybenzamine (an alpha-adrenergic blocking drug) prevented the initial epinephrine and levarterenol vasoconstriction, but did not affect either isoproterenol vasodilatation or the vasodilatation observed with epinephrine and norepinephrine. These workers suggested that there are both sympathetic vasoconstrictor and parasympathetic vasodilator receptors in the coronary vessels. Although it was also observed that dichloroisoproterenol (DCI) completely blocked the coronary vasodilation produced by all three amines (epinephrine, norepinephrine, and isoproterenol), the presence of sympathetic vasodilator receptors in the coronary vessels was considered improbable, since the associated myocardial metabolic effects were also blocked by DCI.

Szentiványi and Juhász-Nagy (1959) and Juhász-Nagy and Szentiványi (1961) have postulated three different types of cardiac sympathetic fibers in cats and dogs. Two of these types are believed to synapse with adrenergic or cholinergic postganglionic neurons, and the third leads only to cardiac acceleration and increased contractility. By using low voltage (0.1–2 volts) stimulation of the cardiac branches from the stellate ganglion, coronary constriction *only* was produced, without associated changes in blood pressure, heart rate, or oxygen consumption of the heart. With high voltage (5–20 volts) stimulation, there was an increased coronary flow associated with increase in blood pressure and oxygen consumption. The alpha-adrenergic blocking agent, dibenamine, abolished the coronary vasoconstriction observed in these experiments. It was therefore concluded that the sympathetic exerted a primary tonic coronary vasoconstrictor effect, but that coronary vasodilation was due only to a compensatory response resulting from adrenergic cardiac stimulation. Szentiványi and Juhász-Nagy (1963a & b) have further suggested that this sympathetic tonic coronary vasoconstrictor effect might be of physiological importance in adjusting coronary flow to provide a greater coronary reserve by limiting the degree of increase in cardiac oxygen consumption associated with increased cardiac work.

Siegel and co-workers (1961) have shown that DCI in anesthetized dogs converted the coronary vasodilator response following stellate ganglion stimulation to a coronary constrictor response, and concomitantly abolished both the chronotropic and inotropic responses. Alanis and his associates (1962) obtained similar results with hypothalamic stimulation in dogs. Using the sympathetic innervated isolated rabbit heart preparation, Hukovíc and Muscholl (1962) have shown that electrical stimulation of cardiac sympathetic nerves leads only to a decrease in coronary flow associated with cardiac stimulation and an increased output of norepinephrine. Yurchak and his colleagues (1964) have also concluded that norepinephrine produces a primary coronary vasoconstrictor action in man, probably acting on alpha-adrenergic or vasoconstrictor receptors, although no clear evidence for this was given by the authors. In conclusion, recent studies by Doutheil and co-workers (1964) and Takenaka (1966), using pronethalol to block "beta-receptors" in the perfused dog heart, would seem to suggest that both alpha- and beta-adrenergic receptor mechanisms might exist in the coronary vascular bed in that species. However, the exact significance of both adrenergic vasoconstriction and adrenergic vasodilatation in the physiological regulation of the coronary blood flow, and whether or not these mechanisms are involved in coronary heart disease, remain to be established.

Results

Adrenergic Drug Responses in Isolated Perfused Monkey Hearts

Although it was reported quite early that epinephrine produces coronary constriction in isolated perfused hearts of rhesus monkeys, and that this effect appeared similar to that observed on isolated human coronary strips, the exact mechanism of this response is still unclear. In the present studies, both rhesus monkeys (*Macaca mulatta,* formerly known as *Macacus rhesus,* weighing 3–4 kg) and vervet or South African green monkeys (*Cercopithecus oethiops,* weighing 2.5–3 kg) were used. Under intraperitoneal (i.p.) pentobarbital sodium (60 mg/kg) anesthesia, the hearts were excised and placed in cold (10° C) oxygenated McEwen (1956) solution for two to three hours prior to use. The rhesus hearts weighed 12.5–15 g, and the vervet hearts weighed approximately the same (10–15 g). All hearts were perfused according to the usual Langendorff method, with oxygenated McEwen solution with a constant perfusion pressure of 60 cm of water and a constant temperature of 37 ± 1° C. Every liter of McEwen solution contains: NaCl, 7.6 g; KCl, 0.42 g; $CaCl_2$, 0.24 g; NaH_2PO_4, 0.143 g; $NaHCO_3$, 2.1 g; dextrose, 2.0 g; and sucrose, 4.5 g; made up with distilled water. Using this solution, it was unnecessary to add serum to the perfusing fluid, as was done in earlier attempts to perfuse primate hearts. Coronary inflow, amplitude or left ventricular contractions, and heart rate (from the ECG) were recorded simultaneously. The rate of coronary flow was measured with a 100 ml per minute maximum-flow capacity rotameter (Wilson) and recorded on a Gilson polygraph. A suitable calibration curve was made by recording the pen deflection corresponding to the volume of perfusion fluid collected over a one-minute period at various known flow rates. Mean coronary flow (milliliters per minute) represents the average of maximum and minimum flow rates recorded. Heart contractions were measured by a Grass Model (FT .03) force-displacement transducer, and recorded concurrently on the Gilson, as millimeters of pen deflection. Heart rate was calculated from the ECG, recorded on a Sanborn Viso-cardiette, from sterling silver wires attached to the aortic stump and to the apex of the left ventricle.

For comparative purposes, responses to isoprenaline (*l*-isoproterenol *d*-bitartrate, 0.04 μg), adrenaline (*l*-epinephrine bitartrate, 1 μg), noradrenaline (levarterenol bitartrate, 1 μg), and calcium chloride (5 mg) were studied before and during beta-adrenergic blockade with pronethalol (Nethalide ®).† The concentration of pronethalol employed was 0.12 μg/ml in McEwen solution, since this concentration was previously observed (Melville and Benfey, 1965) to block completely responses to isoproterenol in isolated rabbit hearts. In each experiment, the blocking agent was given for a period of 30 minutes prior to testing the other agents and continued during the tests for an additional 30 to 40 minutes.

As is evident from FIGURE 2, all four agents studied induced marked increased myocardial contractility in rhesus hearts, but only after isoproterenol was this response associated with increased coronary flow coronary vasodilatation. Epinephrine, levarterenol, and calcium chloride produced only decreased coronary flow (coronary vasoconstriction) in this species. It is also clear that the effects of isoproterenol (coronary vasodilatation and increased contractility) were completely prevented during pronethalol infusion. On the other hand, the other agents still induced some coronary constriction and increased myocardial contractility, although both of these effects were reduced.

FIGURES 3, 4, and 5 show typical examples of the changes in contractile force, coronary flow, heart rates, and ECG, as recorded before and during pronethalol perfusion with isoproterenol, levarterenol, and calcium chloride, respectively. The responses to epinephrine, as already noted, were similar to those observed with levarterenol.

As is evident, isoproterenol led rapidly to increased systolic flow, whereas levarterenol decreased systolic flow. Subsequently, and associated with the increased myocardial contractility, both isoproterenol and levarterenol increased diastolic coronary flow. On the other hand, calcium chloride decreased both systolic and diastolic coronary flow, with increased myocardial contractility. The records also show that isoproterenol led to relatively less tachycardia than did levarterenol in rhesus hearts, but these effects were significantly reduced or abolished by pronethalol.

In the course of these experiments, hearts from South African green or vervet monkeys were similarly investigated for comparative purposes. As shown in FIGURE 6, under identical experimental conditions, isoproterenol, epinephrine, and levarterenol all induced definite coronary dilatation and increased myocardial contractility, whereas calcium produced coronary vasoconstriction but also enhanced contractility. During pronethalol perfusion, the responses to isoproterenol were again completely or almost completely abolished, and both

† Courtesy of Ayerst, McKenna and Harrison Ltd., Montreal, Canada.

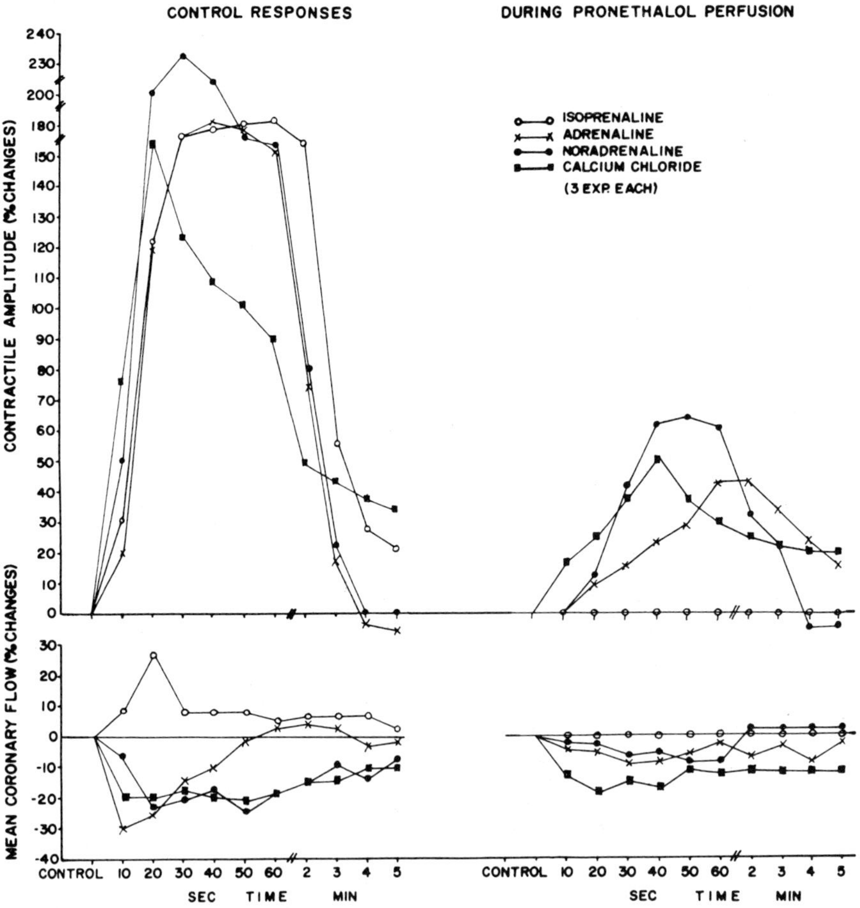

FIGURE 2. Mean coronary flow and mean cardiac contractile changes recorded in isolated perfused hearts of rhesus monkeys. Effects of single doses of isoprenaline (1 μg), adrenaline (1 μg), noradrenaline (1 μg), and calcium chloride (5 mg), before (control responses) and during pronethalol perfusion, as shown.

coronary dilatation and increased contractility following epinephrine and levarterenol were significantly reduced. In striking contrast, however, both the cardiac contractile and coronary constrictor responses to calcium were still in evidence during pronethalol perfusion.

It was also observed that the tachycardia produced by isoproterenol, epinephrine, and levarterenol was more marked in vervet hearts than in the rhesus hearts, but the response was significantly reduced or abolished by pronethalol. Calcium did not significantly affect heart rate in either vervet or rhesus hearts.

Since isoproterenol, epinephrine, and levarterenol, all led *only* to coronary dilatation with tachycardia and increased myocardial contractility in vervet hearts, and since all of these effects are abolished by pronethalol, it would appear that all of these changes are mediated by beta-adrenergic receptors in this species. On the other hand, as already pointed out, only isoproterenol

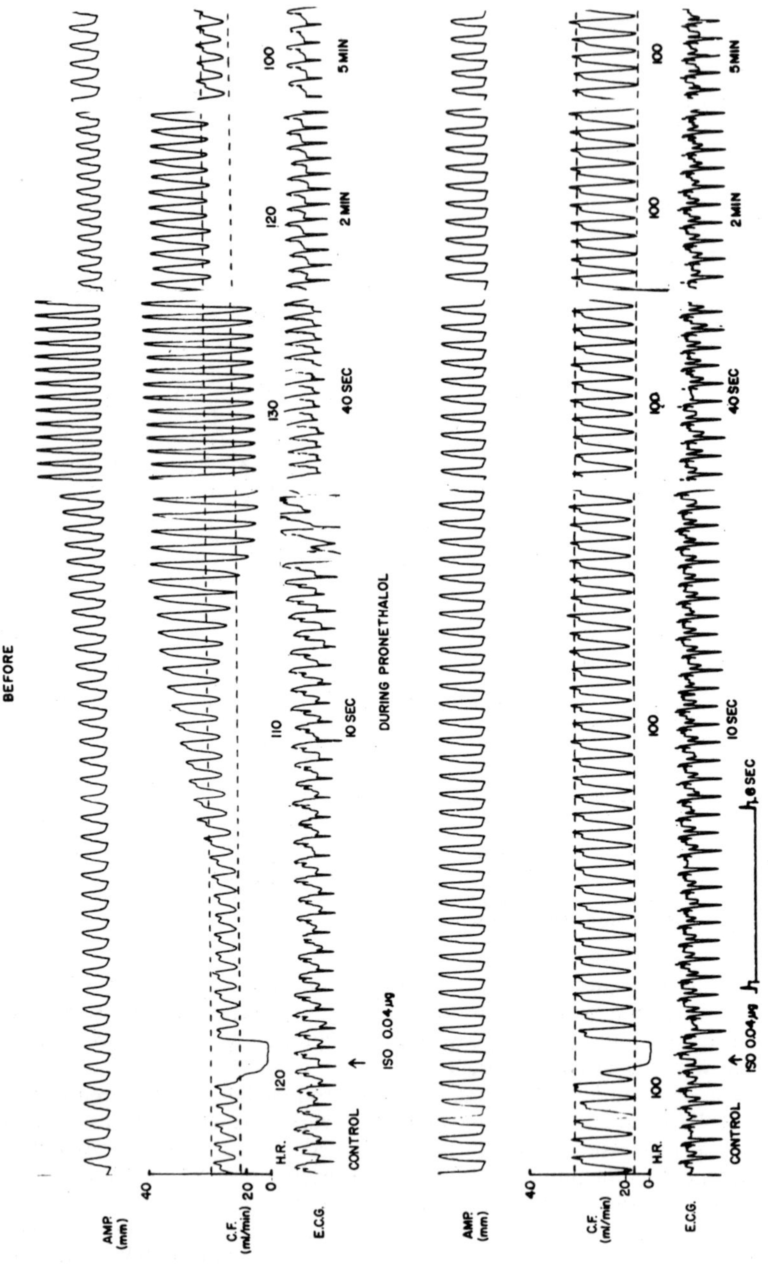

FIGURE 3. Isolated perfused heart of rhesus monkey. Effects of isoprenaline (0.04 μg) on contractile amplitude (AMP), coronary flow (CF), and heart rate (HR) before and during pronethalol perfusion. Broken lines indicate diastolic (above) and systolic (below) flow.

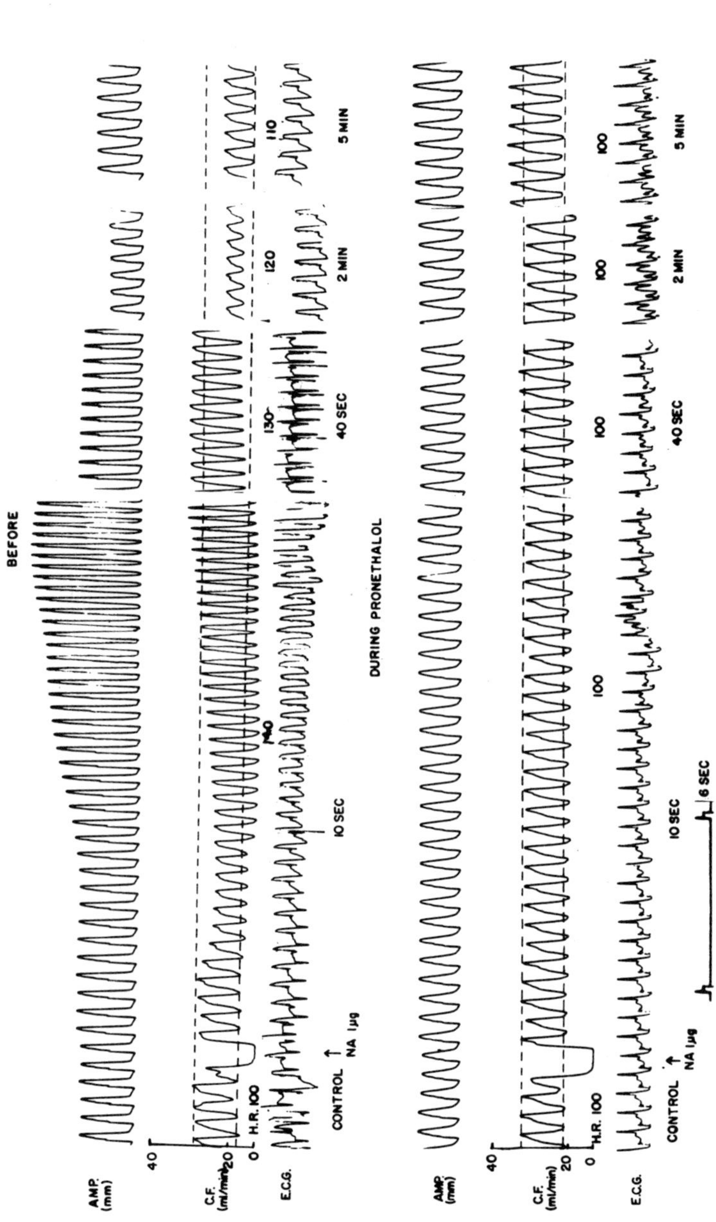

FIGURE 4. Isolated perfused heart of rhesus monkey. Effects of noradrenaline (1 μg) on contractile amplitude (AMP), coronary flow (CF), and heart rate (HR). Broken lines indicate diastolic (above) and systolic (below) flow.

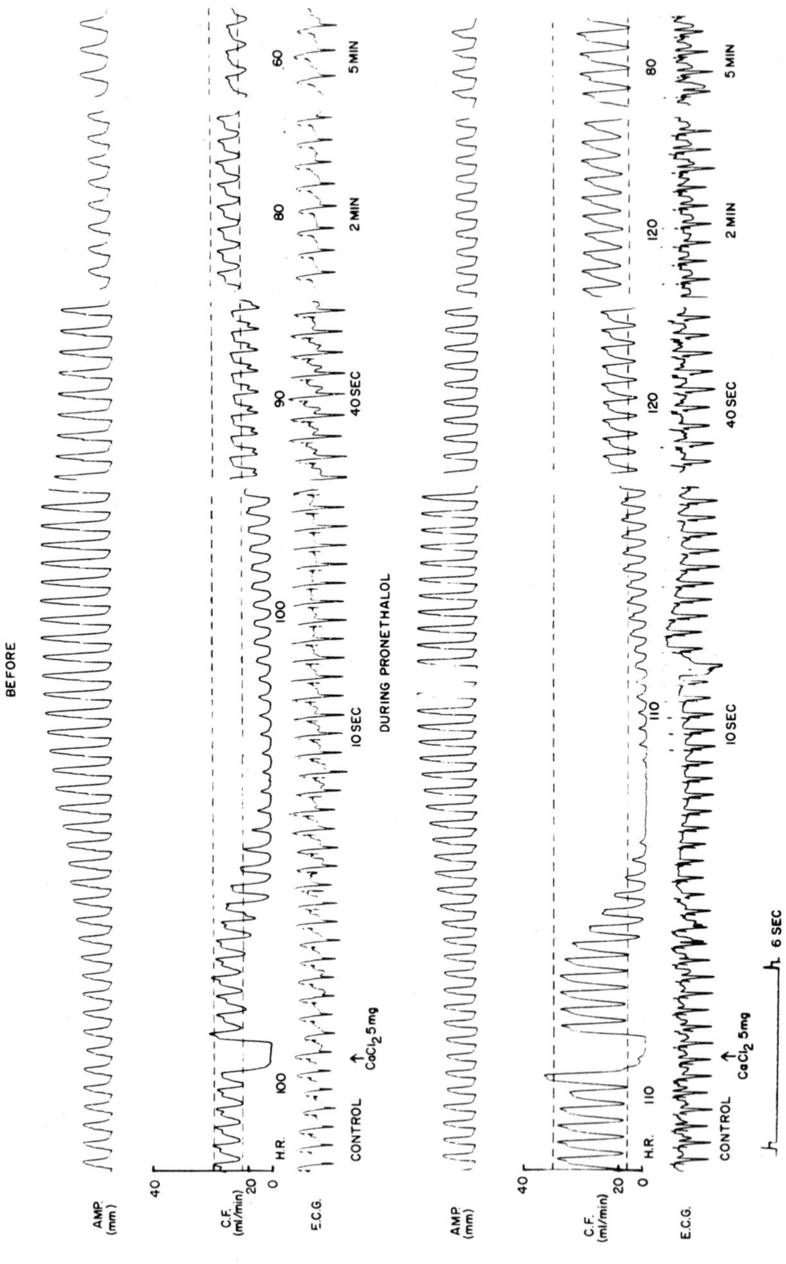

FIGURE 5. Isolated perfused heart of rhesus monkey. Effects of calcium chloride (5 mg) on contractile amplitude (**AMP**), coronary flow (CF), and heart rate (**HR**). Broken lines indicate diastolic (**above**) and systolic (below) flow.

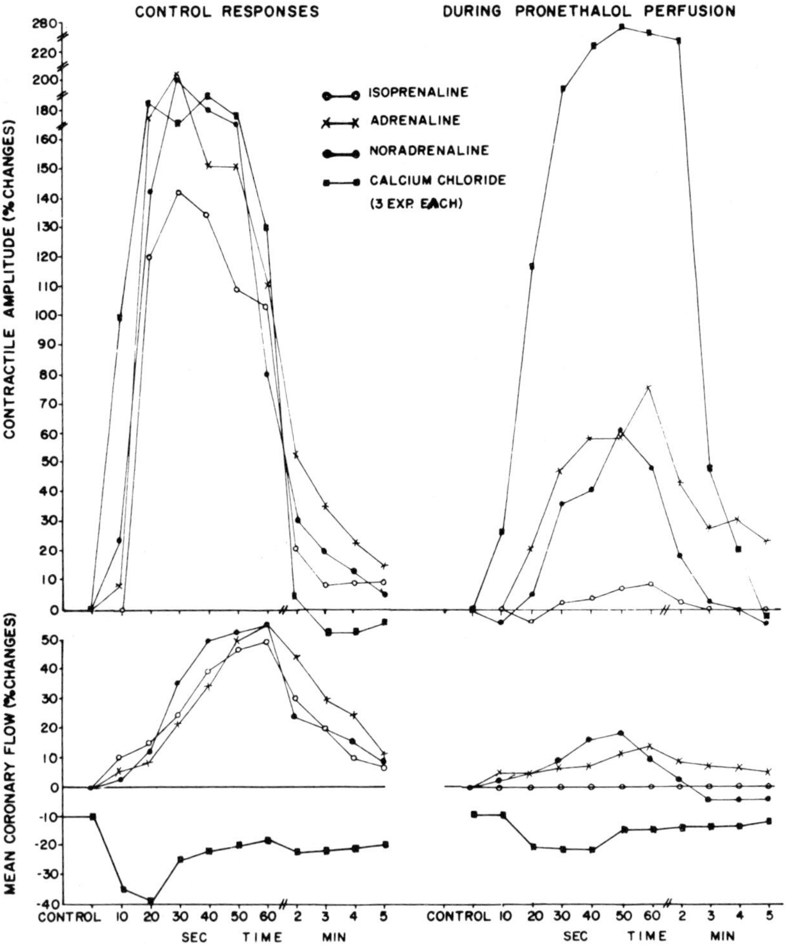

FIGURE 6. Mean coronary flow and mean cardiac contractile changes recorded in isolated perfused hearts of vervet monkeys. Effects of single doses of isoprenaline (1 μg), adrenaline (1 μg), noradrenaline (1 μg), and calcium chloride (5 mg) before (control responses) and during pronethalol perfusion, as shown.

exerts similar effects in the rhesus hearts, and both epinephrine and levarterenol lead mainly to coronary constriction. It is possible, therefore that coronary vasoconstriction might be mediated by some other mechanism, probably alpha-adrenergic receptors in the coronary vessels, as has been suggested. However, further study is necessary before any definite conclusion on this point can be drawn.

As previously indicated, the nonadrenergic agent calcium led to coronary constriction and increased contractility in both rhesus and vervet hearts, but these effects, although definitely reduced in the rhesus heart, were not completely abolished by pronethalol. On the other hand, neither the coronary constriction nor the stimulation induced by calcium in vervet hearts were prevented by beta-blockade with pronethalol. In preliminary experiments, similar results were obtained using the same concentrations of propranolol (Inderal ®)‡ instead of pronethalol.

The fact that both epinephrine and levarterenol lead to coronary vasoconstriction in the rhesus monkey and to coronary vasodilatation in the vervet, but to similar increases in contractility in both species, would not suggest that the coronary constriction observed in these experiments is due to mechanical compression of the coronary vessels nor to any "metabolic" effect. It is therefore postulated that epinephrine and levarterenol either directly or indirectly excite alpha-adrenergic receptor mechanisms, which might also be influenced by calcium in the rhesus hearts, although it is obvious that there are fundamental differences in the responses to the amines and to calcium. This problem requires further study.

Since pronethalol is also known to exert local anesthetic and direct myocardial depressant actions, the reduced degree of coronary constriction following epinephrine and levarterenol in rhesus hearts might be due to these associated effects of pronethalol.

From the above findings, it is concluded: (1) that both alpha-adrenergic coronary vasoconstrictor mechanisms and beta-adrenergic coronary vasodilator mechanisms might be involved to varying degrees in the control of the coronary circulation in different species of hearts; (2) that apparent species differences herein-described or previously reported in the literature might, in fact, be due only to predominance of one or the other type of adrenergic control; and (3) that alpha-adrenergic coronary vasoconstrictor mechanisms might predominate in the rhesus heart, and, presumably, might also be the main effect of cardiac sympathetic functions in the human heart.

Blood Pressure and Cardiac Ischemic Changes Following Lateral Hypothalamic Stimulation in Rhesus Monkeys

In this series of experiments, eight rhesus monkeys (seven males and one female, weighing 2.8–4 kg) were anesthetized with ether followed intravenously (i.v.) by chloralose (80 mg/kg) and succinylcholine (1 mg per minute, as required) and maintained with artificial respiration. Unipolar stimulation was applied with stainless steel electrodes with bare tips of approximately 20 μ in diameter. The electrode was placed stereotaxically into the left lateral hypothalamic area, employing the Horsley-Clarke coordinate system according to the atlas of Olszewski (1952). The exact coordinates employed in each experiment are given in the legends of the figures. As in earlier similar experiments on cats (Melville *et al.*, 1963), it was observed that pressor responses and ischemic-like changes occurred only from discrete areas of stimulation. It was often necessary, therefore, to explore functionally the hypothalamic area by lowering or raising the electrode after using the placements as indicated by the atlas. Final placements of electrodes were verified anatomically and histologically by the method of Hess, as far as possible.

Stimulation of the lateral hypothalamic areas was carried out, using square wave pulses at a frequency of 100 cycles per second (cps) and duration of 1 millisecond (msec). Each period of stimulation lasted for 60 seconds. A Grass stimulator (S4) was used throughout. The stimulus strength employed was 1 milliampere (ma) continuously monitored on an oscilloscope and delivered through an isolation transformer. During and after each period of stimulation,

‡ Courtesy of Ayerst, McKenna and Harrison Ltd., Montreal, Canada.

the femoral arterial blood pressure (recorded with a Statham transducer) and ECG (precordial lead V4, approximately over the apical area with the animal in the left lateral position) were simultaneously recorded on a Sanborn Recorder.

For postmortem histological examinations, the hearts were usually excised 20 to 24 hours after the last of a series of repeated stimulations, or after a similar delay in the control, nonstimulated animals. In order to maintain the preparation for these prolonged periods, artificial respiration and chloralose anesthesia were continued throughout, and 200,000 IU of penicillin procaine mixed with 0.25 g of streptomycin sulfate was injected intramuscularly (i.m.). Immediately after excision, all hearts were placed in a 10% solution of formalin.

FIGURE 7 shows typical examples of the responses recorded during lateral hypothalamic stimulation before and after double cervical vagotomy. Similar results were obtained in three monkeys.

As is evident, before vagotomy (upper records) during stimulation there was a prompt rise in blood pressure, with increases in both systolic and diastolic pressures (from 125/100 to 190/115). This pressor effect persisted throughout almost the entire period of stimulation (60 seconds). Initially (within five seconds), there was also a marked sinus tachycardia (heart rate increasing from 180 to 220 beats per minute) and progressive T wave elevation, with slight sagging of the P-R interval. Within ten seconds, the heart rate decreased to approximately 180 beats per minute, with irregular periods of sinus block associated with transient declines in the blood pressure, but marked T wave elevation persisted. Toward the termination of the stimulation, there was some decline in blood pressure with a distinct bradycardia (90 beats per minute), plus marked diminution of the T wave and sagging of the ST segment. Immediately following stimulation, bradycardia was accentuated, but within two to five minutes there was a progressive restoration of blood pressure and heart rate to control levels.

The above responses were repeatable for three succesive repetitions of the same type of stimulation at five-minute intervals. The vagus nerves in the neck were then sectioned, and stimulation was again repeated (15 minutes later), as shown in FIGURE 7 (lower records). As can be seen, there was again a rapid similar elevation of blood pressure, with a sinus tachycardia (increase in heart rate from 200 to 240 beats per minute) associated with distinct increase in the T wave voltage. These changes persisted for the duration of the stimulation, the heart rate increasing to 260 beats per minute and the T waves showing a slight reduction in height. Following stimulation, the blood pressure gradually returned to normal, but, in contrast with the nonvagotomized animals, tachycardia and T wave elevation persisted for two to five minutes, returning only slowly (within ten minutes) to the control. It is therefore evident that vagotomy enhanced the adrenergic responses induced by lateral hypothalamic stimulation.

When similar stimulations were repeated 24 times at five-minute intervals in this experiment (FIGURE 7), similar blood pressure and ECG changes were recorded with each stimulation. Following a post-stimulation period of 22 hours, the heart was excised and showed grossly pronounced subendocardial hemorrhages over the interventricular septum and papillary muscle. FIGURE 8 shows a microphotograph of the myocardium. On lower magnification (x 100), microscopical foci of necroses (microinfarcts) surrounded by normal tissue

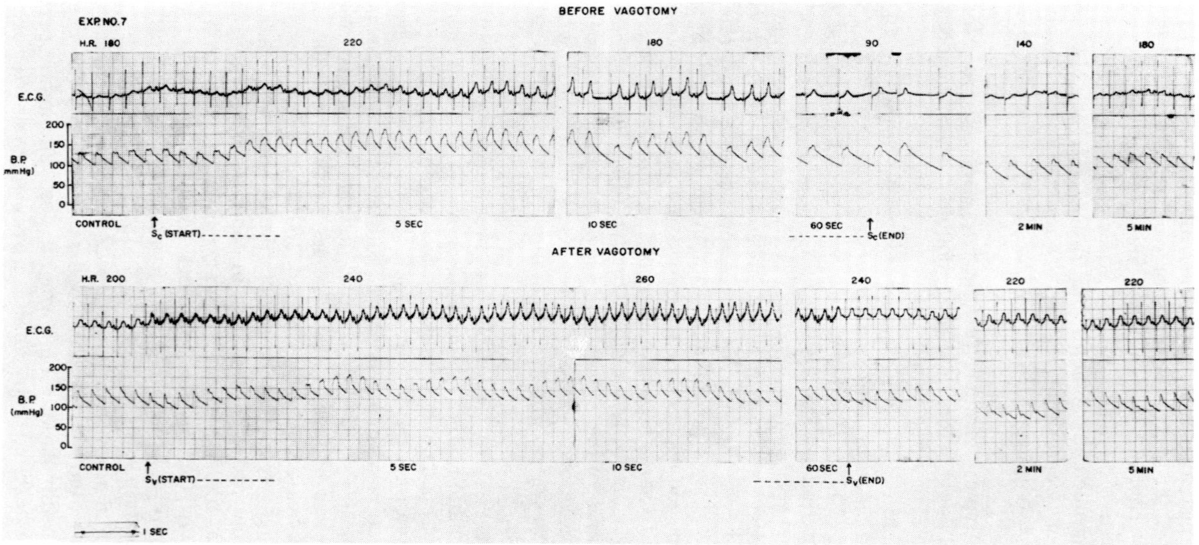

FIGURE 7. Rhesus monkey (2.6 kg) subjected to left lateral hypothalamic stimulation. Simultaneous ECG (lead V4) and blood pressure changes before and after bilateral vagotomy. Stereotaxic coordinates: frontal, 10.5; sagittal, 2.0; and horizontal, 3.0.

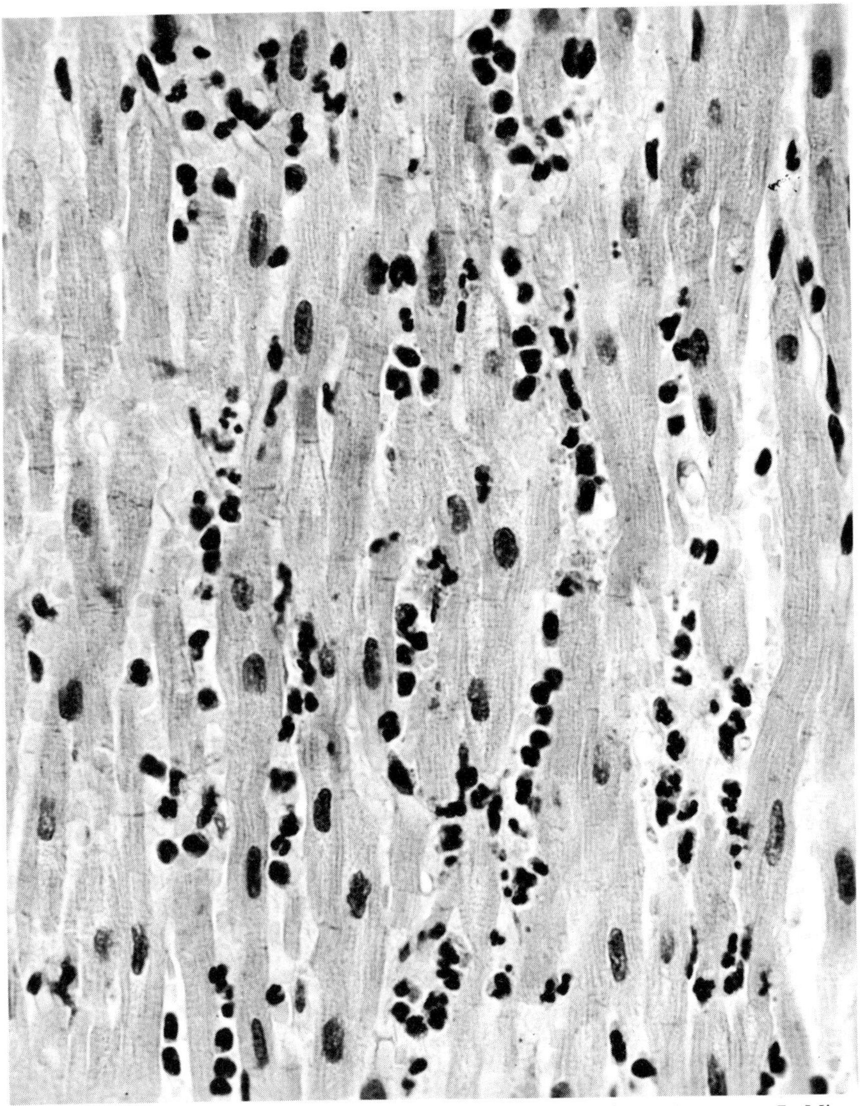

FIGURE 8. Heart from rhesus monkey used in experiment shown in FIGURE 7. Microphotograph of myocardium showing varying stages of necrosis of myocardial fibers with polymorphonuclear leukocyte response. Stain: hematoxylin and eosin. × 400.

could be seen, and at higher magnification (x 400), as shown in FIGURE 8, there were varying stages of necrosis of myocardial fibers, with moderate polymorphonuclear leukocyte response, although many fibers were well preserved. These changes are believed to be ischmic lesions. However, histochemical examinations§ of the heart for lactic acid dehydrogenase (LDH) were inconclusive and showed no clear evidence of any increase.

In one control monkey heart (i.e., a heart excised after a period of 22 hours, during which the animal had been subjected to identical anesthetic and surgical procedures with the electrodes implanted as noted previously, but without stimulation) there was no histological evidence of necrosis of the myocardial fibers, although there was gross evidence of subendothelial hemorrhages, with varying degrees of microscopical interstitial hemorrhages. It is of interest that all hearts excised following the operative procedures employed in these studies consistently showed a similar type of pathology, although necrosis of the myocardium was only observed in the stimulated hearts. Although the exact significance of this observation is not known, these lesions appeared to be similar to those observed postmortem in humans following acute deaths from cerebral injury. It is postulated, therefore, that these cardiac changes might be evidence of some type of nonspecific response of the monkey heart to the "stresses" of the anethetic and operative procedures involved in the implantation of the electrodes into the hypothalamus. This type of response was not seen in earlier similar studies on cats, suggesting that the rhesus monkey is more sensitive to such changes, and possibly therefore a more satisfactory experimental species for this type of investigation.

With the hope of detecting an increase in serum enzymes, determinations of serum glutamic oxalacetic transaminase (SGOT), using the method of Reitman and Frankel (1957), and serum lactic dehydrogenase (SLDH), using the method of Berger and Broida,¶ were made before and after prolonged lateral hypothalamic stimulations. The results obtained were variable and inconclusive. However, contrary to expectations, blood samples taken from one monkey (used for the experiments shown in FIGURES 7 and 8) showed only a decrease in SGOT from a control level of 40 units/ml to 19.5 units/ml (22 hours after stimulation); SLDH also decreased in the same samples from a control value exceeding 1,000 units/ml to 790 units/ml. Control values obtained from blood samples taken from two normal unanesthetized rhesus monkeys gave the following serum enzyme values: SGOT, 58 units/ml and 80 units/ml; SLDH, exceeding, 1,000 units/ml in both cases. It is not clear why these values decreased rather than increased in these experiments, and the problem is being further studied.

Finally, in the course of these experiments, it was also noted that both simple withdrawal of blood (two experiments) or section of the vagus nerves in the neck (two experiments) induced a profound fall in blood pressure and a reversible "shock-like" state in the monkeys. In one other animal, however, these changes were markedly intensified and irreversible, as shown in FIGURE 9.

In this experiment, again, stimulation before vagotomy induced the usual pressor response associated with sinus tachycardia and T wave elevations. After 40 seconds, premature ventricular beats appeared, with aberrant conduction (probably nodal), and toward the end of the stimulation there was a sinus block. Immediately following stimulation, there was an accentuation

§ Courtesy of the Department of Pathology, McGill University, Montreal, Canada.

¶ As described by Sigma Chemical Co., St. Louis, Mo.

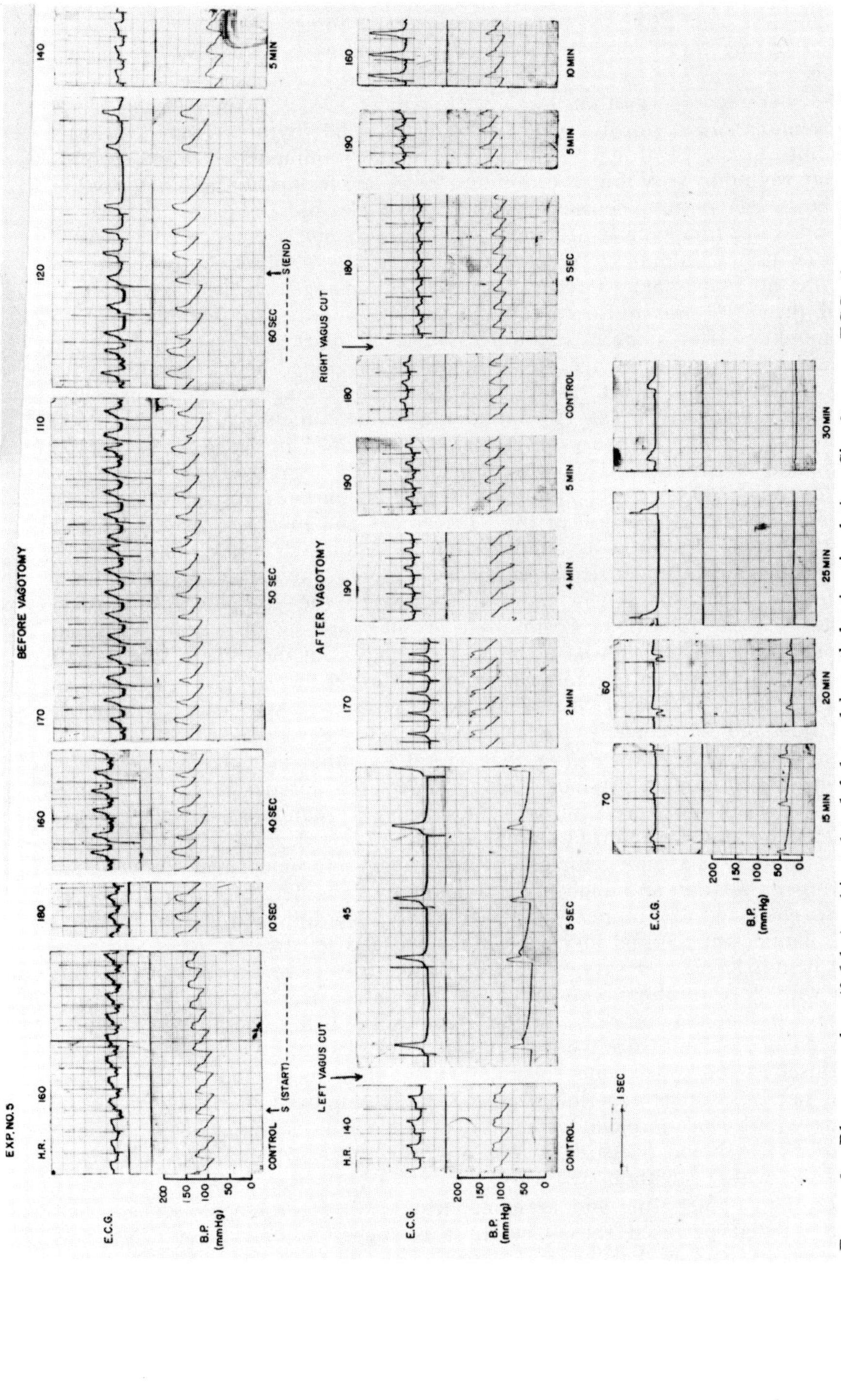

FIGURE 9. Rhesus monkey (3.6 kg) subjected to left lateral hypothalamic stimulation. Simultaneous ECG (lead V4) and blood pressure changes before and after left and right vagotomy. Stereotaxic coordinates: frontal, 9.4; sagittal, 3.0; and horizontal, 3.5.

of bradycardia with increased sinus block, and a progressive restoration of blood pressure and ECG to normal within five minutes. Similar results were recorded during three successive similar stimulations repeated at five-minute intervals.

The lower records (FIGURE 9) show that there was a distinct fall in blood pressure and marked slowing of the heart with nodal rhythm (from 150 beats per minute in the control to 45 beats per minute) immediately (five seconds after left vagotomy). Within two minutes, however, restoration to sinus rhythm (170 beats per minute) ensued, with T wave elevation and an increase in blood pressure, following which there was a progressive return to control conditions (within 15 minutes). When the right vagus was subsequently sectioned, there was no immediate (5 seconds) significant change, and the general pattern of the ECG was quite comparable at five minutes to that observed in other monkeys after bilateral vagotomy. However, marked elevation of the ST segment and increased voltage of the T waves developed at ten minutes, with slight slowing of the heart rate but no significant change in blood pressure. There was subsequently (at 15 minutes) a sudden intense fall in the blood pressure from which recovery never ensued, as shown in the records marked 20, 25, and 30 minutes. This was associated with a marked slowing of the heart to 70 and 60 beats per minute at 15 and 20 minutes, respectively. There was also a distinct depression of the ST segment and inversion of the T wave (at 20 minutes), followed by abnormal QRS complexes, either supraventricular with aberrant intraventricular conduction or an idioventricular rhythm (at 25 minutes), and subsequent reduced voltage of the complexes to cardiac standstill (at 30 minutes). Postmortem examination of the heart removed immediately thereafter showed no gross pathology, but there were some small microscopical interstitial hemorrhages. In this experiment, there was also no change in the SGOT and SLDH in blood samples taken before the initial stimulation and immediately after death.

In summary, it is shown: (1) that lateral hypothalamic electrical stimulations in rhesus monkeys induce striking repeatable adrenergic cardiovascular changes (rise in blood pressure, ischemic-like ST-T changes, and tachycardia), associated (in nonvagotomized animals) with varying degrees of cardiac vagal effects (bradycardia and ectopic rhythm) which are intensified immediately following stimulation and abolished by vagotomy (adrenergic cardiac responses are also enhanced and more sustained following vagotomy); (2) that repeated hypothalamic stimulations in rhesus monkeys lead to striking gross subendothelial hemorrhages and varying degrees of necrosis of myocardial fibers associated with polymorphonuclear leukocyte responses, probably due to ischemic lesions; (3) that the "stresses" of the anesthesia and the operative procedures employed in inserting the hypothalamic electrodes in the rhesus monkey can in themselves induce definite subendothelial hemorrhages, but without myocardial necrosis; other experimental procedures employed in rhesus monkeys, such as withdrawal of blood or section of the vagus nerves, can also induce marked fall in blood pressure and cardiac slowing associated with a "shock-like" state with or without recovery.

Since both epinephrine and norepinephrine induce coronary vasconstriction in the isolated perfused rhesus heart, it is suggested that these deleterious cardiac effects of hypothalamic stimulation might be caused by release of these amines in the body under the conditions employed. It has long been known that norepinephrine is the main amine released by cardiac sympathetic nerve stimulation (Outschoorn & Vogt, 1952), but the possible role of epinephrine released from the adrenal glands in these experiments has not been investigated.

In conclusion, the findings presented also indicate that the coronary vasoconstriction observed following injections of epinephrine or levarterenol in isolated perfused rhesus hearts might be due to alpha-adrenergic receptor excitation in the coronary vessels. These coronary responses in conjunction with the cardiac ischemic changes and other deleterious cardiovascular effects observed in intact rhesus monkeys following hypothalamic stimulation, or the various experimental procedures described above, would also suggest that cardiac adrenergic changes arising from central nervous system excitation or involvement might be of considerable importance in the pathogenesis of human ischemic heart disease. The close similarity between the deleterious experimental cardiac effects observed in the rhesus monkey and the cardiac pathological changes known to occur in man would strongly support this concept.

References

ALANIS, J., E. LOPEZ & O. ROSAS. 1962. Changes in dogs coronary circulation by hypothalamic stimulation. Arch. Inst. Cardiol. Mex. **22**: 743.

BARBOUR, H. G. 1912. The constricting influence of adrenalin upon the human coronary arteries. J. Exp. Med. **15**: 404–414.

BARBOUR, H. G. & A. L. PRINCE. 1915. The influence of epinephrine upon the coronary circulation of the monkey. J. Exp. Med. **21**: 330–337.

BERNE, R. M. 1958. Effect of epinephrine and norepinephrine on coronary circulation. Circ. Res. **6**: 644-655.

BERNE, R. M. 1964. Regulation of coronary blood flow. Physiol. Rev. **44**: 1–29.

BRACHFELD, N., J. BOZER & R. GORLIN. 1959. Action of nitroglycerin in the coronary circulation in normal and mild cardiac subjects. Circulation **19**: 697–704.

CARROL, JR., M. N., R. J. GOLINKO, D. H. FORD, A. GOLFELD & R. BYRD. 1966. CNS-evoked coronary flow changes and other cardiodynamic alterations. Effects of mebutamate and pentobarbital. Proc. 3rd Int. Pharmacol. Congr., July 24–30, Sao Paolo, Brazil. Abstr. no. 524.

DOUTHEIL, U., H. G. TEN BRUGGENCATE & K. KRAMER. 1964. Coronarvasomotorik unter l-Noradrenalin und Isopropyl-noradrenalin nach Blockierung der adrenergischen β-receptoren durch Nethalide. Pflueger. Archiv. Ges. Physiol. **281**: 181–190.

DRILL'S Pharmacology in Medicine, 1965, J. R. Dipalma, Ed., 3rd edit. : 504–623. McGraw-Hill Book Co. New York, N. Y.

GORLIN, R., N. BRACHFELD, C. MACLEOD & P. BOPP. 1959. Effects of nitroglycerin in the coronary circulation in patients with coronary artery disease or increased left ventricular work. Circulation **19**: 705–718.

HASHIMOTO, K., T. SHIGEI, S. IMAI, Y. SAITO, N. TAGO, I. UEI & R. E. CLARK. 1960. Oxygen consumption and coronary vascular tone in the isolated fibrillating dog heart. Amer. J. Physiol. **198**: 965–970.

HUKOVÍC, S. & E. MUSCHOLL. 1962. Die Noradrenalin-Abgabe aus dem isolierten Kaninchenherzen bei sympathischer Nervenreizung und ihre pharmakologische Beeinflussung. Arch. Exp. Path. Pharmak. **244**: 81–96.

HURST, J. W. & R. B. LOGUE. 1966. The Heart. McGraw-Hill Book Co. New York, N. Y.

JUHÁSZ-NAGY, A. & M. SZENTIVÁNYI. 1961. Separation of cardioacceleration and coronary vasomotor fibers in the dog. Amer. J. Physiol. **200**: 125–129.

KATZ, L. N., E. LINDNER, W. WEINSTEIN, D. I. ABRAMSON & K. JOCHIM. 1938. Effects of various drugs on the coronary circulation of the denervated isolated heart of the dog and cat. Arch. Int. Pharmacodyn. **59**: 399–415.

KISIN, I. E. & L. N. SINITSIN. 1963. Prevention of disturbed coronary circulation consequent upon stimulation of the brain cortex effected with pharmacological agents. Bull. Acad. Med. Sci. (Moscow) **1**: 18–23 (in Russian).

LU, F. C. & K. I. MELVILLE. 1951. Effects of noradrenaline on coronary flow and heart contraction as recorded concurrently in isolated rabbit hearts. J. Physiol. (London) **113**: 365–371.

LUEBS, E. D., A. COHEN, E. J. ZALESKI & R. J. BING. 1966. Effects of nitroglycerin, intensain, isoptin and papaverine on coronary blood flow in man. Amer. J. Cardiol. **17**: 535–541.

McEwen, L. M. 1956. The effect in the isolated rabbit heart of vagal stimulation and its modification by cocaine, hexamethonium and ouabain. J. Physiol. (London) **131**: 678–689.

McGregor, M. & W. M. Fam. 1966. Regulation of coronary blood flow. Bull. N. Y. Acad. Med. **42**: 940–950.

Melville, K. I. & B. G. Benfey. 1965. Coronary vasodilatory and cardiac adrenergic blocking effects of iproveratril. Canad. J. Physiol. Pharmacol. **43**: 339–342.

Melville, K. I., B. Blum, H. E. Shister & M. D. Silver. 1963. Cardiac ischemic changes and arrhythmias induced by hypothalamic stimulation. Amer. J. Cardiol. **12**: 781–791.

Melville, K. I. & H. L. Garvey. 1966. Adrenergic drug responses in isolated perfused monkey hearts. Proc. 3rd Int. Pharmacol. Congr., July 24–30, Sao Paulo, Brazil. Abstr. no. 288.

Melville, K. I. & R. A. Gillis. 1965. Cardiac sympathetic activity during experimental rabbit atherosclerosis. Fed. Proc. **24**: 2.

Melville, K. I. & F. C. Lu. 1950. Effects of epinephrine, aminophylline, nitroglycerine and papaverine on coronary inflow and on heart contractions as recorded concurrently. J. Pharmacol. Exp. Ther. **99**: 286–303.

Melville, K. I. & F. C. Lu. 1952. Effects of ephedrine, phenylephrine, isopropylarterenol and methoxamine on coronary flow and heart activity as recorded concurrently. Arch. Int. Pharmacodyn. **92**: 108–118.

Melville, K. I. & N. N. Share. 1963. Cardiovascular responses following injection of picrotoxin into the lateral cerebral ventricle. Rev. Canad. Biol. **22**: 265–273.

Olszewski, J. 1952. The Thalamus of the *Macaca mulatta:* An Atlas for Use with the Stereotaxic Instrument. S. Karger, New York, N.Y.

Outschoorn, A. S. & M. Vogt. 1952. The nature of cardiac sympathin in the dog. Brit. J. Pharmacol. **7**: 319–324.

Reitman, S. & S. Frankel. 1957. A caloric method for the determination of serum glutamic pyruvic transaminase. Amer. J. Clin. Path. **28**: 56–73.

Severs, W. B., A. E. Daniels, H. H. Smookler, W. J. Kinnard & J. P. Buckley. 1966. Interrelationship between angiotensin II and the sympathetic nervous system. J. Pharmacol. Exp. Ther. **153**: 530–537.

Share, N. N. & K. I. Melville. 1963. Centrally mediated sympathetic cardiovascular responses induced by intraventricular norepinephrine. J. Pharmacol. Exp. Ther. **141**: 15–21.

Share, N. N. & K. I. Melville. 1965. Involvement of brain-stem norepinephrine in picrotoxin and tyramine-induced central sympathetic stimulation. Arch. Int. Pharmacodyn. **153**: 267–282.

Siegel, J. H., J. P. Gilmore & S. J. Sarnoff. 1961. Myocardial extraction and production of catecholamines. Circ. Res. **9**: 1336–1350.

Smookler, H. H., W. B. Severs, W. J. Kinnard & J. P. Buckley. 1966. Centrally mediated cardiovascular effects of angiotensin II. J. Pharmacol. Exp. Ther. **153**: 485–494.

Szentivány, M. & A. Juhász-Nagy. 1959. A new aspect of the nervous control of the coronary blood vessels. Quart. J. Exp. Physiol. **44**: 67–79.

Szentiványi, M. & A. Juhász-Nagy. 1963a. The physiological role of the coronary constrictor fibers. I. The effects of the coronary vasomotors on the systemic blood pressure. Quart. J. Exp. Physiol. **48**: 93–104.

Szentiványi, M. & A. Juhász-Nagy. 1963b. The physiological role of the coronary constrictor fibers, II. The role of the coronary vasomotors in metabolic adaptation of the coronaries. Quart. J. Exp. Physiol. **48**: 105–118.

Takenaka, F. 1966. Effects of epinephrine and beta-adrenergic blocking agents on coronary circulation and myocardial metabolism. Arch. Exp. Path. Pharmak. **252**: 407–417.

Varma, D. R., N. N. Share & K. I. Melville. 1961. Cardiovascular responses following injection of picrotoxin into the lateral cerebral ventricle of rabbits. Biochem. Pharmacol. **8**: 451.

Yurchak, P. M., E. L. Rolett, L. S. Cohen & R. Gorlin. 1964. Effects of norepinephrine in the coronary circulation in man. Circulation **30**: 180–187.

FOCAL MYOCYTOLYSIS AND FUCHSINOPHILIC DEGENERATION OF THE MYOCARDIUM OF PATIENTS DYING WITH VARIOUS BRAIN LESIONS

Richard C. R. Connor

Department of Neuropathology, Western Infirmary, and Glasgow Institute of Neurological Sciences, Killearn Hospital, Glasgow, Scotland

It is nearly 30 years since Aschenbrenner and Bodechtel[1] reported abnormalities in the electrocardiograms (ECG) of young patients with brain tumors. Many reports have since appeared on ECG abnormalities associated with intracranial lesions.[2-14] These abnormalities have often been reported as those of myocardial infarction, but only Burch and co-workers[15] and Eichbaum and his associates[16] describe any histological damage in the myocardium.

However, myocardial damage does occur fairly often in humans with brain lesions. Some cases have focal myocytolysis, and others fuchsinophilic degeneration. I have described my findings separately in the sections of this paper.

Material

With one exception, the patients were all seen in the West of Scotland Neurosurgical Unit (now the Neurosurgical Unit of the Glasgow Institute of Neurological Sciences), which treats unselected patients from a population of three million. Details of the patients included in this study are found in TABLES 1 and 2.

Methods

Blocks of heart muscle were fixed in buffered 10% formol-saline and then processed by the rapid double-embedding technique of Russell.[17] Sections were stained with hemalum and eosin, Masson trichrome, and by the acid-fuchsin technique first described by Bajusz:[18] Paraffin sections were rinsed in distilled water and stained for 15 minutes in solution A [50 ml of cresyl violet (1 g in 500 ml of water, filtered after 1 hour), 150 ml of distilled water, and 0.8 ml of a 1% solution of oxalic acid (must be prepared immediately prior to use)]. After another rinsing in distilled water, sections were stained for 8 minutes in solution B (20 ml of 10% phosphomolybdic acid, 20 ml of 10% phosphotungstic acid, 10 ml of 2% acid fuchsin, 0.8 ml of 1% aniline hydrochloride, 2 ml of glacial acetic acid, and 150 ml of distilled water). Sections were then rinsed in 0.5% glacial acetic acid, differentiated in 0.5% glacial acetic acid for 12 minutes, and rinsed in distilled water. After dehydration in 70% alcohol and two changes of absolute alcohol, the sections were cleared in xylol and mounted.

I have confirmed the finding of Bajusz (personal communication) that delay in fixation does not cause false results when using this technique. Bleaching-out of the formalin pigment caused failure of the stain in the one case in which it was used.

Myocytolysis

In the 18-month period during which I collected this material, 231 neurosurgical autopsies were performed. In 18 cases (8%), there were foci of myocytolysis (FIGURES 1 and 2).

The most obvious abnormality was loss of sarcoplasm with retention of the

TABLE 1

SUMMARY OF CASES WITH MYOCYTOLYSIS

Case No.	Sex	Age (years)	Raised Intracranial Pressure or Shift	Survival after Ictus (days)	Coronary Stenosis	Total Lung Weight (g)	Main Clinical and Pathological Findings
121/64	F	61	+	7	+	860	Ruptured vertebral aneurysm; subarachnoid, intraventricular hemorrhage; ECG reported as "anterior infarction"
192/64	F	38	+	5	–	930	Severe hypertension in labor; intracerebral, intraventricular hemorrhage
70/65	M	11	+	2	–	555	Severe brain lacerations following a 50-ft fall
78/65	M	60	+	4	–	1,350	Anterior cerebral aneurysm; subarachnoid, intracerebral, intraventricular hemorrhage
95/65	M	26	+	7	–	1,410	Anterior communicating aneurysm; subarachnoid, intraventricular hemorrhage; postoperative infection; anterior cerebral infarction
98/65	M	21	+	5	–	1,800	Ethmoiditis; cerebral abscess; meningitis; status epilepticus
86/65	F	58	+	4	–	900	Internal carotid aneurysm; subarachnoid hemorrhage
112/65	M	56	+	5	–	1,370	Anterior cerebral aneurysm; subarachnoid, intraventricular, intracerebral hemorrhage
122/65	F	46	+	6	–	990	Posterior communicating aneurysm; subarachnoid hemorrhage; cerebral infarction
125/65	M	16	–	7	–	1,280	Craniopharyngioma; cerebrospinal fluid pressure, 300 mm; 8-mm mid-line shift; hemorrhagic infarction of adrenals
128/65	F	54	+	4	–	750	Hypertensive intracerebral hemorrhage
135/65	M	28	+	5	–	1,400	Hemorrhage into choriocarcinoma deposit from testis
2/66	M	42	–	4	+	2,160	Internal carotid aneurysm clipped four days before death
3/66	F	4	–	16	–	260	Posterior fossa dermoid; post-operative meningitis; fits 16 days before death; hemorrhagic infarction of adrenals
7/66	F	58	+	5	–	1,660	Carotid occlusion; cerebral infarction and swelling
43/66	F	59	+	15	–	980	Pericallosal aneurysm; anterior cerebral infarction; 6-mm mid-line shift
46/66	F	52	+	3	+	1,100	Internal carotid aneurysm; subarachnoid, intracerebral hemorrhage; cerebral infarction; 10-mm mid-line shift
59/66	F	62	+	5	+	1,330	Ruptured aneurysm; large cerebral infarct; 10-mm mid-line shift

TABLE 2

SUMMARY OF CASES WITH FUCHSINOPHILIC DEGENERATION

Case No.	Sex	Age (years)	Raised Intracranial Pressure or Shift	Survival after Ictus (days)	Coronary Stenosis	Total Lung Weight (g)	Main Clinical and Pathological Findings
27/64	F	50	+	3	−	920	Multiple aneurysms; infarction of left middle cerebral territory
103/64	M	60	+	3	−	900	Subarachnoid hemorrhage; postoperative infarction of anterior cerebral territory
115/64	F	48	+	2	+	840	Anterior communicating aneurysm; postoperative infarction of anterior cerebral territory
121/64	F	61	+	7	+	860	Ruptured vertebral aneurysm; subarachnoid, intraventricular hemorrhage
134/64	M	54	+	13	+	1,500	Vascular malformation; intracerebral, intraventricular hemorrhage
161/64	F	23	−	1	−	950	Vertebral aneurysm causing brainstem shift; postoperative hemorrhage
186/64	M	49	+	1	−	990	Hypertensive intracerebral, intraventricular hemorrhage
192/64	F	38	+	5	−	930	Hypertensive intracerebral hemorrhage in labor
37/65	M	42	+	21	+	1,930	Hypertensive intracerebral, intraventricular hemorrhage
70/65	M	11	+	2	−	555	Severe brain laceration
72/65	M	14	+	<½	−	edematous	Vascular malformation; subarachnoid hemorrhage [described in Lancet i: 822 (1965)]
78/65	M	59	+	4	−	1,350	Multiple aneurysms; subarachnoid, intracerebral, intraventricular hemorrhage; anterior cerebral infarction
86/65	F	58	+	4	−	900	Internal carotid aneurysm; subarachnoid hemorrhage
94/65	F	44	+	½	−	810	Multiple aneurysms; subarachnoid and intraventricular hemorrhage
95/65	M	26	+	7	−	1,410	Anterior communicating aneurysm; postoperative infection and anterior cerebral infarction
98/65	M	21	+	5	−	1,800	Cerebral abscess; meningitis due to ethmoid infection
99/65	M	27	+	4	−	750	Brainstem vascular malformation and hemorrhage
101/65	F	38	+	3	−	1,140	Aneurysm clipped three days before death; gross brain swelling
102/65	F	15	+	5	−	460	Tubercular meningitis at 1 year; many operations for drainage; terminal ventriculitis
107/65	F	25	+	1	−	1,090	Puerperal carotid thrombosis; massive cerebral infarction and swelling

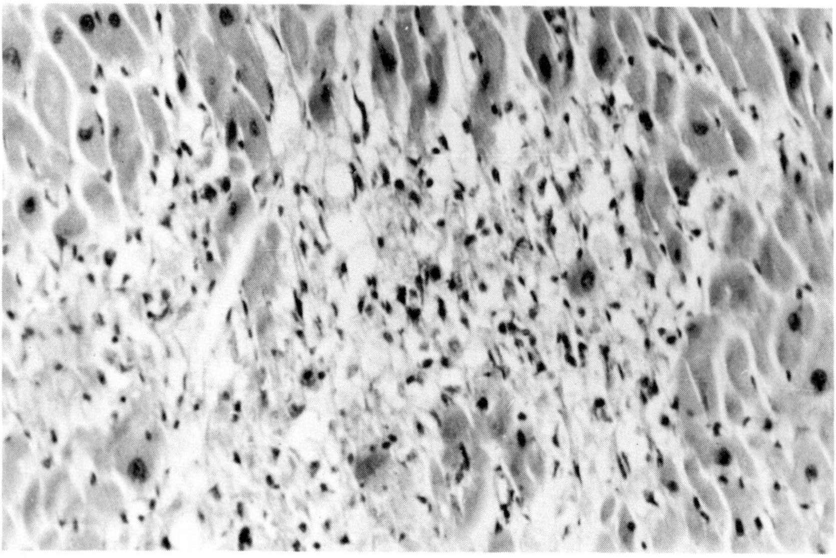

FIGURE 1. Focal myocytolysis in a moderate-sized lesion from the heart of a 61-year-old woman who died with a ruptured cerebral aneurysm. Her ECG was reported to show "anterior myocardial infarction." Coagulative necrosis is not seen, but the sarcolemmal sheaths are visible. Stain: hemalum and eosin. × 112 (orig. mag. × 125).

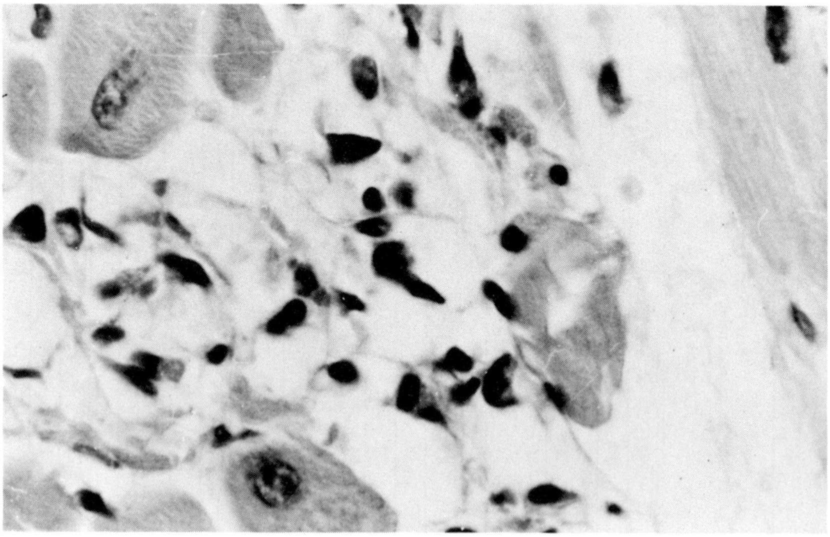

FIGURE 2. Focal myocytolysis. Note the remaining sarcolemma and muscle nuclei and the absence of acute inflammatory cells. Stain: hemalum and eosin. × 470 (orig. mag. × 525).

TABLE 3

INCIDENCE OF MYOCARDIAL PATHOLOGY FOUND IN NEUROSURGICAL AUTOPSIES

Cause of Death	Percent of Total Deaths*	No. of Cases with Focal Myocytolysis	No. of Cases with Fuchsinophilia
Intracranial hemorrhage	35	13	16
Intracranial infection	15	2	1
Head injury (trauma)	20	1	1
Intracranial tumors	25	1	—
Infarction	—	1	1
Others	5	—	1
Total	100	18	20

* Based on a total of 231 deaths. Focal myocytolysis was noted in 8% of the cases, fuchsinophilia in 9%.

TABLE 4

AGE DISTRIBUTION OF MYOCARDIAL PATHOLOGY FOUND IN NEUROSURGICAL AUTOPSIES

Age at Death (years)	Percent of Total Deaths*	No. of Cases with Focal Myocytolysis	No. of Cases with Fuchsinophilia
0–9	8	1	—
10–19	6	2	3
20–29	8	3	5
30–39	6	1	2
40–49	20	2	5
50–59	31	7	4
60–69	18	2	1
Over 70	3	—	—
Total	100	18	20

* Based on a total of 231 deaths.

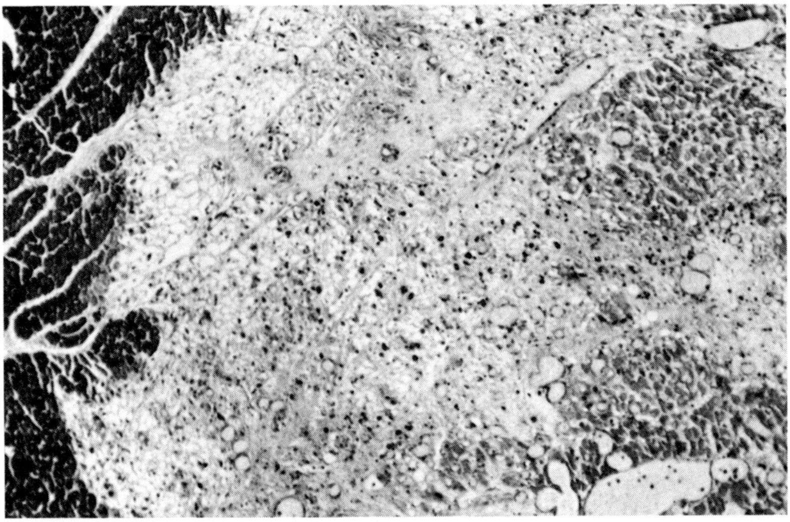

FIGURE 3. Fuchsinophilia in a section from the heart of a man who died with a well-established infarct. On the left is muscle undergoing coagulative necrosis, and the intense red coloration appears as deep black. In the center is young scar tissue, with relatively healthy muscle seen on the right. Stain: acid-fuchsin. × 44.

sarcolemma, muscle nuclei, and lipofuscin. Polymorphs were rarely seen, but histiocytes were present. The sarcoplasm of surrounding fibers could be vacuolated or shredded, but coagulative necrosis was not seen, and the process was therefore basically different from infarction. The lesions were usually small and affect only a few adjacent fibers.

The lesion was not always present in every block. In the 170 blocks examined from these 18 cases, myocytolysis was seen in 101, but some sections contained only one small focus.

The clinical aspects of the 18 cases have been analyzed (TABLES 3 and 4): There was a marked preponderance of patients with spontaneous intracranial hemorrhage, and seven cases occurred in the sixth decade, which provides the highest number. Eight of the patients were male and ten female.

Pulmonary edema was a common finding. Taking a weight of 900 g as the top limit of normal for the combined lung weights,[19] 14 adults had lung edema, as did two children in the series. The average weight of the lungs was 1,270 g in the 16 adults.

Although it has been difficult in these cases to determine the exact date of occurrence of the terminal intracranial lesion, an attempt has been made to estimate the survival time necessary for myocytolysis to develop. The average survival following the ictus was six days, with a minimum of two and a maximum of 16 days; 15 of the cases succumbed between the fourth and seventh days. In only two cases were ECG recordings taken; both showed ischemic changes. Only four cases had some coronary stenosis.

Fuchsinophilic Degeneration

Lesser degrees of heart damage will now be discussed. Human hearts were stained with the cresyl violet-acid fuchsin technique of Bajusz, who used this

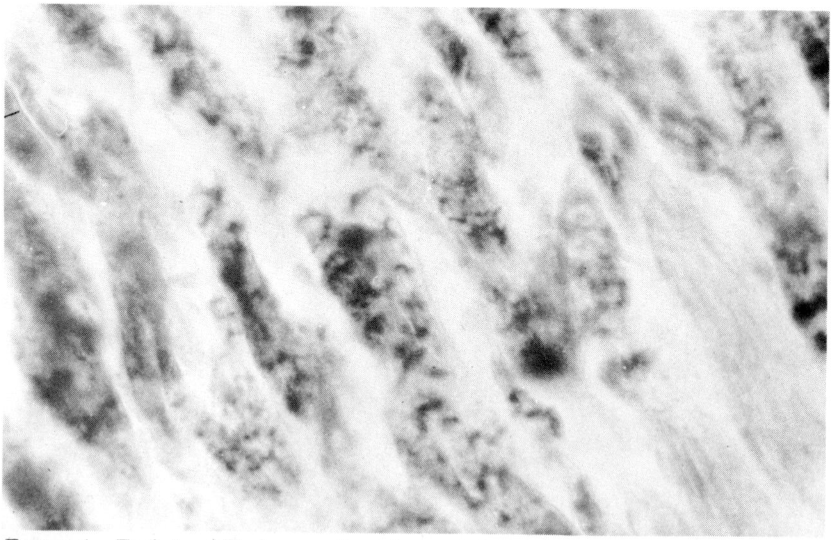

FIGURE 4. Fuchsinophilia in a section of myocardium, showing bands and collections of coagulated sarcoplasm. The patient died rapidly of ischemic heart disease. Stain: acid-fuchsin. × 470 (orig. mag. × 525).

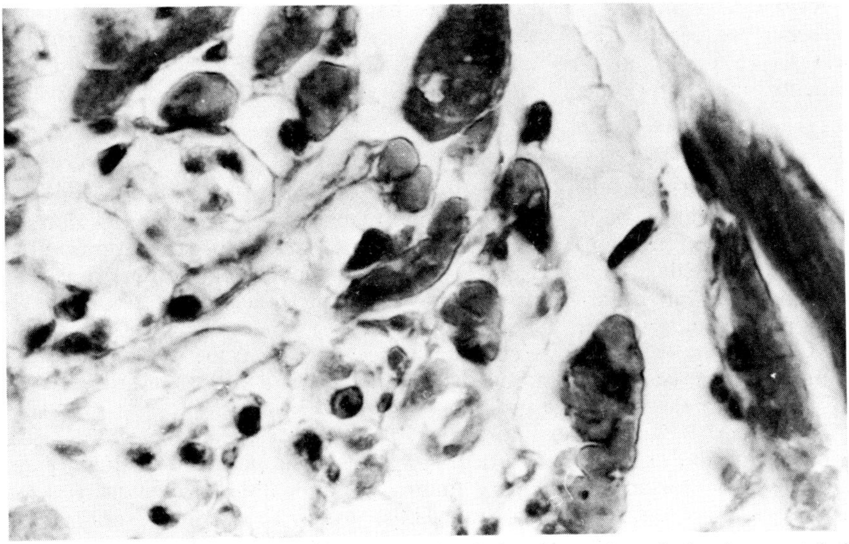

FIGURE 5. Fuchsinophilia. In the lower left of the picture there is focal myocytolysis. Above and to the right are remnants of sarcoplasm which have stained red with the acid-fuchsin (black in the picture) and appear to be undergoing lysis. Stain: acid-fuchsin. × 470 (orig. mag. × 525).

stain to demonstrate prenecrotic myocardial damage in rats subjected to stress.[18] Poley and co-workers[20] have used a similar stain to demonstrate changes in patients dying soon after ischemic heart attacks. My personal studies have confirmed their findings. FIGURE 3 shows the changes seen when this stain is applied to a heart in which ischemic damage has progressed to infarction.

Thus far, I have examined 136 hearts. The two main difficulties encountered in using this stain are obtaining normal heart muscle and assessing the degree of fuchsinophilia. All the hearts examined to date have shown fuchsinophilia of some fibers, but 15 patients without cardiac or brain lesions showed no significant change. I have included in this study only hearts showing fuchsinophilia as severe as that seen in patients dying soon after ischemic heart attacks (FIGURE 4).

Of the 92 hearts from patients with brain lesions, 20 showed significant degrees of change. There were 153 blocks examined from these 20 patients, and 112 showed fuchsinophilia. FIGURE 5 shows the heart of a patient with a subarachnoid hemorrhage who had myocytolysis, with intense fuchsinophilia of muscle fibers preceding complete lysis. FIGURES 6–8 show fuchsinophilia and the coagulated sarcoplasm stained with fuchsin.

The distribution of fuchsinophilia did not correspond to vascular territories; indeed it sometimes ended abruptly at an intercalated disc. This peculiar distribution of damage has been found by others studying "ischemic" lesions in human hearts. As shown in TABLE 3, intracranial hemorrhage was, by far, the most common cause of fuchsinophilic degeneration in the hearts of these patients. The age distribution was more even than in the cases with myocytolysis (TABLE 4), and there was no difference in the sex ratio.

The average survival time in this series (4.7 days) was lower than in the myocytolysis cases. My impression is that fuchsinophilic degeneration may precede lysis of the sarcoplasm, as is suggested by a study of lesions such as that shown in FIGURE 5. Pulmonary edema was a frequent finding in these patients, and the average combined lung-weight for the series was 1,120 g.

Discussion

Two manifestations of myocardial damage associated with brain lesions have been described. In both groups, the most common precipitating lesion was spontaneous intracranial hemorrhage, in most cases due to rupture of an aneurysm, possibly because this is the most acute brain lesion to cause a sudden rise in intracranial pressure and because it frequently occurs in patients with preexisting systemic hypertension.

There are only two significant differences between the two groups. The patients with myocytolysis survived the fatal lesion a little longer and tended to come from the older age groups.

The paper of Schlesinger and Reiner,[21] describing focal myocytolysis, concerns this lesion in ischemic heart disease, but these authors also quote papers that describe the same histological findings in idiopathic cardiomegaly, scleroderma, bacterial endocarditis, poliomyelitis, insulin shock, and excess of sympathomimetic agents, endogenous or administered. The same lesion has also been described in cardiomyopathy of pregnancy.[22] Schlesinger and Reiner[21] note that similar lesions have also been found in animals following oxygen deprivation, adrenaline injections, and hyperthyroidism. Stress following steroid administration[18] and injection of air into the ventricles of rabbit brains[23] have also been associated with myocytolysis of the heart.

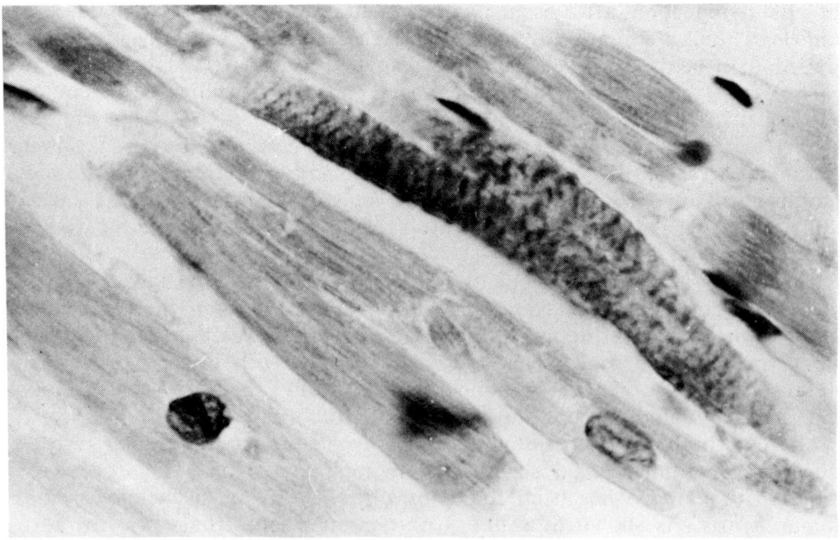

FIGURE 6. Fuchsinophilia. The coagulated sarcoplasm can be seen clearly in the fiber near the center; the fibers above and below show coarsening and fuchsinophilia of the "transverse striations." Stain: acid-fuchsin. × 470 (orig. mag. × 525).

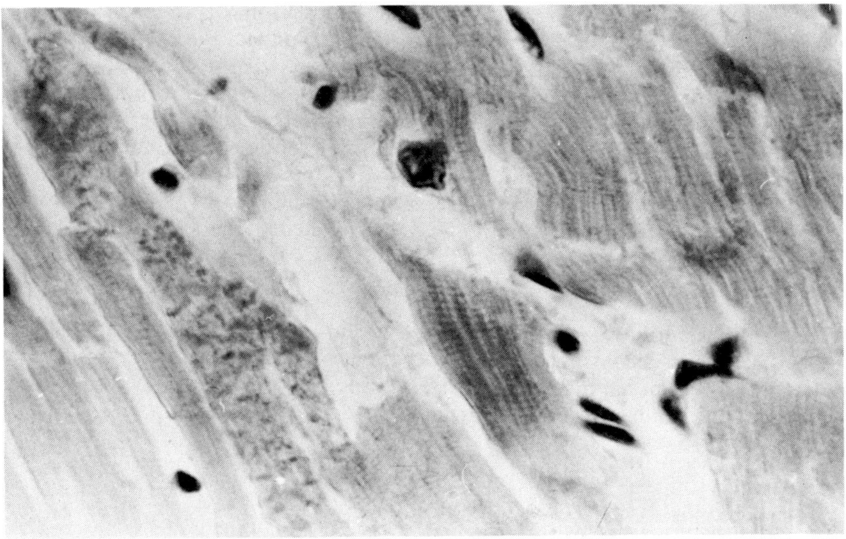

FIGURE 7. Fuchsinophilia in a section from the heart of the same patient as in FIGURE 6, a 25-year-old woman. The coarsening of the "transverse striations" can be seen in the fiber near the center, to the left of which there is a fiber showing coagulation of the sarcoplasm. Stain: acid-fuchsin. × 470 (orig. mag. × 525).

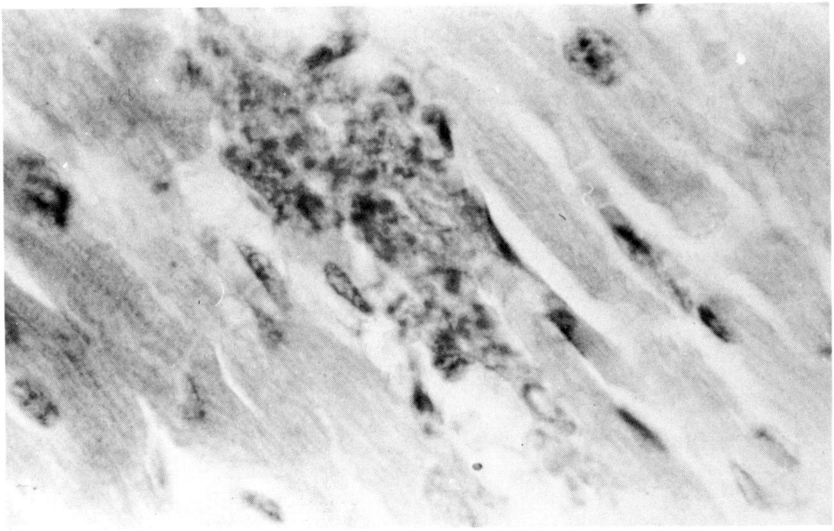

FIGURE 8. Fuchsinophilia in a section from the heart of a 15-year-old girl who died of ventriculitis. Stain: acid-fuchsin. × 470 (orig. mag. × 525).

Two mechanisms by which brain stimulation could cause myocardial damage have been suggested. One is direct neural stimulation of the heart, with a decrease of coronary blood flow. The second is sudden release of hormones from the adrenals.

Shkhvatsabaia and Men'shikov[24] have reported that the catechol content is increased in the heart and decreased in the suprarenals following brain stimulation. A local increase of these substances might increase the metabolism of the sarcoplasm to a level at which the blood supply becomes insufficient. The terminal effect might well be a failure of the mechanism by which a positive potassium:sodium balance is maintained in the heart fibers.[25]

Summary

This paper describes two types of lesion found in the hearts of patients dying with brain lesions. Fuchsinophilic degeneration is probably a precursor of focal myocytolysis. Pulmonary edema is often associated with both types of myocardial damage, and may be due to left ventricular failure.

References

1. Aschenbrenner, R. & G. Bodechtel. 1938. Klin. Wschr. **17:** 298–302.
2. Byer, E., R. Ashman & L. A. Toth. 1947. Amer. Heart J. **33:** 796.
3. Burch, G. E., R. Meyers & J. A. Abildskov. 1954. Circulation **9:** 719.
4. Popov, V. G. 1955. Ter. Arkh. **27:** 45–56.
5. Kung, L. S. 1958. Chin. Med. J. (Peiking) **76:** 445.
6. Schuster, S. 1960. Brit. Heart J. **22:** 316.
7. Alanis, J., E. Lopez & O. Rosas. 1962. Arch. Inst. Cardiol. Mex. **32:** 743–757.
8. Tomatsu, T. 1964. Jap. Circ. J. **28:** 905–912.
9. Hersch, C. 1964. Brit. Heart J. **26:** 785–793.
10. Paci, A. 1960. Riv. Clin. Pediat. **65:** 155.
11. Sulc, J., B. Novak, H. Drahozal & J. Hasa. 1965. Lancet **i:** 1337.
12. Pool, J. L. 1957. Arch. Neurol. Psychiat. **78:** 355.
13. Korenevskaia, T. B. 1958. Ter. Arkh. **30:** 43.
14. Whitby, J. D. 1963. Brit. J. Anaesth. **35:** 624–630.
15. Burch, G. E., N. DePasquale & G. Malaret. 1960. Ann. Intern. Med. **52:** 587.
16. Eichbaum, F. W. & P. C. Bissetti. 1966. Proc. 5th Int. Cong. Neuropath. : 1016–1020. Excerpta Medica Found. Amsterdam, The Netherlands.
17. Russell, N. L. 1956. J. Med. Lab. Techn. **13:** 484-485.
18. Bajusz, E. 1963. Conditioning Factors for Cardiac Necroses. S. Karger, Basel. Switzerland.
19. Weisman, S. J. 1939. Surgery **6:** 722–729.
20. Poley, R. W., C. D. Fobes & M. J. Hall. 1964. Arch. Path. (Chicago) **77:** 325.
21. Schlesinger, M. J. & L. Reiner. 1955. Amer. J. Path. **31:** 443–459.
22. Connor, R. C. R. & J. H. Adams. 1966. J. Clin. Path. **19:** 244–249.
23. Shkhvatsabaia, I. K. & I. V. Postnov. 1964. Atherosclerosis and Thrombosis. : 49–57. Medizina. Moscow, U.S.S.R.
24. Shkhvatsabaia, I. K. & V. V. Men'shikov. 1962. Kardiologia. **2:** 27–30.
25. Bajusz, E., Ed. 1965. Electrolytes and Cardiovascular Diseases. **1:** 274–322. S. Karger. Basel, Switzerland.

CARDIOTOXIC EFFECTS OF ELECTRICAL STIMULATION OF THE STELLATE GANGLIA*

Mary A. Klouda† and G. Brynjolfsson

Departments of Physiology and Pathology
Stritch School of Medicine
Loyola University, Chicago, Ill.

Cardiac lesions induced by various vasoactive substances, as well as by other chemical agents, have been studied extensively for the past several years.[1-11] During a study of cardiovascular response to prolonged electrical stimulation of the stellate ganglion in the dog, the observation was made that many of the hearts revealed subendocardial hemorrhages.[12] Similar hemorrhages have been noted following large doses of epinephrine and norepinephrine,[3, 13, 14] during hemorrhagic shock;[15-17] after occlusion of the main coronary arterial supply to the left ventricle,[18] and in a variety of other conditions.[19, 20]

Our first series of experiments was undertaken in an attempt to elucidate the pathogenesis of these endocardial hemorrhages. The hearts were examined macroscopically. Later, our investigation included a histological examination of the hearts in order to study the effects of stellate ganglion stimulation on the myocardium.

Material and Methods

All experiments were carried out on mongrel dogs under general anesthesia. Some of the dogs were anesthetized with phenylcyclidine hydrochloride (Sernylan®)‡ and α-chloralose and others with sodium pentobarbital (Nembutal®).§ The Sernylan was injected intramuscularly at a dosage of 2 mg/kg. The α-chloralose was sometimes dissolved in polyethylene glycol (100 mg/ml) and injected intravenously at a dosage of 85-90 mg/kg. Otherwise the α-chloralose was dissolved in normal saline and given intraperitoneally at a dosage of 80 mg/kg, since rather large quantities of saline had to be used, the chloralose being poorly soluble in water (1 g in 225 ml of water at 15° C).[21] The Nembutal was given intraperitoneally at a dosage of 25 mg/kg.

For the chronic experiments, bipolar stimulating electrodes were implanted under sterile surgical conditions on the left stellate ganglion. The animals were anesthetized, and positive pressure respiration was initiated. The chest was opened on the left side at the second intercostal space. The second rib was removed to allow easy access to the stellate ganglion. Pieces of insulated Nichrome wire with the insulation removed at both ends served as electrodes. The electrodes were attached at the anterior and posterior sides of the stellate ganglion, the leads were brought out through the incision, and the various layers of tissue were closed around them.

For the acute experiments, the chest was opened bilaterally at the second intercostal space, and the sternum was cut at this point. In some animals the chest remained open, but in others the chest was closed after the electrodes had been applied to the ganglia. A Grass Model S5 stimulator was used to stimulate the ganglia with pulses of 5 volts having a 5-msec duration and a

* This work was supported by United States Public Health Service grant no. HE-08682.

† Present address: Department of Zoology, University of Massachusetts, Amherst, Mass.

‡ Distributed by Parke, Davis & Co., Detroit, Mich.

§ Distributed by Abbott Laboratories, North Chicago, Ill.

frequency of 10 cycles per second. All animals were stimulated for a period of four hours.

The arterial blood pressure (femoral artery for the chronic experiments and carotid artery for the acute experiments) was recorded from a Statham P23Db transducer, and the output was fed into a Grass polygraph recorder. Electrocardiograms (ECG) were recorded on some of the experiments. Heparin was used to prevent coagulation in the arterial catheter.

For the histological examinations, multiple tissue blocks were taken from various parts of the left ventricle (an average of 25), as well as representative sections from the right ventricle and the atria. Sections were also taken from

TABLE 1

MAXIMUM SYSTOLIC PRESSURE IN DOGS SUBJECTED TO STELLATE GANGLION STIMULATION*

Series 1		Series 2	
Lesions	No Lesions	Lesions	No Lesions
275	235	345	210
235		370	240
210			260
250			280
250			230
140			170

* All values in mm Hg.

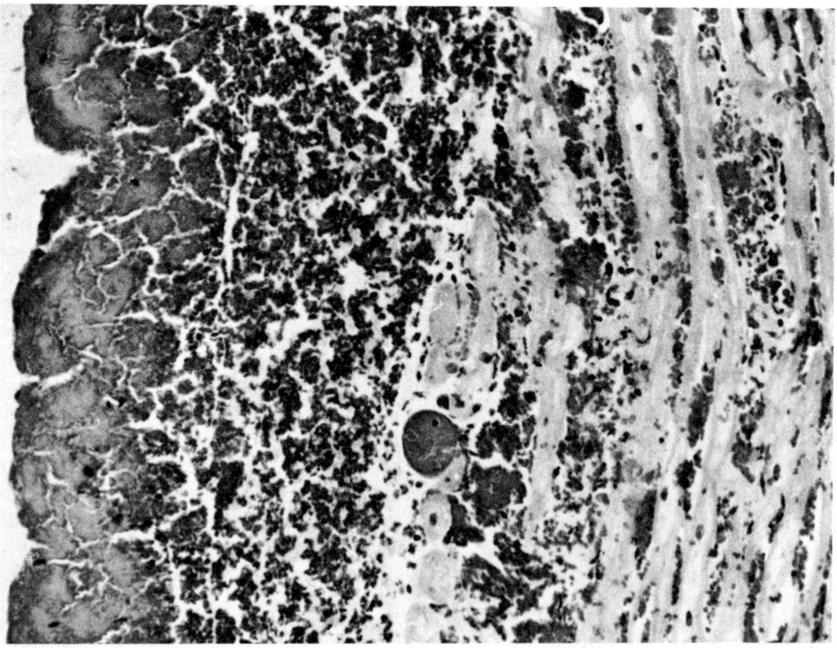

FIGURE 1. Hemorrhage in endocardium and underlying myocardium. Stain: hematoxylin and eosin. × 200.

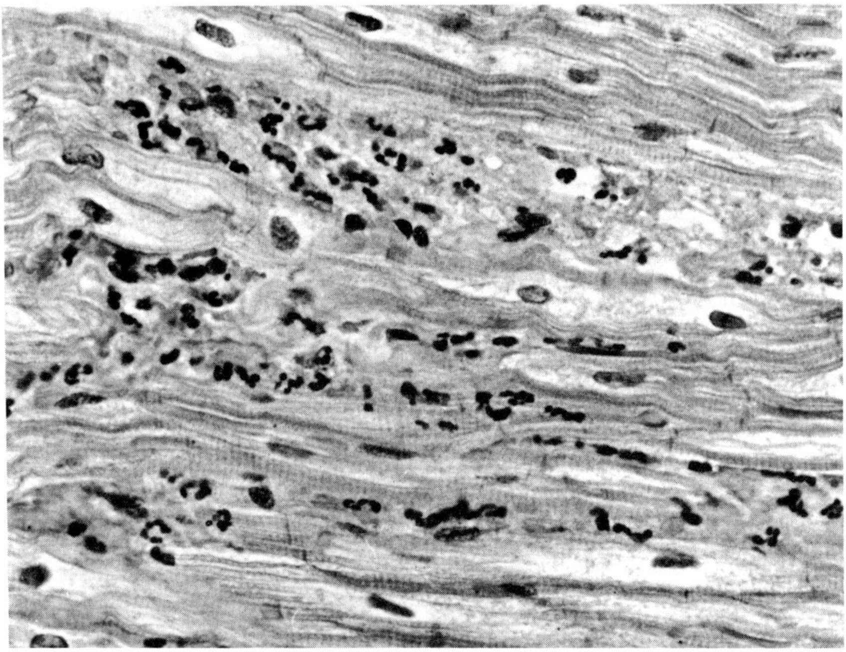

FIGURE 2. Neutrophilic infiltration, edema, and extravasation of a few red blood cells. Dog sacrificed immediately following four hours of stimulation. Stain: hematoxylin and eosin. × 500.

the lungs, liver, spleen, pancreas, intestine, kidneys, adrenals, and voluntary muscle. The tissue was fixed in 10% phosphate-buffered formalin (pH 7.0), and other tissue blocks were quick-frozen in a cryostat. The fixed tissue was embedded in paraffin and sectioned at 5 μ. The sections were stained with hematoxylin and eosin for routine observation and by the periodic acid-Schiff method with and without prior diastase digestion. Frozen as well as formalin-fixed sections of heart were stained with oil-red-O. Selected blocks were stained with phosphotungstic acid hematoxylin. Some of the dogs were sacrificed immediately following four hours of stimulation and others one to eight days later.

Results

The cardiac response to stellate ganglion stimulation consisted of a typical increase in heart rate and an increase in systolic, diastolic, and pulse pressures.[22] There was an increase in the force of contraction of the myocardium which presumably resulted in a reduced end-systolic volume of the ventricle.[23]

In the first series of experiments, the animals were sacrificed immediately following four hours of stimulation. Six out of seven dogs had grossly visible subendocardial hemorrhages, most marked on the papillary muscles and the trabeculae carneae of the left ventricle. Similar lesions were found on the septal wall of the left ventricle, and hemorrhages were also observed in the right ventricle in two of the dogs. No histological examination was carried out on these hearts.

In an attempt to determine the effect of reduction in the end-systolic volume of the left ventricle on the endocardial hemorrhages, our second experiment was devised to keep the end-systolic volume high even during stellate ganglion stimulation.

The stellate ganglia were stimulated in exactly the same manner as the previous group. However, an attempt was made to prevent complete ventricular emptying during stellate stimulation. These animals were continuously infused with large volumes of saline in order to increase the vascular volume. In addition, a ligature was looped around the thoracic aorta just below the aortic arch and then passed through a piece of glass tubing to form a snare. The snare was tightened enough to partially occlude the aorta. Presumably, a combination of these two procedures would prevent the ventricles from emptying during stellate stimulation. The cardiac response of these animals to stellate stimulation was essentially the same as in the preceding group. However, after four hours of stimulation, only two of the nine dogs in this series had any grossly visible subendocardial hemorrhages. The two animals that developed lesions showed systolic pressures of 345-370 mm Hg, respectively (see TABLE 1).

Our third series of experiments consisted of ten dogs stimulated under α-chloralose anesthesia. The α-chloralose was dissolved in polyethylene glycol, and given intravenously, or in normal saline, and given intraperitoneally. Some of the dogs were sacrificed immediately following four hours of stimulation and others one to eight days later. Eight of the ten dogs showed subendocardial hemorrhage ranging from mild to very extensive (FIGURE 1). All of the hearts

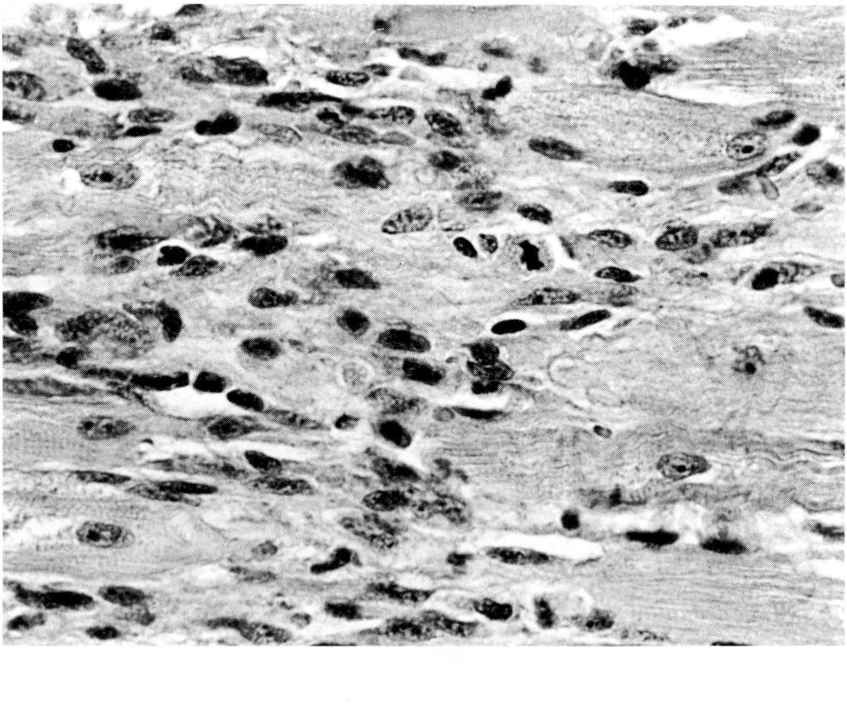

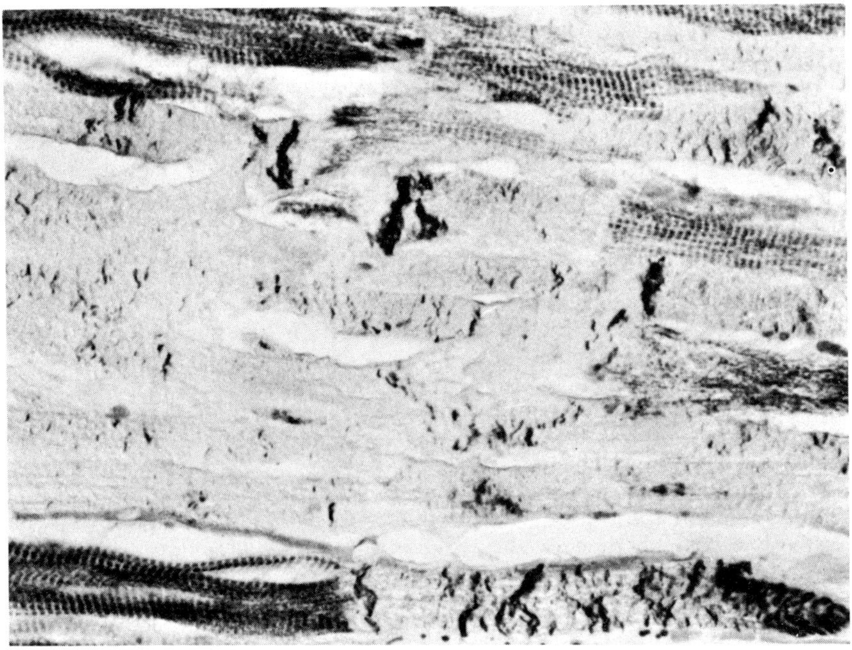

FIGURE 4. Severely damaged muscle fibers. Dog sacrificed 48 hours following stimulation. Stain: phosphotungstic acid hematoxylin. × 500.

showed some myocardial degeneration and necrosis, minimal in some of the dogs but marked in others. Degenerative changes with edema and neutrophilic infiltration were noted immediately following four hours of stimulation (FIGURE 2). Dogs sacrificed a few days following stimulation revealed marked proliferative reaction (FIGURE 3). Some of the necrotic foci showed deposition of calcium. It was felt that the myocardial damage was a synergistic action between the stimulation and the anesthetic, since some of the control dogs also revealed myocardial lesions, although not as early and not as extensive as the stimulated dogs. The effect of α-chloralose on the myocardium is under further study.

In our fourth series of experiments, the dogs were stimulated under Nembutal anesthesia. Four out of six dogs showed multiple small subendocardial hemorrhages in the left ventricle, most marked on the papillary muscles and trabeculae carneae. Hemorrhages were also noted at the base of the mitral valves. In two of the dogs, the inner part of the myocardium showed some poorly defined tan or yellowish-tan areas on gross examination. On microscopical examination, all of the hearts showed focal myocardial degeneration and necrosis (FIGURE 4). The myocardial damage was quite variable from one dog to another: only a few scattered foci of necrosis were found in some, whereas in others, most of the tissue blocks from the left ventricle revealed some muscle damage. Many of the foci were minute, consisting of only one or two muscle cells; other foci were composed of several cells, and some measured 1–2 mm in diameter (FIGURES 5 and 6). In some areas, these foci were numerous and partly confluent. Most of the damaged cells did not contain any stainable glycogen but had periodic acid-Schiff-positive, hyaline cytoplasm after diastase digestion (FIGURE 7). In many of the foci, there was no neutrophilic reaction two days after stellate ganglion stimulation. In other foci, especially when several cells were involved, mild neutrophilic infiltration was noted, as well as some histiocytic reaction and beginning proliferation of fibroblasts. Stain for fat revealed numerous small fat droplets in some of the hyalinized cells, as well as in many of the adjacent muscle cells, which still retained normal cross striation.

Although the damaged cells could be found anywhere in the wall of the left ventricle, they were most prominent in the inner one-third of the wall, particularly in the papillary muscles. Lesions were also found throughout the right ventricle. Only minimal changes were noted in the atria, and there were no pertinent findings in other organs. Although as a rule the cardiac lesions were most marked in dogs that showed the most marked response to the stimulation, the correlation between the cardiac lesions and the increased blood pressure and heart rate was not always very close. No muscle necrosis was found in the control dogs.

In addition to causing systolic hypertension and tachycardia, prolonged stellate stimulation also produces gross changes in the ECG. In the third and fourth series of experiments, the ECG was recorded periodically throughout the four-hour stimulation period and then continuously for four more hours

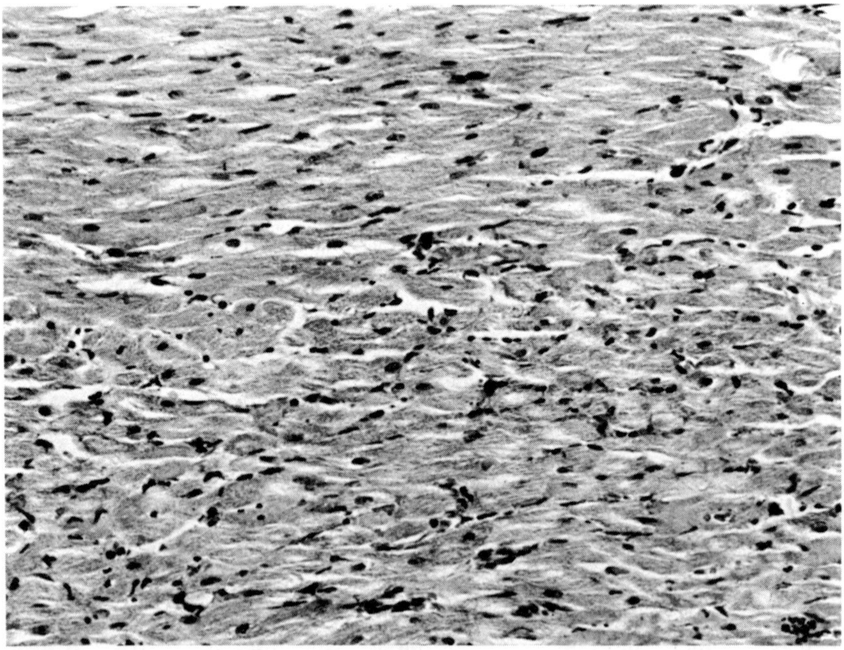

FIGURE 5. Section taken at junction of necrotic and viable myocardium. Scattered nuclear fragments, mild neutrophilic infiltration, and early fibroblastic proliferation in necrotic portion. Myocardial fibers disorganized and smudgy. Dog sacrfiiced 48 hours following stimulation. Stain: hematoxylin and eosin. × 200.

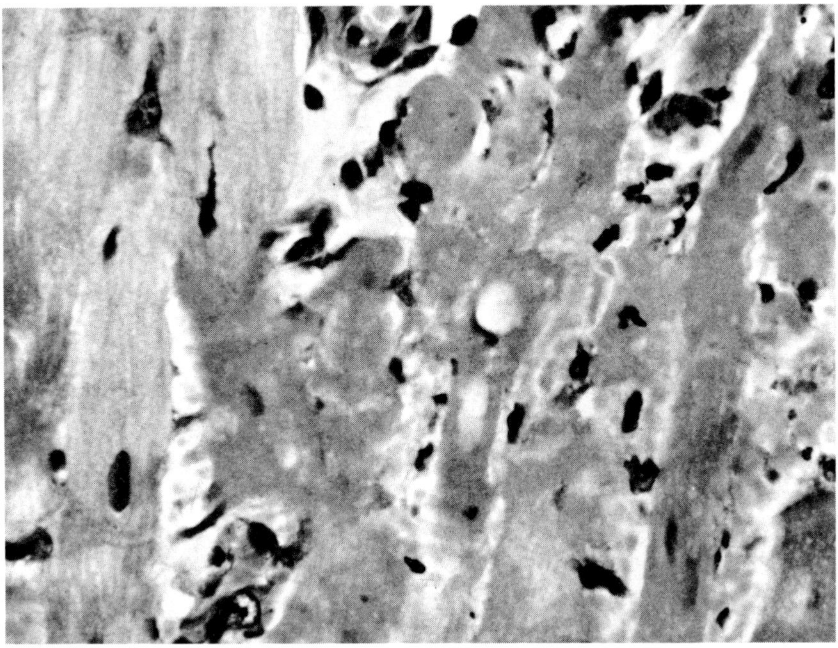

FIGURE 6. Section shown in FIGURE 5, in greater detail. × 550.

after the stimulation was terminated. Since the ECG could not be recorded while the animal was being stimulated, the stimulus was turned off for about 30 seconds approximately once every 30 minutes throughout the stimulation period. By the end of the first hour of stimulation, changes in the ECG were evident. The P wave was usually not much affected. The amplitude of the QRS complex decreased, while the amplitude of the T wave increased. In some experiments, either the negative Q wave or the negative S wave became much larger. The T wave often became inverted. The ST segment was frequently elevated. The ECG aberrations gradually became worse, and, at the end of the four-hour stimulation period, the tracing was usually no longer recognizable as an ECG. About two or three hours after the termination of the stellate stimulation, the ECG began to return slowly to its control configuration. Generally, by the end of the four-hour observation period, the ECG had recovered substantially toward the control configuration.

FIGURE 8 shows the changes that took place during a stimulation period of four hours followed by a post-stimulation period of 200 minutes. The first tracing shows a control recording of the carotid blood pressure and lead II of the ECG. The following six records were obtained during the four-hour stimulation period, and the last five records were taken during the observation period after the end of stimulation.

Discussion

Our second series of experiments indicates that the subendocardial hemorrhages might, at least in part, be due to mechanical causes. With reduction

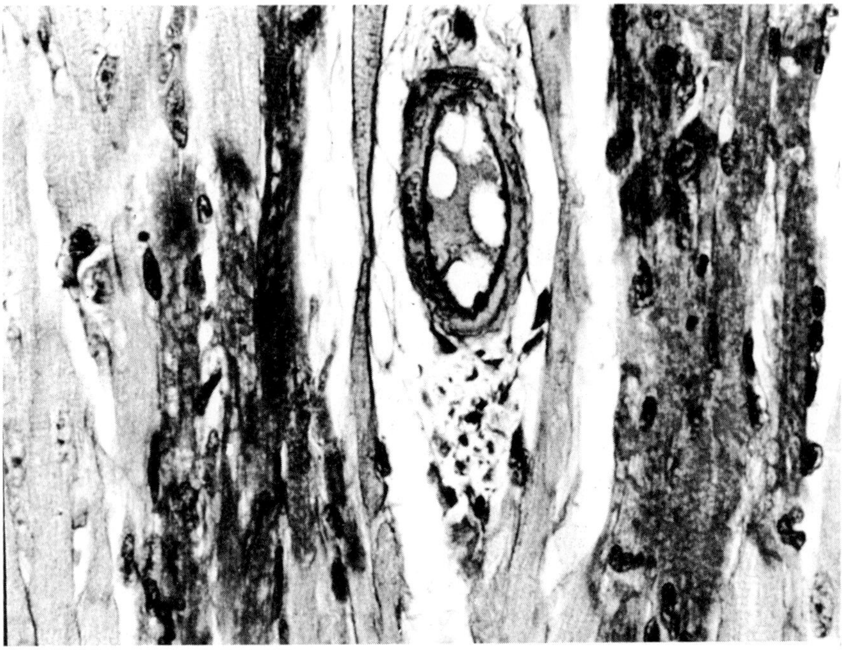

FIGURE 7. The dark muscle fibers are Schiff-positive after diastase digestion. There is beginning proliferation of cardiac histiocytes (myocytes) and fibroblasts. Dog sacrificed 48 hours following stimulation. Stain: periodic acid-Schiff. × 500.

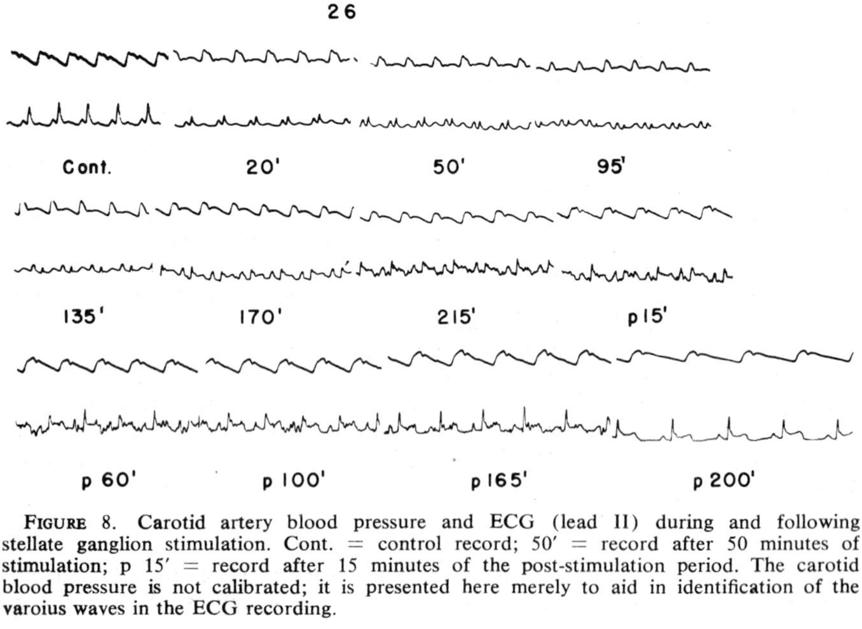

FIGURE 8. Carotid artery blood pressure and ECG (lead II) during and following stellate ganglion stimulation. Cont. = control record; 50′ = record after 50 minutes of stimulation; p 15′ = record after 15 minutes of the post-stimulation period. The carotid blood pressure is not calibrated; it is presented here merely to aid in identification of the varoius waves in the ECG recording.

in the end-systolic volume, the opposing walls of the nearly empty ventricle may come into contact with one another. Such contact would normally be prevented by the end-systolic volume of the ventricles. When the end-systolic volume was elevated during stellate ganglion stimulation, only two out of nine dogs had grossly visible subendocardial hemorrhage, and these two animals had a systolic blood pressure of 345 and 370 mm Hg, respectively. With the development of such high pressures, it seems likely that the ventricles might have emptied in spite of the hypervolemia and partial aortic occlusion. It would appear, therefore, that, if the heart can be prevented from emptying during stellate ganglion stimulation, the development of subendocardial hemorrhages can also be prevented or at least reduced.

The distribution of subendocardial hemorrhages also tends to favor a mechanical origin. The lesions are most prominent on the papillary muscles and on the septal wall of the left ventricle. These are the areas one would expect to be affected if the lesions are indeed caused by a more complete emptying of the heart. Lesions are less frequently found on the areas of the free wall of the left ventricle which lie in between the papillary muscles. The lesions are also found much less frequently in the right ventricle than in the left.

The myocardial damage produced by the stellate ganglion stimulation is histologically nonspecific, and similar lesions have been produced by various other means.[1-20] On the basis of the location of these lesions, predominantly in the inner one-third of the left ventricular wall, and in view of the marked increase in the oxygen demand of the overstimulated heart, it seems most probable that relative ischemia contributes to the formation of these lesions, in spite of demonstrated increase in coronary blood flow during stellate ganglion stimulation.[24] Berne and co-workers[25] have shown that the increase in coronary blood flow which accompanies stellate ganglion stimulation is always associated with a reduction in coronary sinus blood oxygen tension. The rise in the intraventricular pressure, as a result of the forceful systolic contractions, could be expected to interfere with coronary blood flow, especially in the subendocardium.

Summary

Electrical stimulation of the stellate ganglion in the dog causes elevation of the blood pressure, especially the systolic pressure, increased heart rate, and augmentation in pulse pressure. Postmortem examination of the hearts revealed subendocardial hemorrhage and focal myocardial necrosis, most marked in the inner one-third of the left ventricle and in the papillary muscles. Some of the endocardial hemorrhages were prevented by increasing the end-systolic volume of the left ventricle. Relative anoxia, due to augmented myocardial oxygen consumption, is considered likely to play a role in the pathogenesis of the myocardial necrosis.

Acknowledgments

The authors wish to acknowledge the technical assistance rendered by Mr. J. Genovese, Mrs. E. Smith, Mr. M. Fethiere, and Mr. R. Branski.

References

1. Raab, W. 1953. Hormonal and Neurogenic Cardiovascular Disorders. Williams & Wilkins Co. Baltimore, Md.
2. Raab, W. 1956. The adrenergic-cholinergic control of cardiac metabolism and function. *In* Advances in Cardiology. 1: 165. S. Karger. Basel, Switzerland.

3. Szakacs, J. E. & A. Cannon. 1958. l-Norepinephrine myocarditis. Amer. J. Clin. Path. **30:** 425–434.
4. Selye, H. 1958. The humoral production of cardiac infarcts. Brit. Med. J. **1:** 5071–5075.
5. Rona, G., C. I. Chappel, T. Balazs & R. Gaudry. 1959. An infarct-like myocardial lesion and other toxic manifestations produced by isoproterenol in the rat. Arch. Path. (Chicago) **67:** 443–455.
6. Szakacs, J. E., R. M. Dimmette & E. C. Cowart, Jr. 1959. Pathologic implication of the catechol amines, epinephrine and norepinephrine. U. S. Armed Forces Med. J. **10:** 908–925.
7. Szakacs, J. E. & B. Mehlman. 1960. Pathologic changes induced by l-norepinephrine. Amer. J. Cardiol. **5:** 619–627.
8. Raab, W. 1963. Neurogenic myocardial injury (pathogenic mechanism and prevention). *In* Coronary Heart Disease. **:** 82–88. (The Seventh Hahnemann Symposium.) Grune & Stratton. New York, N. Y.
9. Bajusz, E. & G. Jasmin. 1964. Influence of variations in electrolyte intake upon the development of cardiac necrosis produced by vasopressor amines. Lab. Invest. **13:** 757–766.
10. Ferrans, V. J., R. G. Hibbs, W. C. Black & D. G. Weilbaecher. 1964. Isoproterenol-induced myocardial necrosis. A histochemical and electron microscopic study. Amer. Heart J. **68:** 71–90.
11. Highman, B., P. D. Altland & J. Garbus. 1965. Pathological and serum-enzyme changes after epinephrine in oil and adrenergic blocking agent. Arch. Path. (Chicago) **80:** 332–344.
12. Kaye, M., R. McDonald & W. C. Randall. 1961. Systolic hypertension produced by electrical stimulation of the stellate ganglion. Circ. Res. **9:** 1164–1170.
13. Maling, H. M. & B. Highman. 1958. Exaggerated ventricular arrhythmias and myocardial fatty changes after large doses of norepinephrine and epinephrine in unaesthetized dogs. Amer. J. Physiol. **194:** 590–600.
14. Nahas, G. G., J. G. Brunsen, W. M. King & H. M. Cavert. 1958. Functional and morphologic changes in heart lung preparations following administration of adrenal hormones. Amer. J. Path. **34:** 717–730.
15. Melcher, G. W. & W. W. Walcott. 1951. Myocardial changes following shock. Amer. J. Physiol. **164:** 832–836.
16. Hackel, D. B. & B. V. Catchpole. 1958. Pathologic and electrocardiographic effects of hemorrhagic shock in dogs treated with l-norepinephrine. Lab. Invest. **7:** 358–368.
17. Watts, D. T. & C. J. Greever. 1956. Arterial blood epinephrine levels during irreversible hemorrhagic shock in dogs. J. Pharmacol. Exp. Ther. **116:** 60.
18. Wartman, W. B., L. A. Campbell, R. L. Craig & R. B. Jennings. 1955. Effect of ACTH on experimental myocardial infarcts. Circ. Res. **3:** 496.
19. Fassbender, H. G. & H. Wangler. 1952. Zur Ätiologie der subendokardialen Blutung. Virchow. Arch. Path. Anat. **321:** 138–141.
29. Smith, R. P. & B. E. Tomlinson. 1954. Subendocardial hemorrhages associated with intracranial lesions. J. Path. Bact. **68:** 327–334.
21. Monroe, R. R., G. U. Balis & E. Ebersberger. 1963. The hypnotic effects of alpha and beta chloralose in rats. Curr. Ther. Res. **5:** 141–153.
22. Randall, W. C. & W. Rohse. 1956. The augmentor action of the sympathetic cardiac nerves. Circ. Res. **4:** 470–475.
23. Kelso, A. & W. C. Randall. 1959. Ventricular changes associated with sympathetic augmentation of cardiovascular pressure pulses. Amer. J. Physiol. **196:** 731–734.
24. Katz, L. N. & K. Jochim. 1939. Observations on the innervation of the coronary vessels of the dog. Amer. J. Physiol. **126:** 395–401.
25. Berne, R. M., H. DeGeest & M. Levy. 1965. Influence of the cardiac nerves on coronary resistance. Amer. J. Physiol. **208:** 763–769.

PATHOPHYSIOLOGICAL FUNDAMENTALS OF THE ORIGIN AND PREVENTION OF DEGENERATIVE HEART DISEASE

W. Raab

University of Vermont, College of Medicine
Burlington, Vt.

In 1912, Herrick described occlusive coronary thrombosis and the finding of coronary atherosclerosis in most cases of angina pectoris and myocardial infarction; during the following 50 years a mechanistic interpretation of hypoxic degenerative heart disease as being merely a problem of vascular oxygen supply to the heart muscle prevailed. Hardly any attention was paid by pathologists and clinicians to the fact that vital oxygen availability to the myocardial tissue depends not only on vascular oxygen supply but also on metabolic oxygen consumption by the myocardial tissue. Any major discrepancy between these two logically inseparable factors is bound to create local hypoxia and to result in functional and structural alterations that are, in turn, largely mediated by derangements in the cellular electrolyte balance.

Basic Principles of Myocardial Hypoxic Injury

Under normal conditions, coronary vascular dilatability compensates automatically for increased myocardial oxygen consumption, the wide fluctuations of which are largely dominated by autonomic nervous interference. Adrenergic catecholamines (norepinephrine, liberated at the sympathetic nerve endings in the ventricles, and epinephrine, arriving by way of the bloodstream from the adrenal medulla) act directly upon myocardial oxidative metabolism. They cause an "uneconomically" augmented consumption of myocardial oxygen which surpasses the energy requirements of increased external mechanical work performance. This phenomenon apparently is caused by acceleration of the transmembranous exchange of potassium and sodium. The heart rate, being regulated by both adrenergic and cholinergic influences, affects ventricular oxygen economy by inducing either adrenergic increases or cholinergic decreases of oxygen consumption.

Pathogenically hypoxiating disproportions between myocardial oxygen supply and consumption are elicited in vascularly intact hearts by adrenergic catecholamines if they are either spontaneously produced (as in pheochromocytoma) or extrinsically administered in excessive quantities. Electrocardiographic alterations, arrhythmias, necrotizing structural changes, contractile weakness, and, eventually, death are the results.

If coronary compensatory dilatability is impaired by vascular rigidity and narrowing, even moderate or slight augmentations of oxygen-consuming cardiac sympathetic and adrenomedullary activity may produce the manifestations of severe local hypoxia, including micro- and macrofocal necrotic cell destruction. An inadequate flushing-out of accumulating acid metabolites, especially lactic acid, from the affected areas is presumably responsible, in part, for local formation of necroses. In cases of survival, necrosis is gradually replaced by the formation of fibrous scars. These, in conjunction with a weakened contractility of still-functioning myocardial tissue, contribute to the ultimate development of ventricular dynamic failure.

The subendocardial layers of the left ventricle are particularly susceptible to hypoxic damage, presumably because of exposure of their blood vessels to intraventricular hemodynamic pressures and because of the falling pressure gradient between coronary ostia and subendocardium. A decisive pathogenic element in myocardial hypoxia is its detrimental effect upon the delicate intra- and extracellular electrolyte balance, and upon the latter's role in impulse conduction. Oxidative energy is required to maintain the appropriate high intracellular vs. low extracellular potassium concentration and the inversely proportioned sodium concentrations. The energy-yielding so-called "ionic pump" guarantees the active transport of systolically extruded cellular potassium and intruded sodium ions through the cell membranes against their respective gradients during the "phase of restitution." Lack of sufficient oxygen causes loss of intracellular potassium and gain of sodium, conditions that finally become incompatible with myocardial functional and structural integrity.

Coincidence of adrenergic overactivity with an augmented activity of adrenal corticoids, especially of cortisol, greatly intensifies the cardiotoxicity of both of these potassium-depleting agents. It is apt to elicit severe necrotic destruction of myocardial tissue even in the absence of coronary vascular anomalies. Amounts of catecholamines and cortisol which are innocuous by themselves become highly toxic if combined. The common cardiac complications of Cushing's disease may be related to this principle.

Human Pathology

Contrary to still widespread traditional thinking, the pathogenesis of vascular atherosclerosis must be clearly distinguished from that of accompanying myocardial metabolic derangements. To be sure, coronary atherosclerosis constitutes the most ubiquitous and the most important single predisposing and contributory element in myocardial hypoxic pathology. However, one should not overlook the fact that its largely nutritional origin and preventability differ essentially from the neurogenic and hormonal metabolic mechanisms acting upon the heart muscle itself. These neurogenic and hormonal mechanisms appear to be responsible for the degree of myocardial vulnerability and resulting cardiac pathology in the presence (or occasionally even in the absence) of coronary atherosclerosis.

The existence of three long-suspected pathogenic factors with metabolic rather than vascular implications for the myocardium has been confirmed by numerous epidemiological studies of the last decade: (1) lack of physical activity, (2) emotional and environmental stresses, and (3) tobacco smoking. Despite its general heuristic value, the epidemiological approach, as such, contributes little or nothing to the comprehension of underlying basic mechanisms. Consequently, prevailing unfamiliarity with much of the extensive world literature on pathophysiological fundamentals has created a great deal of confusion concerning the nature and preventability of hypoxic degenerative heart disease. This confusion is perpetuated and aggravated by the indiscriminate and misleadingly interchanged use of such terms as "coronary artery disease," "coronary heart disease," "coronary atherosclerosis," "coronary thrombosis," "coronary occlusion," and "ischemic heart disease." These arbitrarily employed designations disregard the nonexistence of thrombi and occlusions in more than one-half of the instances of myocardial infarction, and the blatant discrepancies between the degree and distribution of coronary arterial lesions, on the one hand, and manifestations of myocardial hypoxia and electrolyte imbalance, on the other.

A critical review of available pertinent data permits the conclusion that the three civilization-induced pathogenic factors noted above have one basic feature in common, namely, an absolutely or relatively exaggerated sympathetic-adrenergic activity that interferes with myocardial oxygen economy. This activity is manifested chiefly by an accelerated heart rate and shortened isometric tension period of the left ventricle, in accordance with an augmented catecholamine production.

There are differences between the detailed mechanisms of these types of adrenergic overaction. Lack of exercise causes a deterioration of cardiac sympatho-inhibitory and vagal counterregulation at rest and in response to sensory and mental stresses. Nicotine stimulates the peripheral sympathetic ganglia. Emotional and environmental stresses stimulate the sympatho-adrenomedullary system via hypothalamic pathways. In addition, sensory and emotional stresses and nicotine action are associated with further potassium-depleting and, thus, catecholamine cardiotoxicity-potentiating augmentations of cortisol production.

Principles of Prevention

Preventability of degenerative hypoxic heart disease should be evaluated and preventive action undertaken on the basis of the previously discussed pathogenic principles. There is no adequate proof for the frequently stated claim that muscular exercise retards the development of coronary atherosclerosis. Instead, vigorous physical training is known to produce a beneficial reduction of "oxygen-wasting" cardiac sympathetic tone and stress response (slowing of heart rate and prolongation of isometric tension period). In addition, it seems to accumulate protective potassium reserves in the myocardium, and in predamaged and hypoxic hearts it favors the opening of new collaterals.

Carefully graded exercise training, even in patients who have suffered one or more infarctions, is far better tolerated than was formerly realized, and can lead to remarkable degrees of belated physical fitness. It appears that the risk of potentially hypoxiating and potassium-depleting effects of acute intensive sympathetic stimulation during physical effort is largely offset by the simultaneous massive mobilization of potassium from the contracting skeletal muscles into the circulating blood, and its transfer into the myocardial tissue. It is also noteworthy that, in contrast to emotional excitement, physical exercise is not accompanied by discharges of cortisol.

Abstinence from smoking, mainly by eliminating exaggerated sympathetic ganglionic stimulations and adrenocortical overactivity, produces a demonstrable and immediate reduction in the incidence of myocardial infarctions.

Environmental-emotional relaxation is associated with a decrease in catecholamine and corticoid production and with an improvement or disappearance of "hypoxic" electrocardiographic patterns, as observed in rural reconditioning centers. The ability of the heart muscle to develop a striking resistance to severe destructive stresses by prior exposure to a series of milder ones may possibly be related to neurogenic and hormonal adjustments of the myocardial electrolyte stores. Prevention of experimental myocardial necroses has been effectuated by administration of readily absorbable potassium and magnesium aspartate.

Summary

Contrary to traditional beliefs, degenerative heart disease of the hypoxic type is not attributable solely to coronary atherosclerosis but rather to a bicausal discrepancy between two logically inseparable factors: vascular oxygen supply and myocardial oxygen consumption. The latter, largely dominated by adrenergic sympatho-adrenomedullary activity, and subject to wide fluctuations, is apt to cause critical states of local hypoxia when coronary compensatory dilatability is impaired.

In micro- or macrofocal hypoxic areas, especially in the vascularly handicapped subendocardium, the myocardial cells lose their ability to retain sufficient amounts of potassium and to expel extra sodium. Weakness of contractility and disturbances of impulse formation and conduction, as well as structural disintegration, are the results of myocardial hypoxia.

Three civilization-induced pathogenic factors (lack of exercise, environmental-emotional stresses, and tobacco smoking) share one common, potentially hypoxiating feature, namely, an augmented sympathogenic interference of catecholamines in cardiac oxygen economy. The cardiotoxicity of catecholamines under emotional stress and nicotine action seems to be further aggravated by a simultaneous overproduction of potassium-depleting adrenal corticoids.

Prevention of vascular atherogenesis is possible by dietary adjustments. Counteraction against exaggerated neurogenic and corticoid-induced vulnerability of the heart muscle tissue itself can be achieved by physical training, environmental-emotional relaxation, and abstinence from smoking.

Recommended Readings

BAJUSZ, E. 1963. Conditioning Factors for Cardiac Necroses. S. Karger. Basel, Switzerland.

BAJUSZ, E., Ed. 1965–1966. Electrolytes and Cardiovascular Diseases. Williams & Wilkins. Baltimore, Md.

MYASNIKOV, A. L. 1964. Myocardial necroses of coronary and noncoronary genesis. Amer. J. Cardiol. **13:** 435.

RAAB, W. 1963. The nonvascular metabolic myocardial vulnerability factor in "coronary heart disease." Amer. Heart J. **66:** 685.

RAAB, W. 1966. Emotional and sensory stress factors in myocardial pathology. Amer. Heart J. **72:** 538.

RAAB, W., Ed. 1966. Prevention of Ischemic Heart Disease. Charles C Thomas, Publ. Springfield, Ill.

SELYE, H. 1958. The Chemical Prevention of Cardiac Necroses. The Ronald Press Co. New York, N. Y.

SELYE, H. 1961. The Pluricausal Cardiopathies. Charles C Thomas, Publ. Springfield, Ill.

Part IV. Cardiac Pathology Induced by Isoproterenol and Related Amines

ISOPROTERENOL-INDUCED CARDIAC NECROSIS

D. S. Kahn, G. Rona, and C. I. Chappel

Departments of Pathology, St. Mary's Hospital, Lakeshore Hospital, and McGill University, Montreal, Canada

Isoproterenol [1-(3,4-dehydroxyphenyl)-2-isopropylaminoethanol hydrochloride], a synthetic beta-adrenergic compound, is a potent cardiac stimulant. Compared with other sympathomimetics, it has a stronger inotropic and chromatropic action, resulting in greater oxygen demand by the heart muscle. By means of peripheral vasodilatation, it reduces systemic blood pressure, and, although the drug causes coronary vasodilatation, the reduced systemic blood pressure presumably reduces coronary blood flow.[1, 2]

In 1959, we found that isoproterenol hydrochloride would produce infarct-like cardiac necrosis in various species over a wide dose range.[3] In contrast to the natural catecholamines, epinephrine and norepinephrine, which will also produce myocardial necrosis, isoproterenol does not cause appreciable pulmonary edema, and, even with high doses, the mortality is low. This difference in action makes isoproterenol valuable for the production and study of myocardial necrosis of uniform severity.[3, 4]

For a detailed study of this type of cardiac necrosis, male or female Wistar rats averaging 250 g in weight give the most uniform results.[5] The optimal dose for producing consistent infarct-like myocardial necrosis is 85 mg/kg injected subcutaneously (s.c.) on two consecutive days. Within 20 minutes after each injection the rats become dyspneic, prostrate, and develop tachycardia. The symptoms decrease after six to eight hours, and the mortality rate is less than 10%. Electrocardiographic studies[6, 7] have shown changes consistent with myocardial ischemia or subendocardial necrosis.

Rats sacrificed at 48 hours (24 hours after the second injection) show congestion of the lungs and abdominal viscera. Upon gross examination, the hearts are enlarged and show well-demarcated, pale greyish-yellow areas involving the apex, the adjoining left ventricle, and the apical portion of the right ventricle. On microscopical examination, two types of lesion are found: a nonhomogeneous, confluent type in the area of gross change (FIGURE 1) and a disseminated, focal variety (FIGURE 2) in the papillary muscles and subendocardially in both ventricles and occasionally in the atria. Additional scattered foci may be found throughout the remainder of the ventricular myocardium, and occasionally involving the epicardial aspect of the myocardium at the atrioventricular groove. The basic and earliest lesion would appear to be hyaline necrosis of the muscle fibers; Korb[8] has found that necrosis of some myofibers can be demonstrated with special techniques within two hours after isoproterenol injection. By eight hours, in routine hematoxylin and eosin sections, segments of fibers have become homogeneous, eosinophilic, and periodic acid-Schiff positive. In 24- and 36-hour specimens, in addition to necrotic muscle fibers, scattered areas of capillary dilatation and mucoid edema are found, with scattered polymorphonuclear leukocyte infiltration (FIGURE 3). The acute exudative component of the lesion is fleeting, so that it is much less marked at 48 hours than at 36 hours, and is rarely found much beyond this time.

The evolution of the reaction pattern is remarkably rapid. By 48 hours, marked myocytolysis has already occurred, with the disappearance of many of the affected fibers and the accumulation of large mononuclear cells, presumably histiocytes. In some fibers, the sarcolemma outline remains intact, and the myofiber body seems to be occupied by the histiocytes, superimposed on remnants of the necrotic fibers. In many affected areas, the reticulin framework and capillaries remain intact, although in others they are effaced. By five to six days, the necrotic muscle fibers have all been resorbed, and the involved areas consist of sheets of histiocytes and fibroblasts, producing a granulomatous pattern.[4] These areas are then replaced by fibrous tissue, which ultimately results in either indistinct linear scars or chronic aneurysm formation.[9]

We have found that, on the basis of either single-dose lethality, or absolute amount, isoproterenol is more potent than epinephrine or norepinephrine in producing myocardial necrosis.[1] The "infarct-producing" dose range of isoproterenol in rats is 5.25 to 85 mg/kg on two consecutive days. There are some strain differences: Sprague-Dawley rats are somewhat less sensitive than

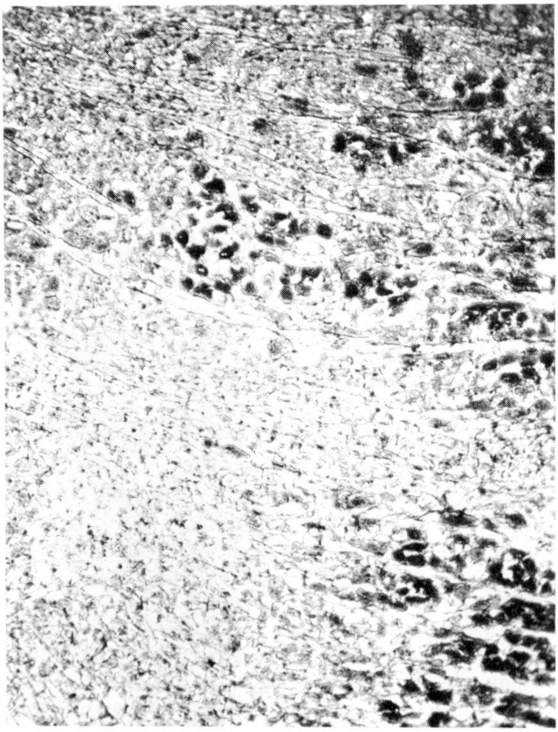

FIGURE 1. Photomicrograph of a section from the apex of the heart of a rat injected with isoproterenol (85 mg/kg) on two consecutive days and sacrificed at 48 hours. There is confluent necrosis of the myocardial fibers, many of which have already been partially resorbed. Stain: Wilder's silver impregnation. × 100.

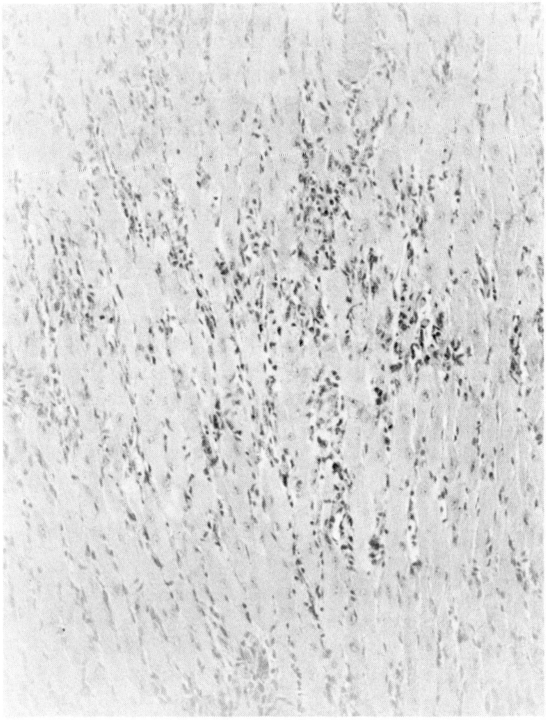

FIGURE 2. Another area of the same heart illustrated in FIGURE 1, showing disseminated focal myocardial necrosis. Stain: hematoxylin and eosin. × 100.

either hooded rats of the Long-Evans strain or Wistar rats.[2] A direct relationship has been found between the severity of the myocardial lesion and the weight of the animal; the slightly greater sensitivity of male rats has been attributed to their faster rate of growth.[5]

Dogs are more sensitive than rats to isoproterenol. In rats, the median lethal dose of a single s.c. injection of isoproternenol is 680 mg/kg. In dogs it is less than 10 mg/kg, and 2.5 mg/kg on two consecutive days produces massive myocardial necrosis; most of the dogs will survive this dose.[2] Other experimental animals are also sensitive to the myocardial-necrosing effect of isoproterenol; mice,[10] rabbits and guinea pigs,[7] hamsters,[11] and reptiles[12] have all been found suitable for this experimental model.

Centrilobular necrosis of the liver, renal cortical necrosis, pulmonary edema, pulmonary hemorrhage, and hydrothorax have been observed with lethal doses of isoproterenol.[5] These could all be the result of severe congestive failure and circulatory collapse. Also, multiple isoproterenol injections have been shown to produce focal nephrocalcinosis, coronary artery hypertrophy with medial hyalinization, aortic aneurysm, and parotid gland enlargement.[13,14]

The pathogenesis of the acute isoproterenol cardiac necrosis is still not completely settled. The basic histological lesion is necrosis of the myocardial fibers, with a later secondary response of the interstitial structures. We did not find occlusion or other significant coronary artery pathology implicating the arterial supply to the myocardium. However, pharmacological studies have shown that isoproterenol has a cardiostimulative effect that greatly increases the oxygen requirements of the myocardial fibers; in addition, as noted previously, it reduces systemic blood pressure by means of peripheral vasodilatation.[5] On the basis of this pharmacological evidence, we have suggested that isoproterenol results in temporary relative ischemia of the myofibers.[3] The electron microscopical studies of early myocardial alterations by Korb[15,16] and by Ferrans and co-workers[17] are also consistent with a hypoxic pathogenesis. Certain drugs, such as monamine oxidase inhibitors[18] and beta-adrenergic compounds,[10,19] which block the cardiostimulative effects of isoproterenol and thus the increased myocardial fiber oxygen requirements, protect against myocardial necrosis.

Handforth[11,20] has suggested, from injection and morphological studies in hamsters and rabbits, that isoproterenol-induced myocardial necrosis is a true ischemic infarct. Its pathogenesis, he feels, is an isoproterenol vasodilatation effect resulting in dilatation of preexisting bypass channels between coronary arteries and veins. This, in turn, would lead to a drop in intramyocardial capillary pressure below that necessary for adequate tissue perfusion. The same author[20] and others[21] have reported segmental coronary arteritis, which they

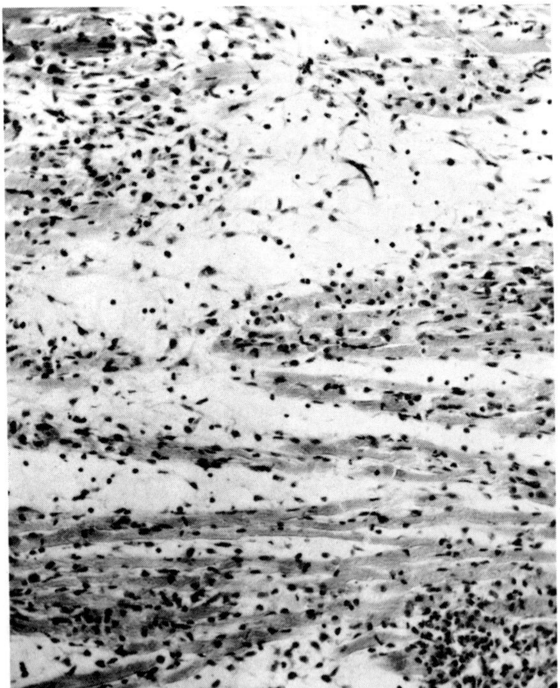

FIGURE 3. Photomicrograph of a heart from a rat injected with isoproterenol (85 mg/kg) on two consecutive days and sacrificed at 36 hours. There is widespread mucinous edema separating the fibers, mild polymorphonuclear infiltration, and coagulation necrosis of some of the myofibers. Stain: hematoxylin and eosin. × 100.

feel might also play a role by causing temporary vasoconstriction. As previously mentioned, we have not found vasculitis or significant arterial, arteriolar, or capillary thrombosis in our studies.

The isoproterenol-induced myocardial necrosis was originally described by us as infarct-like.[3] It has been emphasized in this monograph that, from a morphological point of view, the myocardium has only a few limited ways to react to the many possible agents that can injure it.[22] Thus, the fact that the early isoproterenol-induced myocardial lesion in the rat is not dissimilar to the early changes resulting from ligation of a coronary artery[23] is not enough to suggest a similar pathogenesis for the two lesions. However, as noted previously, in spite of the absence of significant coronary artery pathology, pharmacological studies and the majority of experimental evidence are consistent with an ischemic pathogenesis for the isoproterenol effect.[5,10,11,15-21] This, coupled with the gross and histological features of the myocardial lesion and its location in areas usually affected by ischemic processes, makes us feel that "infarct-like" is still the best designation for the lesion. Objections toward this designation have come from investigators[7,24] who produced only small focal myocardial lesions, which on morphological grounds they felt resembled the lesions seen with metabolic disturbances. These investigators used animals of low weight which are realtively less sensitive to isoproterenol; in addition, they administered small doses of the compound.

The granulomatous reaction in the early healing stage of the isoproterenol-induced lesion is not found after permanent ligation of a coronary artery in the rat.[23] In isoproterenol-induced myocardial necrosis, even though there is minimal polymorphonuclear leukocyte infiltration, there is early and rapid myocytolysis, with infiltration of a large number of mononuclear cells. The observation of Ferrans and co-workers[25] that many of these mononuclear cells are rich in lysosomes would appear to be of some significance in regard to this rapid resorption of the necrotic fibers. We have previously suggested that the rapid evolution of the lesion and the granulomatous-like reaction could have two other explanations.[26] One possibility is that it results from a pharmacological action of the drug on reparative processes; against this interpretation is the fact that a similar reaction is not found in reparative reactions in other tissues in these animals. The second, and we feel the more likely explanation, is that this reaction is related to the persistence of the interstitial tissue, coupled with a retention of the normal blood supply to the injured area during the period of repair. As has already been pointed out, the isoproterenol-induced relative myocardial ischemia is temporary. Focal myocardial necrosis with a granulomatous reaction similar to that found in the present experiment has been produced in the rabbit by a number of agents: group A streptococci,[27] intravenous proteolytic enzymes,[28] and multiple horse serum injections.[29] As in the present experiment, normal coronary circulation was presumably maintained. The granulomas that develop focally around degenerating muscle fibers resemble the "myofiber" Aschoff body described by Murphy and Becker in the rabbit.[30] They also bear some histological similarity to the Aschoff nodules found in acute rheumatic fever. It is possible that some forms of human interstitial myocarditis may represent a reaction to myofiber injury in hearts with a normal blood supply, the initial necrotic stage having passed by the time of necropsy examination.[9] Lesions thought to result from relative or temporary ischemia, such as focal myocytolysis[31] and miliary myocardial infarcts,[32] have also been described in man.

A number of experiments have been carried out in an attempt to influence the severity of isoproterenol-induced necrosis.[10, 19, 33, 34] TABLE 1 summarizes our observations in this line. The results can be divided into three groups. Group I factors had no modifying effect. Group II factors had a protective effect, and group III factors increased the mortality rate and severity of the myocardial necrosis. In addition, our studies have shown that low-potassium diet or deoxycorticosterone acetate (DOCA) pretreatment not only increased the severity of the isoproterenol-induced myocardial necrosis, but modified the reaction of the heart so that bilateral atrial infarct-like myocardial necrosis became prominent.[34-36] Histologically, the findings in the atria resembled the confluent necrosis found in the ventricles; wide areas of atrial myocardial fibers became necrotic and were replaced by mononuclear cells. Supplementary potassium chloride protected the animals against the atrial infarct-like lesions of DOCA pretreatment.

The experiments clearly demonstrate that systemic factors can influence the mortality and severity of experimental myocardial necrosis and illustrate the potential importance of myocardial susceptibility in relation to a subsequent injurious event. Our studies have shown a relationship between salt imbalance in the diet and the resulting isoproterenol myocardial necrosis. A high-potassium

TABLE 1

THE EFFECT OF VARIOUS MODIFYING FACTORS ON ISOPROTERENOL-INDUCED HEART NECROSIS AND MORTALITY RATE*

Factor	Myocardial Necrosis	Mortality
Group I		
Sex	0	0
Premarin	0	0
Progesterone	0	0
ACTH	0	0
Adrenalectomy	0	0
Glucocorticoids	0	0
Group II		
Breed	Sprague-Dawley rats are more resistant	0
Starvation	−1	−3
Hypothyroidism	−3	−2
Low-sodium diet	−2	−2
High-potassium diet	−3	−2
Group III		
Age	+1	+1
Weight	+3	+1
"Isolation stress"	+1	+1
Estrone	+1	+1
Testosterone	+1	+1
Hyperthyroidism	+1	+2
Mineralocorticoids	+3	+3
Low-potassium diet	+2	+2
High-sodium diet	+2	+2

* The + and − grades are in comparison with rats on a normal diet receiving only two doses of 85 mg/kg on two consecutive days. 0 = no effect.

diet afforded some protection, but high-sodium and low-potassium diet or DOCA pretreatment resulted in an aggravation of the cardiac lesions. Lehr[37] found that a shift in myocardial electrolytes (magnesium, calcium, sodium, and phosphate) occurs following administration of alpha- or beta-adrenergic compounds. He suggested that these shifts could result from an effect on ionic transfer at the plasma and subcellular membrane sites of the cell and could be a contributing factor in the initiation of irrversible failure of cell function. Raab and his associates[38] have shown that catecholamines produce a rapid outward transfer of intracytoplasmic potassium through the cell membrane. Thus, in addition to producing relative myocardial ischemia, isoproterenol seems to have a direct effect on myocardial electrolytes. Since anoxia and electrolyte disturbance have a synergistic effect in producing myocardial damage, the isoproterenol-inducd shift in electrolytes probably plays an additive role in the production of the myocardial necrosis. As an explanation for the massive atrial necrosis induced by isoproterenol administration following a low-potassium diet or DOCA pretreatment, we have previously suggested[34,35] that, from an electrolyte standpoint, these pretreatments result in the formation of local handicapped regions that are hypersensitive to subsequent isoproterenol administration.

This experimental model has also been used to study the chronic effect of healed myocardial necrosis in the rat.[39] Of 50 rats receiving the two standard isoproterenol injections, twenty-seven died before the termination of the two-year follow-up; 23 of the deaths were not related to the cardiac status of the animal, although three of these rats had chronic heart aneurysms at the time of death. The other four rats that expired during the course of the experiment died of chronic congestive heart failure. At autopsy, these animals were found to have enlarged hearts with large cardiac aneurysms, pulmonary edema, hydrothorax, ascites, and diffuse hepatic fibrosis. The remaining 23 of the 50 rats survived the two-year observation period. Of these, 15 had normal-size hearts with only thin linear scars. The remaining eight animals had enlarged hearts with large aneurysms. These 23 animals lived out their approximate expected life-span quite happily and comfortably, in spite of their myocardial lesions. Thus, it would appear that the rat, with its good coronary artery supply, has great reserve power to compensate for myocardial damage. Only occasionally was this exceeded, and then it died of congestive heart failure.

Friedberg and Horn[40] did not find any pathological distinction between the myocardial necrosis that developed in man with or without coronary occlusion. Baroldi[41] has recently coined the term "idiopathic coagulation necrosis of the myocardium" for the lesion he found in cases of sudden deaths without evidence of recent coronary artery occlusion. These cases might be explained by the experimental evidence that shows the potential importance of myocardial susceptbility to subsequent relative ischemia. However, in regard to human myocardial infarction, an autopsy study in our department[42] and another recent study[43] found that the majority of acute infarctions are associated with mural coronary artery diseases and recent luminal occlusion.

Myocardial damage in patients who had received large doses of isoproterenol under special circumstances have been reported.[44] It therefore seems worthwhile to remember that, given the right conditions, the human myocardium is also sensitive to the cardiotoxic effects of isoproterenol. However, in view of the widespread use of the drug, the paucity of such reports would seem to indicate that its cardiotoxic effect is negligible in the customary therapeutic dose.

References

1. Chappel, C. I., G. Rona, T. Balazs & R. Gaudry. 1959. Comparison of cardiotoxic actions of certain sympathomimetic amines. Canad. J. Biochem. Physiol. **37:** 35–42.
2. Rona, G., T. Zsoter, C. I. Chappel & R. Gaudry. 1959. Myocardial lesions, circulatory and electrocardiographic changes produced by isoproterenol in the dog. Rev. Canad. Biol. **18:** 83–94.
3. Rona, G., C. I. Chappel, T. Balazs & R. Gaudry. 1959. An infarct-like myocardial lesion and other toxic manifestations produced by isoproterenol in the rat. Arch. Path. (Chicago) **67:** 443–455.
4. Rona, G., D. S. Kahn & C. I. Chappel. 1963. Studies on infarct-like myocardial necrosis produced by isoproterenol: A review. Rev. Canad. Biol. **22:** 241-255.
5. Rona, G., C. I. Chappel, T. Balazs & R. Gaudry. 1959. Severe myocardial necrosis produced by isoproterenol in the rat. Arch. Int. Pharmacodyn. **122:** 123–128.
6. Hill, R., A. N. Howard & G. A. Gresham. 1960. The electrocardiographic appearances of myocardial infarction in the rat. Brit. J. Exp. Path. **41:** 633–637.
7. Mortari, A., F. Piccinini & G. Sioli. 1963. Sull'infarto miocardico sperimentale da isoproterenolo nei piccoli animali: Studio elettrocardiografico. Mal. Cardiov. **4:** 689–707.
8. Korb, G. Personal communication.
9. Rona, G., D. S. Kahn & C. I. Chappel. 1961. Study on the healing of cardiac necrosis in the rat. Amer. J. Path. **39:** 473–489.
10. Zbinden, G. & R. A. Moe. 1967. Pharmacological studies on heart muscle lesions induced by isoproterenol. This monograph.
11. Handforth, C. P. 1962. Isoproterenol-induced myocardial infarction in animals. Arch. Path. (Chicago) **73:** 161–165.
12. Poupa, O. & B. Oštádal. 1967. Experimental cardiomegalies and "cardiomegalies" in free living animals. This monograph.
13. Selye, H., E. Bajusz & R. Veilleux. 1960. Production of dissecting aneurysms by chronic isoproterenol treatment. Cor Vasa **2:** 273–275.
14. Selye, H., R. Veilleux & M. Cantin. 1961. Excessive stimulation of salivary gland growth by isoproterenol. Science **133:** 44–45.
15. Korb, G. 1964. Electronenmikroskopische Befunde am Herzmuskel nach hohen Aludrininjektionen. Verh. Deutsch. Ges. Path. **48:** 245–250.
16. Korb, G. 1965. Electronenmikroskopische Untersuchungen zur Aludrin (Isoproterenolsulfat) Schaedigung des Herzmuskels. Virchow. Arch. Path. Anat. **339:** 136—150.
17. Ferrans, V. J., R. G. Hibbs, W. C. Black & D. G. Weilbaecher. 1964. Isoproterenol-induced myocardial necrosis. A histochemical and electron microscopic study. Amer. Heart J. **68:** 71–90.
18. Zbinden, G. 1961. Effect of anoxia and monamine oxidase inhibitors on myocardial necrosis induced by isoproterenol. Fed. Proc. **21:** 128.
19. Von Breining, H. & O. Strubelt. 1965. Die Bedeutung der adrenergischen Betarezeptoren fur die cardiotoxische Wirkung sympathicomimetischer Amine. Med. Pharmacol. Exp. **13:** 169–176.
20. Handforth, C. D. 1962. Coronary arteritis and myocardial infarction in hamsters produced by isoproterenol (Isuprel). Med. Serv. J. (Canad.). **18:** 506–509.
21. Amelin, A. Z., I. Anshelevick & M. Melzobs. 1963. Experimental infarct-like changes of the myocardium under the influence of isadrine (isopropylnoradrenaline). Arkh. Pat. **25:** 25–29 (in Russian).
22. Wartman, W. B. 1967. Cardiopathy and myocardial degeneration: Problems of terminology in experimental and clinical pathology. This monograph.
23. Dusek, J. & V. Jezdinska. 1965. The course of healing of experimental myocardial infarction in the rat. Cor Vasa. **7:** 136–142.
24. Rosenmann, E., E. Gazenfield, A. Laufer & A. M. Davies. 1964. Isoproterenol-induced myocardial lesions in the immunzied and non-immunized rat. Path. Microbiol. **27:** 303–309.
25. Ferrans, V. J., R. G. Hibbs, J. J. Walsh & G. E. Burch. 1967. Histochemical and electron microscopical studies of the cardiac necroses produced by sympathomimetic agents. This monograph.
26. Rona, G. & D. S. Kahn. 1967. The healing of cardiac necrosis as reflected by experimental studies. *In* Methods and Achievements in Experimental Pathology. E. Bajusz & G. Jasmin, Eds. **3:** 200–249. S. Karger, Basel, Switzerland.

27. MURPHY, G. E. & H. F. SWIFT. 1950. The induction of rheumatic-like cardiac lesions in rabbits by repeated focal injections with group A streptococci: Comparison with the cardiac lesions of serum disease. J. Exper. Med. **91**: 485–498.
28. KELLNER, A. & T. ROBERTSON. 1954. Selective necrosis of cardiac and skeletal muscle induced experimentally by means of proteolytic enzyme solutions given intravenously. J. Exper. Med. **99**: 387–404.
29. MORE, R. H. & H. Z. MOVAT. 1959. Character and significance of the cellular response in the collagen diseases and experimental hypersensitivity. Lab. Invest. **8**: 873–889.
30. MURPHY, G. E. & CARL G. BECKER. 1966. Occurrence of caterpillar nuclei within normal immature and normal appearing and altered mature heart muscle cells and the evolution of Aschoff cells from the latter. Amer. J. Path. **48**: 931–957.
31. SCHLESINGER, M. J. & L. REINER. 1955. Focal myocytolysis of the heart. Amer. J. Path. **31**: 443–459.
32. BARRIE, H. J. & P. G. URBACK. 1957. The cellular changes in myocardial infarction. Canad. Med. Ass. J. **77**: 100–106.
33. BAJUSZ, E. & G. JASMIN. 1962. Protective action of serotonin against certain chemically and surgically induced cardiac necroses. Rev. Canad. Biol. **21**: 51–62.
34. RONA, G., C. I. CHAPPEL & D. S. KAHN. 1962. The pathogenesis of atrial infarction. Amer. J. Path. **41**: 455–466.
35. Rona, G., D. S. KAHN & C. I. CHAPPEL. 1965. The effect of electrolytes on experimental infarct-like myocardial necrosis. *In* Electrolytes and Cardiovascular Diseases. E. Bajusz, Eds. : 181–191. S. Karger. Basel, Switzerland.
36. RONA, G., C. I. CHAPPEL & D. S. KAHN. 1963. The significance of factors modifying the development of isoproterenol-induced myocardial necrosis. Amer. Heart J. **66**: 389–395.
37. LEHR, D. 1967. Tissue electrolyte alteration in disseminated myocardial necrosis. This monograph.
38. RAAB, W., R. J. HUMPHREYS & E. LEPESCHKIN. 1950. Potentiation of pressor effects of nor-epinephrine and epinephrine in man by desoxycorticosterone acetate. J. Clin. Invest. **29**: 1397–1404.
39. RONA, G., C. I. CHAPPEL & D. S. KAHN. 1963. Experimental production of chronic cardiac aneurysm and congestive heart failure in the rat. Exp. Molec. Path. **2**: 40–51.
40. FRIEDBERG, C. K. & H. HORN. 1939. Acute myocardial infarction not due to coronary artery occlusion. J.A.M.A. **112**: 1675–1679.
41. BAROLDI, G. 1965. Acute coronary occlusion as a cause of myocardial infarction and sudden coronary heart death. Amer. J. Cardiol. **16**: 859–880.
42. RONA, G. 1966. The pathogenesis of human myocardial infarction. Canad. Med. Ass. J. **95**: 1012–1019.
43. HARLAND, W. A. & A. M. HOLBURN. 1966. Coronary thrombosis and myocardial infarction. Lancet **ii**: 1158–1159.
44. LOCKETT, M. F. 1965. Dangerous effects of isoprenaline in myocardial failure. Lancet **ii**: 104–106.

PHARMACOLOGICAL STUDIES ON HEART MUSCLE LESIONS INDUCED BY ISOPROTERENOL

Gerhard Zbinden* and Robert A. Moe
Research Division, Hoffmann-La Roche Inc., Nutley, N. J.

Myocardial necrosis produced by isoproterenol has been proposed as a method for testing antianginal drugs (Zbinden, 1962). In order to evaluate the usefulness of this experimental model, morphological and biochemical changes occurring after a single administration of isoproterenol in mice were investigated. Furthermore, various compounds prescribed for the treatment of primary and secondary symptoms of ischemic heart disease and hypertension were tested for their ability to inhibit isoproterenol-induced myocardial necrosis in rats. This method was also used for screening of several new substances. Among these, Ro 5-5340 [*N,N'*-(iminoditrimethylene) di-*p*-toluenesulfonamide hydrochloride] was found to be active and was, therefore, also tested against anoxia-induced changes of the electrocardiogram (ECG) and experimental arrhythmias in dogs. Its cardiovascular effects were compared to those of various other antiarrhythmic and cardioactive agents.

Methods

Biochemical and Histological Studies in Mice

All experiments were conducted in male mice of the CF-1 strain weighing 16–25 g. DL-Isoproternol hydrochloride (Isuprel®)† was injected subcutaneously (s.c.) at a dose of 50 mg/kg. Groups of mice were sacrificed at various time intervals after isoproterenol injection. Glycogen was determined in the heart according to the method described by Seifter and co-workers (1950), and lactic acid was measured in the blood and heart according to the method of Barker and Summerson (1941). For the lactic acid determination, mice were sacrificed with chloroform, and blood was taken by heart puncture at the moment when breathing ceased. The hearts were removed and frozen without washing immediately thereafter. This slight deviation from the preferred sampling method of Dale (1965) accounts for the somewhat higher lactic acid levels in the heart muscle. For the estimation of protein synthesis in the heart, each mouse received an intraperitoneal (i.p.) injection of 2.5 μc (0.8 μmole) of L-valine-1-^{14}C exactly 30 minutes prior to sacrifice. Hearts were rapidly excised, rinsed in an ice-cold solution of 0.9% sodium chloride, blotted, and homogenized in 5% trichloracidic acid with an all-glass, tight-fitting, motor-driven homogenizer. Total heart protein was isolated according to the procedure of Rabinowitz and his associates (1954). Each sample was placed in a 20-ml potassium-free glass vial. To each vial, 1.0 ml of distilled water and 15 ml of scintillation mixture [100 g of naphthalene, recrystallized from ethanol; 7 g of 2,5-diphenyloxazole, 50 mg of 1,4-bis-2-(4-methyl-5-phenyloxazolyl) benzene, and 30 g of thixotropic gel powder (Cab-O-Sil®)‡ per liter of spectroquality dioxane] were added. Radioactivity was measured with a Nuclear Chicago 720 liquid scintillation system. The results were expressed

* Present address: Department of Medicine, University of Cambridge, Cambridge, England.
† Distributed by Winthrop Laboratories, New York, N. Y.
‡ Distributed by New England Nuclear Corp., Boston, Mass.

in disintegrations per minute (dpm) per gram of protein. All samples were corrected for background radiation and for variable degrees of quenching by the channel-ratio method (Bush, 1963). The hearts of other groups of mice also treated with a single injection s.c. of 50 mg/kg of DL-isoproterenol hydrochloride were fixed in Gendre's fluid, embedded in paraffin, and stained with Best's carmine stain and hematoxylin-eosin or fixed in 10% formalin for frozen sections which were stained with Fat-red-7B.§

Drug Effects on Isoproterenol-Induced Myocardial Necrosis in Rats

Rats of both sexes of the Charles River SD strain, weighing 160–220 g, were used. Drugs were administered i.p. on two to seven consecutive days or were given as admixture to the ration for four to nine days. On the last two days of treatment, the rats received 80 mg/kg of DL-isoproterenol hydrochloride s.c. In the case of the monoamine oxidase (MAO) inhibitors and reserpine, drug administration was discontinued 24 hours before the first isoproterenol dose. All rats were sacrificed 24 hours after the second isoproterenol injection. The hearts were removed, washed with saline, and weighed. The left ventricles were fixed in Zenker's or Technicon solution, embedded in paraffin, sectioned, and stained with hematoxylin-eosin. Two sections of each ventricle were examined, and the degree of necrosis was graded 0 to 5+, as described previously (Zbinden, 1962). The degree of myocardial damage was compared to that of a control group which had received the isoproterenol injection at the same time as the treated groups. The 2×2 X^2 test was used for statistical evaluation. The compounds tested are listed in TABLES 1 and 2.

Cardiovascular Studies with Ro 5-5340 in Dogs

Effect on Acute Anoxia

Anesthetized dogs prepared for recording of femoral artery blood pressure and the ECG (lead II) were cannulated for tracheal insufflation. Acute anoxia was produced by substituting 100% nitrogen at the respirator intake for that interval of time required to produce significant arterial blood pressure and ECG changes. The time interval for nitrogen intake was generally between 90 seconds and two minutes, after which room air was again permitted into the pump inlet. Anoxic responses were observed three times prior to drug administration, as well as 30 minutes and one hour after intravenous (i.v.) injection of Ro 5-5340. The effects were compared with those of quinidine sulfate, pronethalol (Nethalide®),¶ sodium lactate, procaine amide, sodium pyruvate, and dextrose.

Antiarrhythmic Effects

Acetylcholine-Induced Auricular Fibrillation. Three dogs anesthetized i.p. with 30 mg/kg of sodium pentobarbital (Nembutal®)|| were prepared for femoral artery blood pressure recording and femoral vein infusion. The trachea was cannulated for positive-pressure respiration. The right thorax was opened, the pericardium cut, and the right auricle, along with the sinus node, exposed. A small cellulose pledget was soaked in 5% acetylcholine and placed directly on the area of the sinus node, resulting in auricular tachycardia. One minute

§ Distributed by Ciba Pharmaceutical Co., Summit, N. J.

¶ Distributed by Imperial Chemical Industries, Ltd., England.

|| Distributed by Abbott Laboratories, North Chicago, Ill.

TABLE 1

EFFECT OF VARIOUS DRUGS ON THE ISOPROTERENOL-INDUCED MYOCARDIAL NECROSIS IN RATS*

Pharmacological Class	Drug	Dose (mg/kg) or % in Ration	Days of Treatment	Route	Isoproterenol (mg/kg, s.c.)	Isoproterenol Hours after Last Treatment	No. of Rats Treated	No. of Rats Controls	Deaths Treated	Deaths Controls	Average Degree of Myocardial Necrosis Treated	Average Degree of Myocardial Necrosis Controls	p
Monoamine oxidase inhibitors	Isocarboxazide	50	7	i.p.	80	24†	28	28	0	1	2.2	4.0	<0.001
	Isocarboxazide	30	7	i.p.	50	24†	8	8	0	0	2.4	3.6	<0.02
Hydrazine type	Iproniazid	50	7	i.p.	80	24†	8	8	0	0	2.5	3.9	<0.05
	Pivaloylbenz-hydrazine	0.2 %	9	p.o.	10	‡	8	12	0	1	2.9	4.3	<0.05
Non-Hydrazine type	Tranylcypromine	25	7	i.p.	80	24†	8	16	0	0	3.8	3.5	>0.05
	Pargyline	25	7	i.p.	80	24†	10	12	0	0	3.6	3.8	>0.05
	Ro 5-7071§	1	2	i.p.	80	24†	12	12	0	0	3.5	3.3	>0.05
Alpha- and beta-adrenergic blocking agents	Azapetine	0.05%	4	p.o.	80	‡	8	14	0	1	4.1	4.5	>0.05
	Propranolol	10	4	i.p.	80	1	12	16	0	0	3.3	3.3	>0.05
	Pronethalol	50	4	i.p.	80	2	12	12	0	2	3.8	3.8	>0.05
Postganglionic blocking agents	Guanethidine	50	3	i.p.	2	4	12	12	0	0	4.0	3.6	>0.05
	Isocaramidine	50	3	i.p.	2	4	12	12	0	0	2.9	3.6	>0.05
	Isocaramidine	15	4	i.p.	80	1	10	15	0	0	3.9	3.9	>0.05

Vasodilators and cardioactive agents	Sodium nitrite	0.2 %	4	p.o.	80	‡	10	10	1	0	3.7	3.7	>0.05
	Aminophylline	2x50	4	i.p.	80	1	10	12	0	0	3.7	3.3	>0.05
	Dipyridamole	2x50	4	i.p.	80	1	10	12	0	0	3.7	3.3	>0.05
	Hexobendine	50	4	i.p.	80	1	12	15	0	0	3.4	3.7	>0.05
Psychotropic drugs	Reserpine	2	2	i.p.	1	24†	10	10	1	1	3.7	3.3	>0.05
	Chlorpromazine	10	4	i.p.	80	2	10	15	0	1	3.4	3.8	>0.05
	Chlordiazepoxide	10	4	i.p.	80	2	10	15	0	1	3.7	3.8	>0.05
	Chlordiazepoxide	0.5 %	7	p.o.	80	‡	8	10	0	1	3.6	4.1	>0.05
	Meprobamate	100	4	i.p.	80	2	10	15	1	1	3.8	3.8	>0.05
	Amitriptyline	10	4	i.p.	80	2	10	15	0	1	3.6	3.8	>0.05
Antithyroid compounds	Thiouracil	50	4	i.p.	80	1	20	24	1	0	3.4	3.7	>0.05
	Thiouracil	0.1 %	7	p.o.	80	‡	10	15	0	1	3.5	3.3	>0.05

* For inactive drugs, only the highest dose levels tested are listed; for active drugs, results of representative experiments are listed.

† Drug administration discontinued 24 hours before first isoproterenol injection.

‡ Drug administration in ration continued until sacrifice.

§ Ro 5-7071 = 4-methyl-5-oxazolecarbamic acid phenyl ester.

TABLE 2

EFFECT OF RO 5-5340, KCl, DEXTROSE, LACTATE, AND PYRUVATE ON THE ISOPROTERENOL-INDUCED MYOCARDIAL NECROSIS IN RATS

Ro 5-5340			Additional Treatment			Isoproterenol		No. of Rats		Deaths		Average Degree of Myocardial Necrosis		
Dose (mg/kg) or % in Ration	Days Treated	Route	Compound	Dose	Route	(mg/kg, s.c)	Hours after Last Treatment	Treated	Controls	Treated	Controls	Treated	Controls	p
5	4	i.p.	—	—	—	80	2	12	12	0	0	3.1	3.7	>0.05
25	4	i.p.	—	—	—	80	1	32	45	1	4	2.6	3.5	<0.01
50	4	i.p.	—	—	—	80	1	44	54	0	1	2.3	3.8	<0.001
50	3	p.o.	—	—	—	80	2	12	12	0	1	3.2	3.6	>0.05
100	3	p.o.	—	—	—	80	2	12	12	0	1	2.5	3.6	<0.05
200	3	p.o.	—	—	—	80	2	12	12	0	1	1.8	3.6	<0.01
25	4	p.o.	—	—	—	80	2	12	15	1	0	2.8	3.9	<0.05
50	4	p.o.	—	—	—	80	2	22	30	1	0	2.5	3.9	<0.05
0.1 %	7	p.o.	—	—	—	80	*	10	15	0	0	3.6	3.5	>0.05
0.25%	7	p.o.	—	—	—	80	*	10	15	0	0	2.8	3.5	>0.05
50	4	i.p.	KCl	1 mM/rat	p.o.	80	1	24	24	1	0	2.2	3.9	<0.001†
50	4	i.p.	—	—	—	80	1	24	24	0	0	3.0	3.9	<0.01
—	—	—	KCl	1 mM/rat	p.o.	80	1	24	24	1	0	3.5	3.9	<0.05
50	4	i.p.	Dextrose	500 mg/rat	p.o.	80	1	12	12	0	0	2.5	3.9	>0.05
50	4	i.p.	—	—	—	80	1	12	12	0	0	3.2	3.9	>0.05
—	—	—	Dextrose	500 mg/rat	p.o.	80	1	12	12	0	0	3.8	3.9	>0.05
—	—	—	Dextrose	180 mg/kg	—	80	—	12	16	1	0	3.5	3.3	>0.05
—	—	—	Sodium lactate	110 mg/kg	—	80	—	12	16	0	0	3.7	3.3	>0.05
—	—	—	Sodium lactate	220 mg/kg	—	80	—	12	16	0	0	3.8	3.3	>0.05
—	—	—	Sodium pyruvate	110 mg/kg	—	80	—	12	16	0	0	3.5	3.3	>0.05
—	—	—	Sodium pyruvate	220 mg/kg	—	80	—	12	16	0	0	3.4	3.3	>0.05

* Drug administration in ration continued until sacrifice.
† Ro 5-5340 + KCl significantly more active than Ro 5-5340 alone.

later, fibrillation was induced by stimulating the apex of the right auricle with several single shocks through a fixed electrode. Two minutes later, when auricular fibrillation was established, the acetylcholine pledget was removed. The auricle then returned to sinus rhythm spontaneously within four to six minutes. At 15-minute intervals over two hours, bursts of auricular arrhythmia were induced to establish a control duration of abnormal rhythm. From two hours on, at the midpoint of the 15-minute interval between fibrillations, RO 5-5340 was administered, starting with 1 mg/kg, i.v. for each subsequent drug administration, the previous dose was doubled until the antiarrhythmic effect was seen.

Effect on Ouabain-Induced Arrhythmia. During the 18 hours prior to the test, all food was withheld from the animals, although water was permitted *ad libitum*. Pentobarbital anesthesia was employed (30 mg/kg, i.v.). The dogs were hydrated with 30 ml/kg of distilled water. Femoral artery blood pressure and lead II of the ECG were recorded. Positive-pressure respiration was carried out through a tracheal cannulation, and the femoral vein was catheterized for i.v. infusions. A single vagus nerve was cleared, tied, and severed in preparation for peripheral stimulation [stimulation of 5 volts at 20 cycles per second (cps) and 0.25 msec per cycle for 1 minute]. The animals were infused through the femoral vein at a constant rate of 3 ml per minute with a solution containing 50 g of dextrose, 450 mg of K_2HPO_4, and 10.7 mg of sodium pentobarbital per kilogram of bodyweight in 1000 ml of distilled deionized water. After a control recording period of about 90 minutes, during which time three to five blood pressure and ECG responses to vagus nerve stimulation were recorded, a loading dose of 60 μg/kg of ouabain was given i.v.; at five-minute intervals thereafter, 4 μg/kg of ouabain were injected until ventricular tachycardia and arrhythmia developed. Stimulation of the vagus nerve at this point failed to elicit a significant parasympathetic response at the auricular level, and dominance of ectopic ventricular beats was apparent. At this time, 0.5 mg/kg of the test drug was infused every five minutes until the onset of sinus rhythm occurred and the number of ventricular escape beats during vagus nerve stimulation approached that of the control level.

Cardiovascular Effects of Ro 5-5340

Four anesthetized, artificially respired, vagotomized dogs were employed. Blood pressure and right ventricular heart force (Boniface *et al.*, 1953) were measured. Blood flow through the femoral artery was measured in two of the animals with a Medicon 3000 flow meter and an electromagnetic flow probe. Cumulative doses of Ro 5-5340 totaled 13 mg/kg in one, 20 mg/kg in the second, and 40 mg/kg in the remaining two animals. The largest single dose was 20 mg/kg, given to two animals over a five-minute period. The effect of the drug on blood pressure, heart rate, heart contractile force, and arterial blood flow was observed. Furthermore, its effect on the cardiovascular responses to norepinephrine, serotonin, isoproterenol, and bilateral occlusion of the carotid arteries and to electrical stimulation of the central portion of a severed vagus nerve was noted.

Results

Biochemical and Histological Studies in Mice

Some of the biochemical events taking place after a single s.c. injection of 50 mg/kg of isoproterenol in mice are shown in FIGURE 1. The glycogen content of the heart decreased rapidly to very low levels, but a rapid increase occurred after 2 hours, and, after ten hours, levels were reached which were about fourfold higher than those found before treatment. After 24 hours, the glycogen levels were back to control values. Lactic acid also decreased initially, with a return to control levels at five hours. It is interesting to note that, at the time of the highest increase of the myocardial glycogen (ten hours after the injection of isoproterenol), the blood glucose levels did not differ from those of control animals sacrificed at the same time. Lactic acid levels in the blood were elevated after one hour and returned to initial values thereafter. Protein synthesis was slightly inhibited one hour after the isoproterenol injection, but showed an increasing trend, as measured by valine-^{14}C incorporation, and was raised above control levels over the following 24-hour period. FIGURE 1 also shows that the standard deviations of the means were quite large, pointing to a considerable variability of the responses, particularly with regard

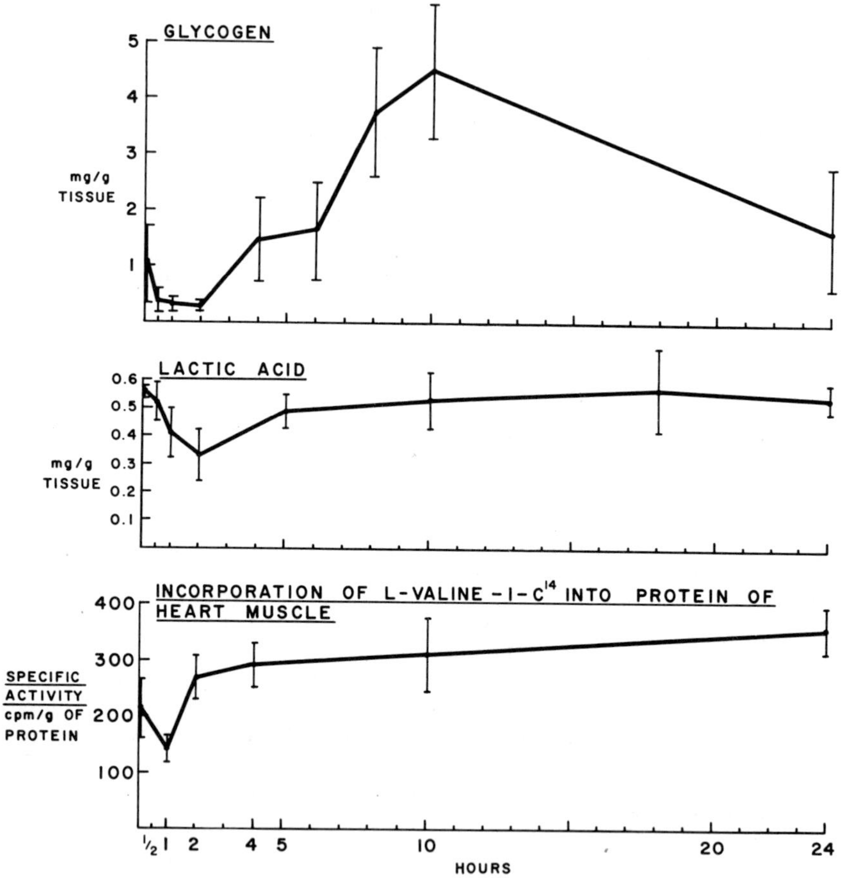

FIGURE 1. Biochemical changes in the heart muscle of mice following a subcutaneous injection of 50 mg/kg of DL-isoproterenol hydrochloride. Standard deviation: ± 1. Glycogen: eight to 18 mice per group; lactic acid: six to eight mice per group; protein synthesis: ten mice per group.

to the increase of glycogen levels and protein synthesis. Histological studies also demonstrated a considerable degree of variability of response to the cardiotoxic effect of isoproterenol. The histochemical reaction for glycogen was weak in control mice, and practically absent in animals sacrificed one or two hours after isoproterenol. It was moderately positive in four out of five animals examined five hours after isoproterenol, and markedly positive in four out of five animals sacrificed after ten hours and in three out of five animals sacrificed after 24 hours. Significant amounts of stainable neutral fat were found in one animal of each of the groups sacrificed one, five, and 24 hours after the isoproterenol injection, and in two out of five mice sacrificed at ten hours after the isoproterenol treatment. Focal degenerative changes of the muscle fibers were first seen in some animals five hours after isoproterenol administration, and in most animals after ten and 24 hours. Swelling and proliferation of interstitial fibroblasts were seen in some animals in the first one to five hours after injection, but were found to be at a maximum after ten and 24 hours. Moderate infiltration of the areas of fiber degeneration with neutrophilic leukocytes was seen only in one out of five mice after ten hours, and in two out of five animals after 24 hours.

Drug Effects on Isoproterenol-Induced Myocardial Necrosis in Rats

TABLE 1 indicates that, of many drugs tested, only the MAO inhibitors of the hydrazine type had a significant and consistent inhibiting effect on isoproterenol-induced damage of the heart. No protection was demonstrated with other potent MAO inhibitors of three different chemical classes. None of the alpha- and beta-adrenergic and postganglionic blockers, vasodilators, psychotropic, or antihydroid drugs showed any protective effect at the doses tested. From a large number of new compounds, Ro 5-5340 emerged as the most potent inhibitor of isoproterenol-induced myocardial necroses. TABLE 2 shows that the drug markedly reduced the degree of necrosis after repeated oral or parenteral administration of doses of 25 mg/kg or more. Isoproterenol causes swelling of the heart, which is directly related to the extent of the necrosis. As a consequence, the protective effect of Ro 5-5340 could often also be demonstrated by the difference in the average absolute and relative heart weights of treated and untreated rats. TABLE 2 also indicates that administration of potassium chloride had a pronounced protective effect and significantly potentiated the effect of Ro 5-5340. No such effects could be demonstrated with dextrose.

Cardiovascular Studies with Ro 5-5340 in Dogs

Effect on Acute Anoxia

FIGURE 2 demonstrates that nitrogen-induced anoxia produced a considerable increase in systolic blood pressure and a marked elevation of the ST segment and the T wave in the ECG. Both effects were prevented by Ro 5-5340. As shown in TABLE 3, the same effect was noted with quinidine sulfate and pronethalol and in two of six dogs with sodium lactate; procaine amide, sodium pyruvate, and dextrose were without effect at the doses tested.

Antiarrhythmic Effects

Acetylcholine-Induced Auricular Fibrillation. The i.v. administration of Ro 5-5340 significantly suppressed the acetylcholine-induced arrhythmia at a cumulative dose of 2–7 mg/kg, i.v. This effect lasted for 45 to 60 minutes.

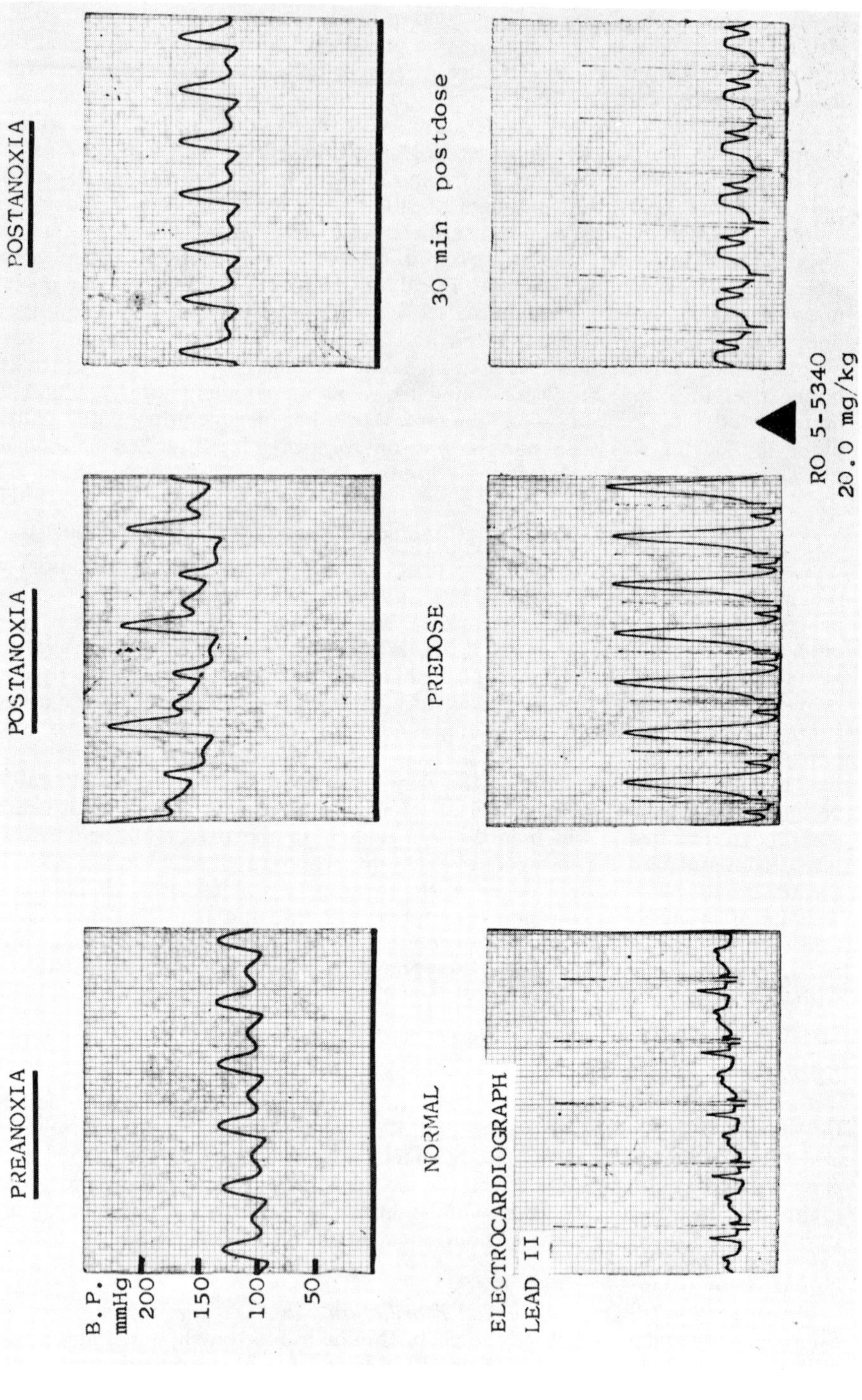
PREANOXIA
POSTANOXIA
POSTANOXIA
B.P.
mmHg
200
150
100
50
NORMAL
PREDOSE
30 min postdose
ELECTROCARDIOGRAPH
LEAD II
RO 5-5340
20.0 mg/kg

TABLE 3

EFFECT OF VARIOUS DRUGS ON THE BLOOD PRESSURE AND ECG RESPONSES TO NITROGEN-INDUCED ANOXIA IN ANESTHETIZED DOGS

Drug*	Dose (mg/kg, i.v.)	No. of Trials	Effect on Responses to Nitrogen-Induced Anoxia† Blood Pressure Rise	T Wave Elevation in ECG (lead II)
Ro 5-5340/1	20	9	9, Moderate to marked inhibition	9, Moderate to marked inhibition
Quinidine sulfate	20	1	1, Marked inhibition	1, Marked inhibition
Procaine amide	20	1	1, No effect	1, No effect
Sodium lactate	20	6	2, Slight inhibition 4, No effect	2, Moderate to marked inhibition 4, No effect
Sodium pyruvate	20	4	4, No effect	1, Moderate inhibition 3, No effect
Dextrose	20	3	3, No effect	3, No effect
Pronethalol	5	1	1, Marked inhibition	1, Marked inhibition

* All drugs prepared as a 1% solution in buffered diluent.
† 30 minutes after drug administration.

Effect on Ouabain-Induced Arrhythmia. FIGURE 3 summarizes the effects of peripheral vagus nerve stimulation (PVS) in a dog before and after ouabain administration. Prior to ouabain, PVS led to lowered blood pressure, cessation of auricular beats, and development of a limited number of ventricular escape beats (about 35 per minute). Following ouabain, the number of escape beats during PVS was increased to approximately 175 per minute. FIGURE 3 also demonstrates that Ro 5-5340 led to rhythmicity and slowing of the heart. This occurred in eight of 11 dogs tested at dose levels of 4–14 mg/kg, i.v.; 4–5 mg/kg of quinidine sulfate had the same effect.

Cardiovascular Effects of Ro 5-5340

After administration of cumulative doses of Ro 5-5340, blood pressure was either not affected or was slightly reduced, at higher doses. Even with the largest cumulative dose, the blood pressure response to i.v. administration of norepinephrine (1 μg/kg), isoproterenol (2 μg/kg), or bilateral occlusion of the carotid arteries was not altered significantly. The response to serotonin appeared to be inhibited to a moderate degree, and arterial blood flow was slightly reduced.

DISCUSSION

The parenteral administration of isoproterenol to small rodents leads to a chain of cardiovascular events that are followed with regularity by focal myocardial necroses (Rona *et al.*, 1959a). The biochemical changes taking place prior to and during the development of the heart-muscle lesions are dramatic:

FIGURE 2. Effect of Ro 5-5340 on blood pressure and ECG changes from nitrogen-induced anoxia in an anesthetized dog. Recording speed, 25 mm per second.

glycogen phosphorylase is stimulated (Mohme-Lundholm & Svedmyr, 1964; Satchell *et al.*, 1964), and heart glycogen falls to very low levels. There is a slight drop of the lactic acid content of the heart and a considerable decrease of protein synthesis. Oxygen consumption is increased (Waterman, 1949), and lactic acid levels in the blood are elevated (Lei & McCutcheon, 1964). In rats and mice, blood glucose shows little change (Ellis, 1956); however, the calcium content of the heart is significantly increased, whereas phosphate and magnesium are somewhat depleted (Lehr *et al.*, 1966). After the acute effects of isoproterenol are over, the myocardial glycogen increases markedly, reaching very high levels after ten hours. Blood and myocardial lactic acid return to normal values, and protein synthesis in the heart is activated. Myocardial degeneration and necrosis become histologically demonstrable after about eight hours (Rosenblum *et al.*, 1965), but slight changes of the mitochondria and the sarcoplasm can be detected with the electron microscope within 30 minutes after isoproterenol injection (Ferrans *et al.*, 1964). Mobilization of free fatty

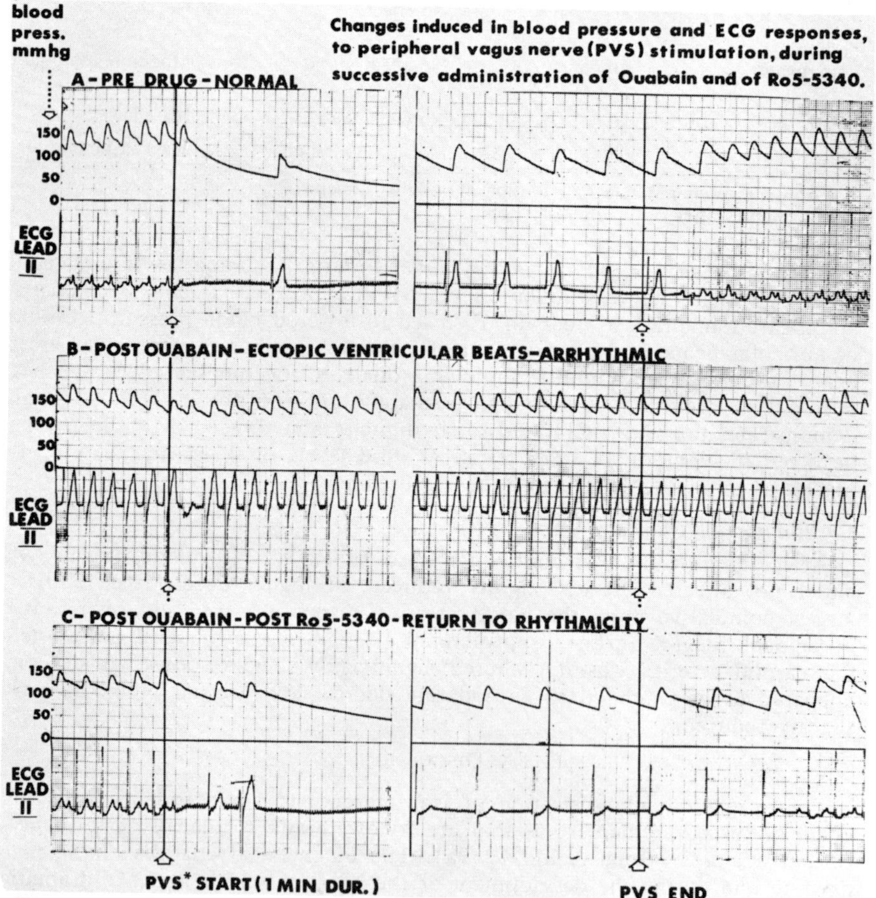

FIGURE 3. Effects of Ro 5-5340 on ouabain-induced arrhythmias in a male dog (no. 14), weighing 9.5 kg, anesthetized with pentobarbital. Stimulation of 5.6 volts at 22 cps and 0.25 msec per second; recording speed, 25 mm per second.

acids takes place within minutes after the isoproterenol injection (Barrett, 1965). Histologically diffuse deposition of lipid droplets occurs in myocardial fibers which reaches moderate proportions only after 12 hours, particularly in the areas of fiber necrosis. It is characteristic that the degree of fiber degeneration varies considerably from animal to animal; consequently, many of the biochemical changes also show marked variations.

In later stages of the isoproterenol-induced syndrome, when myocardial necroses are established, additional biochemical changes can be demonstrated, e.g. decrease of adenosine triphosphate (ATP) and creatinin (Kako, 1965), loss of enzymes such as succinic dehydrogenase and cytochrome oxidase (Ferrans *et al.*, 1964), and an increase of sodium (Lehr *et al.*, 1966).

Many of the early changes observed in the electron microscopical preparations are compatible with the notion that the myocardial damage after isoproterenol is due to acute anoxia (Ferrans *et al.*, 1964; Korb, 1965), which may occur as a result of hemodynamic coronary insufficiency (Rona *et al.*, 1959b; Handforth, 1962) or a marked stimulation of the myocardial metabolism and heart work (Raab, 1963). If this were indeed the case, the isoproterenol-induced myocardial necrosis would be a good experimental model for ischemic heart disease in man despite its very complex mechanism and its profound interference with the biochemical equilibrium of the heart. Pharmacological studies conducted to date indicate that certain drugs having a beneficial clinical effect in angina pectoris can significantly reduce the severity of the cardiotoxic effect of isoproterenol. Among these agents are MAO inhibitors of the hydrazine type, such as isocarboxazide (Zbinden, 1960), iproniazid and pivaloylbenzhydrazine (Zbinden, 1962; Müller, 1966), and nialamide (Bajusz and Jasmin, 1962). The mechanism of this inhibition is not known, but it is probably not due to MAO inhibition, since three potent inhibitors of different chemical structure (TABLE 1) were inactive.

Myocardial necrosis is also inhibited by beta-adrenergic blocking agents (Ehringer & Gögel, 1963; Lehr *et al.*, 1966), antithyroid compounds (Chappel *et al.*, 1959), and potassium ions (Rona *et al.*, 1963). The usefulness of beta-adrenergic blockers and antithyroid agents in angina pectoris is clinically proven, and the potential of potassium ions should be further investigated (Lehr *et al.*, 1966). In the present study, no protective effect was seen with two beta-adrenergic blocking agents and thiouracil at the doses tested. This, however, is not surprising, since minor experimental details may greatly influence the outcome of the pharmacological assays. No effect was seen with sodium nitrite; however, Scriabine and Strebbins (1966) were able to demonstrate protection of rats with trolnitrate phosphate if treatment was given for five days and small doses of isoproterenol (2 mg/kg) were given. The predictive value of the isoproterenol experiment is further supported by the finding that a large number of compounds having a purely symptomatic effect on angina pectoris in man, e.g. tranquilizing and hypotensive drugs, are completely inactive against the necrotizing properties of the catecholamine. On the other hand, thyroxine, a compound that aggravates the symptoms of ischemic heart disease, also potentiates significantly the isoproterenol effect on the rat heart (Rona *et al.*, 1961).

Based on these observations, a substantial number of new chemical substances were screened against the isoproterenol-induced myocardial necrosis in rats. Ro 5-5340 (TABLE 2) was found to be quite active and was therefore studied further. The compound lacked significant cardiovascular properties in intact animals but was able to protect dogs against anoxia-induced ECG changes and blood pressure rise. It shares this remarkable property with the beta-adrenergic blocker pronethalol, and with quinidine sulfate and sodium lactate. It also showed potent antiarrhythmic properties in various experimental procedures in the dog, including the acetylcholine-induced auricular fibrillation, the ouabain-induced arrhythmia, and the ventricular tachycardia observed in the Harris (1950) dog preparation (Osborne, 1966). Since beta-adrenergic blockers have no effect in the latter experimental procedure (Moran *et al.*, 1962), and since Ro 5-5340 lacked significant blocking effects against isoproterneol-induced blood pressure changes in the dog, it is probable that the protective effect of Ro 5-5340 against the cardiotoxic effect of isoproterenol is not due to beta-blockade. Experimental evidence to date indicates that Ro 5-5340 and quinidine sulfate have similar antiarrhythmic properties, both of which can be mimicked with a potassium ion infusate. Furthermore, the protective effect of Ro 5-5340 against isoproterenol-induced myocardial necrosis was significantly potentiated by potassium ion supplementation. This suggests that both Ro 5-5340 and quinidine sulfate may be effective antiarrhythmic agents by virtue of cardiac potassium ion retention properties. Further experiments must be conducted to determine whether Ro 5-5340 may also act via an effect on carbohydrate metabolism. Based on the findings with Ro 5-5340, it may be concluded that isoproterenol-induced myocardial necrosis is a useful experimental model that permits the demonstration of interesting cardioactive properties of drugs which have no direct cardiovascular effects in normal animals and which might therefore be missed in the conventional pharmacological assay procedures.

Summary

The usefulness of isoproterenol-induced myocardial necrosis as an experimental model for the pharmacological evaluation of antianginal and antiarrhythmic drugs has been investigated. Cardiotoxic doses of isoproterenol injected into mice and rats produce a large number of profound biochemical changes in heart muscle, affecting carbohydrate and fat metabolism, protein synthesis, and electrolyte balance. Myocardial necroses appear with regularity after one or two injections. From this study and from reports in the literature, it appears that, of the many pharmacological agents tested, only MAO inhibitors of the hydrazine type, antithyroid drugs, potassium ions, beta-adrenergic blocking agents, and trolnitrate phosphate were able to reduce the severity of the necrosis. During the screening of many new chemicals, Ro 5-5340 [*N,N'*-(iminoditrimethylene)di-*p*-toluenesulfonamide hydrochloride] was found to be a potent inhibitor of isoproterenol-induced myocardial necrosis in rats. This compound also inhibited anoxia-induced changes of the ECG and blood pressure in dogs and had potent antiarrhythmic properties in various experimental preparations. In normal animals, no significant cardiovascular effects were noted. It is concluded that isoproterenol-induced myocardial necrosis is a useful pharmacological test which permits the assay of interesting cardioactive properties of new drugs that could not be demonstrated in normal animals.

Acknowledgments

The authors wish to thank Dr. H. Bates for his contribution of biochemical data on the effects of isoproterenol on myocardial glycogen and protein synthesis. Thanks are also due to Mr. V. Augulis, Mr. P. Gattanell, Mr. Z. Palkoski, and Mr. L. Czyzewski for technical assistance.

REFERENCES

BAJUSZ, E. & G. JASMIN. 1962. Protective action of serotonin against certain chemically and surgically induced cardiac necroses. Rev. Canad. Biol. **21**: 51–62.

BARKER, S. B. & W. H. SUMMERSON. 1941. The colorimetric determination of lactic acid in biological material. J. Biol. Chem. **138**: 535–554.

BARRETT, A. M. 1965. The mobilization of free fatty acids in response to isoprenaline in the rat. Brit. J. Pharmacol. **25**: 545–556.

BONIFACE, K. J., O. J. BRODIE & R. P. WALTON. 1953. Resistance strain gauge arches for direct measurement of heart contractile force in animals. Proc. Soc. Exp. Biol. Med. **84**: 263–266.

BUSH, E. T. 1963. Technical Bulletin No. 13. Nuclear Chicago Corp. Des Plains, Ill.

CHAPPEL, C. I., G. RONA & R. GAUDRY. 1959. Relationship between thyroid function and cardiotoxic properties of isoproterenol. Endocrinology **65**: 208–215.

DALE, R. A. 1965. Effects of sampling procedures on the contents of some intermediate metabolites in glycolysis in rat tissues. J. Physiol. (London) **181**: 701–711.

EHRINGER, H. & H. GÖGEL. 1963. Zur Wirkung von Nethalide auf eine experimentelle Myocardnecrose der Ratte. Naunyn-Schmiedeberg. Arch. Exp. Path. **246**: 47–48.

ELLIS, S. 1956. The metabolic effects of epinephrine and related amines. Pharmacol. Rev. **8**: 485–562.

FERRANS, V. J., R. G. HIBBS, W. C. BLACK & D. G. WEILBAECHER. 1964. Isoproterenol-induced myocardial necrosis. A histochemical and electron microscopic study. Amer. Heart J. **68**: 71–90.

HANDFORTH, C. G. 1962. Isoproterenol-induced myocardial infarction in animals. Arch. Path. (Chicago) **73**: 161–165.

HARRIS, A. S. 1950. Delayed development of ventricular ectopic rhythms following experimental coronary occlusion. Circulation **1**: 1318–1328.

KAKO, K. 1965. Biochemical changes of the rat myocardium induced by isoproterenol. Canad. J. Physiol. Pharmacol. **43**: 541–549.

KORB, G. 1965. Elektronenmikroskopische Untersuchungen zur Aludrin (Isoproterenol-sulfat)-Schädigung des Herzmuskels. Virchow. Arch. Path. Anat. **339**: 136–150.

LEHR, D., M. KRUKOWSKI & R. COLÓN. 1966. Correlation of myocardial and venal necrosis with tissue electrolyte changes. J.A.M.A. **197**: 105–112.

LEI, B. W. & R. S. MCCUTCHEON. 1964. Influence of adrenergic receptors on blood sugar and lactic acid levels in the rat. J. Pharm. Sci. **53**: 503–506.

MOHME-LUNDHOLM, E. & N. SVEDMYR. 1964. Influence of nethalide on the phosphorylase activating effects of adrenaline and isoprenaline in experiments on isolated rat diaphragm. Acta Physiol. Scand. **61**: 192–194.

MORAN, N., J. MOORE, A. HOLCOMB & G. MUSKET. 1962. Antagonism of adrenergically-induced cardiac arrhythmias by dichloroisoproterenol. J. Pharmacol. Exp. Ther. **136**: 327–335.

MÜLLER, E. 1966. Histochemical studies on the experimental heart infarction in the rat. Naunyn-Schmiedeberg. Arch. Exp. Path. **254**: 439–447.

OSBORNE, M. W. 1966. Personal communication.

RAAB, W. 1963. Neurogenic multifocal destruction of myocardial tissue (pathogenic mechanism and its prevention). Rev. Canad. Biol. **22**: 217–239.

RABINOWITZ, M., M. E. OLSON & D. M. GREENBERG. 1954. Independent antagonism of amino acid incorporation into proteins. J. Biol. Chem. **210**: 837–849.

RONA, G., C. I. CHAPPEL, T. BALAZS & R. GAUDRY. 19^59a. An infarct-like myocardial lesion and other toxic manifestations produced by isoproterenol in the rat. Arch. Path. (Chicago) **67**: 443–445.

RONA, G., T. ZSOTER, C. I. CHAPPEL & R. GAUDRY. 1959b. Myocardial lesions, circulatory and electrocardiographic changes produced by isoproterenol in the dog. Rev. Canad. Biol. **18**: 83–94.

RONA, G., C. I. CHAPPEL & R. GAUDRY. 1961. Effect of dietary sodium and potassium content on myocardial necrosis elicited by isoproterenol. Lab. Invest. **10**: 892–897.

RONA, G., C. I. CHAPPEL & D. S. KAHN. 1963. The significance of factors modifying the development of isoproterenol-induced myocardial necrosis. Amer. Heart J. **66**: 389–395.

ROSENBLUM, I., A. WOHL & A. A. STEIN. 1965. Studies in cardiac necrosis. I. Production of cardiac lesions with sympathomimetic amines. Toxic. Appl. Pharmacol. **7**: 1–8.

SCRIABINE, A. & R. B. STREBBINS. 1966. Protection of rats from isoproterenol-induced myocardial necrosis by trolnitrate phosphate (Metamine®). Experientia **22**: 106–107.

SATCHELL, D. G., K. D. CAIRNCROSS & S. E. FREEMAN. 1964. The effect of amitriptyline on glycogen phosphorylase in cardiac muscle. Biochem. Pharmacol. **13**: 1683–1685.

SEIFTER, S., S. DAYTON, B. NOVIC & E. MUNTWYLER. 1950. The estimation of glycogen with anthrone reagent. Arch. Biochem. **25:** 191–200.

WATERMAN, F. A. 1949. Relationship between spontaneous activity and metabolic rate as influenced by certain sympathomimetic compounds. Proc. Soc. Exp. Biol. Med. **71:** 473–475.

ZBINDEN, G. 1960. Inhibition of experimental myocardial necrosis by the monoamine oxidase inhibitor isocarboxazid (Marplan). Amer. Heart J. **60:** 450–453.

ZBINDEN, G. 1962. Beeinflusung der experimentellen durch Isoproterenol hervorgerufenen Myocardnekrose durch Aminooxydasehemme, gefässerweiternde und tranquilisierende Arzneimittel. Arzneimittelforschung. **12:** 635–638.

HISTOCHEMICAL AND ELECTRON MICROSCOPICAL STUDIES ON THE CARDIAC NECROSES PRODUCED BY SYMPATHOMIMETIC AGENTS*

Victor J. Ferrans, Richard G. Hibbs, John J. Walsh, and George E. Burch

Departments of Medicine and Anatomy, Tulane University School of Medicine, and Seamen's Memorial Research Laboratory United States Public Health Service Hospital, New Orleans, La.

The histopathology of myocardial lesions produced by large doses of sympathomimetic amines has been the subject of detailed study in recent years.[1-7] Few reports are available, however, on the histochemical and electron microscopical features of such lesions.[8-14] The present studies of the histochemical and electron microscopical changes induced in the heart muscle by overdoses of isoproterenol, epinephrine, and norepinephrine were undertaken in the hope of providing a better understanding of the responses of myocardium to various types of injury.

Materials and Methods

Three groups of adult male rats, weighing 200–250 g each, were used in these studies. Animals of each group were respectively treated with one subcutaneous (s.c.) injection of isoproterenol (50 mg/kg), norepinephrine (2 mg/kg), or epinephrine (1 mg/kg). Animals were sacrificed at 30 minutes and one, two, four, six, eight, ten, 16, 24, 48, and 72 hours after injection. Samples from each heart were processed immediately for histochemical and electron microscopical study. In order to be sure of the validity of results, samples of normal rat heart were processed simultaneously in all experiments.

The following staining procedures were used on paraffin sections of formalin-fixed tissues: hematoxylin-eosin; periodic acid-Schiff (PAS), before and after amylase digestion; alcian blue; alcian blue-PAS; toluidine blue, and the mixed diamine and iron-diamine methods of Spicer[15] for the demonstration of mucosubstances. Cryostat sections postfixed in formalin were stained with benzyprene-caffeine for the fluorescence microscopy of lipids.[8] Unfixed cryostat sections were stained by tetrazolium-mediated methods for the demonstration of the activity of the following enzymes: succinic, malic, lactic, β-hydroxybutyric, α-glycerophosphate, ethanol, and glutamate dehydrogenases and NAD and NADP diaphorases.[16] Unfixed frozen sections were stained by the method of Burstone for cytochrome oxidase activity.[17] Nonspecific esterase and acid phosphatase activity were studied in frozen sections fixed overnight in the cold with 10% formalin containing 1% calcium chloride. For nonspecific esterase, sections were incubated for 15 minutes at room temperature in the α-naphthyl acetate-hexazotized *p*-rosaniline medium of Barka and Anderson.[18] In order to demonstrate lysosomal esterase, cytoplasmic esterase activity was inhibited by treatment of the sections with 0.01 M sodium fluoride for 30 minutes prior to incubation, followed by addition of 0.01 M sodium fluoride to the incubating medium.[19] For the demonstration of acid phosphatase activity, sections were incubated for 30 minutes at 37° C, using a modified Gomori[20] technique or the method of Burstone.[21]

* Supported by United States Public Health Service research grants nos. HE-6100, HE-2490, and 5-PO1-HE-06769 and by career development award no. 9-K3-HE-15, 281-07 (Doctor Hibbs).

For electron microscopy, 0.5 mm^3 blocks of left ventricular myocardium were fixed for two hours in cold 3% glutaraldehyde in 0.1 M phosphate buffer (pH 7.4) and washed in several changes of 5% sucrose in 0.1 M phosphate buffer (pH 7.4). The blocks were then postfixed for two hours in 1% osmium tetroxide in 0.1 M phosphate buffer (pH 7.4), dehydrated in graded alcohols, and embedded in Maraglas according to the method of Freeman and Spurlock.[22] Sections were cut with an LKB Ultrotome and examined with an RCA EMU 3C electron microscope. Some of the sections were stained with lead citrate and uranyl acetate.

RESULTS

Histological Observations

Cardiac lesions were found in all animals of each group. At the dose levels used, isoproterenol produced the most severe lesions and epinephrine the mildest. Larger doses of epinephrine could not be used, since they resulted in rapid death of most of the animals.

The lesions produced by isoproterenol consisted of large infarct-like areas of myocardial necrosis with hyalinization and/or vacuolization of the muscle fibers, interstitial and intracellular edema, and extensive inflammation. Such changes were particularly extensive in subendocardial areas of the free wall of the left ventricle. Focal necrosis was also found in the left atrium. Lesions were less prominent in the right ventricle and right atrium. The inflammatory response, first evident from six to ten hours after injection, was characterized by the presence of various types of mononuclear cells, including histiocytes, macrophages, lymphocytes, plasmocyte-like cells, Anitschkow cells, and occasional polymorphonuclear leukocytes and mast cells. Mitotic figures were seen in some inflammatory cells and fibroblasts. An increase in the amount of cytoplasm of the perivascular cells (pericytes and fibroblasts) was a consistent finding, even in areas in which the muscle fibers showed no alterations.

Norepinephrine produced less extensive myocardial necrosis than isoproterenol. Other changes, such as interstitial edema and cellular infiltration, were almost as severe as those seen in the isoproterenol-treated animals. Epinephrine caused some focal myocardial necrosis, but interstitial edema and inflammation were relatively more prominent than the alterations of the muscle fibers.

Histochemical Observations

Carbohydrate Stains

As shown by the PAS reaction, before and after amylase digestion, the muscle fibers of the normal rat heart contain variable amounts of glycogen. The basement membrane of the capillaries, the sarcolemma, Z lines, intercalated discs, the ground substance, and fibrillar components of the connective tissue of normal myocardium show an amylase-resistant PAS reaction.[23]

Three types of carbohydrate alterations were seen in this series of studies: loss of glycogen, the accumulation of a PAS-positive material in injured myocardial fibers, and the deposition of a metachromatic substance in areas of inflammation and necrosis. Glycogen loss was most pronounced in the epinephrine-treated animals. The accumulation of the PAS-positive material and the deposition of the metachromatic substance were most marked in isoproterenol-treated animals, and least evident in those given epinephrine.

Loss of stainable glycogen was evident 30 minutes after the administration of sympathomimetic agents. After 24 hours, glycogen began to reappear in many fibers, and by 72 hours, the glycogen content of most non-necrotic areas of myocardium was again normal.

A PAS-positive, amylase-resistant material appeared in some of the injured myocardial fibers one hour after injection. The number of involved fibers and the amount of this material increased gradually during the first 24 hours (FIGURE 1a). This material was still present in some fibers after 72 hours. It did not stain with alcian blue, toluidine blue, or with the diamine methods of Spicer. Phase contrast and polarization microscopy indicated that the accumulation of this material was associated with loss of normal striations. Clear vacuoles were seen in some of the affected fibers, which otherwise showed homogeneous cytoplasmic staining. Granules containing a material histochemically similar to that just described were found in the cytoplasm of macrophages.

A PAS- and Alcian blue-positive, diamine-negative substance that stained metachromatically with toluidine blue (FIGURE 1b) was present in areas of interstitial edema and inflammation, particularly in the subendocardium. This material was often seen on the sarcolemma of adjacent muscle fibers.

Lipids

In benzpyrene-stained preparations of normal rat heart, a pale-blue fluorescence, indicative of phospholipids, was observed in the mitochondria, sarco-

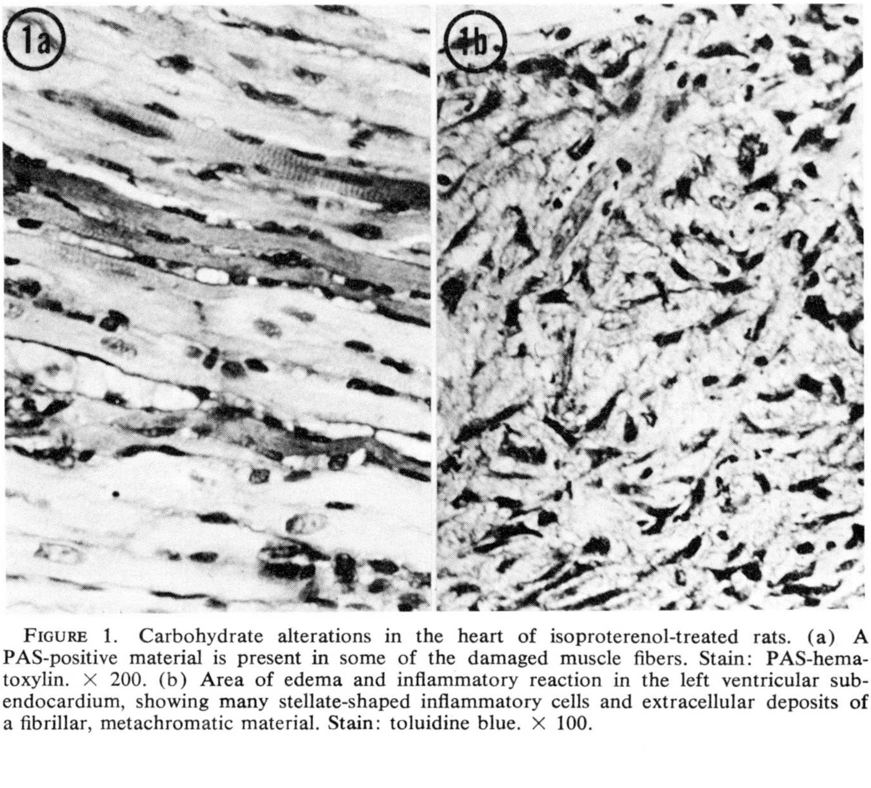

FIGURE 1. Carbohydrate alterations in the heart of isoproterenol-treated rats. (a) A PAS-positive material is present in some of the damaged muscle fibers. Stain: PAS-hematoxylin. × 200. (b) Area of edema and inflammatory reaction in the left ventricular subendocardium, showing many stellate-shaped inflammatory cells and extracellular deposits of a fibrillar, metachromatic material. Stain: toluidine blue. × 100.

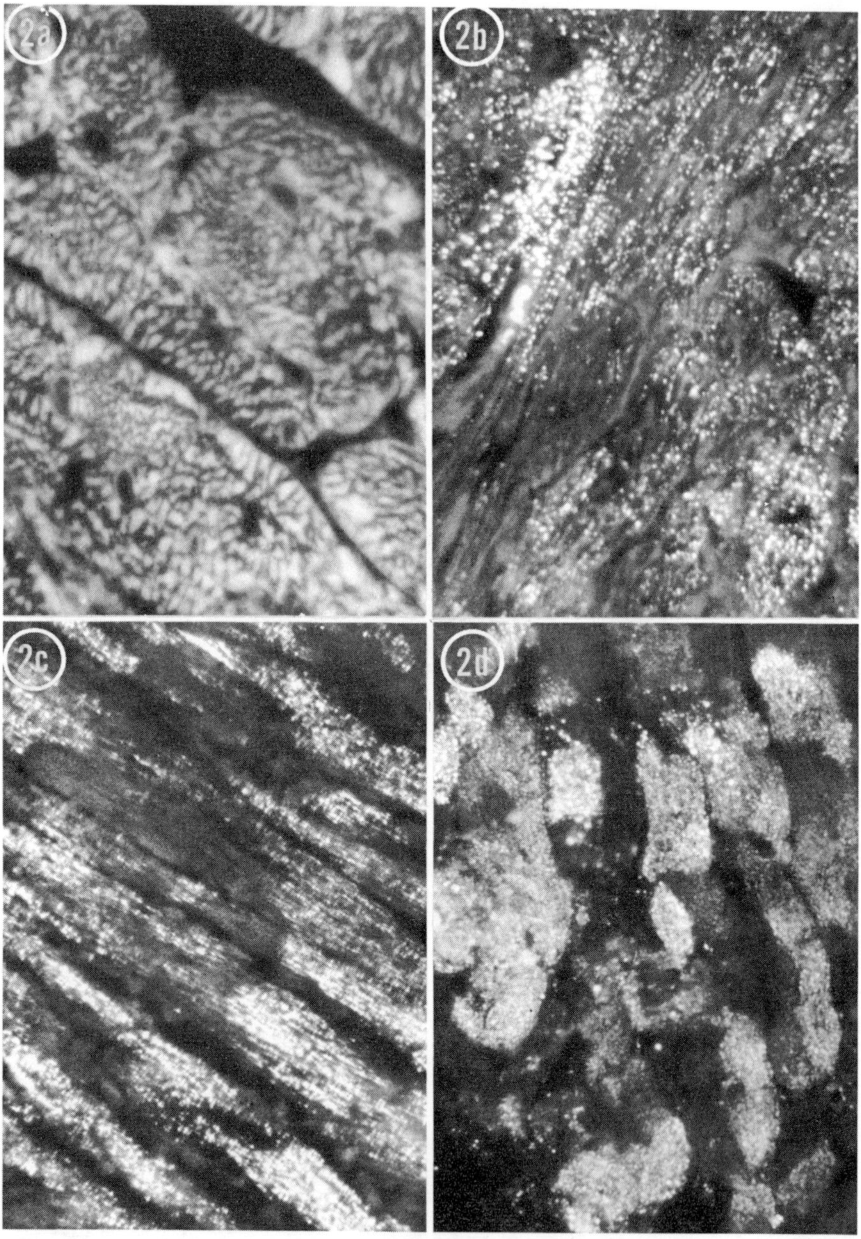

FIGURE 2. Preparations of normal and catecholamine-treated rat heart stained with benzpyrene for the fluorescence microscopy of lipids. (a) Normal heart. The normal pattern of interfibrillary fluorescence is seen in the muscle fibers. × 1,000. (b) 8 hours after isoproterenol. Numerous lipid droplets are present in the muscle cells. × 400. (c) 16 hours after isoproterenol. Fatty change is now more pronounced in many muscle fibers. × 200. (d) 20 hours after epinephrine. Marked fatty change is seen in area of muscle necrosis. × 300.

plasm, and intercalated discs of the cardiac muscle cells (FIGURE 2a). A similar fluorescence was seen in the cytoplasm of endothelial and connective tissue cells. Some muscle cells contained small numbers of minute, brightly fluorescent lipid droplets.

The pattern of lipid staining underwent similar alterations in all groups of experimental animals. An increase in the number of lipid droplets was evident, particularly in the subendocardial fibers, 30 minutes after injection. Fat continued to accumulate (FIGURE 2b and c) up to 24 hours, at which time most myocardial fibers were affected to some degree. In non-necrotic fibers, the fat deposition subsided after 24 hours, and by 72 hours, most of these fibers again contained normal amounts of lipid. In areas of necrosis (FIGURE 2d), the muscle cells contained numerous large lipid droplets that fluoresced intensely. The normal pattern of phospholipid fluorescence was lost from such cells. Isoproterenol resulted in the most pronounced and consistent alterations in all stages. The degree of fatty change produced by epinephrine was least marked.

Tetrazolium-Mediated Methods for Oxidative Enzymes

Tetrozolium-mediated methods for the detection of oxidative enzymes produce mitochondrial staining (FIGURE 3a). The activity of these enzymes in normal cardiac muscle can be graded on a scale of 0 to 4+: succinic dehydrogenase and NAD diaphorase, 4+; lactic and isocitric dehydrogenase, 3+; malic dehydrogenase, 2+, and β-hydroxybutyric and α-glycerophosphate dehydrogenase, 1+. Glutamic and ethanol dehydrogenases, which give weaker reactions, produce only faint homogeneous staining of the cytoplasm.

The sympathomimetic agents produced a biphasic change in the activity of all these enzymes: an initial diffuse increase, followed by a gradual decrease, and finally a complete loss of the activity in damaged muscle fibers. In each case, the degree of change was proportional to the normal level of activity of the enzyme involved.

The initial increase was discernible 30 minutes after injection of the drug and was characterized by the appearance of dark formazan deposits. After six to ten hours, the enzymatic activity began to return to normal in most areas, resulting in an irregular pattern of staining (FIGURE 3b and c). The enzymatic activity of damaged muscle fibers continued to decrease gradually (FIGURE 3c and d), and at 24 and 48 hours, the areas of necrosis were unreactive. The dense formazan deposits in partially necrotic fibers often formed clusters around lipid droplets. This pattern was not seen in fibers undergoing hyaline necrosis without fatty change. The severity of the preceding changes was proportional to the degree of myocardial necrosis.

Mononuclear inflammatory cells gave a relatively intense reaction for lactic dehydrogenase (FIGURE 3d and e), and many of the stellate-shaped histiocytes showed both coarsely granular and diffuse cytoplasmic staining. The activities of isocritric and malic dehydrogenases were less intense, and the reaction for succinic dehydrogenase (FIGURE 3f) was very faint.

Cytochrome Oxidase

The distribution of cytochrome oxidase in normal myocardium is similar to that of succinic dehydrogenase. The deposits formed by this reaction, however, are smaller and more granular than those observed with the tetrazolium methods. In contrast to the latter, no change was seen in cytochrome oxidase

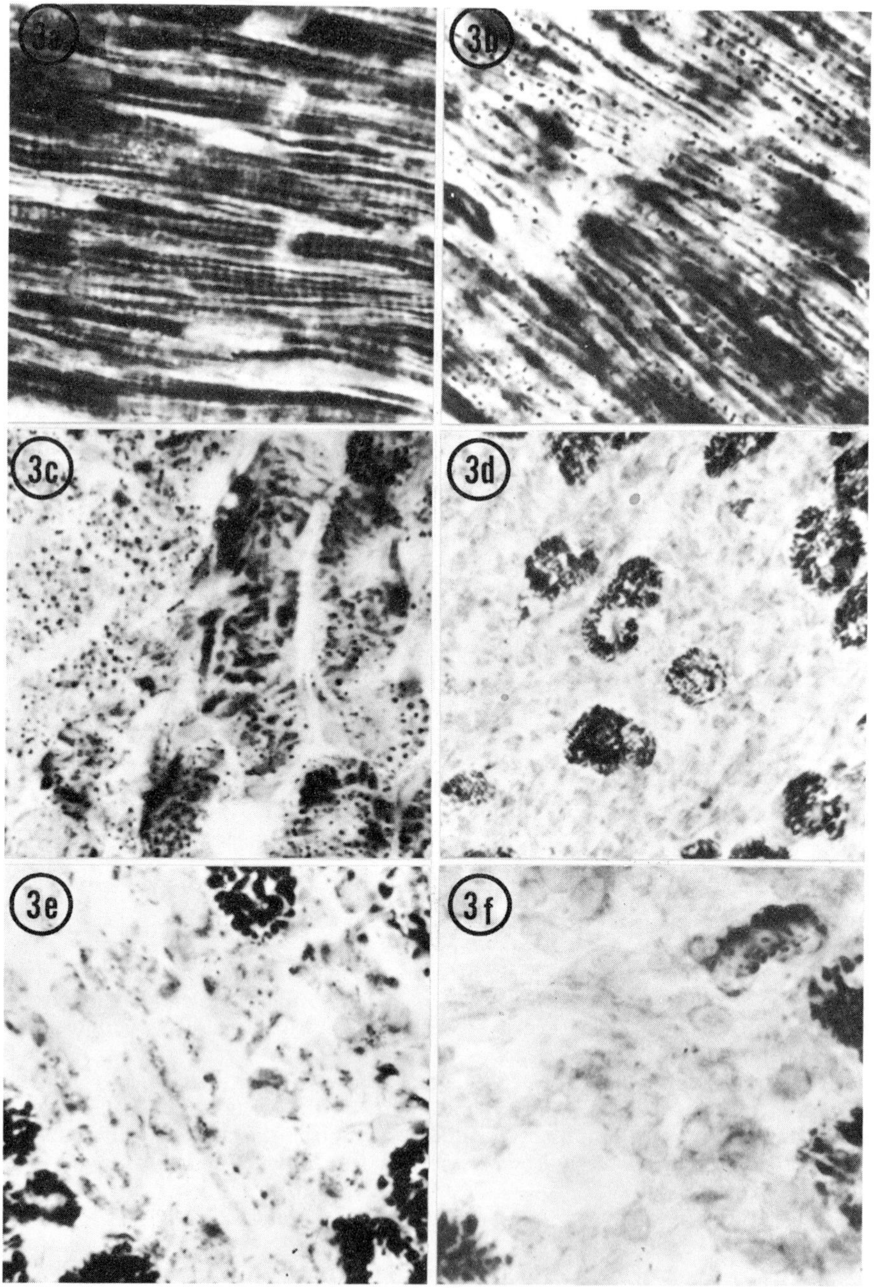

FIGURE 3. Stains for the demonstration of oxidative enzymes in the heart of normal and catecholamine-treated rats. (a) Normal heart. Succinic dehydrogenase. Enzymatic activity is localized in the mitochondria of the cardiac muscle cells. × 1,000. (b) 8 hours after

activity until myocardial necrosis began to develop. There was then a marked decrease in the intensity of the reaction. Cytochrome oxidase activity was low in the inflammatory cells.

Esterase

In normal rat myocardium, the α-naphthyl acetate-hexazotized *p*-rosaniline technique results in faint diffuse staining of the sarcoplasm. The lysosomes of the muscle fibers, usually very small in size and localized in the perinuclear area, show a weak but distinct reaction. The cytoplasm and lysosomes of the perivascular cells, i.e., pericytes, macrophages, histiocytes, and fibroblasts, react intensely (FIGURE 4a). Pretreatment of the sections with 0.01 M sodium fluoride abolishes the diffuse staining, thus permitting the selective demonstration of the esterase activity of the lysosomes (FIGURE 4b).

All three drugs caused a slight irregular increase in the cytoplasmic esterase activity of some of the injured muscle fibers. The perivascular cells, which often had an increased amount of cytoplasm, also showed increased cytoplasmic esterase activity. In addition, many of the inflammatory cells in areas of necrosis showed high esterase activity (FIGURE 4c), which made their differentiation from the perivascular cells difficult. Many of the inflammatory cells (FIGURE 4c, d, and e), particularly the elongated and stellate-shaped histiocytes, contained large amounts of cytoplasmic esterase. The more rounded macrophages contained primarily the lysosomal type of esterase (FIGURE 5a). Other cells, presumably transitional, showed both types of enzymatic activity. The stellate-shaped cells predominated in the earlier stages of inflammation, whereas the macrophages were most abundant in later stages.

Acid Phosphatase

In normal heart, acid phosphatase activity is restricted to the lysosomes of the muscle fibers and perivascular cells. In the muscle fibers, the reaction is faint and of limited value in the study of pathological changes. In the treated animals, a strong acid phosphatase reaction was seen in the inflammatory cells (FIGURE 5b), showing the same distribution as the lysosomal type of esterase.

Electron Microscopical Observations

Electron microscopical observations on the cardiac muscle cells showed quantitative changes in glycogen and lipids, as well as structural changes in the sarcoplasmic reticulum, mitochondria, and myofibrils. While these changes were of a similar nature in the three groups of animals, their severity and rate of progression were different in each group.

Glycogen

A marked reduction in the number of glycogen granules was apparent in all groups of animals during the first 24 hours after treatment (FIGURES 6–10), but was most marked in the epinephrine-treated group. After 24 hours, the

norepinephrine. Succinic dehydrogenase. Note the patchy character of the reaction and the dark dense formazan deposits. × 1,000. (c) 16 hours after norepinephrine. Lactic dehydrogenase. The reaction has returned to normal in some fibers; in others there is only a weak reaction. × 800. (d) 48 hours after norepinephrine. Lactic dehydrogenase. Numerous inflammatory cells are seen surrounding muscle fibers that show a normal reaction. × 200. (e) As in (d). Lactic dehydrogenase. The inflammatory cells show a moderately intense reaction. × 800. (f) As in (d) and (e). Succinic dehydrogenase. The reaction is very weak in the inflammatory cells. × 800.

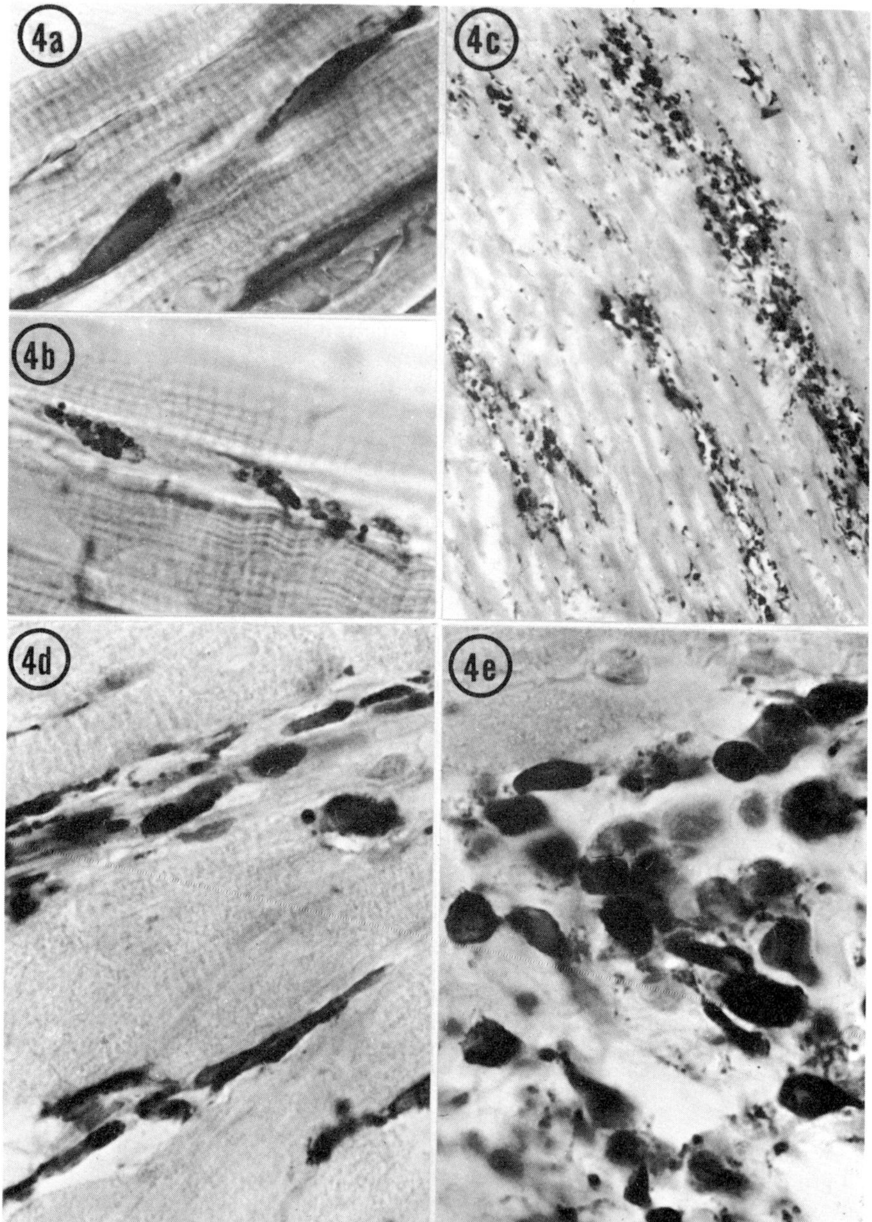

FIGURE 4. Exterase activity in the heart of normal and catecholamine-treated rats. (a) Normal heart. There is intense activity in the perivascular cells. × 1,000. (b) As in (a), after inhibition with 0.01 M sodium fluoride. Lysosomal staining is seen in the cytoplasm of a perivascular cell. × 1,000. (c) 24 hours after isoproterenol. Areas of inflammatory reaction show an intense reaction. × 100. (d) As in (c). Elongated and rounded esterase-positive cells are seen in an area of interstitial inflammatory reaction. × 1,000. (e) 48 hours after isoproterenol. Area of muscle necrosis with numerous esterase-positive macrophages. × 1,000.

number of glycogen granules began to return to normal in non-necrotic fibers. Necrotic fibers usually regained little or no glycogen.

Lipid Droplets

The presence of lipid droplets was observed as in the light microscopical preparations (FIGURES 9 and 10). The average diameter of droplets present in non-necrotic fibers was between 0.5 and 1.0 μ. A few droplets were enclosed by single-layered membranes; the remainder were free in the sarcoplasm, often in close proximity to the mitochondria.

Sarcoplasmic Reticulum

The ordinarily flattened vesicles of the sarcoplasmic reticulum were swollen in all stages subsequent to 30 minutes after treatment (FIGURE 8). In the isoproterenol-treated group, and, to a lesser extent, in the norepinephrine group, the swelling progressed gradually for the first 24 hours. In epinephrine-treated animals, swelling was less pronounced, except in areas of necrosis, where there was also extensive fragmentation and vesiculation of the sarcoplasmic reticulum.

Myofibrils

Alterations of the contractile elements were most pronounced in the isoproterenol-treated animals. A marked thickening of the lines was evident at 30 minutes (FIGURE 7). After six to 12 hours, the Z lines had become less osmiophilic in some areas, and the myofilaments and striations had become

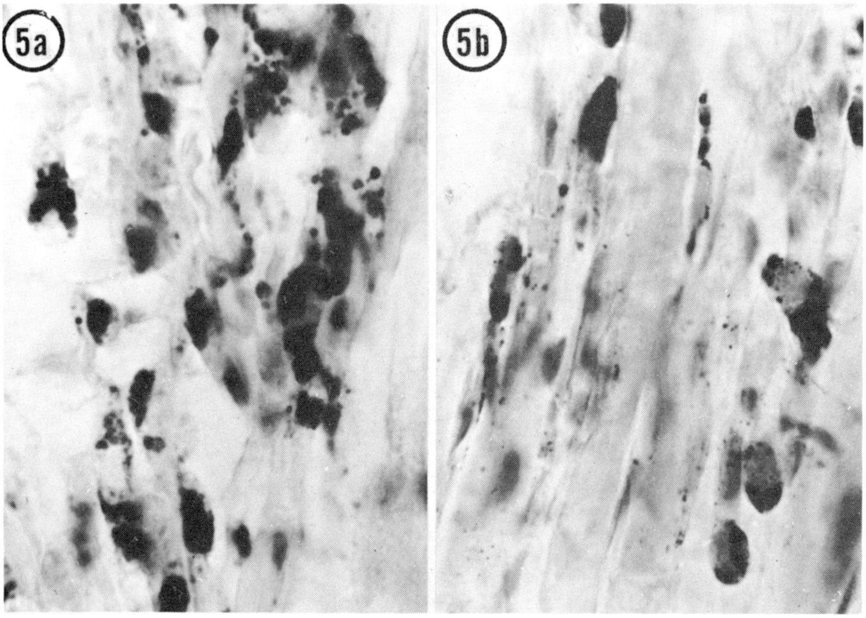

FIGURE 5. Lysosomal enzymes in the heart of catecholamine-treated rats. (a) 16 hours after norepinephrine. Esterase reaction after inhibition with 0.01 M sodium fluoride. Large numbers of lysosomes are seen in the cytoplasm of the inflammatory cells. × 1,000. (b) As in (a), but stained for acid phosphatase by a modified Gomori method. The pattern of staining is similar to that shown in (a). × 1,000.

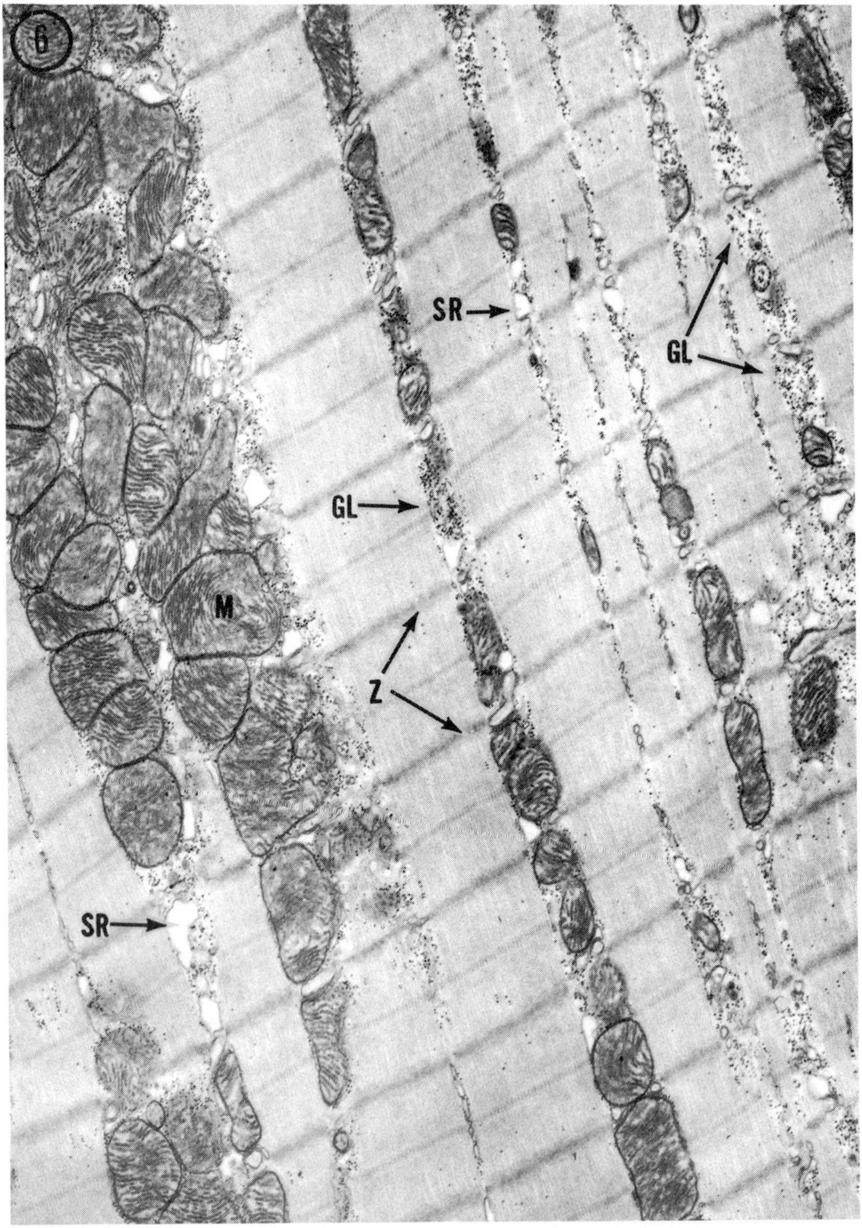

FIGURE 6. Electron micrograph of normal cardiac muscle cells. Note the abundant glycogen granules (GL) in the interfibrillary spaces, the closely packed cristae within the mitochondria (M), and the normal appearance of the sarcoplasmic reticulum (SR) and the Z lines (Z). × 11,000.

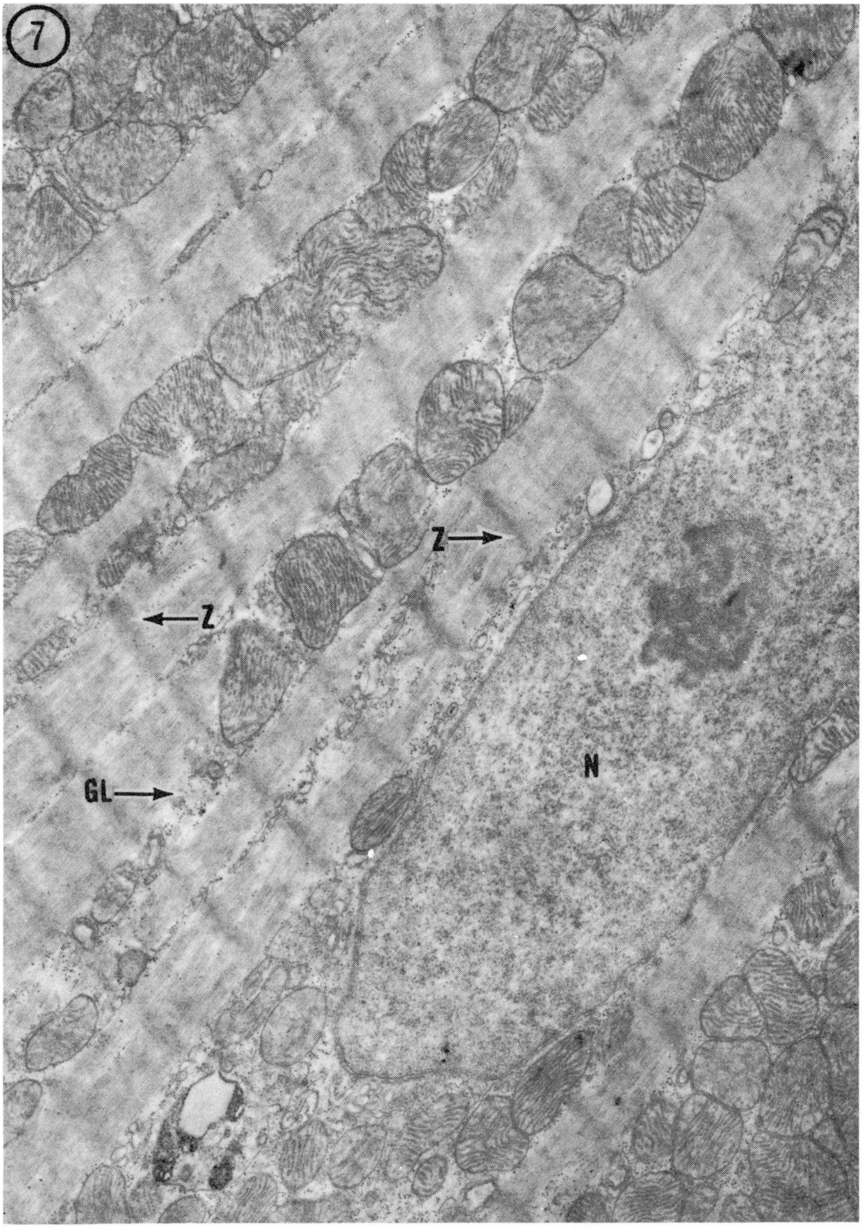

FIGURE 7. Electron micrograph of rat ventricular myocardium, 30 minutes after epinephrine. Thickening of the Z lines (Z) is evident in this longitudinal section of a muscle fiber. Glycogen granules (GL) are scarce. Other than these changes, the fiber is normal. N = nucleus. × 10,500.

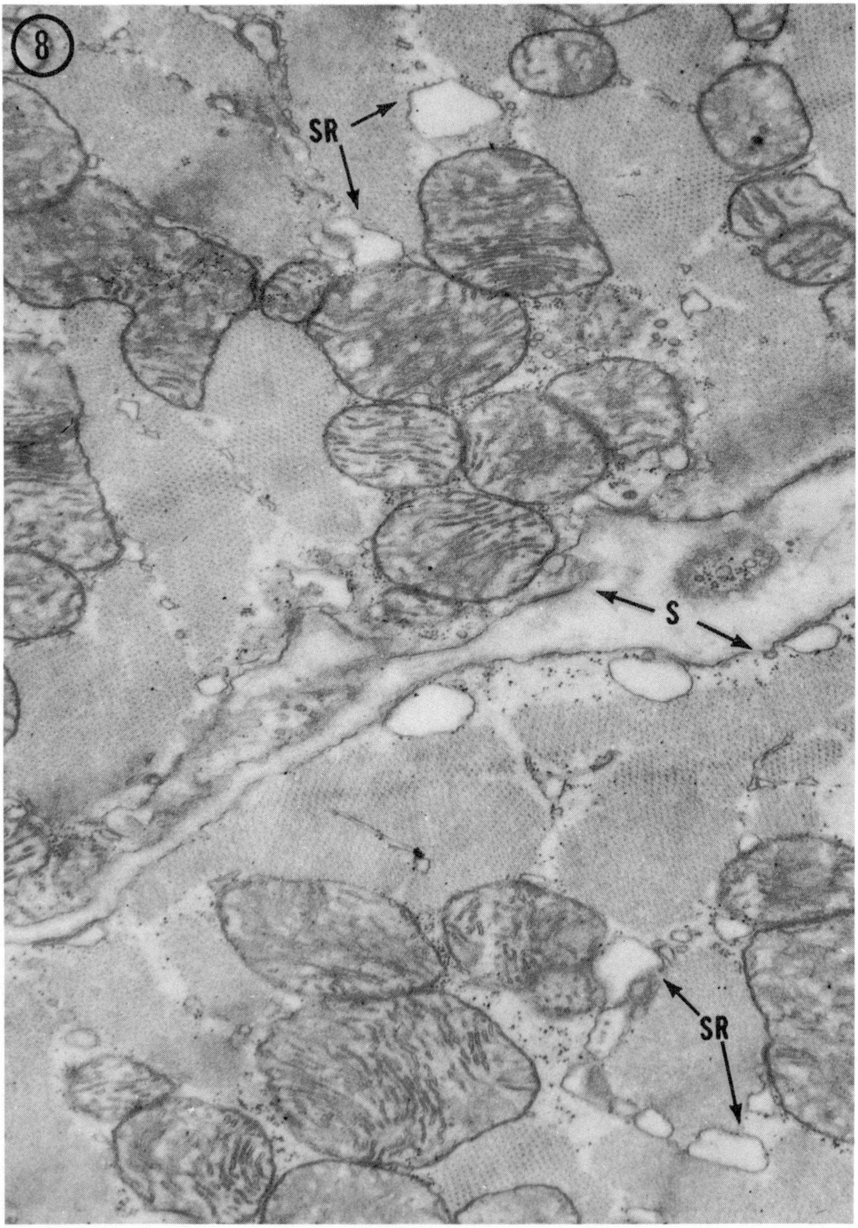

FIGURE 8. Electron micrograph of rat ventricular myocardium 30 minutes after epinephrine. Cross-sectional view of two adjacent muscle fibers. There is swelling of the sarcoplasmic reticulum (SR) and slight intracellular edema. S = sarcolemma. $\times$ 20,000.

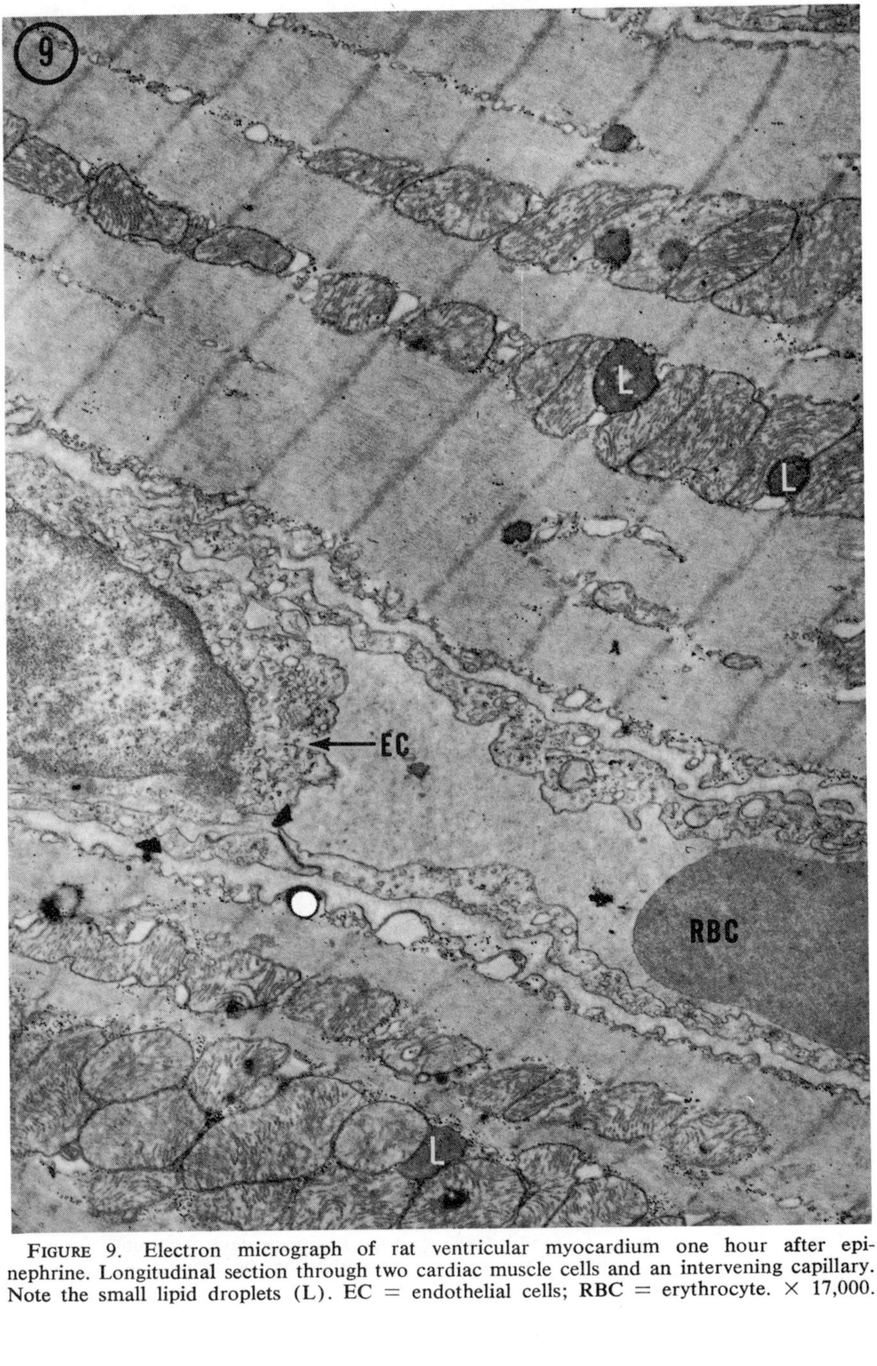

FIGURE 9. Electron micrograph of rat ventricular myocardium one hour after epinephrine. Longitudinal section through two cardiac muscle cells and an intervening capillary. Note the small lipid droplets (L). EC = endothelial cells; RBC = erythrocyte. × 17,000.

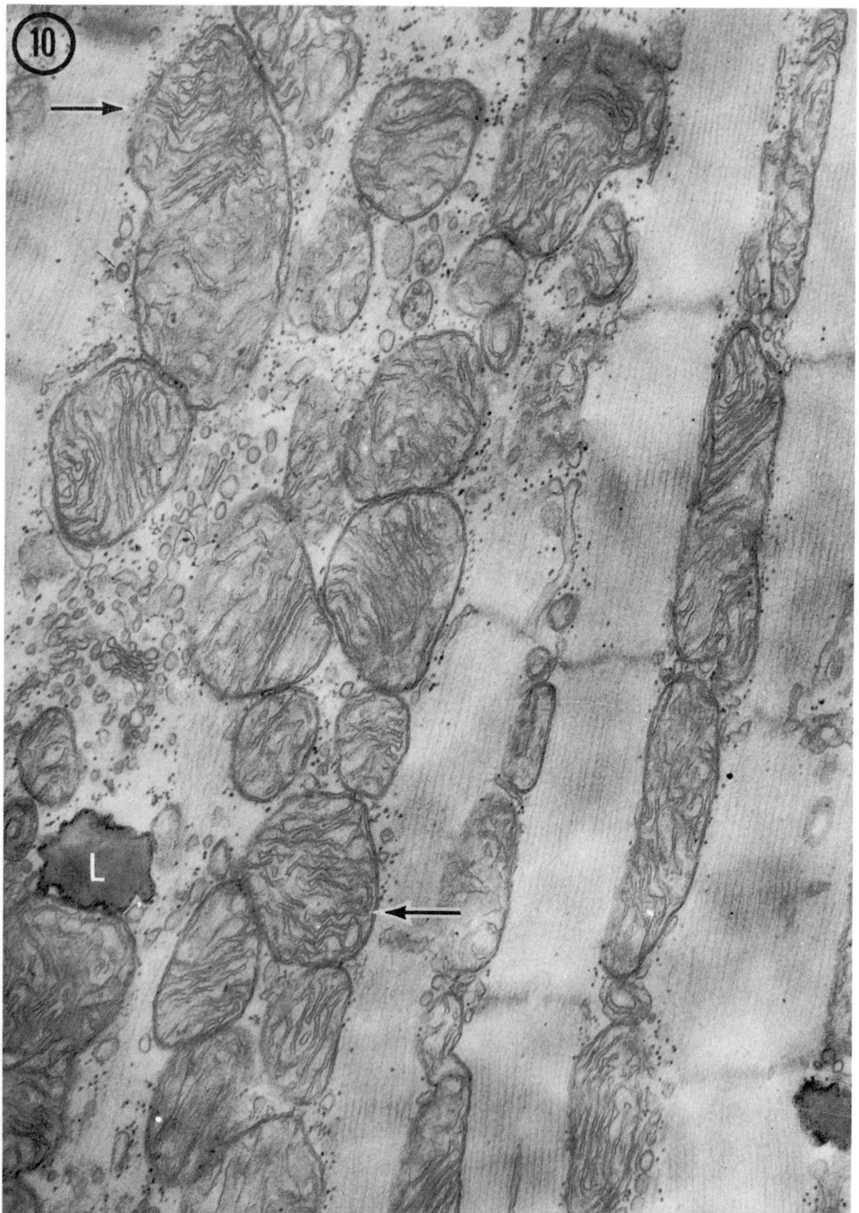

FIGURE 10. Electron micrograph of rat ventricular myocardium one hour after epinephrine. Longitudinal section of a myocardial fiber showing the peculiar zig-zag appearance of many of the mitochondrial cristae (arrows). L = lipid. × 32,000.

indistinct (FIGURES 11–14). The same changes occurred, but to a lesser degree, in the animals treated with epinephrine and norepinephrine.

Mitochondria

Mitochondrial swelling and loss of the cristae was observed in all three groups of animals; however, mitochondrial changes appeared earlier and were more pronounced in the isoproterenol group. In all three groups, the mitochondria of necrotic fibers were markedly damaged (FIGURE 12). It was not uncommon to find normal fibers adjacent to fibers with pronounced mitochondrial damage.

In addition to the alterations just described, a peculiar change was often found in the mitochondria of epinephrine-treated animals. During the first few hours after treatment, the mitochondrial cristae became closely packed, and their usually straight, parallel profiles developed angulations, so that they followed zig-zag courses across the mitochondria (FIGURE 10). In some fibers, this change persisted for 72 hours. This phenomenon did not occur in the isoproterenol-treatment animals, but was occasionally seen in those given norepinephrine.

Lysosomes

All animals sacrificed 24 or more hours after treatment showed an increase in the number of lysosomes in the cardiac muscle cells. This increase was observed throughout the myocardium, but was especially prominent in cells adjoining the necrotic areas. Although no attempt was made to quantitate these changes, it was obvious that the number of lysosomes was greatest in the later stages, particularly in the more severely damaged hearts.

Inflammatory Cells

As observed by light microscopy, the inflammatory cells varied greatly in size and morphology; most of them, however, were of two general types. The first was characterized by the abundance of rough-surfaced endoplasmic reticulum. The reticulum was often in the form of swollen vesicles, the contents of which was more osmiophilic than the surrounding cytoplasm (FIGURE 14). A well-developed Golgi apparatus was usually present in the perinuclear area. Many of these cells closely resembled plasma cells. The second type of cells, presumably macrophages, contained little rough-surfaced endoplasmic reticulum. The cytoplasm contained a few small, smooth-surfaced vesicles, granules of various sizes, a well-developed Golgi apparatus, and numerous lysosomes and residual bodies (FIGURE 14). Most of the cells of both types were closely associated with the capillaries. Other cells were also observed, some of which were intermediate in form between the two types just described; others had little in common with either type. Further studies of the morphology and function of these cells are now under way.

Discussion

The relationship between the known pharmacological properties of sympathominetic amines and their ability to induce cardiac necrosis remains unclear. It should be emphasized that these agents produce myocardial necrosis only when given in extremely large doses, far in excess of those used for clinical purposes. The comparative studies of Rosenblum and his colleagues[24] on the cardiovascular effects of lesion-producing doses of sympathomimetic

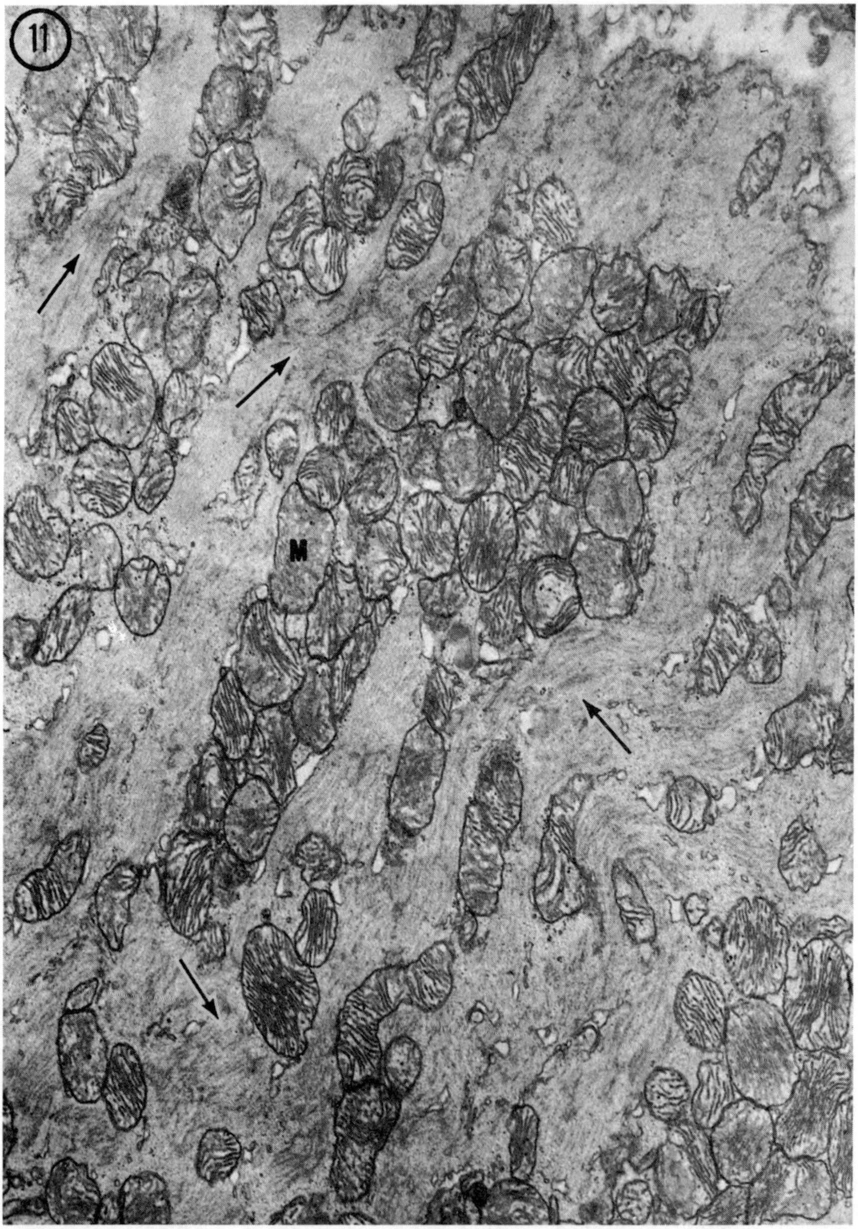

FIGURE 11. Electron micrograph of rat ventricular myocardium, 20 hours after epinephrine. Longitudinal section showing severe myofibrillar damage (arrows). The mitochondria (M) are less severely altered. × 15,000.

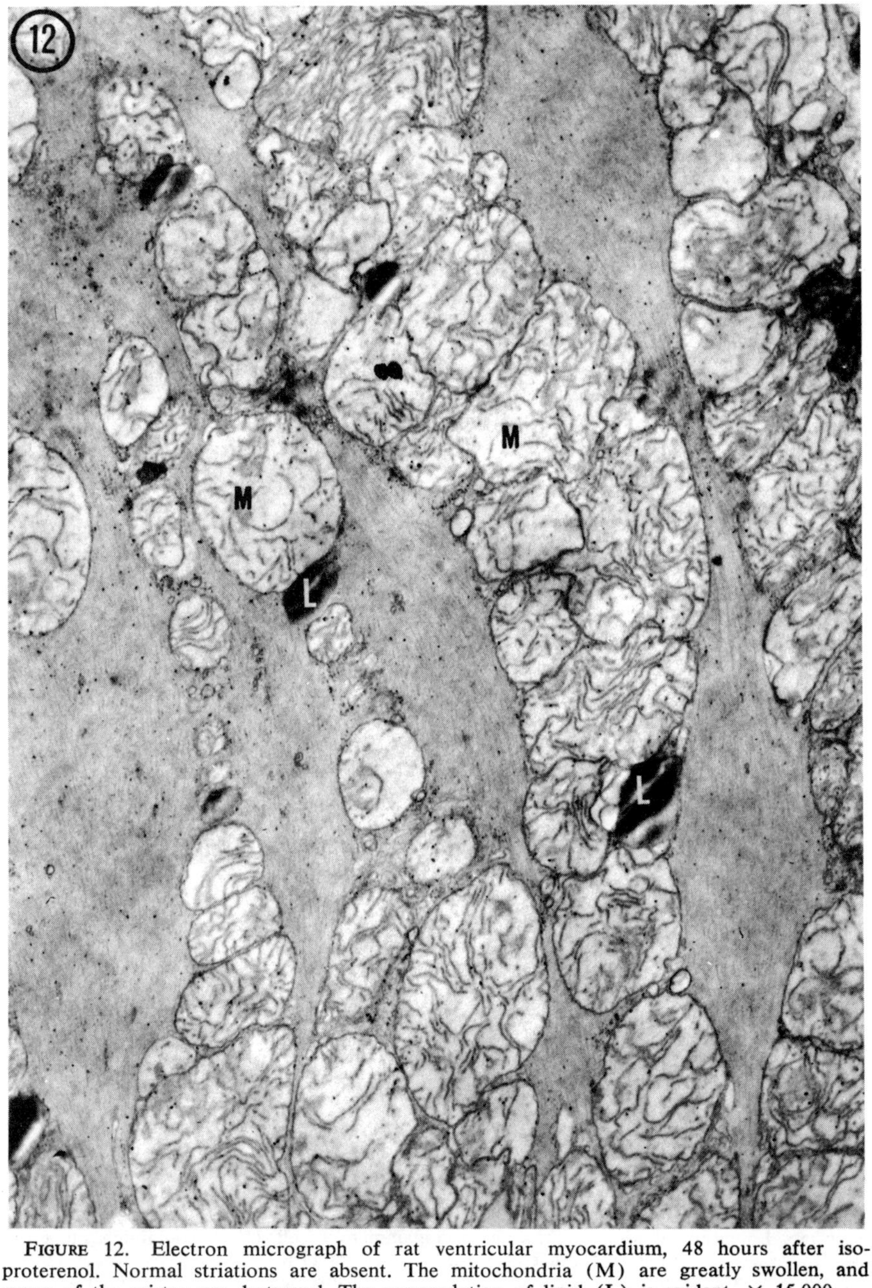

FIGURE 12. Electron micrograph of rat ventricular myocardium, 48 hours after isoproterenol. Normal striations are absent. The mitochondria (M) are greatly swollen, and many of the cristae are destroyed. The accumulation of lipid (L) is evident. × 15,000.

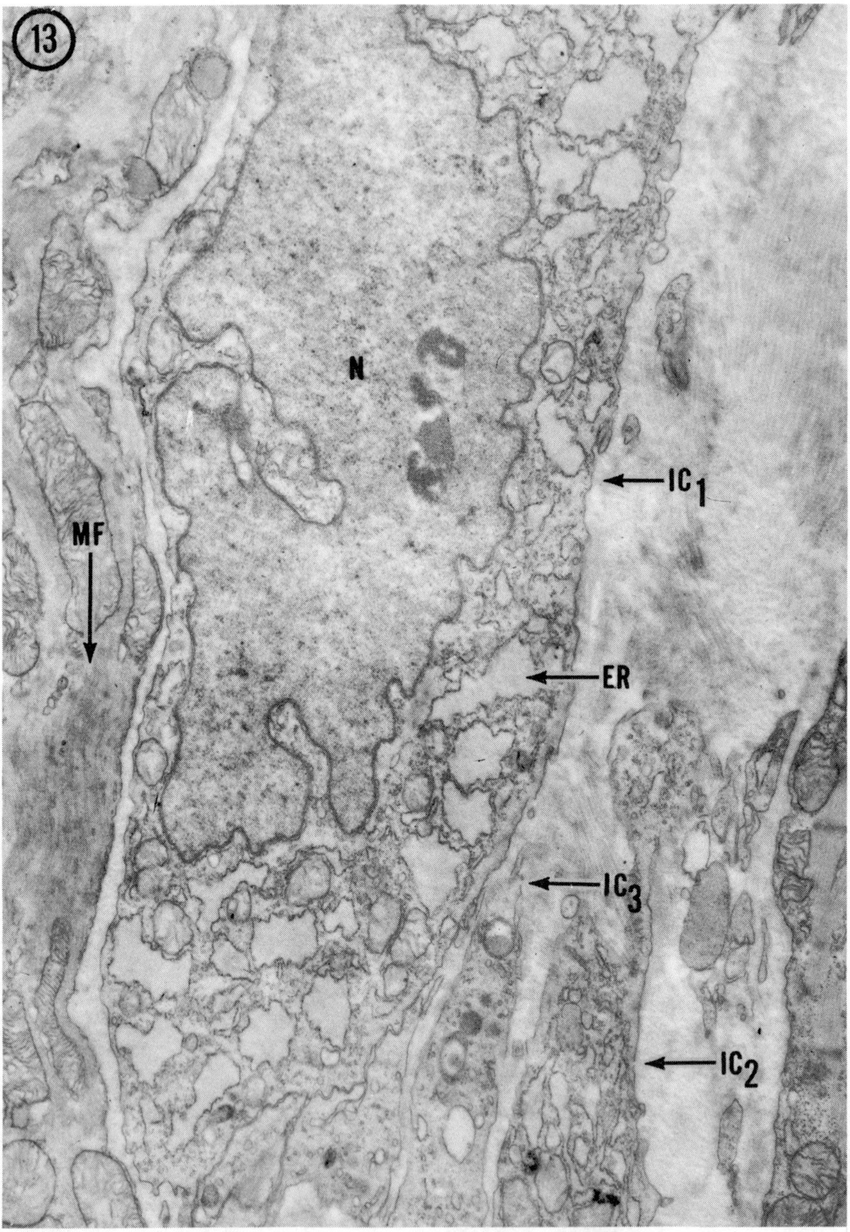

FIGURE 13. Electron micrograph of rat ventricular myocardium, 72 hours after epinephrine. Longitudinal section showing an inflammatory cell (IC_1) containing numerous swollen vesicles of rough-surfaced endoplasmic reticulum (ER). Parts of two other inflammatory cells are seen. One (IC_2) also contains rough-surfaced endoplasmic reticulum; the other (IC_3) has several lysosomes. Note the damaged myofilaments (MF) in the cardiac muscle cell on the left. N = nucleus. × 10,000.

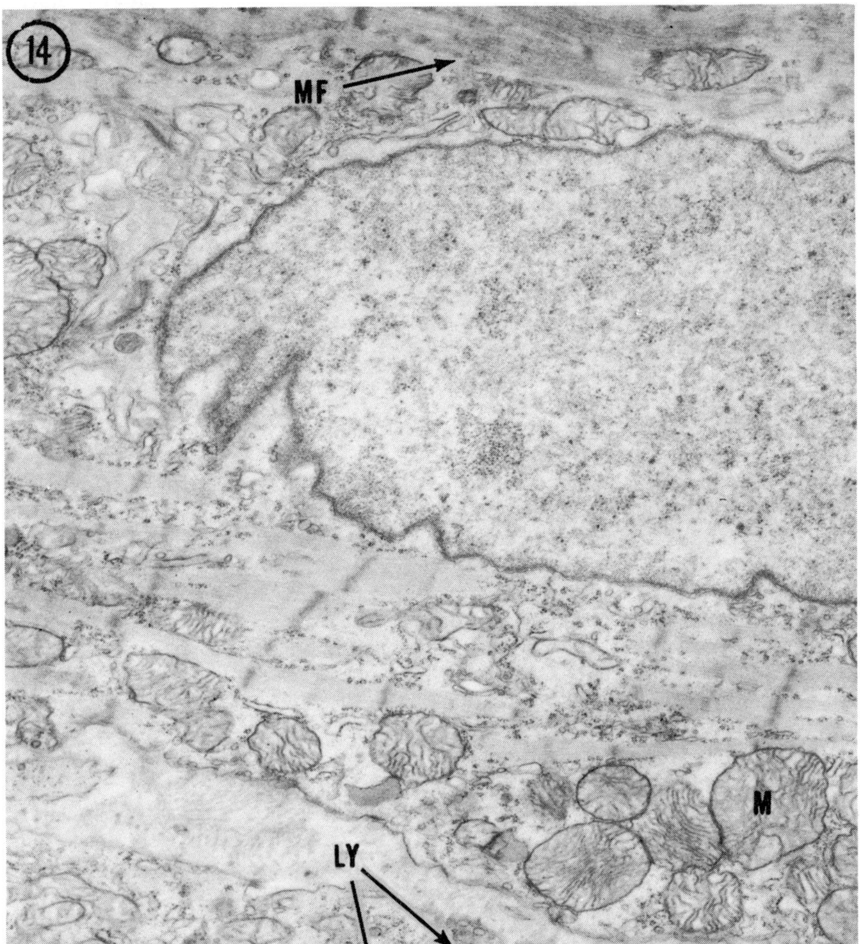

FIGURE 14. Electron micrograph of rat ventricular myocardium, 72 hours after epinephrine. Longitudinal section of a cardiac muscle cell with an adjacent inflammatory cell. Note the swelling of the mitochondria (M) and the damaged myofilaments (MF). The inflammatory cell contains numerous lysosomes (LY). × 11,000.

agents have led to the recognition of three types of pathogenetic mechanisms: metabolic changes, hemodynamic disturbances, and myogenic alterations related to a reduction in myocardial contractile force. This multiplicity of effects is also evident in the present studies. However, the complexity of the relationships between the inotropic and biochemical effects of catecholamines[25-29] and the relative hypoxia produced by overdoses of these agents[3, 8] makes it difficult to estimate their relative importance in the production of myocardial necrosis. Comparison of the results obtained in our three groups of experimental animals suggest that sympathomimetic amines may exert separate and distinct influences on the muscle fibers and on other cellular components of the heart.

Changes in the Muscle Fibers

Some of the metabolic effects of catecholamines on cardiac muscle were clearly demonstrated during the first few hours after injection. The three groups of animals showed loss of myocardial glycogen, accumulation of neutral lipid, increased evidence of oxidative metabolism, and focal hypoxic changes. The rapid depletion of glycogen appeared to be related to the known activation of phosphorylase by sympathomimetic agents.[30,31] Loss of glycogen has also been described in various types of myocardial injury,[8, 16] in which it is possibly mediated through the local release of catecholamines.[31]

Factors related to the accumulation of lipids in myocardial cells have been discussed in detail elsewhere.[8, 16] Biochemical studies suggest that the diffuse fatty change induced by catecholamines in the heart and other organs[32, 33] is primarily due to the increased lipid mobilization produced by these agents.[34, 35] The transport of lipids into myocardial cells may also be increased.[36] The relative hypoxia that results from overdoses of catecholamines[3, 8] plays an important role in the lipid accumulation and mitochondrial alterations seen in damaged muscle cells.[8]

Dense formazan deposits similar to those observed in this study have been described by Cox and co-workers[37] in ischemic myocardium at the periphery of areas of infarction and by Carlson and his associates[32] and by Maunsbach and Wirsén[33] in myocardium, kidney, and skeletal muscle of norepinephrine-treated dogs. The presence of these deposits has been considered evidence of increased mitochondrial oxidative activity; however, their presence may also have resulted from an increase in the permeability of mitochondria to tetrazolium salts. There is still some question as to the intramitochondrial localization of such deposits, and this problem is now the subject of an electron microscopical study in our laboratory.

After the initial increase, the activity of the oxidative enzymes returned to normal levels in most fibers. In others, however, this initial increase was followed by progressive loss of activity, with the development of changes similar to those seen in ischemia and infarction. Comparison with data available on various types of hypoxic injury[8, 10, 14, 16, 37-48] showed that the changes produced by catecholamines, including the swelling of the mitochondria and the sarcoplasmic reticulum, develop more slowly than those caused by temporary or permanent coronary occlusion.

The alterations of the mitochondria and contractile elements were similar to those observed by Sommers and Jennings[45] and by Herdson and co-workers[48] after restoration of blood flow to ischemic areas of dog myocardium. The myofibrillar alterations were also similar to those observed by Reichenbach and Benditt[49] in a variety of circumstances. Although their relationship to the changes in contractile force observed by Rosenblum and co-workers[24] is unknown, they are of particular interest because of their association with the deposition of a PAS-positive material in the muscle fibers. This material appears to be associated with plasma proteins that diffuse into damaged cardiac muscle cells.[50] It differs histochemically from the metachromatic substance that was present in areas of edema and inflammation, presumably in the altered ground substance of connective tissue.

The angular configurations of the mitochondrial cristae, seen primarily in epinephrine-treated animals, are of uncertain significance. They are similar to the mitochondrial cristae normally seen in other cell types[51] and in the heart muscle of the canary.[52] Such alterations result in an increased surface area of the cristae, which in turn may enable the mitochondria to cope better with increased metabolic demands by providing a larger reaction area. This change may be responsible for the relative mildness of the myocardial lesions seen in the epinephrine experiments.

The increased numbers of lysosomes and related cytoplasmic components seen in the cardiac muscle after the administration of catecholamines are considered to represent a nonspecific response to cellular injury. These observations have been discussed in detail elsewhere.[53]

Changes in the Inflammatory Cells

Our histochemical data on the cellular components of the inflammatory reaction show the same changes seen by Hecht[54] in his studies of myocardial infarction. Our studies also indicate that the severity of the inflammatory response is not always directly related to the degree of myocardial necrosis. This conclusion is supported by the data of Rosenblum and his colleagues,[6] and Rona and co-workers.[3] Rosenblum and his colleagues found that, with the exception of isoproterenol, which induced severe myocardial necrosis, a variety of sympathomimetic agents caused primarily interstitial myocarditis. Rona and co-workers[3] observed swelling, increased cytoplasmic basophilia, and proliferation of fibroblasts in the hearts of isoproterenol-treated rats; these changes occurred independently of myocardial necrosis, particularly when low doses of the drug were used. The present studies confirm these observations. In addition, we have found that, after administration of sympathomimetic amines, many of the interstitial cells of the rat heart (fibroblasts, histiocytes, and pericytes) acquire increased amounts of esterase, lactic dehydrogenase, and rough-surfaced endoplasmic reticulum. This suggests that some of these changes may represent a direct cellular response to the drugs. The effects of sympathomimetic agents on cell growth and proliferation have received little attention. However, isoproterenol produces considerable proliferation of the acinar cells of the rat submaxillary gland, presumably through a direct effect,[55] and the possibility that the interstitial cells of the rat heart may show a similar response to catecholamines is now under study.

Summary

Histochemical and electron microscopical studies were made on the heart of rats treated with large doses of isoproterenol, epinephrine, and norepinephrine. Some of the changes observed were similar to those produced by ischemia; others are attributed to the metabolic effects of these agents on cardiac muscle, and some may be caused by actions of these drugs on cellular growth and proliferation.

References

1. VISHNEVSKAYA, O. P. 1956. Reflex mechanisms in the pathogenesis of adrenaline myocarditis. Biull. Eksp. Biol. Med. **41**: 307–310.
2. SZAKÁCS, J. E. & A. CANNON. 1958 1-Norepinephrine myocarditis. Amer. J. Clin. Path. **30**: 425–430.
3. RONA, G., C. I. CHAPPEL, T. BALAZS & R. GAUDRY. 1959. An infarct-like myocardial lesion and other toxic manifestations produced by isoproterenol in the rat. Arch. Path. (Chicago) **67**: 443–455.
4. CHAPPEL, C. I., G. RONA, T. BALAZS & R. GAUDRY. 1959. Comparison of cardiotoxic actions of certain sympathomimetic amines. Canad. J. Biochem. Physiol. **37**: 35–42.
5. SZAKÁCS, J. E., R. M. DIMMETTE & E. C. COWART. 1959. Pathologic implication of the catecholamines, epinephrine and norepinephrine. U. S. Armed Forces Med. J. **10**: 908–925.
6. ROSENBLUM, I., A. WOHL & A. A. STEIN. 1965. Studies in cardiac necrosis. I. Production of cardiac lesions with sympathomimetic agents. Toxic. Appl. Pharmacol. **7**: 1–8.
7. VAN VLIET, P. D., H. B. BURCHELL & J. L. TITUS. 1966. Myocarditis and pheochromocytoma. New Eng. J. Med. **274**: 1102–1108.
8. FERRANS, V. J., R. G. HIBBS, W. C. BLACK & D. G. WEILBAECHER. 1964. Isoproterenol-induced myocardial necrosis: a histochemical and electron microscopic study. Amer. Heart J. **68**: 71–90.
9. CLEMENTI, F., J. NIDIRI & C. PERACCHIA. 1964. Electron microscopic study of myocardial cells in relation to different types of myocardial infarct-like lesions. Panminerva Med. **6**: 420–428.
10. BAJUSZ, E. & G. JASMIN. 1965. Observations on histochemical differential diagnosis between primary and secondary cardiomyopathies. Behavior of monoamine oxidase, phosphorylase and glycogen in heart muscle. Amer. Heart J. **69**: 83–92.
11. KORB, G. 1965. Elektronenmikroskopische Untersuchungen zur Aludrin (Isoproterenolsulfat)-Schädigung des Herzmuskels. Virchow. Arch. Path. Anat. **339**: 136–150.
12. HAUSAMEN, T. U. & R. POCHE. 1965. Elektronenmikroskopische Untersuchungen über die Wirkung von Alupent auf die Ultrastruktur des Herzmuskels der Ratte. Virchow. Arch. Path. Anat. **339**: 225–233.
13. RAAB, W. & E. BAJUSZ. 1965. Epinephrine-induced, early prenecrotic disturbances of myocardial potassium, glycogen, and phosphorylase. Circulation **32**: (Suppl. II): 174.
14. FERRANS, V. J., R. G. HIBBS, H. S. WEILY, D. G. WEILBAECHER, J. J. WALSH & G. E. BURCH. A histochemical and electron microscopic study of epinephrine-induced myocardial necrosis. In preparation.
15. SPICER, S. S. 1965. Diamine methods for differentiating mucosubstances histochemically. J. Histochem. Cytochem. **13**: 211–234.
16. FERRANS, V. J., R. G. HIBBS, D. G. WEILBAECHER, W. C. BLACK, J. J. WALSH & G. E. BURCH. 1965. Alcoholic cardiomyopathy. A histochemical study. Amer. Heart J. **69**: 748–765.
17. BURSTONE, M. S. 1961. Modifications of histochemical techniques for the demonstration of cytochrome oxidase. J. Histochem. Cytochem. **9**: 59–68.
18. BARKA, T. & P. J. ANDERSON. 1963. Histochemistry. Theory, Practice and Bibliography. : 257–277. Hoeber. New York, N. Y.
19. HEGAB, E. S. & V. J. FERRANS. 1966. A histochemical study of the esterases of the rat heart. Amer. J. Anat. **119**: 235–262.
20. GOMORI, G. 1952. Microscopic Histochemistry. University of Chicago Press. Chicago, Ill.
21. BURSTONE, M. S. 1962. Enzyme Histochemistry and its Application to the Study of Neoplasms. : 276–277. Academic Press, Inc. New York, N. Y.
22. FREEMAN, J. & B. SPURLOCK. 1962. A new epoxy embedment for electron microscopy. J. Cell Biol. **13**: 437–443.
23. YOKOYAMA, H. O., R. B. JENNINGS, G. F. CLABAUGH & W. B. WARTMAN. 1955. Histochemical studies of early experimental myocardial infarction. Periodic acid-Schiff method. Arch. Path. (Chicago) **59**: 347–354.
24. ROSENBLUM, I., A. WOHL & A. A. STEIN. 1965. Studies in cardiac necrosis. II. Cardiovascular effects of sympathomimetic amines producing cardiac lesions. Toxic. Appl. Pharmacol. **7**: 9–17.

25. Ellis, S. 1959. Relation of biochemical effects of epinephrine to its muscular effects. Pharmacol. Rev. **11:** 469–479.
26. Weissler, A. M., F. A. Kruger & J. K. Gallimore. 1963. Ventricular performance and epinephrine response in the glycogen-depleted heart. Circulation **28:** 824.
27. Winterscheid, L. C., R. A. Bruce, J. B. Blumberg & K. A. Merendino. 1963. Effect of isoproterenol on carbohydrate metabolism of isolated canine heart. Circ. Res. **12:** 76–84.
28. Drummond, G. I., Valladares, J. R. E. & L. Duncan. 1964. Effect of epinephrine on contractile tension and phosphorylase activation in rat and dog hearts. Proc. Soc. Exp. Biol. Med. **117:** 307–309.
29. Williamson, J. R. 1964. Metabolic effects of epinephrine in the isolated, perfused rat heart. I. Dissociation of the glycogenolytic from the metabolic stimulatory effect. J. Biol. Chem. **239:** 2721–2729.
30. Haugaard, N. & M. E. Hess. 1965. Action of autonomic drugs on phosphorylase activity and function. Pharmacol. Rev. **17:** 27–69.
31. Haugaard, N. & M. E. Hess. 1966. The influence of catecholamines on cardiac function and phosphorylase activity. Pharmacol. Rev. **18:** 197–204.
32. Carlson, L. A., S. O. Liljedahl & C. Wirsén. 1965. Acta Med. Scand. **178:** 81–102.
33. Maunsbach, A. B. & C. Wirsén. 1966. Ultrastructural changes in kidney, myocardium and skeletal muscle of the dog during excessive mobilization of free fatty acids. J. Ultrastruct. Res. **16:** 35–54.
34. Bogdonoff, M. D., J. W. Luiharts, R. J. Klein & E. H. Estes, Jr. 1961. The specific structure of compounds effecting fat mobilization in man. J. Clin. Invest. **40:** 1993–1996.
35. Mueller, P. S. & D. Horwitz. 1962. Plasma free fatty acid and blood glucose responses to analogues of norepinephrine in man. J. Lipid Res. **3:** 251–255.
36. Regan, T. J. 1963. Vasopressin, catecholamines and serotonin as possible causes of myocardial ischemia. *In* The Etiology of Myocardial Infarction. T. N. James & J. W. Keyes, Ed. : 375–387. Little, Brown & Co. Boston, Mass.
37. Cox, J. L., V. W. McLaughlin, N. C. Flowers & L. G. Horan. 1966. Changes in cellular dehydrogenase enzymes in acute myocardial infarction. Circulation **34** (Suppl. III): 80.
38. Wachstein, M. & E. Meisel. 1955. Succinic dehydrogenase activity in myocardial infarction and induced myocardial necrosis. Amer. J. Path. **31:** 353–365.
39. Bryant, R. E., W. A. Thomas & R. M. O'Neal. 1958. An electron microscopic study of myocardial ischemia in the rat. Circ. Res. **6:** 699–709.
40. Caulfield, J. & B. Klionsky. 1959. Myocardial ischemia and early infarction: an electron microscopic study. Amer. J. Path. **35:** 489–523.
41. Hölscher, B., O. H. Just & H. J. Merker. 1961. Studies by electron microscope on various forms of induced cardiac arrest in dog and rabbit. Surgery **49:** 492–499.
42. Hecht, A., G. Korb & H. David. 1961. Vergleichende histochemische, fluorescenzmikroskopische und elektronenoptische Untersuchungen zur Frühdiagnose des Herzinfarktes der Ratte. Virchow. Arch. Path. Anat. **334:** 267–284.
43. Shnitka, T. K. & M. M. Nachlas. 1963. Histochemical alterations in ischemic heart muscle and early myocardial infarction. Amer. J. Path. **42:** 507–527.
44. Poche, R. & H. G. Ohm. 1963. Lichtmikroskopische, histochemische und elektronenmikroskopische Untersuchungen des Herzmuskels vom Menschen nach induziertem Herzstillstand. Arch. Kreislaufforsch. **41:** 86–135.
45. Sommers, H. M. & R. B. Jennings. 1964. Experimental acute myocardial infarction. Histologic and histochemical studies of early myocardial infarcts induced by temporary or permanent occlusion of a coronary artery. Lab. Invest. **13:** 1491–1503.
46. Hecht, A. 1964. Fermenthistochemische Frühveränderungen beim experimentellen Herzinfarkt. Virchow. Arch. Path. Anat. **337:** 414–424.
47. Hibbs, R. G., V. J. Ferrans, W. C. Black, D. G. Weilbaecher, J. J. Walsh & G. E. Burch. 1965. Alcoholic cardiomyopathy. An electron microscopic study. Amer. Heart J. **69:** 766–779.
48. Herdson, P. B., H. M. Sommers & R. B. Jennings. 1965. A comparative study of the fine structure of normal and ischemic dog myocardium with special reference to early changes following temporary occlusion of a coronary artery. Amer. J. Path. **46:** 367–386.
49. Reichenbach, D. & E. P. Benditt. 1966. Myofibrillar degeneration. A new category of myocardial cellular reaction of injury. Amer. J. Path. **48:** 32a.

50. Kent, S. P. 1966. Intracellular plasma proteins : a manifestation of cell injury in experimentally produced myocardial ischemia in the dog. Amer. J. Path. **48:** 31a.
51. Revel, J. P., D. W. Fawcett & C. W. Philpott. 1963. Observations on mitochondrial structure. Angular configurations of the cristae. J. Cell Biol. **16:** 187–195.
52. Slautterback, D. B. 1965. Mitochondria in cardiac muscle cells of the canary and other birds. J. Cell Biol. **24:** 1–22.
53. Hibbs, R. G., V. J. Ferrans, J. J. Walsh & G. E. Burch. 1965. Electron microscopic observations on lyosomes and related cytoplasmic components of normal and pathological cardiac muscle. Anat. Rec. **153:** 173–186.
54. Hecht, A. 1964. Fermenthistochemische Befunde am Granulationsgewebe des experimentellen Herzinfarkts. Virchow. Arch. Path. Anat. **338:** 5–15.
55. Barka, T. 1966. A model of induced cell proliferation: the effect of isoproterenol on salivary glands. J. Cell Biol. **31:** 9A.

FACTORS INFLUENCING THE PRODUCTION OF CARDIOMYOPATHIES BY METHOXAMINE AND METARAMINOL*

G. Jasmin†

Department of Pathology, University of Montreal
Montreal, Canada

The diversity of tissue response to pharmacologically related vasoactive substances is a peculiar phenomenon that has attracted my attention ever since my colleagues and I began a study of the toxic effects of synthetic or naturally occurring amines.[1-4] Whereas some pharmacological properties are evidenced through *in vitro* assays on isolated tissue or organ preparations, the evaluation of morphological effects can only be achieved by *in vivo* studies.

Most sympathomimetic amines, when injected at a sufficiently high dose, cause ischemic lesions whose severity and distribution vary with the animal species, age, sex, dietary conditions, and hormonal state.[5-7] The differences in the nature and location of the degenerative changes are particularly evident after prolonged administration of maximally tolerable doses in laboratory animals.

Previous studies carried out in rats on the production of experimental cardiopathies with two potent vasopressors, methoxamine and metaraminol, served to strengthen my belief that the anoxic tissue changes elicited by certain adrenergic drugs are largely attributable to circulatory failure.[8] The experimental animals invariably exhibit signs of shock, with extreme renal and pulmonary congestion and a drop in the systemic blood pressure, an account of which is outlined under "Observations." The similarity of these histopathological changes with those arising from partial ligature of the heart, kidney, and pulmonary efferent vessels is most striking.[9] Isoproterenol-induced heart lesions, on the other hand, markedly differ from those elicited by methoxamine and metaraminol.

With the object of further elucidating the pathogenesis of heart lesions produced by sympathomimetic amines, the influence of certain conditioning factors and some adrenergic blocking agents was studied in a comparative manner in isoproterenol-, metaraminol-, and methoxamine-treated rats.

Methods

The investigations reported here were carried out in female Sprague-Dawley rats averaging 135 g in body weight. The vasoactive substances were injected subcutaneously, twice daily, at doses varying between 2 and 3 mg/100 g of body weight, for two or more days. Other data pertaining to dosage and duration of treatment are given in TABLES 1–3. Blood pressure determinations were made by inserting, into the common carotid artery, a polyethylene or metal cannula filled with heparin in saline and connected to a mercury manometer. All determinations were performed under ether anesthesia. The procedure followed for the coronary ligature and the forced restraint was similar to that previously described by Selye.[10] Histological studies were carried out with the same methods and reading criteria reported previously.[6]

* These investigations were supported by a grant from the Medical Research Council of Canada.

† Research associate of the Medical Research Council of Canada.

Observations

At the doses utilized, there were no clinical signs of intolerance in isoproterenol-treated rats throughout the experiments; methoxamine and metaraminol, on the other hand, caused respiratory distress and cyanosis, especially during the hours following the first injection, which proved to be most critical for survival. FIGURE 1 illustrates the sharp drop in blood pressure after isoproterenol administration and the tendency to return to a normal level after three hours; following methoxamine, there is a transient rise with a progressive fall toward low values, which remain unchanged for up to 24 hours. When the treatment is repeated, however, the tolerance to both methoxamine and metaraminol markedly improves, and the dosage can be progressively raised up to 19 mg, which approximates six times the acute lethal dose.

The comparative effects of vasoactive drugs given to rats for periods of two to 14 days are outlined in TABLE 1. The heart lesions produced by isoproterenol were constant and severe; they were easily detectable by gross examination and were usually located in the apical region. Histologically, the affected myocardial fibers had a hyaline appearance and were surrounded by granulation tissue; areas of fibrosis developed from healing of the inflammatory lesion (FIGURE 2A). Methoxamine- and metaraminol-induced cardiopathies were less conspicuous; the regressive changes consisted of a hydropic vacuolar degeneration of isolated muscle fibers, with subsequent disintegration of the sarcoplasm and of the myofibrils. Residual myotubes eventually collapsed with little or no connective tissue scarring (FIGURES 2B and C).

Kidney changes occurred in both methoxamine- and metaraminol-treated rats, but very seldom in animals receiving isoproterenol. The infarcted areas were well delineated from the renal parenchyma and usually involved the corticomedullary region with some encroachment of the renal cortex or the papilla. The degenerative process was more characteristic of venous occlusion, with

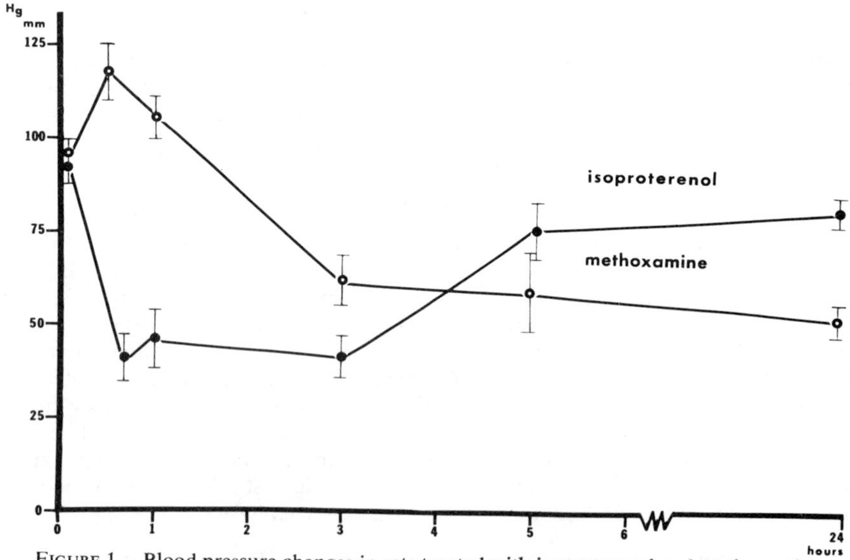

FIGURE 1. Blood pressure changes in rats treated with isoproterenol and methoxamine.

TABLE 1

COMPARATIVE ACTION OF VASOACTIVE DRUGS GIVEN TO RATS AT HIGH DOSAGE

Drug*	Tissue Changes					Cardiovascular Dynamics†			
	Kidney	Heart	Aorta	Lung	Other	Arterial Pressure	Venous Pressure	Venous Return	Inotropic Action
Isoproterenol (3 mg, twice daily)	Transient ischemia	Extensive necrosis	Dilation and occasional aneurysm	Congestion	Hypertrophy of submaxillary glands	↓	0	↑	+++
Metaraminol (3 mg, twice daily)	Tubular necrosis	Focal myolysis	Dilation and occasional aneurysm	Congestion and edema	—	↓	↑	0	+
Methoxamine (3 mg, twice daily)	Tubular and occasional glomerular necrosis	Extensive myolysis	Dissecting aneurysm	Multiple infarcts	Skeletal and visceral muscle degeneration	↓	↑	↓	0

* Injected subcutaneously for periods of two to 14 days.

† ↓ = decrease; ↑ = increase; 0 = no effect; + = mild effect; +++ = marked effect.

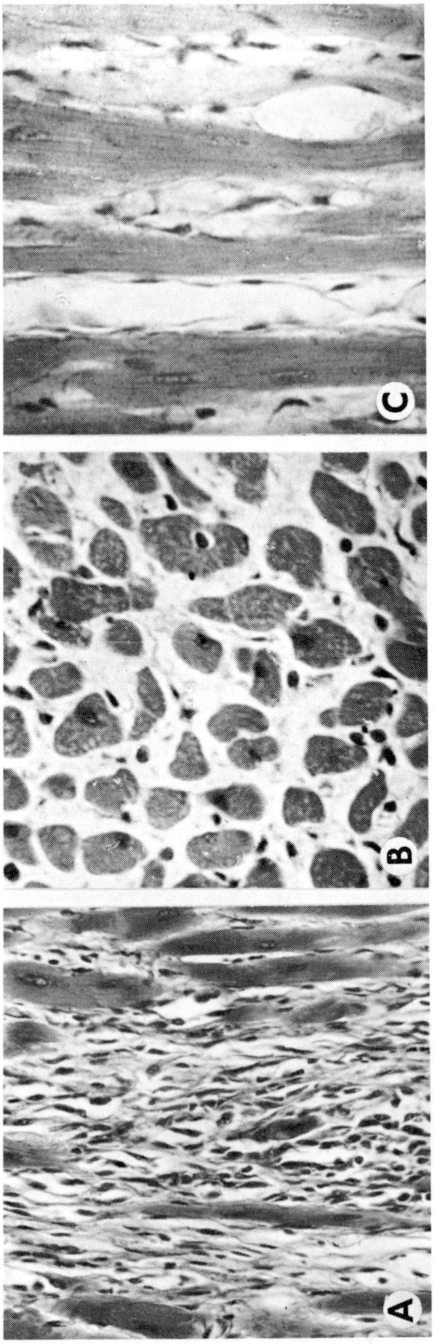

FIGURE 2. Myocardial degenerative changes induced by different vasoactive drugs injected into rats for eight consecutive days. (A) Following isoproterenol, the degenerative process leads to connective tissue proliferation with a cellular infiltrate. (B) Following metaraminol, the myofibers, shown here in cross-section, are surrounded by edema fluid with no stromal reaction. (C) Following methoxamine, the alterations, which are shown here at a more advanced stage than in A and B, consist of a complete dissolution of fibers, with residual emptied endomysium and absence of inflammatory cells: Stain: hematoxylin-phloxine-saffron. × 320 (orig. mag. × 400).

early involvement of epithelial cells of the nephron and partial glomerular destruction (FIGURE 3A); as the congested parenchyma increased in consistency, there was a progressive fibrosis replacement of the destroyed elements, dilation of kidney tubules, and thickening of the basement membrane, which was lined by flat epithelial cells (FIGURE 3B).

Aortic and pulmonary infarct lesions were commonly found after ten to 15 days of treatment with methoxamine and metaraminol. The genesis of aortic aneurysms has been described elsewhere,[8] and the stages of development are illustrated in FIGURE 4. Microscopically, the pulmonary necrotic foci appeared as a lattice of alveolar septa filled with blood cells, proteinaceous material, and other exudative cells, including large macrophages laden with hemosiderin. The necrotic area underwent fibrosis and often calcification, especially in the sub-pleural region. Another interesting and rather constant finding was the presence of cavities lined by epithelial cells containing rectangular-shaped crystals (FIGURE 5A), the exact nature of which remains to be determined; they are resistant to lipid solvents used for histological processing. Similar histological features were also encountered after partial ligation of the pulmonary vein (FIGURE 5B).

Differences in the reactivity of animals to the potentially nephrotoxic and cardiotoxic amines are shown in TABLE 2. The ischemic changes evoked by methoxamine and metaraminol were more severe after adrenalectomy and potassium deficiency; conversely, a low-sodium diet had an opposite effect. In

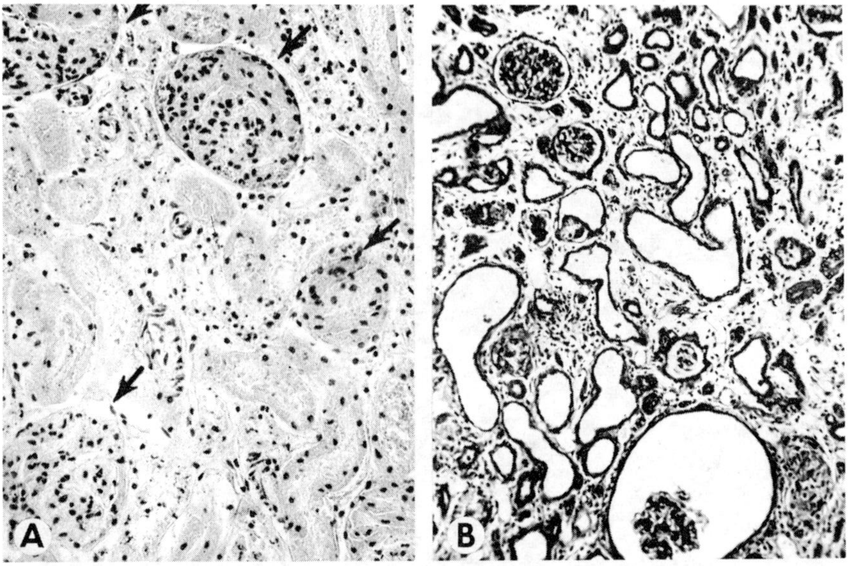

FIGURE 3. (A) Intussusception of the infraglomerular portion of the epithelium of the proximal tubule into the Bowman space (arrows). These changes are demonstrable during the first 12 hours following administration of methoxamine to rats in high dosage. Stain: hematoxylin-phloxine-saffron. × 160 (orig. mag. × 200). (B) Interstitial fibrosis with formation of cyst-like cavities as a result of extreme tubular and glomerular dilation. These sclerotic changes invariably occur in rats after 20 days of sustained treatment with methoxamine. Stain: periodic acid-Schiff. × 95 (orig. mag. × 120).

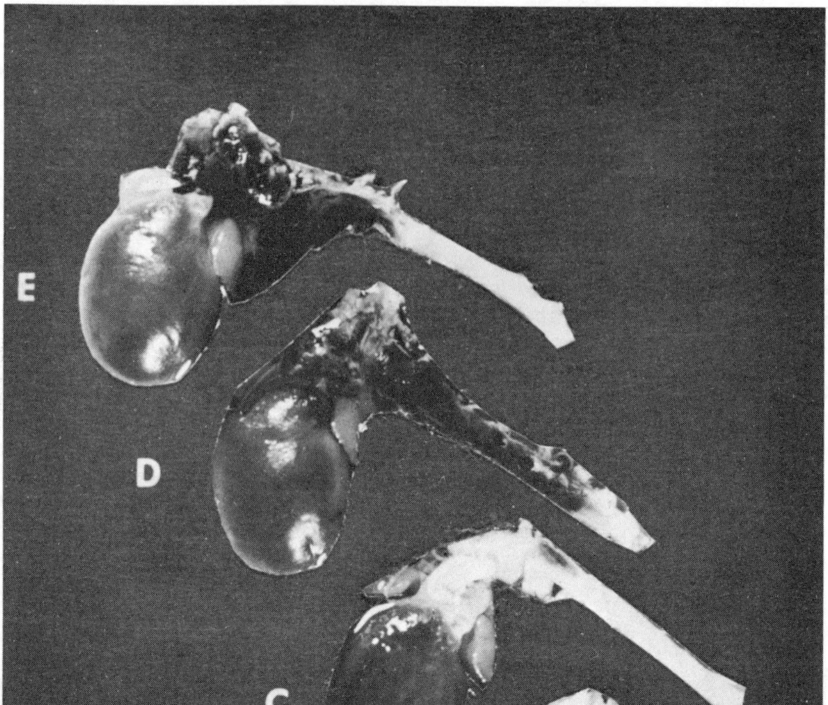

FIGURE 4. Morphogenesis of aortic aneurysms at different time intervals of methoxamine administration. (A) Normal arciform appearance of the aorta in a control rat. (B) Dilation of the arch segment, with evidence of a loss of flexibility observed after eight days of sustained treatment. (C) Focal disruption of the aortic wall, as seen by the spotty infiltration of blood cells in the descending portion of the arch. This lesion developed on the 14th day. (D) Intensive hemorrhage of the periadventitial tissue of the entire aortic arch, as seen on

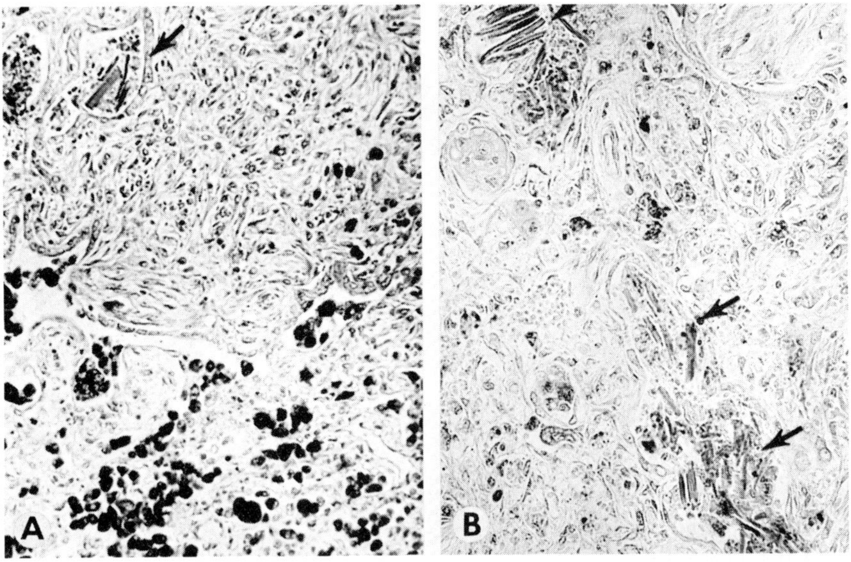

FIGURE 5. Histological aspect of infarcted lungs 20 days after (A) administration of methoxamine and (B) partial ligature of the right pulmonary vein. The arrows in both figures indicate the rectangular-shaped crystals present in epithelial-lined cavities. Note the presence of macrophages laden with hemosiderin in the lower half of part A. Stain: Turnbull blue and hematoxylin-phloxine-saffron. × 150 (orig. mag. × 200).

methoxamine- and metaraminol-treated rats, the renal infarcts were found to be aggravated by forced restraint, coronary ligature, and histamine and serotonin liberators. The genesis of myocardial lesions, on the other hand, was not similarly influenced: Following restraint and coronary ligature, the ischemic effects of isoproterenol were not evident, and those of methoxamine and metaraminol were unchanged.

Quantitative results pertaining to the interaction of vasoactive amines and different antagonists are given in TABLE 3. These observations are based on microscopical studies of the kidney and heart from rats receiving the vasoactive drugs for two consecutive days. The incidence and severity of isoproterenol-induced heart necroses were little modified by the test drugs. Interestingly, some blocking agents such as Dibenamine®, chloropromazine, and hydralazine proved to be efficient in reducing the severity and, to a certain extent, the incidence of methoxamine- and metaraminol-induced heart lesions as well as the kidney infarcts. This reduction, however, was not obtained with the beta-adrenergic antagonists, i.e., dichloroisoproterenol and pronethalol, which had no influence upon the development of the cardiomyopathies, except when dichloroisoproterenol was given in association with methoxamine. Other drugs tested, such as guanethidine and Persantin® (dipyridamole), exerted no significant effect on the methoxamine-induced infarcts.

---

the 21st day; spontaneous rupture often occurs at this stage. (E) Intramural thrombus involving the descending aorta, observed in an animal that survived 28 days of methoxamine treatment.

TABLE 2

INFLUENCE OF SURGICAL, DIETARY, AND PHARMOCOLOGICAL FACTORS ON THE SEVERITY OF RENAL AND CARDIAC LESIONS INDUCED BY VASOACTIVE DRUGS*

Modifying Factor	Renal Lesions			Cardiac Lesions		
	Isoproterenol	Methoxamine	Metaraminol	Isoproterenol	Methoxamine	Metaraminol
Adrenalectomy (deoxycorticosterone acetate administered)	0	↑	↑	0	↑	↑
Potassium deficiency (seven days)	0	↑	0	↑	↑	0
Sodium deficiency (seven days)	0	↓	0	↓	↓	0
Restraint (24 hours)	0	↑	↑	↓	0	↑
Coronary ligature (seven days previously)	0	0	↑	↓	0	0
Histamine and serotonin liberators (0.5 mg 48/80 or reserpine administered four days previously)	0	↑	↑	↑	↑	0

* Vasoactive drugs were injected subcutaneously twice daily at a dose of 2.5 mg/100 g of body weight for two consecutive days to groups of six rats or more. ↓ = decrease or prevention; ↑ = increase; 0 = no effect.

TABLE 3

INTERACTION OF VASOACTIVE AMINES AND INFLUENCE OF DIFFERENT DRUGS ON CARDIAC AND RENAL LESIONS

Treatment*	Dosage (mg/kg)	No. of Rats	Cardiac Lesions		Renal Lesions	
			Grade (0–3)	Incidence (%)	Grade (0–3)	Incidence (%)
Isoproterenol	50	6	1.6 ± 0.29	100	0	0
+ Dibenamine®	50 + 10	6	1.1 ± 0.24	100	0	0
+ Dichloroisoproterenol	50 + 25	6	1.7 ± 0.29	100	0	0
+ Hydralazine	20 + 20	6	1.5 ± 0.19	100	0	0
+ Pronethalol	50 + 25	6	1.3 ± 0.09	100	0	0
+ Methoxamine	5 + 5	10	1.8 ± 0.08	100	0	0
+ Metaraminol	5 + 5	6	1.6 ± 0.17	100	0.8 ± 0.11	66
Metaraminol	20	12	2.1 ± 0.33	100	0.8 ± 0.24	50
+ Dibenamine®	25 + 10	6	0	0	0.4 ± 0.19	33
+ Dichloroisoproterenol	25 + 25	6	2.2 ± 0.27	100	1.5 ± 0.21	100
+ Chlorpromazine	10 + 10	8	0.6 ± 0.15	100	0.1 ± 0.06	25
+ Hydralazine	20 + 30	8	0.7 ± 0.12	100	0.2 ± 0.11	50
+ Pronethalol	25 + 25	6	1.6 ± 0.21	100	0.8 ± 0.16	50
Methoxamine	30	20	1.3 ± 0.22	90	1.9 ± 0.18	100
+ Dibenamine®	30 + 10	6	0.9 ± 0.14	83	1.7 ± 0.29	100
+ Dichloroisoproterenol	30 + 25	6	0.8 ± 0.19	50	1.1 ± 0.24	33
+ Chlorpromazine	25 + 10	6	0	0	0.3 ± 0.03	33
+ Pronethalol	30 + 25	6	1.4 ± 0.12	100	1.3 ± 0.14	50
+ Guanethidine	30 + 10	6	1.6 ± 0.11	100	2.2 ± 0.22	100
+ Persantin®	30 + 25	6	1.1 ± 0.14	100	1.7 ± 0.26	100

* Administered subcutaneously twice daily on two consecutive days.

Discussion and Conclusion

These experiments emphasize the important role of hemodynamics in the production of myocardial lesions by sympathomimetic amines. The cardiovascular and renal alterations of methoxamine and metaraminol were enhanced by adrenalectomy and by forced restraint, most probably as a result of an increase and prolongation of the visceral circulatory stasis. Similar adverse effects were not noted in isoproterenol-treated rats. In the latter animals, restraint and coronary ligature actually afforded protection, as previously reported by other workers.[10] However, heart lesions induced by any one of the sympathomimetic amines were aggravated equally by potassium deficiency and by histamine and serotonin liberators. Most probably, the modifying action of these stimuli primarily involves the myocardium.

Two mechanisms may be proposed regarding the production of myocardial lesions by sympathomimetic amines. The first is exemplified by the strong inotropic action of isoproterenol, with its resultant greater oxygen demand by the heart muscle, as was suggested by Rona and his colleagues.[11] The second is typical of methoxamine and metaraminol and similar vasopressors; their toxic effects are derived mainly from localized or generalized hemodynamic changes, with alterations in the metabolism of the myocardial fibers, as was previously shown through histoenzymatic studies;[12] the lesions are wholly regressive in nature. Hence, we are inclined to believe that the ability of certain adrenergic blocking agents to prevent anoxic tissue changes is a reflection of their favorable systemic action upon vascular resistance.

Summary

Experiments on factors influencing the development cardiopathies induced by isoproterenol, methoxamine, and metaraminol in rats have been described. Results of these studies emphasize the importance of hemodynamic changes in the pathogenesis of the heart lesions.

Acknowledgments

The drugs used in these investigations were generously supplied by Ayerst, McKenna & Harrison Limited, Canada (pronethalol); Burroughs Wellcome & Co. (Canada) Ltd. (methoxamine); Ciba Company Limited, Canada (hydralazine, guanethidine); Geigy Pharmaceuticals, Division of Geigy (Canada) Limited (Persantin®); Merck Sharp & Dohme of Canada Limited (metaraminol); Poulenc Limited, Canada (chlorpromazine); Smith Kline & French, Inter-American Corporation (Dibenamine®); Winthrop Laboratories (isoproterenol).

References

1. Jasmin, G. 1956. Étude de l'inflammation anaphylactoïde. Rev. Canad. Biol. **15:** 107.
2. Jasmin, G. & P. Bois. 1959. Influence des libérateurs d'histamine sur la production et la prévention des ulcères gastriques chez le rat. Rev. Canad. Biol. **18:** 367.
3. Jasmin, G. & P. Bois. 1960. Effect of various agents on the development of kidney infarcts in rats treated with serotonin. Lab. Invest. **9:** 503.
4. Jasmin, G. & R. Gareau. 1961. Histopathological study of muscle lesions produced by paraphenylenediamine in rats. Brit. J. Exp. Path. **42:** 592.
5. Jasmin, G. & E. Bajusz. 1964. Étude pathogénique des lésions cardiaques rénales et musculaires provoquées chez le rat par la méthoxamine et le métaraminol. Rev. Canad. Biol. **23:** 67.

6. Bajusz, E. & G. Jasmin. 1964. Influence of variations in electrolyte intake upon the development of cardiac necrosis produced by vasopressor amines. Lab. Invest. **13:** 757.
7. Rona, G., D. S. Kahn & C. I. Chappel. 1963. Studies on infarct-like myocardial necrosis produced by isoproterenol: A Review. Rev. Canad. Biol. **22:** 241.
8. Jasmin, G. 1965. Cardiac, aortic and pulmonary lesions induced by vasopressors. Vasc. Dis. **2:** 115.
9. Jasmin, G. 1966. Morphologic effects of vasoactive drugs. Canad. J. Physiol. Pharmacol. **44:** 367.
10. Selye, H. 1961. The Pluricausal Cardiopathies. : 114. Charles C Thomas. Springfield, Ill.
11. Rona, G., C. I. Chappel, T. Balazs & R. Gaudry. 1959. An infarct-like myocardial lesion and other toxic manifestations produced by isoproterenol in the rat. Arch. Path. (Chicago) **67:** 443.
12. Bajusz, E. & G. Jasmin. 1964–65. Enzyme histochemistry of some chemically induced cardiac necroses. II. Myocardial lesions induced by methoxamine. Z. Vitamin. Hormon. Fermentforsch. **14:** 43.

TISSUE ELECTROLYTE ALTERATION IN DISSEMINATED MYOCARDIAL NECROSIS*

David Lehr

Department of Pharmacology
New York Medical College
Flower and Fifth Avenue Hospitals
New York, N. Y.

An entire section of this monograph is devoted exclusively to myocardial injury induced by sympathomimetic amines. It seems pertinent, therefore, to explain that omission of this specific identification from the title of my presentation was deliberate and intended to emphasize that the myocardial changes to be described are not limited to damage induced by adrenergic amines, but appear to be a characteristic and perhaps stereotyped expression of cellular injury.

There is little doubt that tissue response to an injurious stimulus may be as uniform and as specific as that to physiological activation. Thus, cardiac muscle, for instance, which contracts in the same way, irrespective of the nature of the eliciting stimulus, apparently responds to a great variety of noxious agents with the development of disseminated necrosis and mononuclear cell infiltration. This point was emphasized by Dr. Wartman in his opening remarks to this monograph; he stated that there are only a few possible morphological reactions to injury, and since there are numerous injurious agents, many will cause the same morphological changes. Drs. Laufer and Davis put it even more succinctly when they said that the myocardium may be damaged in many ways, but reacts in very few.

The findings to be reported in this paper will demonstrate that the similarity is not limited to the morphological appearance of the injury, but probably encompasses a number of other parameters. In fact, it would seem that the morphological changes are the late expression of a series of characteristic metabolic alterations inherent in cell degeneration which may participate in the initiation of irreversible failure of cell function.

It was with this concept in mind that my associates and I became interested several years ago in the significance of shifts of the tissue electrolyte content which accompany the development of disseminated myocardial necrosis induced by a variety of unrelated procedures. We wanted to know, in particular, whether some of these electrolyte shifts contribute to the causation of myocardial injury or whether all such derangements are solely the consequence of necrosis.

In favor of a causative influence of electrolyte imbalance, one may cite the fact that cardiac necrosis can be induced by dietary deficiency of potassium or magnesium, and that the severity of this injury can be enhanced by sodium loading and by mineralocorticoids and inhibited by the administration of magnesium and potassium chloride. Against a causative role of electrolyte derangements, on the other hand, one may cite the well-documented findings that necrotic tissue invariably manifests substantial deviations of the electrolyte content.

It will be demonstrated in this paper that similar sequential alterations of the myocardial electrolyte pattern accompany the evolution and healing of disseminated myocardial necrosis from unrelated noxae. The observations to be

* Supported by United States Public Health Service research grant no. HE-00890-16 from the National Heart Institute, National Institutes of Health, Bethesda, Md.

reported add considerable weight to the concept of a specific tissue response to injury and indicate that, in the case of the myocardium, initial lesions of the myofibers may entail changes in permeability at cellular and subcellular membrane sites, which, in turn, may be responsible for the creation of electrolyte imbalance. Such a sequence of events would lend support to our view that early ionic shifts probably occur in the living cell and that electrolyte derangements thus created may contribute to the initiation of irreversible failure of cell function.

Results

For the purpose of this study, two apparently unrelated procedures were utilized for the production of severe disseminated myocardial necrosis. One consists in oral NaH_2PO_4 loading of parathyroidectomized rats (Lehr *et al.*, 1967), and the other is based on the injection of excessive amounts of adrenergic amines, first described by Rona and his colleagues (1963) for isoproterenol and subsequently amplified in various laboratories to include a number of additional adrenergic amines (Bajusz & Jasmin, 1962; Rosenblum *et al.*, 1965; Wenzel & Chau, 1966).

Myocardial Necrosis Produced by Sodium Phosphate Loading of Parathyroidectomized Rats

Severe myocardial and renal necrosis can be readily produced in parathyroidectomized rats by a simple procedure developed in our laboratory which has been described in detail elsewhere (Lehr *et al.*, 1967). To recapitulate briefly: parathyroidectomized rats given 4 cc of a 15% aqueous solution of NaH_2PO_4 twice daily by gavage, succumb in a maximum of three days with signs of hypocalcemic tetany. They invariably develop extensive disseminated myocardial necrosis and renal tubular necrosis within 48 hours of NaH_2PO_4 loading. The procedure was found to be foolproof in properly parathyroidectomized rats. When phosphate loading was stopped after the fourth intubation, most animals survived and apparently recovered fully within a few days. This modification of the procedure was utilized for the study of healing of cardiac and renal necrosis (Krukowski & Lehr, under publication).

The consistency of the appearance of severe cardiorenal injury obtainable in parathyroidectomized rats by NaH_2PO_4 loading and the protective effect of the animal's own parathyroid gland are illustrated in Table 1. Whereas the 12 intact rats seemed to suffer no ill effects except for moderate degrees of nephrocalcinosis, even after three full days of NaH_2PO_4 administration, all 14 parathyroidectomized rats exhibited advanced degrees of myocardial and renal necrosis. These animals invariably manifested lethargy, weakness, spasticity, and dyspnea, and seven were moribund at the time of sacrifice.

Morphology of Cardiorenal Injury

Heart

To the naked eye, the foci of necrosis appeared as multiple, often slightly elevated, grayish areas, varying in size from barely visible dots and streaks to patches occupying substantial parts of the epicardial surface, and surrounded by purple-red, apparently normal, myocardial tissue. On cross-section, many of these foci were seen to extend deep into the wall of both ventricles and often to link with grayish streaks and dots on the endocardial surface, including papillary muscles, thus forming a reticulum of disintegrating muscle fibers. Confluence of such foci accounted for the presence of larger patches of necrosis which were often seen to accompany the course of smaller branches of the coronary vasculature over considerable distances. Most lesions were clearly visible to the naked eye.

Under the microscope, numerous muscle fibers in affected areas showed loss of cross-striation, homogenization or fine and coarse granular disintegration, and, finally, rupture. These foci of necrosis often contained, in addition to the muscular debris, accumulations of a homogeneous material positive to periodic acid-Schiff (PAS). The lesions were invaded by primarily mononuclear inflammatory cells having vesicular ovoid nuclei that contained many nucleoli (FIGURES 1 and 2). Interspersed between the mononuclear cells in some areas there were considerable numbers of polymorphonuclear leukocytes, which frequently exhibited an eosinophilic cytoplasm and were grouped around the edges of fragmented muscle fibers. Some of these muscle fragments still showed cross-striation and contained pale swollen nuclei (FIGURE 3). There was no

TABLE 1

CARDIORENAL INJURY INDUCED BY PHOSPHATE LOADING IN PARATHYROIDECTOMIZED RATS*

Group	Autopsy No.	Time before Sacrifice (days)†	Foci of Necrosis in Heart	Kidney: Calcium Casts in Papilla	Kidney: Tubules Degeneration in Medulla
Intact plus NaH_2PO_4	4852	2.5	−	++	++
	4853	2.5	−	++	+++
	4854	2.5	−	+	++
	4855	2	−	++	++
	4856	2	−	++	++
	5025	3	−	−	−
	5026	3	−	++	+
	5027	3	−	++	++
	5028	3	−	+	+
	5029	3	−	++	−
	5099‡	2.5	−	−	−
	5102‡	2.5	−	−	−
					Necrosis in Cortex
Parathyroidectomized plus NaH_2PO_4	4843	2 (m)	+++	−	++++
	4844	2.5 (s)	++++	−	++++
	4847	2 (m)	++++	−	+++
	4849	2 (m)	+++	−	+++
	4850	2 (m)	++++	−	++++
	4851	2 (m)	++++	−	++++
	4893	1.5 (m)	+++	−	+++
	4896	2 (m)	++++	−	+++
	4899	2.5 (s)	+++	−	++++
	4900	2.5 (s)	++++	−	++++
	4901	2.5 (s)	++++	−	++++
	4902	2.5 (s)	+++	−	++++
	4944	2.5 (s)	++++	−	++++
	5023	2.5 (s)	++++	−	++++

* From Lehr *et al.* (1967).
† (m) = moribund condition at time of sacrifice; (s) = animal appeared very sick.
‡ Sham parathyroidectomized.

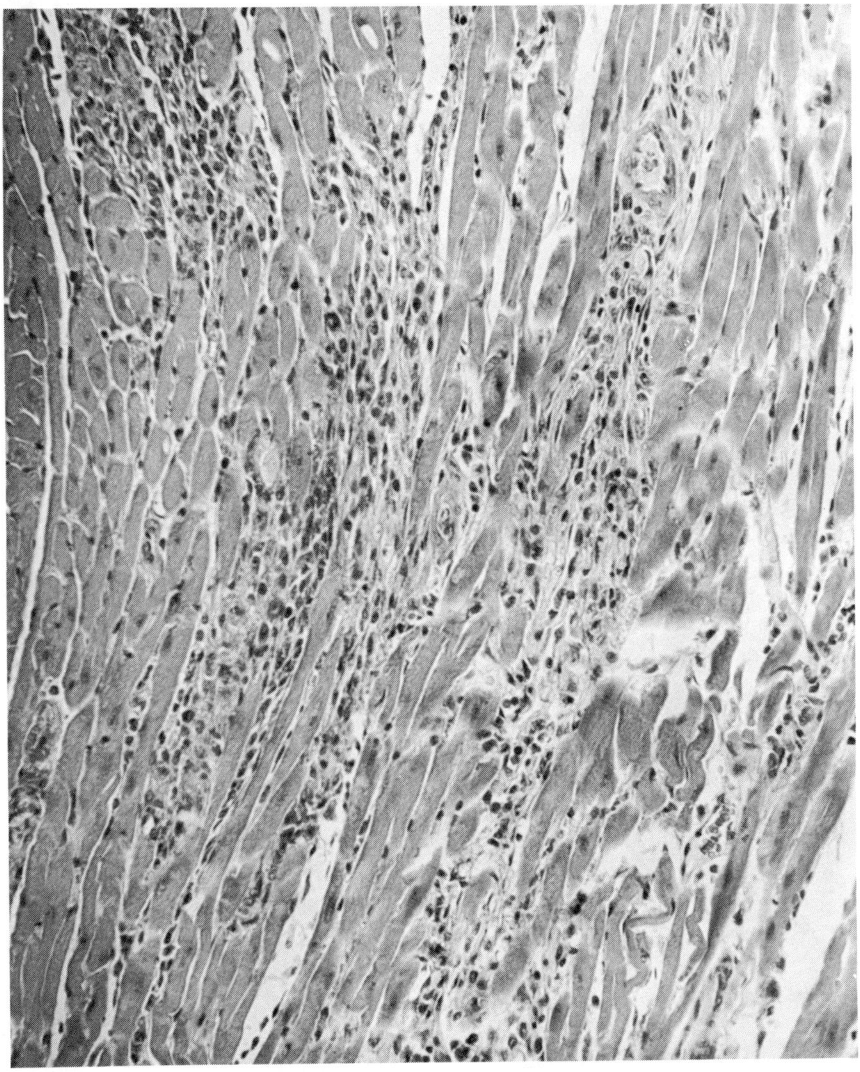

FIGURE 1. Myocardium of parathyroidectomized albino rat after five NaH_2PO_4 loads. Note the typical wide dissemination and confluence of necrotic foci containing disintegrating myocardial fibers and muscular debris, usually adjacent to or surrounding small blood vessels. All areas of necrosis are invaded by mostly mononuclear inflammatory cells. Stain: hematoxylin-eosin. × 70 (orig. mag. × 120). (From Lehr *et al.*, 1967. Reproduced by permission of the publisher.)

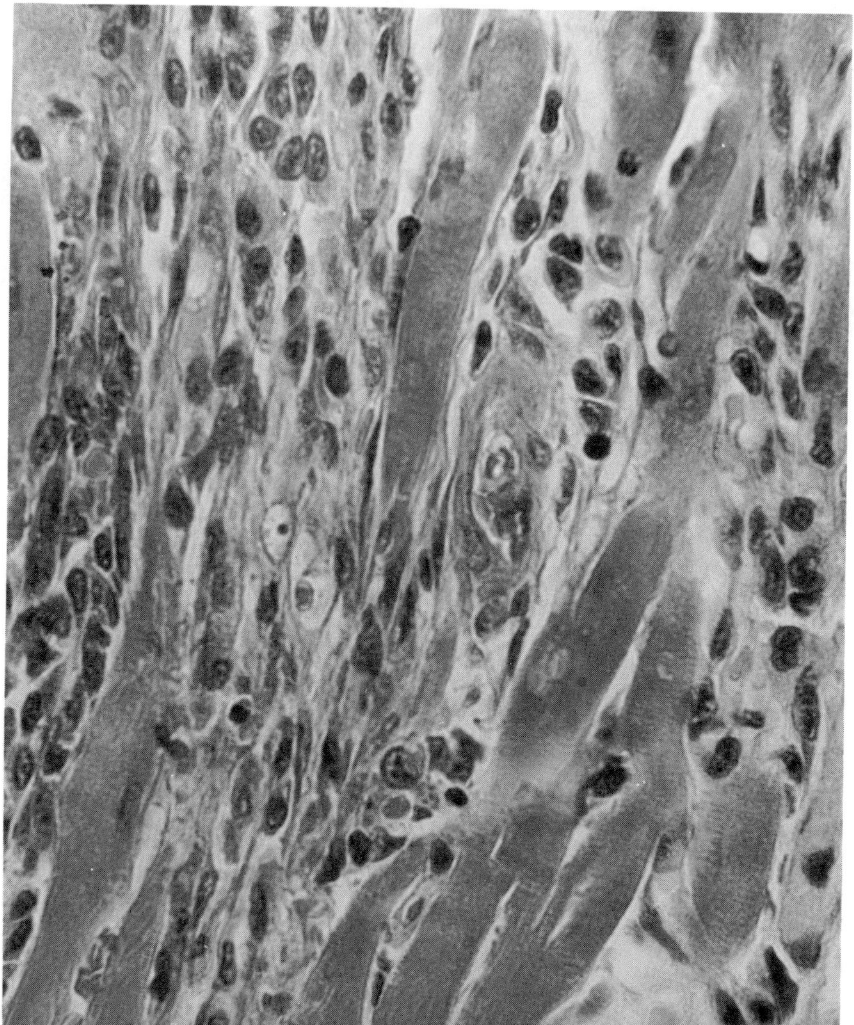

FIGURE 2. Detail from the center of FIGURE 1, examined under higher power. Note the partial loss of nuclei and of cross-striation in disintegrating muscle fibers, and swelling and homogenization of the wall of the small blood vessel in the center of the photograph; several Anitschkow type nuclei are near the right margin of the photograph. A single segmented polymorphonuclear leukocyte can be seen in the center (lower half) of the photograph. Stain: hematoxylin-eosin. × 250 (orig. mag. × 400). (From Lehr *et al.*, 1967. Reproduced by permission of the publisher.)

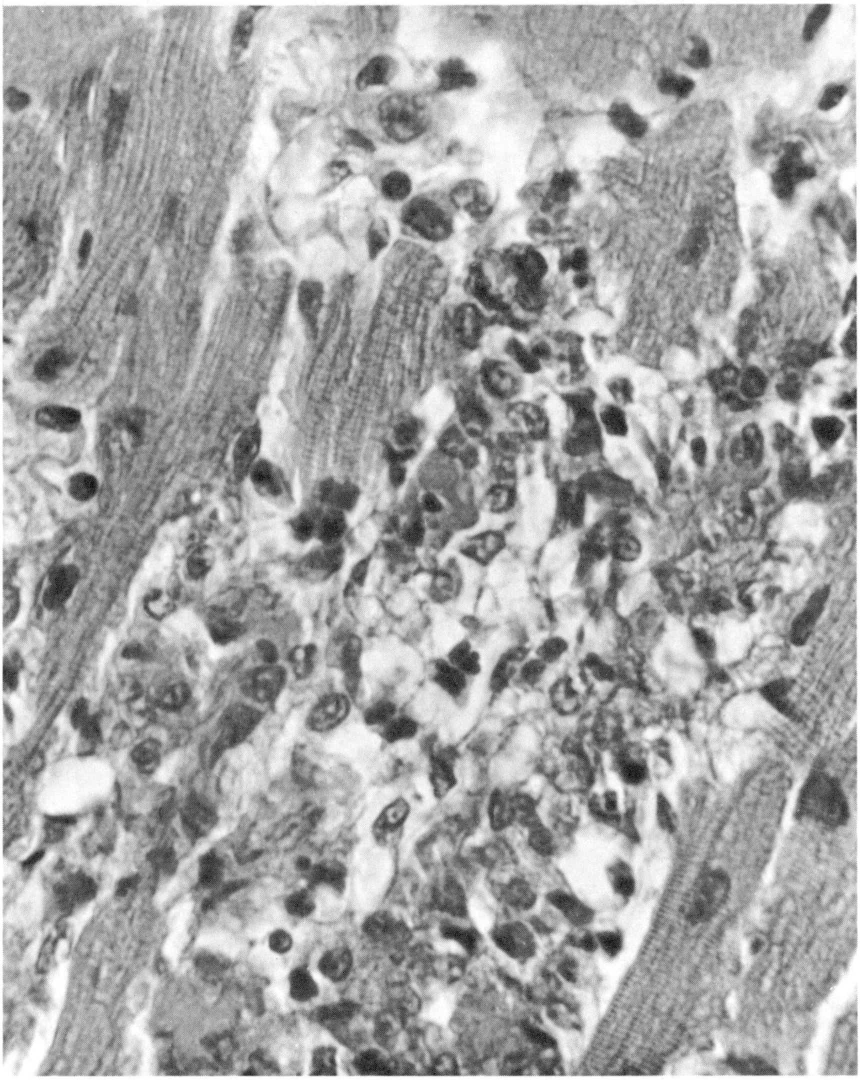

FIGURE 3. Myocardium of parathyroidectomized albino rat sacrificed after four NaH_2PO_4 loads. Note, particularly in the right lower corner, the fragmentation of myocardial fibers, which in many areas clearly show cross striation and contain swollen nuclei. The lower center of the photograph depicts coarse granular, as well as homogeneous, muscular debris, and infiltration with mononuclear inflammatory cells. The muscle fragment in the upper center of the photograph is surrounded by polymorphonuclear eosinophilic leukocytes. Stain: hematoxylin-eosin. × 235 (orig. mag. × 400).

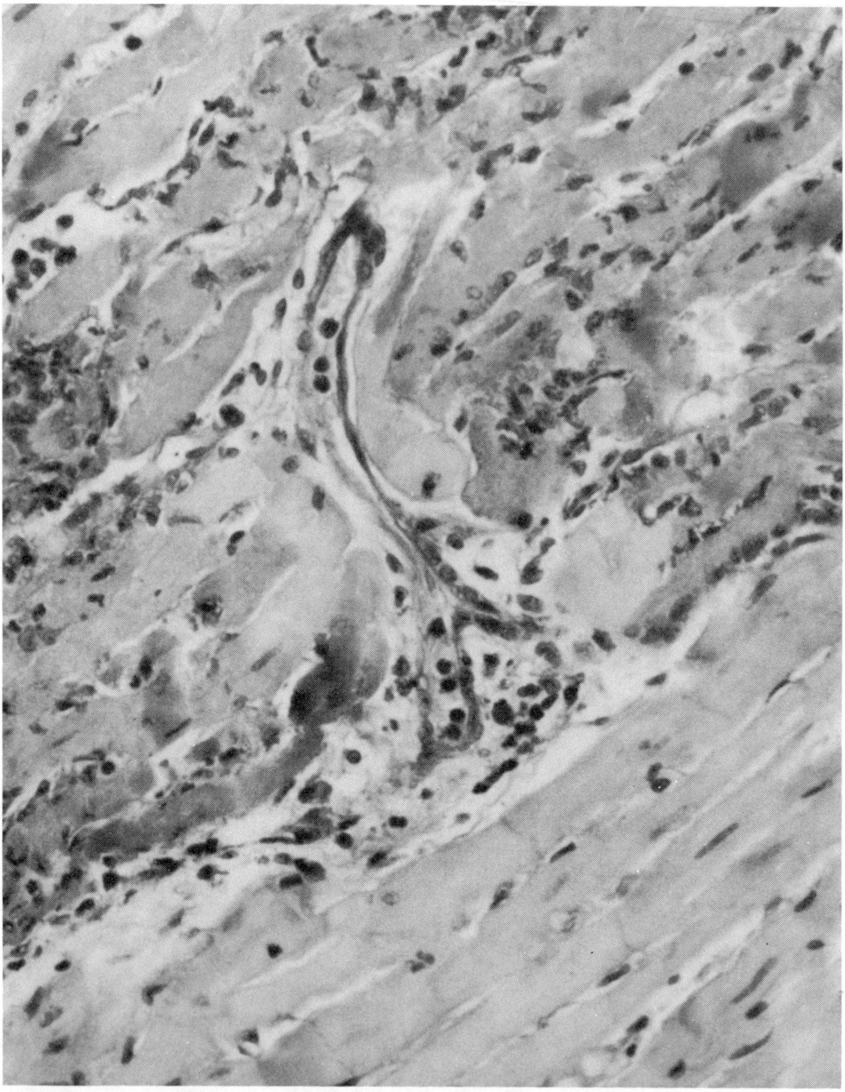

FIGURE 4. Myocardium of parathyroidectomized albino rat exposed to NaH_2PO_4 loading for two and one-half days. In the center of the photograph is a branching coronary arteriole, cut longitudinally, which exhibits loss of normal architecture and rather intense infiltration of its wall with PAS-positive material. The myocardial fibers surrounding this vessel are necrotic and exhibit imbibition with PAS-positive material and invasion by mononuclear inflammatory cells. The purple appearance of this focus in the original stain provides a sharp contrast to the pale pink of intact myocardial fibers at the left top and right bottom of the photograph. Stain: periodic-acid-Schiff. × 75 (orig. mag. × 120). (From Lehr, *et al.*, 1967. Reproduced by permission of the publisher.)

inflammatory border offsetting the necrotic regions from surrounding intact myocardium. Such foci sometimes covered large areas of the epicardial or endocardial surface.

The microcirculation of the heart was invariably damaged. Many arterioles exhibited a loss of the normal architecture of the media, with disintegration of the muscle fibers and appearance of smudgy, homogeneous, PAS-positive masses that frequently engulfed the entire circumference of the wall over considerable distances (FIGURE 4). Material of similar staining characteristics was seen in the thickened walls of precapillaries and capillaries and in areas of myocardial necrosis, particularly adjacent to damaged vessels. The perivascular localization of PAS-positive material suggests possible seepage through damaged blood vessel walls into the myocardium proper.

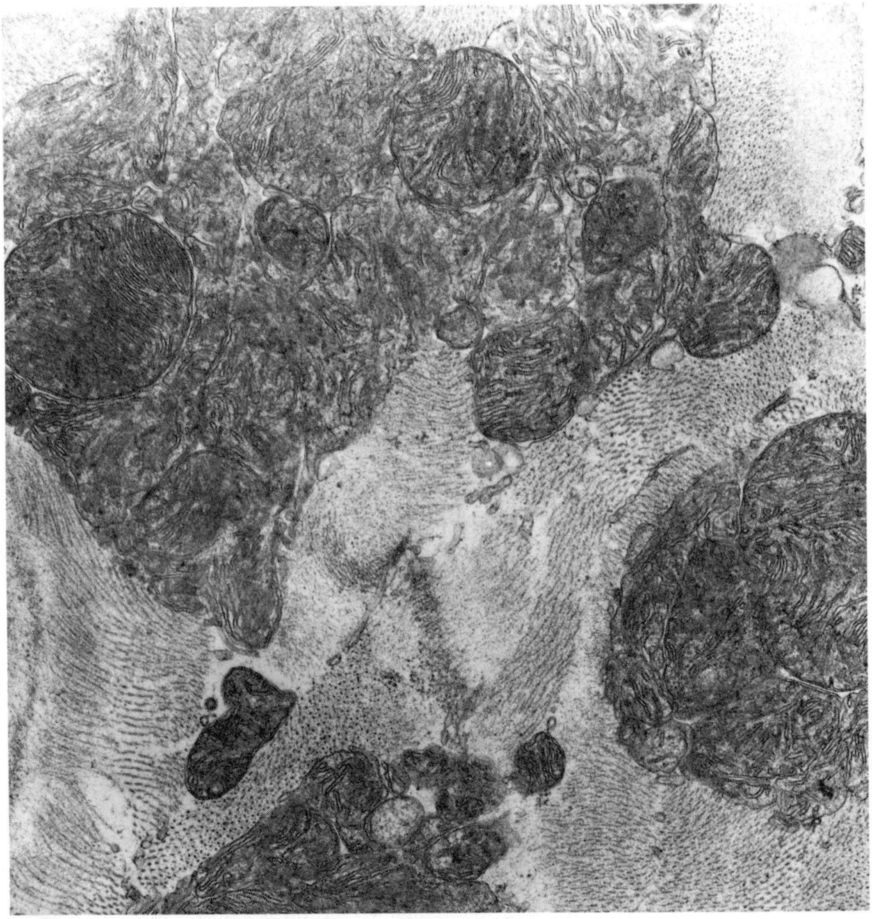

FIGURE 5. Rat myocardium 18 hours after single NaH_2PO_4 load. Note the swelling and clumping of sarcosomes and loss of normal architecture of sarcosomal cristae and of myofibrils. Stain: uranyl acetate. Orig. mag. × 13,000. (From Lehr, 1967. Reproduced by permission of the publisher.)

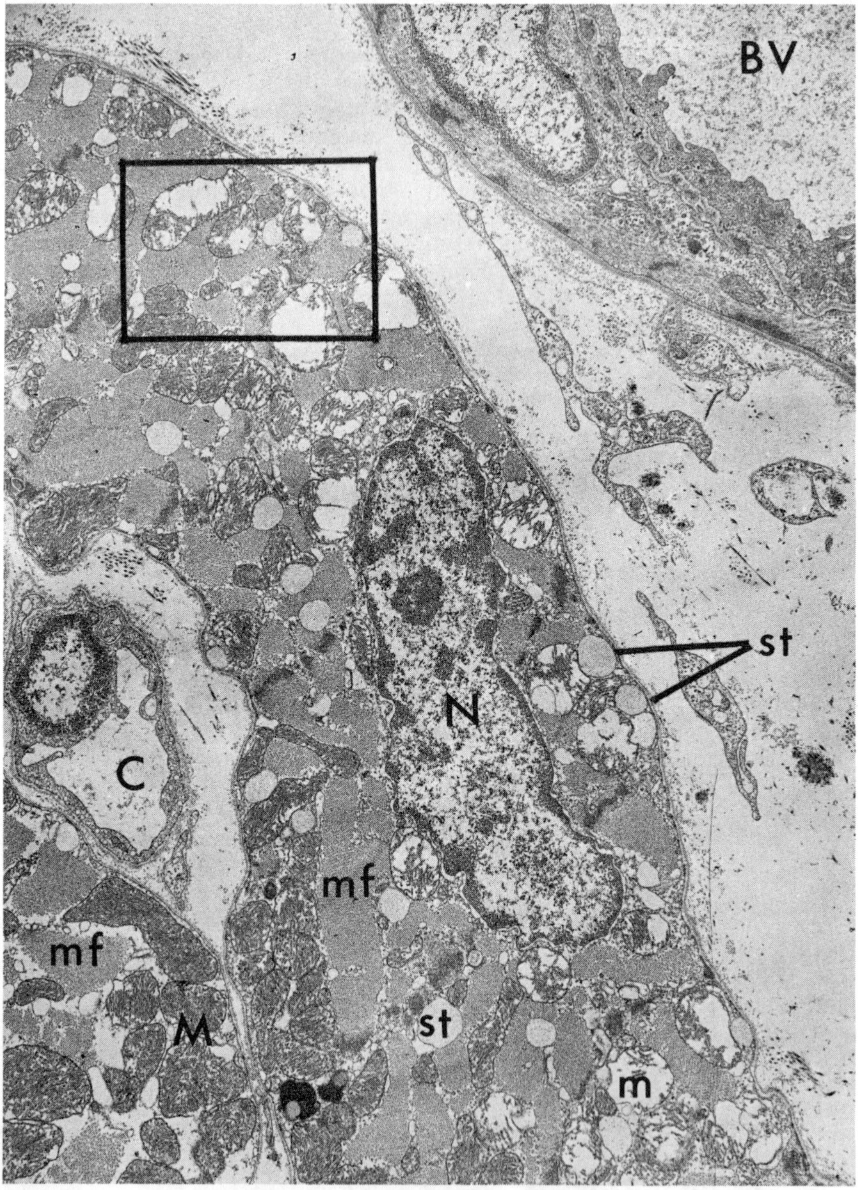

FIGURE 6. Myocardium of parathyroidectomized albino rat after two NaH_2PO_4 loads. BV = large blood vessel; C = capillary; N = nucleus of muscle cell, showing margination of chromatin; mf = intact myofibrils; M = clumps of swollen mitochondria; m = swollen cystic mitochondrion (most cristae have disappeared); st = swollen sarcotubules appearing spherical rather than flat. In lower left corner, myofibrils and mitochondria are pushed apart by edema fluid. Stain: uranyl acetate. Orig. mag. × 2,500. (From Lehr *et al.*, 1966. Reproduced by permission of the publisher.)

After a single NaH_2PO_4 load (total experimental period, 18 hours), clumping of sarcosomes and disturbances in the normal myofibrillar pattern could be seen under the electron microscope in some areas of the myocardium (FIGURE 5), as well as considerable edema, which produced wide interspaces between sarcolemma and myofibrils. After two NaH_2PO_4 loads (total experimental period, 24 hours) one could see, in parts of the myocardium which had not undergone necrosis, that the myofibrils were intact but pushed apart by edema fluid. The nuclei of muscle cells often showed margination of chromatin. The mitochondria were swollen and exhibited various degrees of disintegration of the normal architecture, with disappearance of cristae and the formation of granular debris. All that remained of the sarcosomes in advanced instances were large ovoid cystic structures. The sarcotubules were greatly enlarged and filled with a fine granular material (FIGURES 6 and 7).

After four intubations of NaH_2PO_4 within a two-day period, necrotic areas of the myocardium showed homogenization of myofibrils with complete loss of their characteristic structure, clumping and shrinkage of damaged mitochondria, and enlarged sarcotubules (FIGURE 8). In addition, one could frequently observe intensely electron-dense fibrillar material that was structurally quite distinct from the appearance of myofibrils, although in some instances it seemed as if material of this same electron density had coated disintegrating

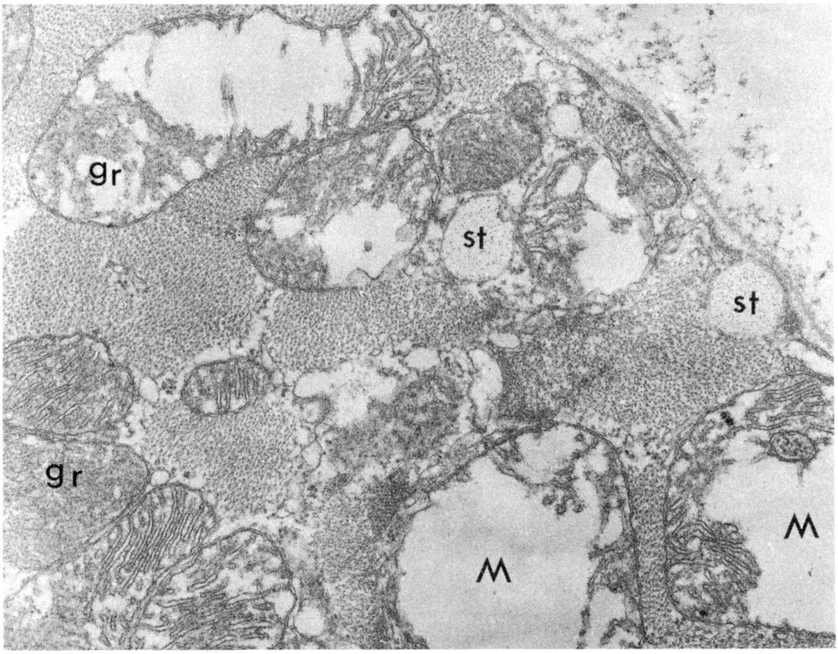

FIGURE 7. Detailed section from the upper left portion of FIGURE 6. Note swelling of all mitochondria and disintegration of cristae with formation of granular debris (gr) and cystic degeneration (M). Swollen sarcotubules (st) can be distinguished from cystic mitochondria by absence of cristae and presence of homogeneous stippling. Myofilaments are intact. Stain: uranyl acetate. Orig. mag. × 12,000. (From Lehr *et al.*, 1966. Reproduced by permission of the publisher.)

myofibrils, or condensed upon them as a matrix (FIGURE 9). It was noted further that this same substance was predominantly present in the vicinity of damaged capillaries. The capillary basement membrane was not always distinct. Fibrin-like electron-dense material was prominent at the capillary wall and appeared to ooze in strands into the pericapillary space (FIGURES 10 and 11). It seemed as if conglomeration of these fine pericapillary strands resulted in the formation of thick electron-dense globs and bands. With higher resolution, the typical structured appearance of fibrin was unmistakable (FIGURE 12). It was considered likely that this material was identical with the PAS-positive substance seen in light microscopical sections which seemed to ooze through

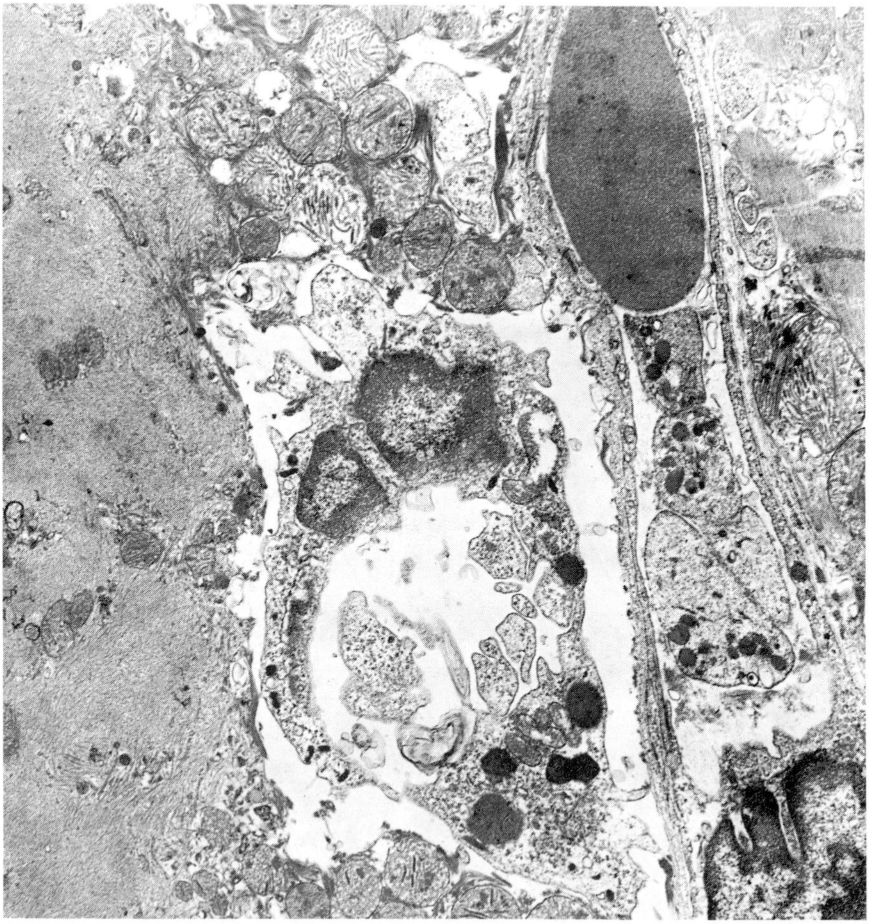

FIGURE 8. Myocardium of parathyroidectomized albino rat after four NaH_2PO_4 loads. In the center is an inflammatory cell flanked on the left by part of a necrotic myocardial cell exhibiting homogenized myofibrils and shrunken sarcosomes; on the right is a capillary sectioned longitudinally. Note at the height of the red blood cell intensely electron-dense material in the pericapillary space in the immediate vicinity of the capillary wall and also engulfing a clump of damaged sarcosomes. Stain: uranyl acetate. Orig. mag. × 4,000.

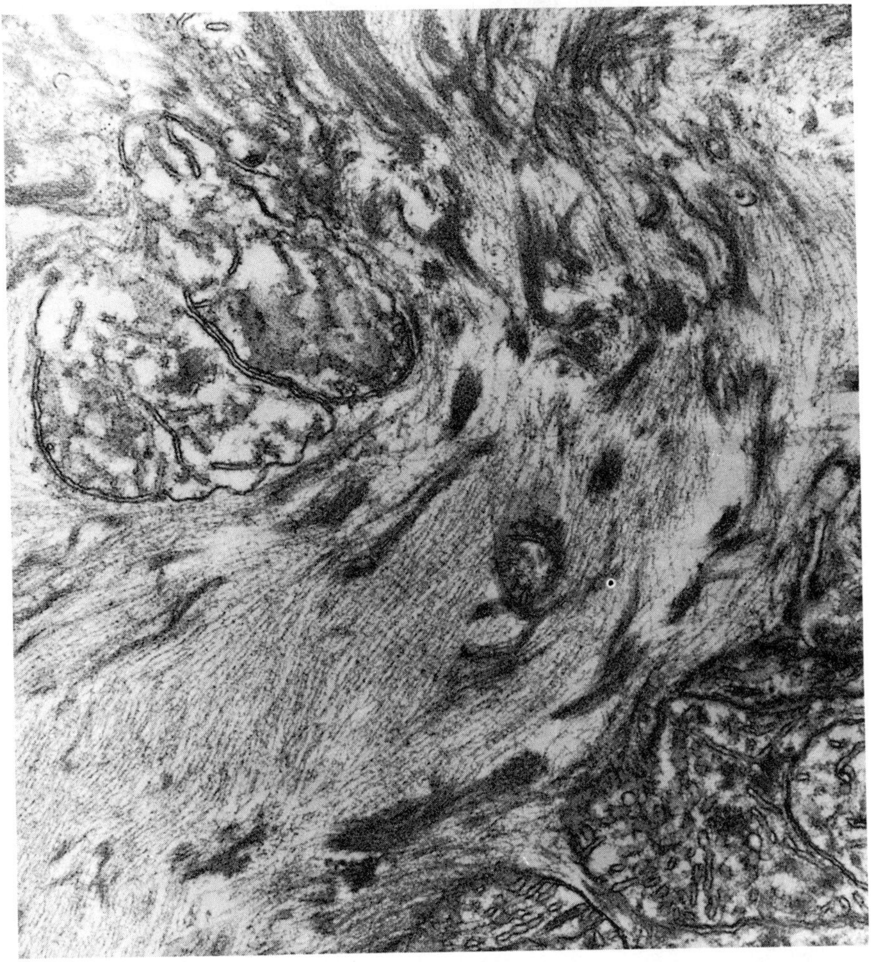

FIGURE 9. Same heart as shown in FIGURE 8. Strands of electron dense material appear to coat some of the disintegrating myofibrils. Severely damaged sarcosomes are in evidence. Stain: uranyl acetate. Orig. mag. × 20,000. (From Lehr, 1967. Reproduced by permission of the publisher.)

the wall of damaged components of the microcirculation and to infiltrate perivascular foci of myocardial necrosis. The endothelial cells contained an abundance of large and frequently confluent cytoplasmic vesicles and were often loaded with intensely electron-dense cytoplasmic granules (FIGURES 13).

Kidney

Except for enlargement and pallor, due to parenchymatous swelling and edema, there was no particularly characteristic alteration in the gross appearance of the kidneys. On cross-section, the entire surface was usually pale olive green. The cortex was distinctly paler than the medulla and contained a sharply demarcated, extremely pale-gray zone, about 2–3 mm in width, at the cortico-medullary junction.

Under the microscope, one could observe widespread and severe damage affecting most parts of the nephron. In the glomeruli, there was swelling of the tufts and capsular thickening. In the tubules, one noted various degrees of degeneration which, in the proximal convolution, had reached complete necrosis with sloughing off of the epithelium, whereas the cells of the basement membrane had remained intact (FIGURE 14). Thus, wide areas of the cortex were seen to contain tubular channels filled with eosinophilic, granular, or smudgy epithelial debris. The flushing out of this necrotic proteinaceous material apparently created numerous partially denuded and empty tubules, and resulted in a peculiar embroidery-like pattern of the kidney cross-section under low magnification (FIGURE 15).

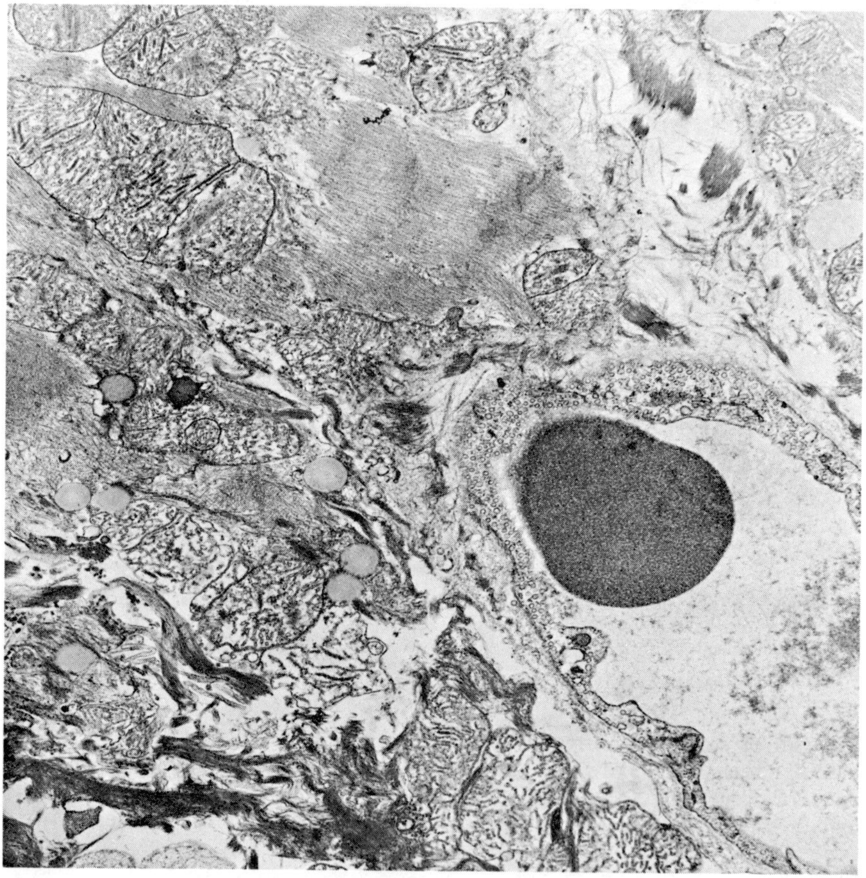

FIGURE 10. Myocardium of parathyroidectomized albino rat after four NaH_2PO_4 loads. Fine strands of electron-dense material which form a network in the pericapillary space appear to condense into thick globs and bands as they infiltrate the disintegrating myocyte. The sarcosomes of the muscle cell are severely damaged, and the myofibrils have lost their normal architecture. Stain: uranyl acetate. Orig. mag. × 4,000.

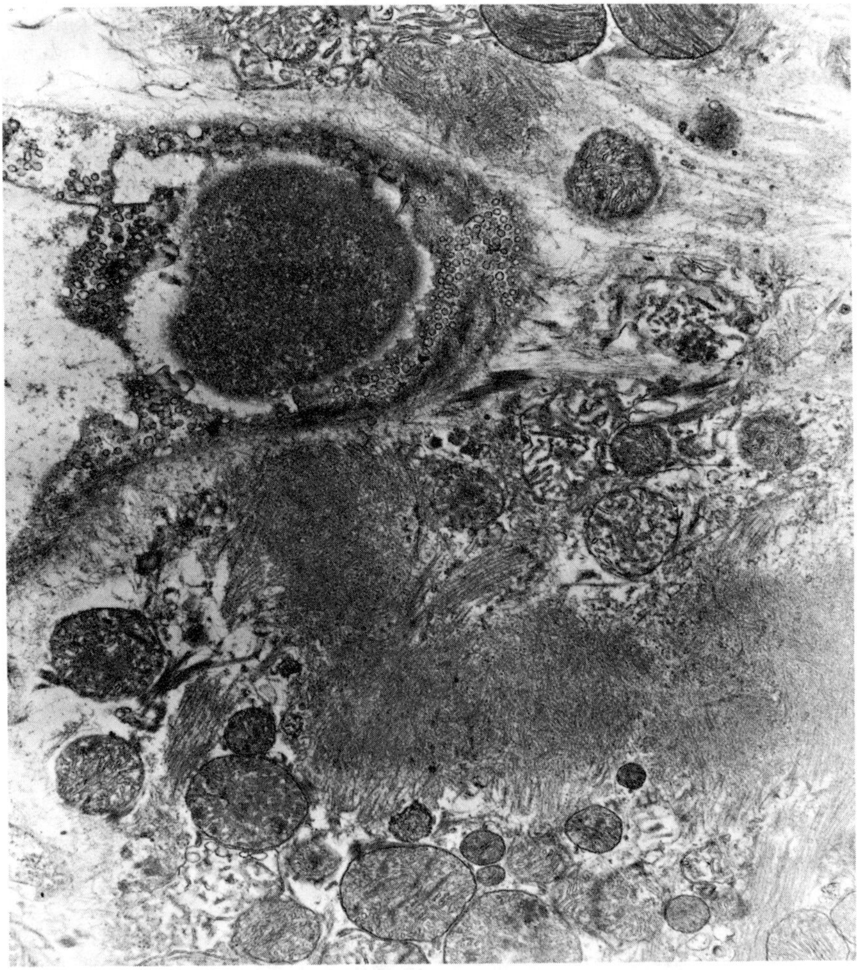

FIGURE 11. Myocardium of parathyroidectomized albino rat after four NaH_2PO_4 loads. Grazing cut through myocardial capillary. There is an abundance of cytoplasmic vesicles and strands of fibrin-like electron-dense material at and near the damaged capillary wall. The fibrin-like strands appear to ooze from the endothelial cell into the pericapillary space. The sarcosomes of the muscle cell are damaged, and the myofibrils are necrotic. Stain: uranyl acetate. Orig. mag. × 9,000.

PAS-stained sections revealed that considerable amounts of a PAS-positive substance were present in the glomerular loops and from there had found their way into Bowman's space, convoluted tubules, and collecting ducts (FIGURE 16), suggesting the abundant presence of PAS-positive material in the bloodstream.

Alterations of the Tissue Electrolyte Content in the Development and Healing of Cardiorenal Necrosis

Development of Necrosis

The emergence of morphological alterations was found to be associated with pronounced and specific shifts in the electrolyte content of hearts and kidneys. For the purpose of close correlation with pathological anatomical findings, determination of electrolytes was carried out in individual tissue samples by automated chemical analysis. It can be seen from TABLE 2 that NaH_2PO_4 loading of intact rats did not damage the heart, but did induce moderate nephrocalcinosis. Accordingly, there was no significant shift in the cardiac electrolyte content, which remained in the range of the normal control animals,

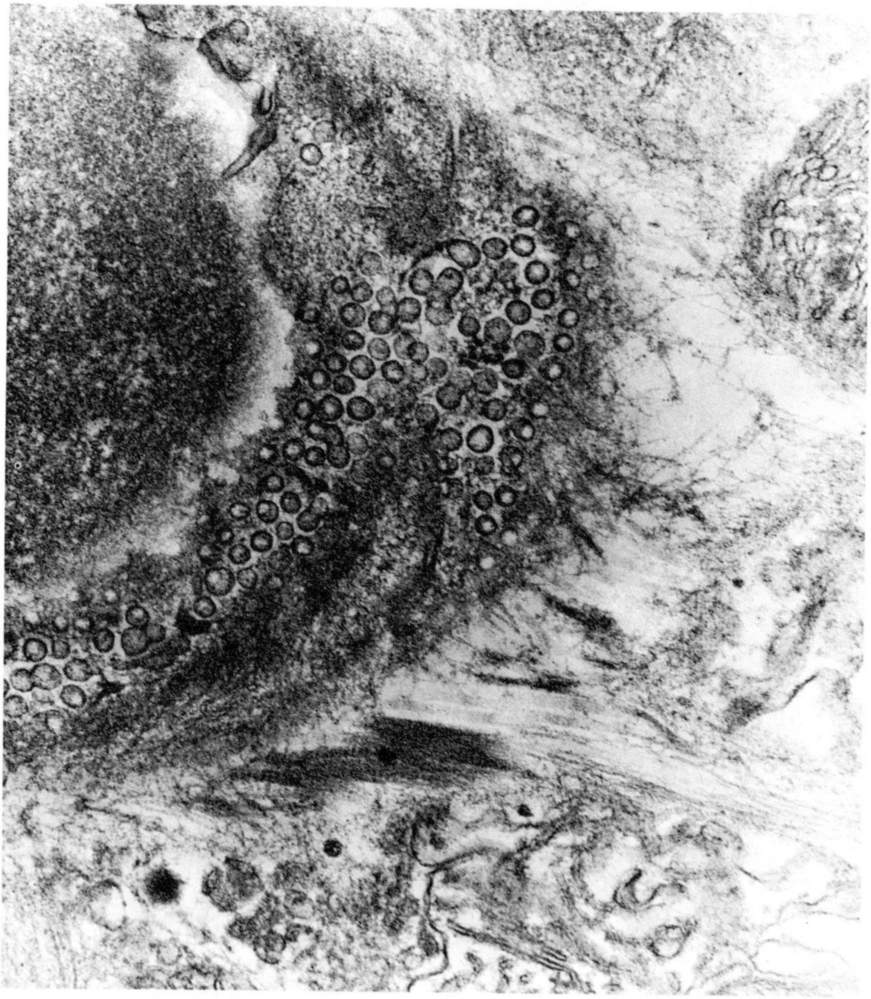

FIGURE 12. Detail from the center of FIGURE 11, at higher magnification. The typical structured appearance of fibrin strands is unmistakable. Note also the abundance of large and partly confluent cytoplasmic vesicles in the endothelial cell of the capillary. Stain: uranyl acetate. Orig. mag. × 31,000. (From Lehr, 1967. Reproduced by permission of the publisher.)

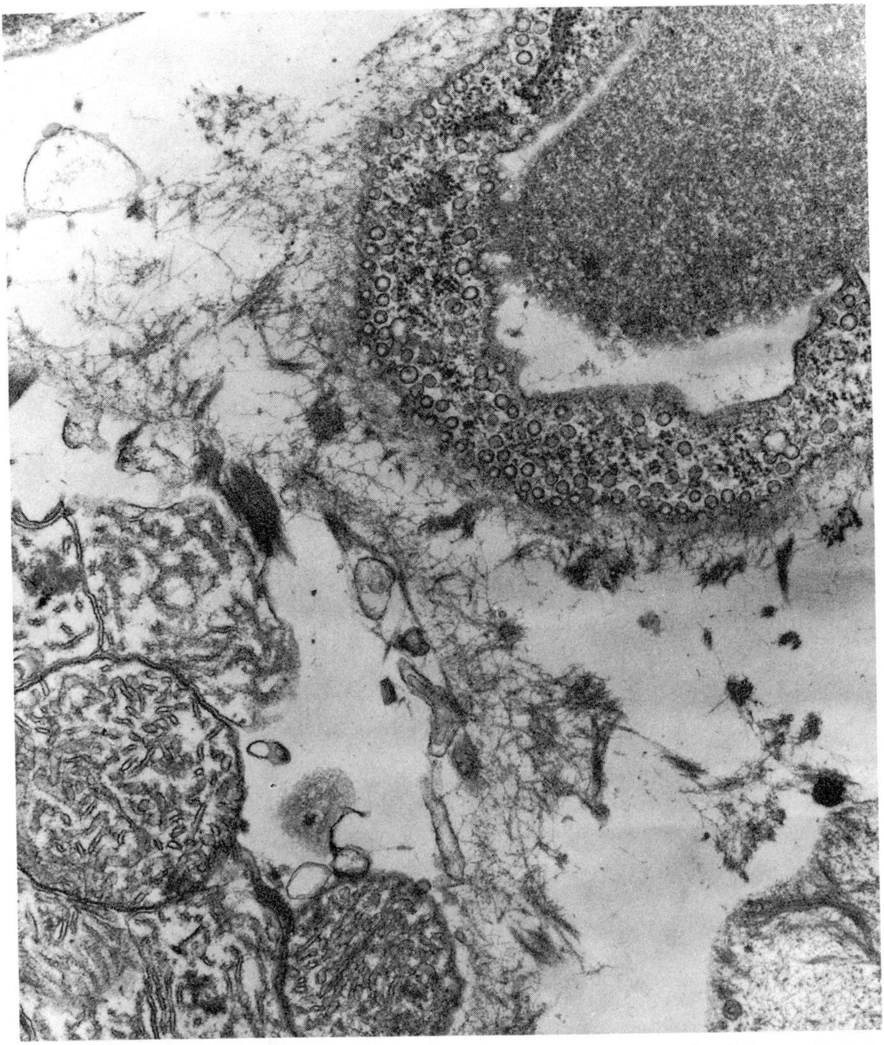

FIGURE 13. Same heart as shown in FIGURE 11. The endothelial cell of the capillary is loaded with electron-dense granules that are outside of the cytoplasmic vesicles. Electron-dense material appears to surround the capillary wall and to condense into fuzzy conglomerates or to form a fine web in the pericapillary space. Damaged sarcosomes may be seen at the lower left. Stain: uranyl acetate. Orig. mag. × 11,000.

whereas the renal calcium and phosphate values reflect the calcium salt deposition in this organ.

Parathyroidectomized rats, which were moribund after only two days of NaH_2PO_4 loading, invariably developed severe myocardial necrosis and characteristic changes of the electrolyte content, consisting of a decrease in magnesium and phosphate and an accumulation of sodium. Electrolyte alterations in the kidneys of these animals, which manifested extensive tubular necrosis rather

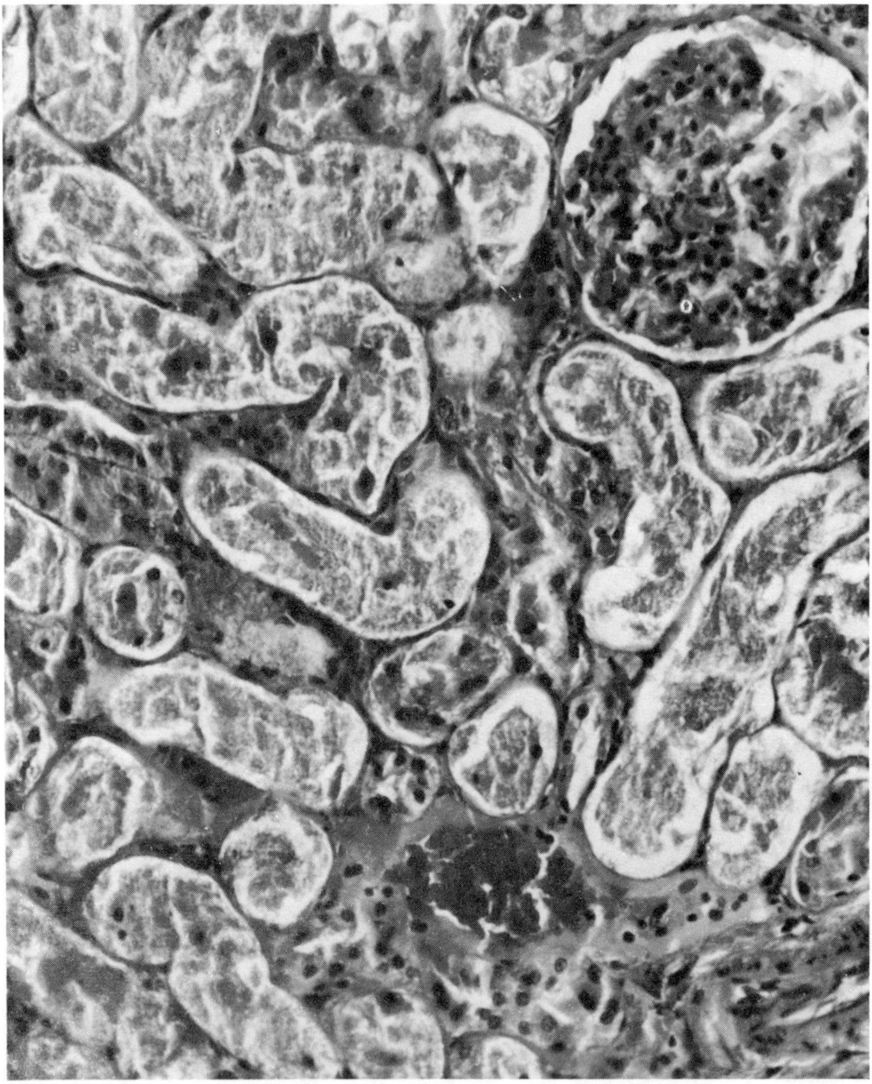

FIGURE 14. Kidney of parathyroidectomized albino rat after five NaH_2PO_4 loads. Note complete necrosis of epithelium of proximal convoluted tubules down to basement membrane. The tubular lumen is filled with proteinaceous epithelial eosinophilic debris. The glomerulus in the right upper corner of the photograph exhibits a thickened capsule and swollen, partly coalescing glomerular tufts. There is some dilatation of Bowman's space. Stain: hematoxylin-eosin. × 70 (orig. mag. × 120). (From Lehr *et al.*, 1967. Reproduced by permission of the publisher).

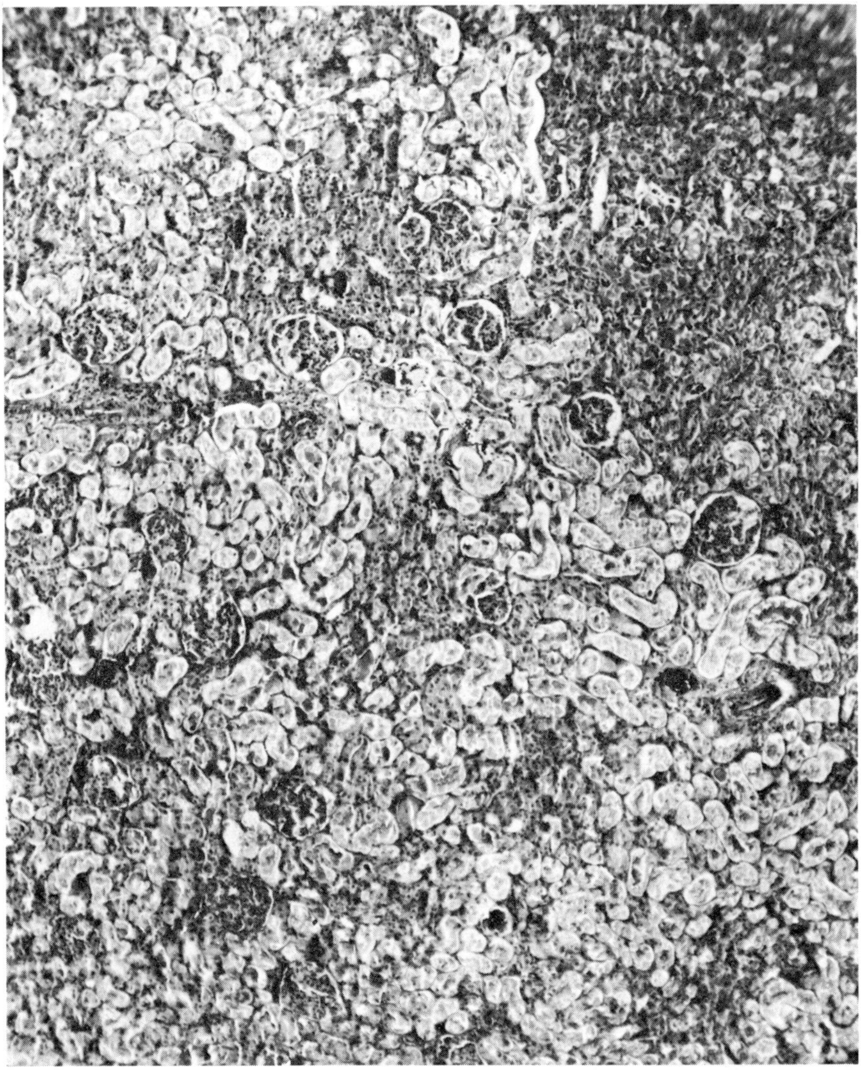

FIGURE 15. Kidney shown in FIGURE 14, at lower magnification. Note the embroidery-like pattern created by the extensive necrosis of proximal convoluted tubules and the partial flush-out of necrotic debris. Stain: hematoxylin-eosin. × 20 (orig. mag. × 35). (From Lehr *et al.*, 1967. Reproduced by permission of the publisher.)

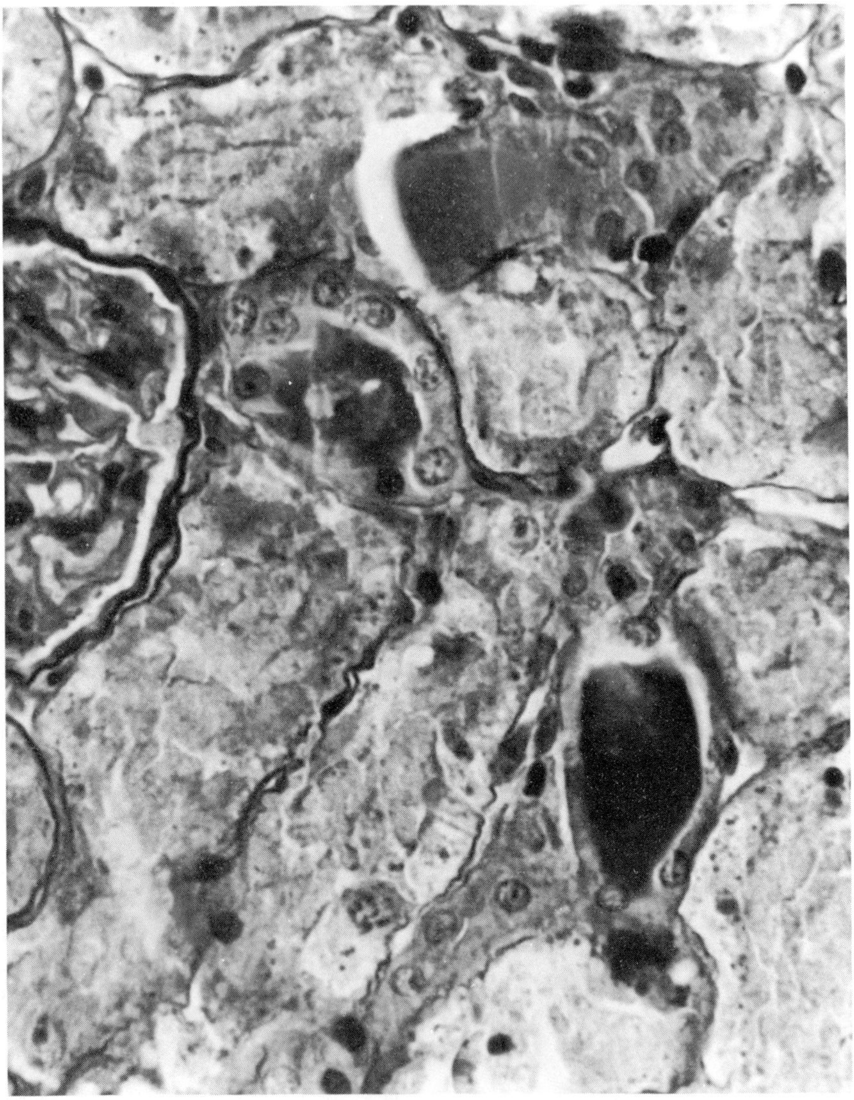

FIGURE 16. Kidney of parathyroidectomized albino rat after five NaH_2PO_4 loads. Note the PAS-positive material in glomerular tufts, Bowman's capsule, and lumen of some of damaged tubules appearing dark in the photograph, deep red in original stain. Stain: periodic-acid-Schiff. × 250 (orig. mag. × 400). (From Lehr *et al.*, 1967. Reproduced by permission of the publisher.)

TABLE 2

PROTECTIVE EFFECT OF PARATHYROID EXTRACT (PTE) AGAINST MYOCARDIAL NECROSIS PRODUCED BY SODIUM PHOSPHATE LOADING OF PARATHYROIDECTOMIZED RATS*

	No. of Rats	Incidence and Type of Cardiac Injury	Heart Electrolytes [Mean mEq/kg ± S.E. (wet weight)]					Incidence and Type of Renal Injury	Kidney Electrolytes [Mean mEq/kg ± S.E. (wet weight)]				
			Ca	P	Mg	Na	K		Ca	P	Mg	Na	K
Untreated Controls	15		2.8 ± 0.2	57.6 ± 1.0	19.1 ± 0.3	44.1 ± 0.6	83.6 ± 0.8		3.7 ± 0.2	64.0 ± 2.1	17.7 ± 0.2	69.2 ± 1.3	74.4 ± 1.1
Intact + NaH_2PO_4	12	—	3.5 ± 0.3	61.1 ± 1.2	19.2 ± 0.3	42.4 ± 0.7	82.1 ± 1.1	100% calcinosis	12.9 ± 2.2	76.9 ± 2.4	18.4 ± 0.5	68.6 ± 2.1	71.7 ± 0.9
Parathyroidectomized + NaH_2PO_4	15	100% necrosis	3.2 ± 0.2	53.5† ± 1.2	15.7‡ ± 0.4	49.0† ± 0.8	81.3 ± 0.8	100% necrosis	3.4† ± 0.2	56.6† ± 2.3	13.2† ± 0.4	86.3† ± 2.2	60.7‡ ± 2.7
Parathyroidectomized + NaH_2PO_4 + PTE (30 units)	20	23% necrosis		60.3 ± 1.2		47.3‡ ± 1.0	82.4 ± 0.8	45% necrosis	3.4† ± 0.2	67.6‡ ± 1.7		77.6‡ ± 2.1	71.3 ± 2.3
Parathyroidectomized + NaH_2PO_4 + PTE (50 units)	12	—	3.2 ± 0.1	61.4 ± 1.2	18.4 ± 0.3	43.8 ± 1.0	82.9 ± 0.5	50% calcinosis	5.7‡ ± 0.7	70.4 ± 1.8	16.6‡ ± 0.1	73.6 ± 1.3	70.2 ± 1.4
Parathyroidectomized + NaH_2PO_4 + PTE (100 units)	11	—	3.0 ± 0.3	66.2 ± 2.2	18.6 ± 0.2	44.1 ± 1.4	85.4 ± 1.0	56% calcinosis	9.5 ± 2.2	80.6 ± 3.3	17.8 ± 0.5	72.1 ± 1.8	69.6 ± 1.4

* From Lehr *et al.* (1966).
† Significance compared with intact rats + NaH_2PO_4: $p < 0.001$.
‡ Significance compared with intact rats + NaH_2PO_4: $p < 0.01$.

than calcinosis, were similar to those in the heart except for the additional lowering of the potassium content. It is of particular interest that the heavy loss of inorganic phosphate from myocardial and renal tissue occurred in the presence of pronounced hyperphosphatemia (serum inorganic phosphate levels of around 35 mg%) which caused hypocalcemic tetany (serum calcium levels of around 4.5 mg%) in all unprotected parathyroidectomized rats.

It can be seen further that the occurrence of these severe morphological and electrolyte disturbances are readily inhibited or totally obviated by the administration of parathyroid extract (PTE)† to parathyroidectomized rats during the period of NaH_2PO_4 loading. It should be emphasized that the entire range, from incipient preventive activity to full protection against cardiorenal necrosis, was encompassed by a dosage differential of only 20 units of PTE per rat daily. Animals treated with fully protective dosages of PTE were actually indistinguishable from the intact rats. Such animals were found to tolerate NaH_2PO_4 loading with impunity over extended periods of time.

Repair of Necrosis

The phenomena associated with healing of this particular type of cardiorenal necrosis were studied by my research associate, Dr. M. Krukowski. The analysis entailed correlation of morphological alterations at successive stages of repair with simultaneously occurring changes of the myocardial and renal electrolyte content and with abnormalities of the electrocardiogram (ECG). The tissue electrolyte pattern in hearts and kidneys of rats killed at the height of injury and at five predetermined stages of recovery, along with control values of intact and parathyroidectomized animals, are listed in TABLE 3.

It can be seen that, in the heart, the decreased inorganic phosphate and magnesium content and the increased sodium concentration observed at the peak of injury (no recovery) are still in evidence 24 hours after discontinuation of NaH_2PO_4 loading (one day of recovery). However, there is a distinct indication of return toward normal values for both sodium and phosphate, whereas magnesium is depressed still further and associated with a significant decrease in the myocardial potassium content.

After three days of recovery, the concentration of sodium has returned to normal and remains unaltered from this time on. Inorganic phosphate is in a low-normal range, magnesium stays significantly depressed, and there is a further marked depletion of potassium.

Two days later (fifth day of recovery), there is a substantial rise of phosphate, potassium, and magnesium levels, pointing toward rapid progression of healing. However, complete return to control values is not achieved for all electrolytes even one week later (12 days of recovery), since the concentration of myocardial magnesium at this time is still in a significantly subnormal range ($p < 0.001$). No further change in the electrolyte pattern is noted three months following injury.

The kidneys of animals sacrificed immediately following NaH_2PO_4 loading (no recovery) show, like the heart, significant alterations of inorganic phosphate, magnesium, and sodium. Compared with the myocardium, the derangement of these electrolytes is of much greater magnitude. However, the most outstanding distinction at this time, referred to earlier, is the presence of significant depletion of renal potassium (Lehr, 1965). By the third day, all

† Liberal supplies of PTE (injection parathyroid) were made available by Eli Lilly and Co., Indianapolis, Ind.

TABLE 3

ALTERATIONS IN THE TISSUE ELECTROLYTE PATTERN ASSOCIATED WITH VARIOUS PHASES OF REPAIR OF DISSEMINATED MYOCARDIAL NECROSIS

Group	No. of Rats	Heart Electrolytes [Mean mEq/kg ± S.E. (wet weight)]					Kidney Electrolytes [Mean mEq/kg ± S.E. (wet weight)]				
		Ca	P	Mg	Na	K	Ca	P	Mg	Na	K
Normal controls	15	2.8 ± 0.2	57.6 ± 1.0	19.1 ± 0.3	44.1 ± 0.6	83.6 ± 0.8	3.7 ± 0.2	64.0 ± 2.1	17.7 ± 0.2	69.2 ± 1.3	74.4 ± 1.1
Parathyroidectomized only	13	2.9 ± 0.2	58.4 ± 1.6	19.7 ± 0.3	43.1 ± 0.8	83.8 ± 0.8	4.1 ± 0.2	65.8 ± 1.5	17.8 ± 0.3	70.9 ± 1.3	76.8 ± 1.0
No recovery	16	2.9 ± 0.2	53.2* ± 1.1	17.3* ± 0.5	48.7* ± 1.7	81.7 ± 1.1	3.6 ± 0.2	53.4* ± 1.5	14.5* ± 0.3	83.5* ± 1.8	59.3* ± 1.7
One day of recovery	14	2.9 ± 0.2	54.4† ± 1.1	16.3* ± 0.2	45.8† ± 1.0	79.4* ± 1.0	3.5 ± 0.2	51.0* ± 2.1	14.1* ± 0.4	81.0* ± 2.6	64.1* ± 1.9
Three days of recovery	14	2.5 ± 0.2	54.6 ± 1.5	16.8* ± 0.3	44.0 ± 0.7	75.0* ± 1.1	3.3 ± 0.2	59.2 ± 3.7	15.8* ± 0.5	77.4† ± 2.1	67.2* ± 2.1
Five days of recovery	24	2.4† ± 0.1	56.8 ± 0.7	18.1* ± 0.1	44.9 ± 0.9	77.9* ± 0.8	3.0† ± 0.2	59.4† ± 1.5	16.2* ± 0.4	77.6† ± 2.0	72.6† ± 1.1
12 days of recovery	18	2.3† ± 0.1	55.8 ± 0.9	17.7* ± 0.2	43.1 ± 0.6	82.6 ± 0.5	3.0† ± 0.2	61.8 ± 1.5	16.1* ± 0.4	72.1 ± 1.9	74.8 ± 1.3
Three months of recovery	13	2.4 ± 0.2	55.9 ± 0.9	17.9* ± 0.2	44.0 ± 0.9	81.1 ± 1.0	3.5 ± 0.3	66.6 ± 0.9	16.9† ± 0.3	71.7 ± 0.9	76.4 ± 1.1

* Significance compared with parathyroidectomized rats: $p < 0.01$.
† Significance compared with parathyroidectomized rats: $p < 0.05$.

TABLE 4

SUCCESSIVE STAGES IN REPAIR OF DISSEMINATED MYOCARDIAL NECROSIS: CORRELATION OF MORPHOLOGICAL CHANGES WITH ALTERATIONS OF THE ELECTROLYTE PATTERN AND THE ELECTROCARDIOGRAM*

Group	Myocardial Electrolytes†				Microscopical Cardiac Pathology	Electrocardiography				Serum Range (mg%)	
	P	Mg	Na	K		Prolonged Q-at	High Take-off of T Wave	T Wave Ending in Negative Trough	Flat T_1	Ca	P
No recovery	↓↓	↓↓	↑↑	—	Degeneration necrosis inflammation	70%	100%	0%	0%	3–5	18–40
One day of recovery	↓	↓↓	↑	↓↓	Removal of muscular debris	100%	100%	100%	0%	4–6	16–40
Three days of recovery	—	↓↓	—	↓↓	Granulation tissue	100%	0%	60%	60%	5–7	12–16
Five days of recovery	—	↓↓	—	↓↓	Loose young scars	70%	0%	0%	67%	5–8	11–15
12 days of recovery	—	↓↓	—	—	Young contracting scars	50%	0%	0%	100%	5–7	11–15
Three months of recovery	—	↓↓	—	—	Focal and/or diffuse fibrosis	50%	0%	0%	60%	6–8	11–14

* All data based on a minimum of ten animals per group.

† Deviation from baseline values: ↓↓ = highly significant; ↓ = significant.

deranged electrolyte levels have shifted considerably in the direction of normal. The concentrations of inorganic phosphate and potassium continue to rise, whereas sodium declines, so that normal concentrations of these electrolytes have been reestablished by the 12th day of recovery. The magnesium content, on the other hand, rises only slightly, and, as in the myocardium, remains significantly depressed, even three months after injury.

Analyses of the electrolyte pattern in samples of stomach wall and diaphragm, done to ascertain whether or not there were simultaneously occurring electrolyte shifts in smooth and skeletal muscle, failed to reveal any significant alterations in the electrolyte content of these tissues, at any of the stages studied.

TABLE 4 contains a correlation of all significant deviations from the norm of the myocardial electrolyte content at the various stages of recovery, with the specific morphological status of repair at each stage as well as ECG changes and the range of calcium and inorganic phosphate levels in the serum. (It should be emphasized that sodium and potassium serum levels remained within normal limits at all stages of observation.)

It is apparent that the substantial return to normal of the electrolyte pattern coincided with the disappearance of muscular debris and the development of scar tissue. Lack of early potassium depletion was thought to be caused by myocardial infiltration with potassium-rich inflammatory cells, and the persistence of a subnormal magnesium content in the fully healed myocardium was attributed to "dilution" of the myocardium with collagen fibers of scar tissue which are known to be poor in magnesium (Manery, 1954).

The most significant early ECG abnormalities, consisting of a high take-off of the T wave and a prolonged Q-aT interval, were thought to be caused primarily by the severe derangement of the electrolyte pattern, whereas persistence of a flat T wave in the healed myocardium was interpreted as signifying considerable myocardial fibrosis. The correlation of all parameters will be discussed in greater detail elsewhere (Krukowski & Lehr, under publication).

Myocardial Necrosis Produced by Adrenergic Amines

The sympathomimetic amines appeared ideally suited as cardiotoxic agents for comparative studies involving the myocardial electrolyte content, since they are known to cause disseminated myocardial necrosis when used in excess and have, in fact, been implicated by Raab (1953) in such cardiac injury of human beings. Moreover, it is believed that the activity of the catecholamines released at the effector site as well as of exogenous compounds of this series is mediated through cation exchanges, and that adrenergic blocking agents may exert their antagonistic action by countering these ionic fluxes.

We selected isoproterenol at the start because Rona and his associates (1963), in extensive studies, had demonstrated the high efficacy of this compound as a cardiotoxic agent and had perfected a simple and well-standardized method for the production of myocardial necrosis with this catecholamine. Furthermore, these same Canadian workers had presented evidence for the beneficial influence of a high potassium diet and the deleterious effect of a high sodium diet and of mineralocorticoids in isoproterenol-induced myocardial necrosis. Finally, the gross and microscopical appearance of the injury closely resembled the lesions produced by our method of NaH_2PO_4 loading of parathyroidectomized rats, and Ferrans and co-workers (1964) had demonstrated that, within two hours of isoproterenol injection, the mitochondria and the sarcotubular system of myocardial cells may show changes that are likewise similar in appearance to early lesions encountered with our method (FIGURES 6 and 7).

Development of Necrosis

The gross and light microscopical appearance of myocardial necrosis produced by isoproterenol has been described in detail elsewhere in this monograph (Kahn *et al.*, 1968) and is, therefore, omitted from this paper. The data correlating cardiac electrolyte values with the incidence of myocardial necrosis under the influence of isoproterenol,‡ propranolol,§ or the combination of these two compounds after three, seven, and 24 hours are summarized in TABLE 5. The beta-adrenergic blocking agent propranolol was administered in an equimolecular dosage five minutes prior to the injection of isoproterenol. The subcutaneous route was used throughout.

One is impressed by the similarity in alterations of the electrolyte pattern occurring in isoproterenol-induced myocardial necrosis and the changes illustrated earlier in NaH_2PO_4-loaded parathyroidectomized rats (TABLE 2), except that with isoproterenol-induced necrosis there is an additional increase in the calcium content. It is interesting that calcium accumulation and the depletion of magnesium and phosphate, all of a highly significant degree, are encountered as early as three and seven hours after isoproterenol injection. In the three-hour group, no morphological alterations could be discerned under close inspection with a binocular loupe, but a 60% incidence of myocardial necrosis was encountered after the seven-hour exposure to isoproterenol. A significant sodium increase is noted only at the 24-hour interval, when severe myocardial injury was present in every single animal. Additional experiments, carried out recently, indicate that magnesium depletion can be demonstrated as early as one hour after isoproterenol injection.

Another aspect that stands out dramatically is the constancy in the total myocardial potassium content, despite the substantial alterations of all the other electrolytes tested. This fact deserves emphasis in view of the important role ascribed to this ion by many authors in the production and prevention of experimental myocardial necrosis. A shift of potassium between compartments can, of course, not be excluded by our method.

It can be seen further that propranolol is highly effective in inhibiting the emergence of isoproterenol-induced myocardial necrosis. Although calcium accumulation is not fully prevented by the beta-adrenergic blocking agent, there is a significant rise, rather than a fall, of phosphate after seven and 24 hours, and a significant drop in sodium, rather than a rise, at the 24-hour interval. The reason for the overshoot in the case of these two electrolytes is under study. Moreover, there is no deviation from the norm in the magnesium content of these animals. Finally, propranolol alone caused no morphological alterations and no changes whatsoever from the normal in the tissue electrolyte content. It is noteworthy that no abnormalities of the electrolyte content and no morphological changes were observed in striated muscle (diaphragm) and smooth muscle (stomach wall) of animals belonging to any of the three experimental groups.

Since isoproterenol is primarily a beta-adrenergic agent, the myocardial necrosis produced by this drug was compared with similar injury following injection of predominantly alpha-adrenergic agents, metaraminol and phenyl-

‡ Isoproterenol was generously supplied by Winthrop Laboratories, New York, N. Y.
§ Propranolol was generously supplied by the Ayerst Laboratories, New York, N. Y.

TABLE 5

TISSUE ELECTROLYTE PATTERN IN ISOPROTERENOL-INDUCED MYOCARDIAL NECROSIS AND THE EFFECT OF BETA-ADRENERGIC BLOCKADE*

Drugs Injected	No. of Rats	Time after Injection (hours)	Heart Electrolytes [Mean mEq/kg ± S.E. (wet weight)]					Incidence of Lesions (%)
			Ca	P	Mg	Na	K	
Normal controls	15		2.8 ± 0.2	57.6 ± 0.1	19.2 ± 0.3	44.1 ± 0.6	83.6 ± 0.8	
Isoproterenol	12	3	3.8† ± 0.1	53.9† ± 0.6	17.0† ± 0.8	42.4 ± 0.9	83.0 ± 1.5	0
	10	7	4.8† ± 0.1	53.6 ± 1.9	16.3† ± 0.3	47.1 ± 1.7	83.0 ± 1.5	60
	14	24	4.3† ± 0.3	48.1† ± 1.5	15.6† ± 0.3	53.0† ± 1.3	81.3 ± 1.0	100
Isoproterenol plus propranolol	12	3	4.3† ± 0.2	57.4 ± 0.8	20.8 ± 0.5	42.1 ± 1.6	84.9 ± 0.9	0
	10	7	3.3 ± 0.1	61.0‡ ± 0.6	19.9 ± 0.4	46.2‡ ± 0.7	82.3 ± 1.3	0
	12	24	3.8‡ ± 0.4	62.1† ± 1.0	19.6 ± 0.3	41.9‡ ± 0.7	81.9 ± 1.3	25
Propranolol	5	7	2.9 ± 0.1	58.4 ± 1.1	19.8 ± 0.3	43.9 ± 1.5	79.5 ± 1.4	0
	10	24	3.1 ± 0.2	59.9 ± 1.8	19.6 ± 0.4	42.9 ± 1.9	82.2 ± 1.8	0

* Modified from Lehr *et al.* (1966).
† Significance compared with normal controls: $p < 0.01$.
‡ Significance compared with normal controls: $p < 0.05$.

ephrine, and also with epinephrine, which possesses both alpha- and beta-adrenergic activity. In addition to propranolol, the alpha-adrenergic antagonist tolazoline was used to test the specific protective effectiveness against the necrotizing action of equimolecular amounts of either alpha- or beta-agonists.

TABLE 6 depicts the number of survivors among groups of albino rats, 24 hours after a single subcutaneous injection of one of several adrenergic amines, with and without pretreatment with specific antagonists. In addition, it relates changes of the myocardial electrolyte content of the surviving rats to the incidence of morphological lesions encountered in these animals.

It is apparent that the myocardial electrolyte imbalance created by the alpha-adrenergic agent metaraminol is similar to that caused by isoproterenol (see TABLE 5), except for more pronounced calcium accumulation. Phenylephrine and epinephrine likewise induced magnesium depletion and even more conspicuous increases in the calcium and sodium content, but no significant losses of inorganic phosphate. There were, thus, both similarities and differences in the derangement of the electrolyte pattern produced by these three adrenergic amines; this finding pointed toward a considerable degree of specificity, since the lack of similarity could not be accounted for solely by the variation in degree and incidence of lesions.

Interestingly, there were distinct differences also in the electron microscopical picture of the myocardial injury produced by these adrenergic amines when injected in the dosages shown in TABLE 6. These morphological differences will be depicted elsewhere in detail, but it should be emphasized that the basic features of the injury were similar in all instances, consisting of swelling of sarcosomes and severe structural damage to their cristae, rupture and complete disintegration of myofibrils, pronounced swelling of the sarcotubular system, and, finally, intracellular edema.

The lower half of TABLE 6 illustrates the effect of pretreatment with autonomic blocking agents. It is of interest that the beta-adrenergic antagonist propranolol, which sharply reduced the incidence and also the degree of myocardial lesions caused by isoproterenol, and completely obviated the emergence of tissue electrolyte changes characteristic of necrosis, failed to show any protective effect against the injurious action of the alpha-adrenergic agent phenylephrine. The alpha-adrenergic antagonist tolazoline, on the other hand, readily and completely prevented phenylephrine-induced necrosis. Finally, simultaneous blocking of both alpha- and beta-adrenergic receptors was needed to obviate the toxic sequelae of epinephrine injection. (The values for calcium were unfortunately lost in this instance through a technical error.)

In recent studies not depicted in TABLE 6, it was found that metaraminol-induced injury was likewise effectively blocked by tolazoline and partially also by the alpha-adrenergic antagonist dibozane, whereas propranolol was again without effect in this instance.

Healing of Necrosis

Studies on the influence of repair of catecholamine-induced necrosis upon the alteration of the myocardial electrolyte pattern are presently in progress. Information available at this writing justifies the statement that the findings are in line with those reported on the healing of myocardial injury produced by our method of NaH_2PO_4 loading in parathyroidectomized rats. Thus, it was found that three as well as five days after injection of necrosis-producing amounts of an alpha- or beta-adrenergic amine (phenylephrine or isoproterenol),

TABLE 6

ALTERATIONS OF MYOCARDIAL ELECTROLYTE PATTERN INDUCED BY ADRENERGIC AMINES AND THE EFFECT OF ADRENERGIC BLOCKADE

Group	Dose (mg/kg)	No. of Rats (survived/total)	Heart Electrolytes [Mean mEq/kg ± S.E. (wet weight)]					Incidence of Lesions (%)
			Ca	P	Mg	Na	K	
Control		17	2.9 ± 0.3	60.6 ± 1.2	19.6 ± 0.3	40.3 ± 0.7	75.9 ± 0.9	
Phenylephrine	15.0	18/24	7.8* ± 1.7	58.5 ± 1.9	17.0† ± 0.3	57.0† ± 2.2	78.5 ± 1.0	78
Epinephrine	4.0	15/22	14.0† ± 2.2	57.9 ± 1.3	15.6† ± 0.3	54.5† ± 1.4	72.3 ± 1.6	100
Metaraminol	10.0	24/25	6.3† ± 0.7	54.6† ± 1.1	17.3† ± 0.3	50.2† ± 1.6	75.9 ± 2.1	80
Phenylephrine + propranolol	15.0 14.75	13/16	6.2* ± 1.2	54.7* ± 1.2	17.5† ± 0.3	45.8‡ ± 2.9	75.3 ± 1.0	76
Phenylephrine + tolazoline	15.0 17.1	10/10	4.0 ± 0.4	63.7 ± 1.8	20.1 ± 0.4	42.2 ± 1.1	78.9 ± 1.6	0
Epinephrine + tolazoline + propranolol	4.0 17.1 14.75	7/7		61.3 ± 1.7	18.9 ± 0.2	41.1 ± 1.2	82.1† ± 1.1	0

* Significance compared with control group: $p < 0.01$.
† Significance compared with control group: $p < 0.001$.
‡ Significance compared with control group: $p < 0.05$.

the inorganic phosphate and potassium content of the myocardium was still significantly below normal, whereas the sodium content had returned into the physiological range.

Discussion

Perusal of the literature reveals a surprising dearth of experimental studies in which major efforts were made to correlate myocardial necrosis with alterations of the tissue electrolyte content. Some information is available on one particular injury of this type, designated as electrolyte-steroid cardiac necrosis (ESCN) by Selye (1958). In 1959, du Ruisseau and Mori found a marked depletion of magnesium and an increase in the sodium and calcium content. This was accompanied by an increase of sodium and calcium in the abdominal muscle. Mishra (1960) likewise reported magnesium depletion. Nickerson and co-workers (1961), who determined only the potassium concentration in ESCN, observed a significant decrease of this ion in the heart, and postulated that the necrosis resulted from intracellular potassium depletion, and that it was, moreover, histologically indistinguishable from myocardial lesions induced by potassium deficiency. Prioreschi (1962), on the other hand, showed that, in the ESCN method, potassium loss occurred in hearts irrespective of the development of necrosis, and that substantial potassium depletion, as well as a rise in sodium, was observed only after necrosis was established. He therefore did not accept the hypothesis that potassium loss causes myocardial necrosis.

Based on the many studies of the electrolyte pattern in acute myocardial necrosis carried out in our laboratory, we are inclined to agree with Prioreschi's view, since the potassium content remained initially unchanged in the face of highly significant depletion of magnesium and phosphate and an increase in sodium content (Lehr *et al.*, 1966). It was only later, in fully developed necrosis and in the early stages of repair, that the potassium content began to drop. A similar observation was made by Cameron and Spector (1961) in the livers of dietetically deficient rats.

There is little doubt that some of the alterations of the electrolyte content encountered in chronic experiments, such as depletion of myocardial potassium in ESCN, are secondary in nature. This seems to apply equally to the substantial simultaneous rises in calcium and phosphate which usually denote secondary calcification.

It is of interest, in this connection, that, according to D'Agostino (1964), the ESCN lesion produced in rats by the combined administration of 9α-fluorocortisol and sodium phosphate is characterized by the appearance of granular and crystalline inclusions in mitochondria which morphologically resemble hydroxyapatite. D'Agostino suggests that the mitochondrial inclusion may represent calcium phosphate and that a functional alteration of mitochondria induced by the mineralocorticoid and sodium phosphate results in an accumulation of minerals. He refers to biochemical evidence which indicates that the accumulation of calcium and phosphate within mitochondria can substitute for the formation of adenosine triphosphate (ATP) and thus interfere with certain steps of oxidative phosphorylation. Prolongation of such an insult to mitochondria could then result in cell degeneration and necrosis. Such an interpretation may, in his view, also be applicable in the mechanism of cell death produced by other interferences with phosphorylation reactions, as in magnesium deficiency. Magnesium is an activator ion in various transphosphorylation reactions, and similar mitochondrial inclusions have been described in magnesium deficiency.

It is our view that certain consistently occurring early shifts in the tissue electrolyte pattern which accompany the emergence of cellular necrosis produced by a number of unrelated methods are not merely a consequence of cellular impairment and death, but may, in fact, play a contributory role in the initiation of cellular dysfunction. The remarkably similar pattern starting with magnesium and phosphate depletion and followed by sodium accumulation, in similar organic injuries produced by different and apparently unrelated means, suggests that these electrolyte changes are a specific expression of deranged cellular function. Since the ionic shifts precede morphological alterations readily detectable under the light microscope, they would seem to constitute a more sensitive parameter for the discovery of cellular derangement than histological examinations.

It is possible that these electrolyte alterations are the result of interference with ionic transfer at the plasma membrane and at important subcellular sites (mitochondria), and that the resulting ionic imbalance contributes to the initiation of a state of irreversible failure of cell function. In favor of a causative role of electrolyte disturbances, one may cite the production of myocardial necrosis by diets that exclude magnesium and potassium, and the well-known enhancing effect of mineralocorticoids and of sodium loading in the development of cardiovascular injury. Mention should also be made of the well-documented observations that changes of the intracellular electrolyte content which encompass a decrease in potassium and magnesium and an increase in sodium, chloride, and calcium are not the consequence but rather the cause of hypoxic heart failure (Hochrein & Lossnitzer, 1968).

Further support for a contributing role of electrolyte shifts in the mechanism of cellular injury can be derived from the remarkable protection that can be achieved against the emergence of disseminated myocardial and cardiorenal necrosis by the administration of electrolyte solutions containing either chloride, magnesium, or potassium (Selye, 1958; Tucker *et al.,* 1963; Lehr *et al.,* 1966). This protection has been accomplished even in necrosis ostensibly not produced or suspected to be based on depletion of these ions.

With regard to experimental data presented in this paper, it should be emphasized that both parathyroid hormone and the heart-active catecholamines are known to exert profound effects upon electrolyte movements and ionic homeostasis at the cellular and probably also at the subcellular level. Recent investigations with isolated mitochondria infer a fundamental and general function of parathyroid hormone. It has been proposed that this hormone effects ionic distribution across subcellular as well as cellular membranes, and that the plasma membrane and mitochondrial membrane probably possess basically similar mechanisms for transporting calcium and phosphate. In accordance with this view, the primary effect of parathyroid hormone is on the cellular accumulation and transport of calcium and phosphate in a variety of tissues. Although the movement of calcium ions across membranes requires the additional presence of vitamin D, the translocation of inorganic phosphate is dependent solely upon parathyroid hormone (Rasmussen & DeLuca, 1963).

The singular importance ascribed to parathyroid hormone in the transport of phosphate is fully supported by our findings that parathyroidectomized animals, under heavy NaH_2PO_4 load, exhibited marked phosphate depletion in the myocardium and kidneys in the face of pronounced accumulation of this anion in the blood, and that the disturbance could be readily obviated by adequate substitution with PTE. Thus, there is no doubt that, in special stress situations, parathyroid hormone may be vital for the preservation of cardiac and renal integrity. It appears likely that a similar situation may be found to exist in a number of other organs.

The lack of phosphate transfer into the cell interior, together with a substantial loss of myocardial magnesium, would seem to fit well with the picture of massive disintegration of mitochondrial structures observed in the myocardial fibers of these animals. Mitochondria are known to contain large quantities of magnesium and phosphate (Thiers & Vallee, 1957).

Regarding the possible role of electrolyte shifts in the mechanism of action of catecholamines upon the heart, it has been proposed that sympathomimetic amines affect permeability for sodium and possibly other ions, thus tending to depolarize the membrane and to increase excitability (Hutter, 1957), and that adrenergic blocking agents may exert their antagonistic action by specifically countering these ionic fluxes (Sréter & Friedman, 1961; Zaimis, 1964). Major and sustained electrolyte shifts in the presence of toxic concentrations of heart-active catecholamines might therefore be explained on the basis of a direct and specific action, rather than as the sequelae of other eliciting factors, such as absolute or relative oxygen deficiency. In fact, even the chief proponents of the hypoxia theory of catecholamine-induced myocardial necrosis do not fail to emphasize the important contributory influence of sodium and the protective effect of potassium, as well as the deleterious contribution of mineralocorticoids, which may cause both sodium accumulation and potassium depletion.

With regard to the prevention of catecholamine-induced myocardial necrosis by adrenergic blocking agents, it was indicated earlier that the antagonists may exert their beneficial effect by interfering with ionic shifts associated with the depolarization and repolarization of the muscle membrane. An additional explanation relates to the enzyme phosphorylase. Accumulation of this enzyme is needed for the breakdown of glycogen, and is promoted by adenosine 3,5-phosphate (cyclic 3,5-AMP). It has been shown (Sutherland, 1963) that almost all adenyl cyclase, the enzyme system which forms cyclic 3,5-AMP from ATP, is located in the cell membrane of various tissues and that catecholamines (isoproterenol, epinephrine, and norepinephrine) have a catalytic effect on the formation of cyclic 3,5-AMP which is blocked by the beta-adrenergic antagonist dichloroisoproterenol. On the basis of these observations, it was proposed (Zaimis, 1964) that the "therapeutic" effect of the beta-adrenergic blocking agents may result from their ability to inhibit certain metabolic effects of the catecholamines, which may include the regulation of the "recovery" process of the cell after activation. On the other hand, the inability of the beta-adrenergic antagonist propranolol to prevent the emergence of myocardial necrosis induced by alpha-adrenergic stimulants suggests a high specificity of antagonistic action.

In the face of this multiplicity of theories, the depletion of the intracellular ion magnesium, representing an early and consistent change in the development of myocardial necrosis produced by two unrelated procedures, emerges as a finding that deserves closer scrutiny in view of the known significance of magnesium in vital enzymatic and energy processes of the cell. On the basis of our experimental findings to date, including preliminary results with magnesium-excluding diets (unpublished data), and the known importance of the magnesium ion, we are inclined to believe that magnesium loss, in particular, may contribute to the initiation of cellular injury, and that this event may, perhaps, play a role in many apparently unrelated experimental situations that result in cellular dysfunction and necrosis in the heart and in other organs.

It is of particular interest, in this connection, that the similarity in disturbance of the tissue electrolyte pattern was reflected in striking similarities of the electron microscopical changes (as indicated previously). Mention should be made of the thorough work of Heggtveit (1965) with myocardial injury resulting from magnesium depletion and the studies of Rona and co-workers (1963) and of Ferrans and his associates (1964) with adrenergic amines.

It should be kept in mind that the term necrosis, as used by the pathologist, implies cellular death and disintegration. It is based on observations of morphological alterations with the naked eye or the microscope. From the point of view of cell function, necrosis represents the terminal structural expression of an irreversible process that had undoubtedly reached the "point of no return" and, in fact, inexorable progression long before the ultimate morphological signs of cell death have made their appearance.

For the purpose of devising prophylactic and therapeutic measures in the many clinical conditions that may lead to cardiovascular necrosis, in particular, and cellular necrosis, in general, it would be of vital importance to be able to distinguish the stages of progression from reversible to irreversible injury as early as possible and, preferably, in other than purely morphological terms. On the basis of our studies to date, it seems that analysis of progressive alterations of the tissue electrolyte pattern offers one such possibility, particularly if studied in conjunction with examination of morphological alterations at the cellular and subcellular level (electron microscope), and perhaps also with the observations of electrical phenomena at the membrane and the interior of the cell (electrogram, transmembrane potential), which we are conducting at present.

Finally, in the face of the apparent rapidity of major changes in the myocardial electrolyte content induced by adrenergic amines, one wonders whether certain ionic shifts are necessary for the specific pharmacological effect of many drugs active in the cardiovascular system and elsewhere, and, if so, whether noticeable alterations of the tissue electrolyte pattern could be uncovered with dosages lying within the therapeutic range. If, on the other hand, such changes were to constitute concomitant untoward reactions, merely contributing to the toxicity of the drug in question, proper corrective measures could be instituted without interference with the therapeutic aims.

It should be pointed out, that, although the determination of the total tissue electrolyte content does not make it possible to distinguish between extra- and intracellular positions of ions, the electrolyte composition of interstitial fluid is known to be similar to that of serum. Hence, substantial alterations of the tissue electrolyte content, which are not reflected in corresponding changes of simultaneously determined serum electrolyte concentrations, can be assumed to constitute evidence for the participation of the cell interior. Thus, our finding of magnesium depletion, phosphate depletion, and sodium accumulation in damaged tissues could be explained only by the involvement of intracellular compartments.

In conclusion, there were close similarities in the alterations of the electrolyte content in myocardial necrosis produced by two unrelated procedures, and a definite sequence of events appeared to govern the emergence and recession of electrolyte imbalance in the evolution and healing of this injury. The emphasis upon a possible contributory role of substantial electrolyte shifts in the pathogenesis of cellular injury is not intended to detract from the importance of oxygen deficiency and other disturbances as the prime eliciting factors. Nevertheless, our data do not rule out the possibility that certain early electrolyte shifts might occur as independent primary events, e.g. as a result of interference with important transport mechanisms in situations of special stress, or as the sequelae of exaggerated pharmacological responses at specific cellular receptor sites.

Finally, as was pointed out elsewhere (Lehr *et al.*, 1966), with all due consideration of differences between species and between experimental and clinical conditions, the demonstration of early loss of magnesium in the evolvement of experimental myocardial necrosis might prove of considerable importance for the prophylaxis and treatment of human myocardial failure and necrosis, whether produced by vascular occlusion or otherwise. In this connection, greater emphasis should perhaps be given to the possibility that large dosages of sympathomimetic amines, often used in shock due to myocardial infarction, may aggravate electrolyte depletion of the heart, enhance necrosis, and initiate dangerous arrhythmias. In this situation, the judicious simultaneous employment of "beneficial" electrolytes (e.g., $MgCl_2$ or KCl) may lessen or obviate these dangers. Moreover, the use of such electrolytes alone may aid the failing heart and limit the spread of necrosis by restoring partially damaged cells to full function. The "polarizing" treatment, introduced by Sodi-Pallares and his associates (1962) in Mexico and by Laborit and his associates (1958) and Weber and his co-workers (1958) in France, represents convincing evidence of the experimental and clinical effectiveness of electrolyte solutions in the treatment of heart failure and myocardial infarction. These so-called polarizing solutions make use of the beneficial effects of potassium, magnesium, and chloride. Confirmation of the effectiveness of this therapy has since come from many laboratories (Larcan, 1966; Nieper and Blumberger, 1966; Hochrein & Lossnitzer, 1968).

Summary

In studies on disseminated myocardial necrosis produced in the parathyroidectomized albino rat by oral sodium phosphate loading, attention was focused upon correlation of changes in morphology at successive stages of evolvement and repair of the injury with alterations of the myocardial electrolyte content.

The earliest discernible submicroscopical changes in myocardial cells consisted of swelling and degeneration of sarcosomes and enlargement of the sarcotubular reticulum. These alterations preceded disintegration of myofibrils and were associated with significant deviations from the norm of the myocardial electrolyte content, consisting of a decrease in magnesium and inorganic phosphate and an increase in sodium, whereas potassium remained initially remarkably constant, and calcium stayed within the physiological range throughout.

The kidneys of such animals exhibited extensive tubular necrosis and similar changes of the electrolyte pattern, except for an additional early decrease of the potassium content.

Despite the severity of the organic injury, timely discontinuation of sodium phosphate loading usually led to full recovery. In the heart, the elevated sodium concentration declined to normal in the initial phase of healing, whereas a decreased inorganic phosphate level was maintained during the first three to five days of repair. The potassium content dropped to a low level around the third day of repair and stayed in this range for several additional days. The magnesium concentration remained below normal for extended periods (three months.)

A similar picture of ultramicroscopical changes and shifts in electrolyte content, except for an additional early elevation of the calcium content, was encountered in the development and healing of disseminated myocardial necrosis produced in the albino rat by the subcutaneous injection of adrenergic amines in excessive dosage. The characteristic sequence and pattern of electrolyte deviations in the myocardium were encountered irrespective of whether the beta-adrenergic agonist isoproterenol or the alpha-adrenergic amines metaraminol and phenylephrine were utilized as the necrosis-eliciting agents. The same results were achieved with epinephrine, which has both alpha- and beta-adrenergic activity, except for a far more pronounced elevation of the myocardial calcium content.

The morphological and electrolyte alterations could be readily obviated by pretreatment with the beta-adrenergic blocking agent propranolol, in the case of isoproterenol, or with the alpha-adrenergic antagonist tolazoline, in the case of metaraminol and phenylephrine, whereas complete prevention of epinephrine-induced myocardial injury necessitated combined alpha- and beta-adrenergic blockade.

No abnormalities were found in the anatomical appearance of skeletal muscle (diaphragm) and smooth muscle of the gut (stomach wall) as a result of either of the two procedures employed, nor were there any deviations from the norm in the electrolyte content of these structures.

It is thought that the described early changes of the myocardial electrolyte content could have been initiated by abnormalities of ionic transfer at the plasma membrane and subcellular membrane sites of the living cell, and that the resulting ionic derangement might have contributed to initiation of irreversible failure of cellular function.

References

Bajusz, E. & G. Jasmin. 1962. Protective action of serotonin against certain chemically and surgically induced cardiac necrosis. Rev. Canad. Biol. **21:** 51–62.

Cameron, R. & W. G. Spector. 1961. The Chemistry of the Injured Cell. Charles C Thomas, Publ. Springfield, Ill.

D'Agostino, A. N. 1964. An electron microscopic study of cardiac necrosis produced by 9α-fluorocortisol and sodium phosphate. Amer. J. Path. **45:** 633–644.

du Ruisseau, J. P. & K. Mori. 1959. Biochemical studies on experimental cardiopathy electrolyte in rat tissues. Brit. J. Exp. Path. **40:** 250–254.

Ferrans, V. J., R. G. Hibbs, W. C. Black & D. G. Weilbaecher. 1964. Isoproterenol-induced myocardial necrosis. A histochemical and electron microscopic study. Amer. Heart J. **68:** 71–90.

Heggtveit, H. A. 1965. The cardiomyopathy of magnesium-deficiency. *In* Electrolytes and Cardiovascular Diseases. E. Bajusz, Ed. **1:** 204–220. S. Karger. Basel, Switzerland.

Hochrein, H. A. & K. Lossnitzer. The interrelation between myocardial metabolism and heart failure. This monograph.

Hutter, O. F. 1957. Mode of action of autonomic transmitters on the heart. Brit. Med. Bull. **13:** 176–180.

Kahn, D. S., G. Rona & C. I. Chappel. 1968. Isoproterenol-induced necrosis. This monograph.

Laborit, H., B. Weber, P. Niaussat, J. M. Jouany, G. Guiot, J. Zawadowski & C. Baron. 1958. Note préliminaire sur l'étude expérimentale de quelque sels de l'acide D, L-aspartate. Anesth. Analg. (Paris) **15:** 480–494.

Larcan, A. 1966. Pathophysiological basis and practical application of a 'metabolic' therapy of myocardial infarction. *In* Electrolytes and Cardiovascular Diseases. E. Bajusz, Ed. **2:** 277–301. S. Karger. Basel, Switzerland.

LEHR, D. 1965. The role of certain electrolytes and hormones in disseminated myocardial necrosis. *In* Electrolytes and Cardiovascular Diseases. E. Bajusz, Ed. **1:** 248–273. S. Karger, Basel Switzerland.

LEHR, D. 1967. About the pathogenesis of perivascular myocardial necrosis. 4th European Conf. Microcirc., Cambridge, 1966. Bibl. Anat. **9:** 355–362.

LEHR, D., M. KRUKOWSKI & R. COLÓN. 1966. Correlation of myocardial and renal necrosis with tissue electrolyte changes. J.A.M.A. **197:** 105–112.

LEHR, D., M. KRUKOWSKI & R. COLÓN. 1967. A simple method for the production of acute cardiorenal necrosis. Arch. Int. Pharmacodyn. **168:** 251–277.

MANERY, J. F. 1954. Water and electrolyte metabolism. Physiol. Rev. **34:** 334–417.

MISHRA, R. K. 1960. Studies on experimental magnesium deficiency in the albino rat. I. Functional and morphological changes associated with low intake of Mg. Rev. Canad. Biol. **19:** 122–135.

NICKERSON, M., G. W. KARR & P. E. DRESEL. 1961. Pathogenesis of "electrolyte-steroid-cardiopathy". Circ. Res. **9:** 209–217.

NIEPER, H. A. & K. BLUMBERGER. 1966. Electrolyte transport therapy of cardiovascular diseases. Experimental and clinical basis. *In* Electrolytes and Cardiovascular Diseases. E. Bajusz, Ed. **2:** 141–173. S. Karger. Basel, Switzerland.

PRIORESCHI, P. 1962. Role of potassium in the pathogenesis of the electrolyte-steroid-cardiopathy with necrosis". Circ. Res. **10:** 782–785.

RAAB, W. 1953. Hormonal and Neurogenic Cardiovascular Disorders. Williams & Wilkins Co. Baltimore, Md.

RASMUSSEN, H. & H. F. DELUCA. 1963. Calcium homeostasis. Ergebn. Physiol. **53:** 108–173.

RONA, G., D. S. KAHN & C. I. CHAPPEL. 1963. Studies on infarct-like myocardial necrosis produced by isoproterenol: A review. Rev. Canad. Biol. **22:** 241–255.

ROSENBLUM, I., A. WOHL & A. A. STEIN. 1965. Studies in cardiac necrosis. I. Production of cardiac lesions with sympathomimetic amines. Toxic. Appl. Pharmacol. **7:** 1–8.

SELYE, H. 1958. Chemical Prevention of Cardiac Necroses. The Ronald Press. New York, N. Y.

SODI-PALLARES, D., M. TESTELLI, B. FISHLEDER, A. BISTENI, G. MEDRANO, C. FRIEDLAND & A. DE MICHELI. 1962. Effects of an intravenous infusion of K-glucose-insulin solution on the ECG signs of myocardial infarction. Am. J. Cardiol. **9:** 166–181.

SRÉTER, F. A. & S. M. FRIEDMAN. 1961. The effects of adrenergic blockade on cationic exchanges in contracting muscle. J. Pharmacol. Exp. Ther. **131:** 158–166.

SUTHERLAND, E. 1963. In discussion. 2nd Int. Pharmacol. Meeting, Prague. Biochem. Pharmacol. **12** (Suppl): 144.

THEIRS, R. E. & B. L. VALLEE. 1957. Distribution of metals in subcellular fractions of rat liver. J. Biol. Chem. **266:** 911–930.

TUCKER, V. L., H. HANNA, C. J. KAISER & D. C. DARROW. 1963. Cardiac necrosis accompanying potassium deficiency and administration of corticosteroids. Circ. Res. **13:** 420–431.

WEBER, B., H. LABORIT, J. M. JOUANY, P. NIAUSSAT & C. BARON. 1958. Modifications des signes électrocardiographiques de l'infarctus du myocarde expérimental chez le lapin par l'injection de sels de l'acide aspartique. C. R. Soc. Biol. (Paris) **152:** 431–436.

WENZEL, D. G. & R. Y. P. CHAU. 1966. Effect of adrenergic blocking agents on reduction of myocardial aspartate amino-transferase activity by sympathomimetics. Toxic. Appl. Pharmacol. **9:** 514–520.

ZAIMIS, E. 1964. Drug-induced myopathies. *In* Cardiomyopathies. Ciba Found. Symp. G. E. W. Wolstenholme & C. M. O'Connor, Eds. : 214–233. Little, Brown & Co. Boston, Mass.

Part V. Progress in Studies on Cardiac Hypertrophy, Valvular Lesions, and Cardiac Failure

EFFECTS OF HEART FAILURE, VENTRICULAR HYPERTROPHY, AND ALTERATIONS IN THE THYROID STATE ON THE CONTRACTILITY OF ISOLATED CARDIAC MUSCLE

Eugene Braunwald, Edmund H. Sonnenblick, James F. Spann, Jr., and Robert A. Buccino

Cardiology Branch, National Heart Institute, Bethesda, Md.

The investigations described in this report were undertaken to determine the manner in which the intrinsic contractile state of isolated myocardium is altered by the development of ventricular hypertrophy and failure, by norepinephrine depletion, and by changes in the thyroid state. Several recent developments have made it possible to examine these questions. The mechanics of isolated cat papillary muscles from the normal heart have been described in a manner similar to that employed for skeletal muscle.[1] Further, it has been shown that these mechanical functions can be quantitatively measured and norms established, that the variability of function is small among muscles from groups of similar animals, and that the function of muscles from different groups of animals can therefore be compared in a quantitative and meaningful manner.[2]

In order to study the effects of ventricular hypertrophy and heart failure on myocardial contractility, papillary muscles were obtained from normal cats and cats with right ventricular hypertrophy, with or without overt congestive heart failure produced by chronic constriction of the main pulmonary artery, a procedure described in detail elsewhere.[3, 4] A circular clip with an internal diameter (I.D.) of 3.5 mm or 2.8 mm was placed around the proximal main pulmonary artery under sterile conditions. Between 21 and 90 days later, the cats were anesthetized with pentobarbital, and right-heart catheterization was carried out; the hearts were then excised rapidly, and the papillary muscles were removed and studied in a myograph at 30° C and at a contraction frequency of 12 per minute.[2]

Heart failure occurred after constriction of the lumen of the pulmonary artery with the 2.8-mm I.D. clip. The presence of heart failure was defined on the basis of the existence of one or more of the following findings: (1) pleural effusion, (2) ascites, and (3) an abnormally elevated right ventricular end-diastolic pressure in combination with either an abnormally low cardiac index or a high arterio-mixed venous oxygen difference. In the 11 cats with heart failure, the average right ventricular weight was increased from a normal value of 0.55 g/kg to 1.33 g/kg. Right ventricular hypertrophy without heart failure occurred in cats in which the lumen of the pulmonary artery had been reduced to 20% of normal by the application of the 3.5-mm I.D. clip. Cats were included in this group only if there was no pleural fluid or ascites and if values for right ventricular end-diastolic pressure, cardiac index, and arterio-mixed venous oxygen difference were within the range of normal. The right ventricular weight was almost double the normal in this group and averaged 1.05 g/kg.

In the muscles removed from both of these groups of animals, the actively developed tension was less than normal (FIGURE 1). Maximum isometric tension in the muscles from animals with right ventricular hypertrophy was slightly, but not significantly, reduced, averaging 5.3 ± 0.6 g/mm[2] [standard error of the mean (S.E.)] compared with the normal value of 6.2 ± 0.7 g/mm[2], whereas the maximum isometric tension of the muscles from the cats with heart failure was markedly reduced, averaging 2.4 ± 0.4 g/mm.[2] The velocity of shortening at a small preload (0.5 g/mm[2]) was used to estimate the maximum isotonic velocity of contraction, i.e., the V_{max}. This variable averaged 0.90 ± 0.08 l_0/sec in normal muscles and was significantly lower ($p < .01$), averaging 0.65 ±

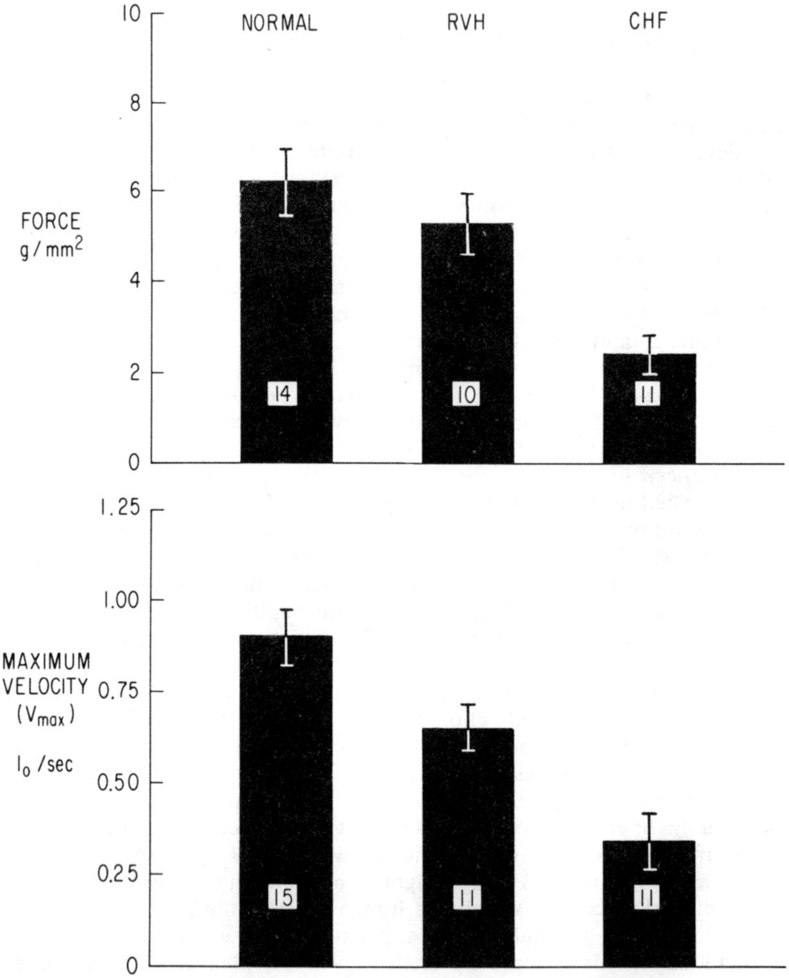

FIGURE 1. (Top) Average values (± S.E.) for the isometric force developed by papillary muscles at the peak of their length-active tension curves. The absolute force developed was corrected for the cross-sectional area of the muscles and expressed in g/mm.[2] RVH = muscles removed from cats with right ventricular hypertrophy; CHF = muscles removed from cats with heart failure. The numbers in each bar represent the number of muscles in each group. (Bottom) Velocity of shortening of muscles contracting isotonically against a small preload (0.5 g). The velocity of shortening was corrected for the initial length of the muscle and was expressed in muscle lengths per second (l_0/sec).

0.06 l_0/sec, in the muscles from cats with right ventricular hypertrophy. The V_{max} was significantly lower in the muscles from the cats with heart failure than in either of the other two groups ($p < 0.01$), averaging 0.34 ± 0.06 l_0/sec. The norepinephrine concentration was markedly reduced in the right ventricles of both of these experimental groups, from an average value of 2.13 μg/g in normal cats to 0.18 μg/g in cats with right ventricular hypertrophy and 0.24 μg/g in cats with heart failure.

Although delineation of the intrinsic contractile properties of the myocardium in hypertrophied and failing hearts is essential to an understanding of the basic processes underlying ventricular compensation and failure, relatively little experimental data concerning this problem have previously been available. It was observed in the present investigation that a profound depression of the intrinsic contractile state exists in cardiac muscle removed from the hearts of animals with overt congestive heart failure. This depression was characterized by a downward shift of the force-velocity curve, with substantial reductions of the intrinsic speed of contraction (V_{max}). The reduction in the intrinsic speed of contraction was further manifested by a decrease in the rate of force development (df/dt). These findings indicate that the intensity of the active state is depressed, and can be interpreted as a reduction in the rate of interactions at contractile sites in these muscles.[5] Of considerable interest, also, was the finding that muscles removed from animals without heart failure but with ventricular hypertrophy exhibited qualitatively similar depressions of contractile function, although of lesser magnitude. It should be emphasized that these abnormalities were intrinsic to the cardiac muscle of the failing heart and the hypertrophied nonfailing heart, since they were present *in vitro,* where the chemical and physical conditions in which the muscles were examined were controlled and identical with the conditions under which the normal muscles were studied.

From these findings, it appears that the initial response of a ventricle chronically stressed by increased impedance to emptying is to increase its total muscle mass. This increase in muscle mass, operating perhaps in conjunction with the Frank-Starling mechanism and increased sympathetic stimulation, maintains overall circulatory compensation, despite the fact that the intrinsic contractile state of each unit of myocardium is depressed.[4] This depression is manifested, in the mildest form, by a reduction in the intrinsic velocity of myocardial fiber shortening (V_{max}), but by only a minimal decrease in the isometric force development. As the intrinsic contractile state of each unit of myocardium is further depressed, more extensive reductions in V_{max} occur, accompanied by marked decreases in maximal isometric force. At this point, circulatory compensation can no longer be maintained despite maximal utilization of the compensatory mechanisms provided by cardiac dilatation and increases in muscle mass, and overt congestive heart failure occurs. The depletion of cardiac norepinephrine stores in the overloaded heart removes the ability of the circulation to derive significant benefit from the activity of the sympathetic nervous system.[4, 6-8]

Cardiac tissues contain substantial quantities of norepinephrine which appear to be localized almost exclusively within the terminations of the sympathetic nerves, in close apposition to the myocardial fibers. An increase in sympathetic activity augments myocardial contractility, and loss of the cardiac sympathetic neurons or removal of their norepinephrine stores abolishes that aspect of myocardial regulation which is provided by this system. However, there has been no agreement concerning the importance of these nerves and their norepinephrine stores in maintaining the basal contractile state of the myocardium and its ability to respond to various inotropic interventions. It has been proposed that intact norepinephrine stores are required to maintain the basal contractile state of heart muscle[9] and its contractile responses to changes in the frequency of contraction;[10] however, these hypotheses have been questioned.[2, 11, 12] The profound depletion of cardiac norepinephrine stores found in clinical heart failure and in experimental ventricular overload, as outlined above, has raised the question of a possible causal relationship between cardiac norepinephrine depletion and myocardial failure.

In order to assess the role played by endogenous norepinephrine stores on the intrinsic contractile state of cardiac muscle, the right ventricular papillary muscles from 15 normal cats, 14 cats with cardiac norepinephrine depletion produced by chronic cardiac denervation, and eight cats that had undergone reserpine pretreatment and norepinephrine depletion were studied, in the same manner as that utilized for the muscles obtained from cats with right ventricular hypertrophy and heart failure outlined above, and described in detail elsewhere.[2] Neither the maximum isometric force nor the maximum velocity of isotonic shortening were significantly depressed in either group of catecholamine-depleted muscles (FIGURE 2). In addition, it was observed that the entire length-resting tension curves, length-active tension curves, force-velocity curves, and augmentation of isometric tension achieved by paired electrical stimulation and by increasing frequency of contraction were not depressed in either group of norepinephrine-depleted muscles. Similarly, no changes in the absolute refractory period and electrical excitability were observed.

On the basis of these studies, it can be concluded that cardiac stores of norepinephrine are not fundamental for maintaining the intrinsic contractile state of the myocardium. Furthermore, release of endogenous norepinephrine from cardiac muscle does not appear to play an essential role in the mediation of the positive inotropic effects of increasing frequency of contraction or of sustained postextrasystolic potentiation. When the results of these studies are extrapolated to the failing heart, it would appear that the norepinephrine depletion occurring in congestive heart failure might impair cardiac performance, not by altering the intrinsic contractile state of the myocardium but by interfering with the augmentation of contractility provided by the adrenergic nervous system.[8]

It is well known that alterations in thyroid activity result in profound changes in cardiovascular function. In the intact organism, these alterations in cardiovascular function have been interpreted as being secondary to the changes in the peripheral metabolic requirements and in the autonomic nervous system induced by the abnormal thyroid state.[13] However, the possibility that thyroid hormone exerts a direct effect on the intrinsic properties of the myocardium and that the changes in the circulation result, at least in part, from such a direct effect warrants consideration. Accordingly, effects of hyper- and hypothyroidism upon the intrinsic contractile properties of the myocardium were studied.[14] The basic experimental plan was to compare the behavior of papillary muscles obtained from thee groups of cats: (1) 24 untreated (i.e., euthyroid) cats; (2) 13 cats in which hypothyroidism had been induced by the administration of ^{131}I (1 mc/kg) three months prior to the study; and (3) 13 cats rendered hyperthyroid by daily intraperitoneal injections of *l*-thyroxine (1

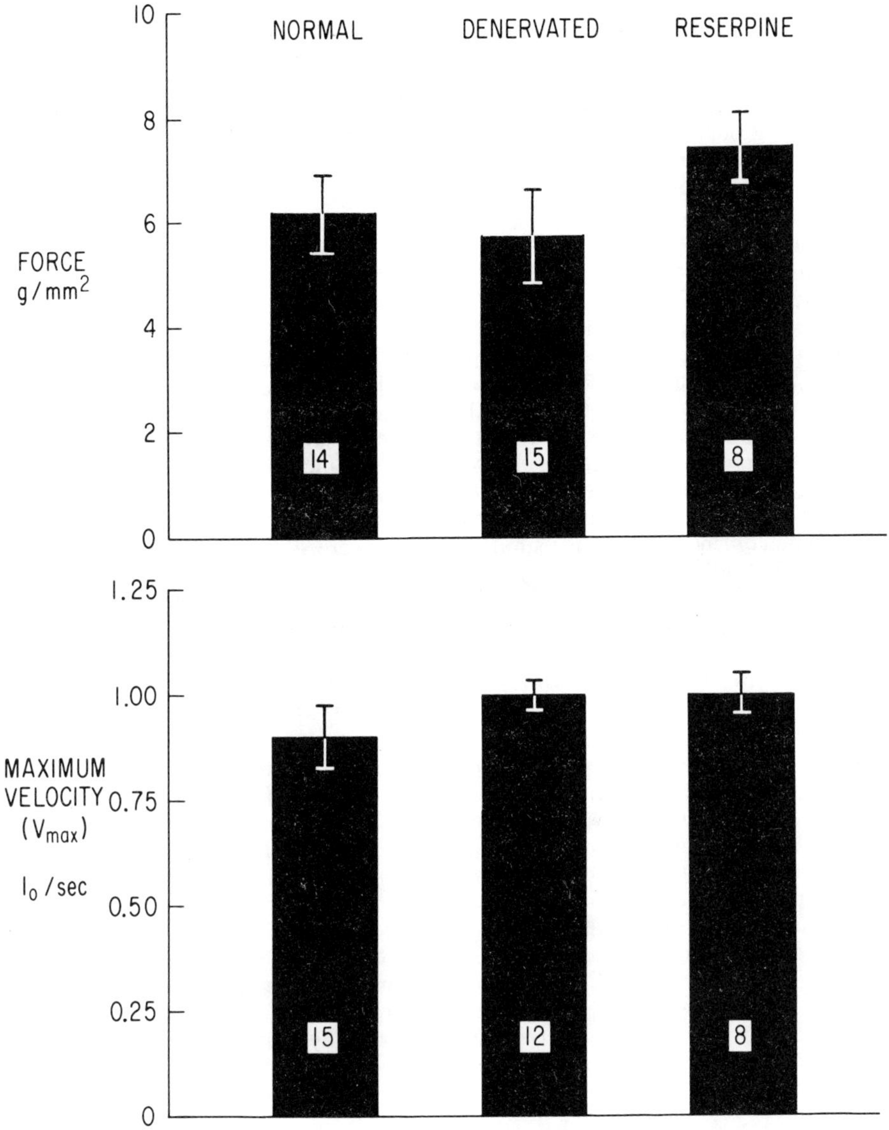

FIGURE 2. Effects of catecholamine depletion produced by chronic cardiac denervation and reserpine pretreatment on myocardial force development (top) and the velocity of shortening (bottom).

mg/kg) for eight to 17 days. Two additional groups of animals were studied to define the relationship between norepinephrine stores and hyperthyroidism: one group subjected to catecholamine depletion with reserpine, administered prior to and concurrent with induction of the hyperthyroid state, and the other treated with the same schedule of reserpine alone.

Changes in the thyroid state resulted in only slight changes in the maximum isometric tension developed by these muscles. Maximum active tension averaged 6.8 ± 0.3 g/mm^2 in muscles from 24 euthyroid animals, 7.7 ± 0.5 g/mm^2 in muscles from 11 hyperthyroid animals, and 5.4 ± 0.7 g/mm^2 in muscles from 13 hypothyroid animals (FIGURE 3). Although neither the hyper- nor hypothyroid groups differed significantly from the euthyroid, the maximum isometric tension in the hyperthyroid muscles was significantly ($p < .02$) greater than that of the hypothyroid group.

However, the rate of tension development differed significantly and markedly in all three groups, averaging 17.6 ± 2.8, 29.8 ± 3.9, and 44.6 ± 3.6 g/mm^2/sec for the hypothyroid, euthyroid, and hyperthyroid groups, respectively. The maximum velocity of isotonic shortening (V_{max}) was also found to vary directly with the level of the thyroid state (FIGURE 3). At a load of 0.5 g/mm^2, the V_{max} averaged 0.90 ± 0.08 l_0/sec in muscles from 12 euthyroid cats, was significantly lower ($p < .01$) in muscles obtained from 12 hypothyroid cats, averaging 0.58 ± 0.12 l_0/sec, and was significantly higher ($p < .01$) in muscles from 13 hyperthyroid cats, averaging 1.67 ± 0.12 l_0/sec. These profound increases in the V_{max} of isotonic contractions and the rate of force development of isometric contractions, both of which are characteristic of muscles removed from hyperthyroid animals, were not dependent on intact norepinephrine stores, since similar changes were seen in muscles obtained from hyperthyroid cats in which catecholamine stores had been obtained from hyperthyroid cats in which catecholamine stores had been depleted with reserpine.[14] The increments in isometric force produced by the addition of strophanthidin (1.0 μg/ml) were greatest in hypothyroid muscles (3.6 ± 1.0 g/mm^2), intermediate in euthyroid muscles (2.2 ± 0.3 g/mm^2), and least in hyperthyroid muscles (1.1 ± 0.4 g/mm^2), raising absolute tension to similar levels in all three groups.

On the basis of these observations, it may be concluded that the thyroid state profoundly affects the intrinsic contractile state of cardiac muscle, primarily by altering the rate of interaction at the contractile sites, as reflected in the V_{max} of isotonic contractions and the rate of tension development of isometric contractions. These findings suggest strongly that the alterations in cardiovascular dynamics observed in the intact organism with hyper- or hypothyroidism do not result merely from the changes in the load placed upon the myocardium by the induced alterations in the metabolism of the extracardiac tissues. Instead, they indicate that the observed variations in cardiac output, mean systolic ejection rate, and myocardial fiber-shortening rate result, at least in part, from the direct effects of the thyroid hormone on the intrinsic contractile behavior of the myocardium.

Summary

The effects of cardiac hypertrophy, cardiac failure, norepinephrine depletion, and hyper- and hypothyroidism on the intrinsic contractility of the myocardium and papillary muscles were studied. These conditions were created in cats, and their papillary muscles were excised and studied in a myograph. Heart failure depressed both the isometric force developed by the isolated muscle and the velocity of isotonic shortening. Cardiac hypertrophy reduced the velocity of shortening but had little effect on isometric tension. Catecholamine depletion did not affect the intrinsic contractile state of the myocardium. Hypothyroidism reduced the velocity of isotonic shortening and the rate of tension develop-

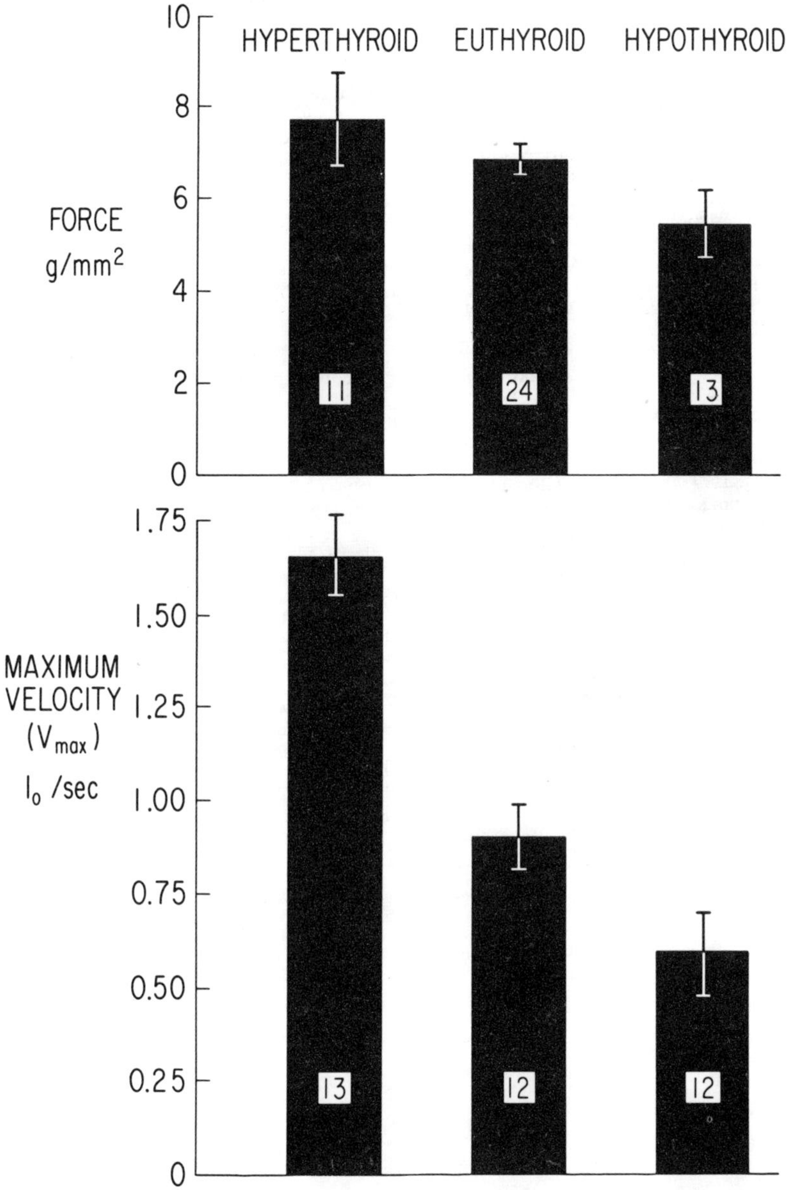

FIGURE 3. Effects of hyperthyroidism and hypothyrodism on myocardial force development (top) and the velocity of shortening (bottom).

ment, whereas hyperthyroidism exerted the opposite effect. The latter changes were not dependent upon the norepinephrine stores of the heart.

References

1. SONNENBLICK, E. H. 1962. Force-velocity relations in mammalian heart muscle. Amer. J. Physiol. **202:** 931.
2. SPANN, JR., J. F., E. H. SONNENBLICK, T. COOPER, C. A. CHIDSEY, V. L. WILLMAN & E. BRAUNWALD. 1966. Cardiac norepinephrine stores and the contractile state of heart muscle. Circ. Res. **19:** 317.
3. SPANN, JR., J. F., R. A. BUCCINO & E. H. SONNENBLICK. Production of right ventricular hypertrophy with and without congestive heart failure in the cat. Proc. Soc. Exp. Biol. Med. Submitted for publication.
4. SPANN, JR., J. F., R. A. BUCCINO, E. H. SONNENBLICK & E. BRAUNWALD. The contractile state of cardiac muscle in ventricular hypertrophy and heart failure. In preparation.
5. PODOLSKY, R. J. 1962. Mechano-chemical basis of muscular contraction. Fed. Proc. **21:** 964.
6. CHIDSEY, C. A., E. BRAUNWALD & A. G. MORROW. 1965. Catecholamine excretion and cardiac stores of norepinephrine in congestive heart failure. Amer. J. Med. **39:** 442.
7. CHIDSEY, C. A., G. A. KAISER, E. H. SONNENBLICK, J. F. SPANN, JR. & E. BRAUNWALD. 1964. Cardiac norepinephrine stores in experimental heart failure in the dog. J. Clin. Invest. **43:** 2386.
8. COVELL, J. W., C. A. CHIDSEY & E. BRAUNWALD. 1966. Reduction of the cardiac response to postganglionic sympathatic nerve stimulation in experimental heart failure. Circ. Res. **19:** 51.
9. LEE, W. C. & F. E. SHIDEMAN. 1959. Role of myocardial catecholamines in cardiac contractility. Science **129:** 967.
10. WHALEN, W. J., N. FISHMAN & R. ERICKSON. 1958. Nature of the potentiating substance in cardiac muscle. Amer. J. Physiol. **194:** 573.
11. MAXWELL, R. A., J. J. KELLEY, JR. & E. T. ECKHARDT. 1964. Effect of catecholamine depletion on an index of myocardial contractility in isolated rabbit hearts. Proc. Soc. Exp. Biol. Med. **116:** 672.
12. FURCHGOTT, R. F., T. DE GUBAREFF & A. GROSSMAN. 1959. Release of autonomic mediators in cardiac tissue by suprathreshold stimulation. Science **129:** 328.
13. THEILEN, E. O. & W. R. WILSON. 1967. Hemodynamic effects of peripheral vasconstriction in normal and thyrotoxic subjects. J. Appl. Physiol. **22:** 207.
14. BUCCINO, R. A., J. F. SPANN, JR. P. E. POOL, E. H. SONNENBLICK & E. BRAUNWALD. Influence of the thyroid state on the intrinsic contractile properties and energy stores of the myacordium. In preparation.

THE INTERRELATION BETWEEN MYOCARDIAL METABOLISM AND HEART FAILURE*

Hans A. Hochrein and Klaus Lossnitzer

Department of Medicine, University of Würzburg, Würzburg, Germany

Heart failure must be considered when the function and load capacity of the heart are disturbed. This event may occur in different pathological and experimental conditions. The two most frequent causes of heart failure are hypoxia and overload of the cardiac muscle. Both result in disturbances of the myocardial metabolism and, because of a metabolic deficiency of energy, a consequent imbalance of electrolytes in the intra- and extracellular compartments of myocardial tissue.[1] The experiments discussed in this paper were carried out in guinea pigs, whose hearts were examined *in situ* or as heart-lung preparations.

Hypoxic heart failure occurs when the oxygen supply is decreased below a critical level. The disturbed myocardial metabolism is characterized by an increased supply of glycogen,[2] an accumulation of lactate,[3-6] and an inhibition of aerobic glycolysis via the Krebs cycle. As a result, there is a decreased accumulation of energy-rich phosphates which, in turn, influences the intracellular environment of ions.[7] Besides the intracellular accumulation of inorganic phosphate, a decrease of potassium and magnesium and an increase of sodium, chloride, and water in the myocardial cells have been noted. Thus, the intracellular volume increases, and myocardial edema develops (FIGURE 1).

With the development of overload insufficiency, there is initially an increased lactate consumption[8] and an intensified glycolysis and synthesis of adenosine triphosphate (ATP), followed by a decrease of phosphocreatine[9] and an intensified splitting of ATP, with a higher turnover of chemical energy. In contrast to hypoxic insufficiency, in heart failure as a result of mechanical overload the total glycolytic metabolism is inhibited.[10] The chemical stores of energy are exhausted; consequently, there is a disturbance of extra- and intracellular electrolytes, with an increased outflow of potassium and magnesium and an increased inflow of sodium, chloride, and water (FIGURE 2).

This inflow of water into the myocardial cells during heart failure can be calculated by a measured decrease of the myocardial extracellular fluid space and an increase of myocardial water content. In relation to 100 g (wet weight) of myocardial tissue, the extracellular fluid space, as measured by inulin incubation, decreases from 8.6 ml (11%) to 5.8 ml (7.1%). The intracellular fluid space increases from 69.4 ml (89%) to 76.3 ml (92.9%) when the functional state of the heart changes from normal to failure.[11] These changes are the consequences of a disturbed energy-electrolyte metabolism and reflect the direct connection between the metabolism of a failing heart muscle and failing mechanical function.

From a biochemical point of view, however, heart failure is a disturbance of the production of metabolic energy, and it seems unlikely that heart failure caused by hypoxia has the same metabolic genesis as that caused by overload. Our investigations of myocardial glycolytic metabolism, done by analysis of substrates, actually showed a considerable difference. With increasing pressure load and more so in overload, as a consequence of an increased substrate con-

*This work was supported by the German Research Society (Deutsche Forschungsgemeinschaft).

sumption, a decline of myocardial glucose content was found (FIGURE 3), whereas the myocardial glucose uptake did not increase under these conditions. In contrast with lactate, myocardial glucose uptake depends on extracellular glucose concentration.[8] The myocardial content of lactate initially increases in the high load state, because the cardiac muscle takes up more lactate with increasing load.[12] In overload, lactate decreases again to a normal level, because in this state the myocardium loses the ability to take up lactate. On the other hand, the myocardial lactate content in hypoxia caused by asphyxia of guinea pigs shows a rapid increase, beginning after 1 minute of asphyxia. The glucose content, after a slight increase initially, remains unchanged. TABLE 1 shows that myocardial glucose content in overload heart failure is decreased as significantly as in mono-iodine-acetate intoxication. Myocardial lactate content increases significantly only in hypoxic heart failure, because anaerobic substrate metabolism continues after aerobic metabolism stops. In myocardial hypoxia, there is a reduced energy production from anaerobic glycolysis, with a continuing utilization of glucose and glycogen. In mechanical overload of the

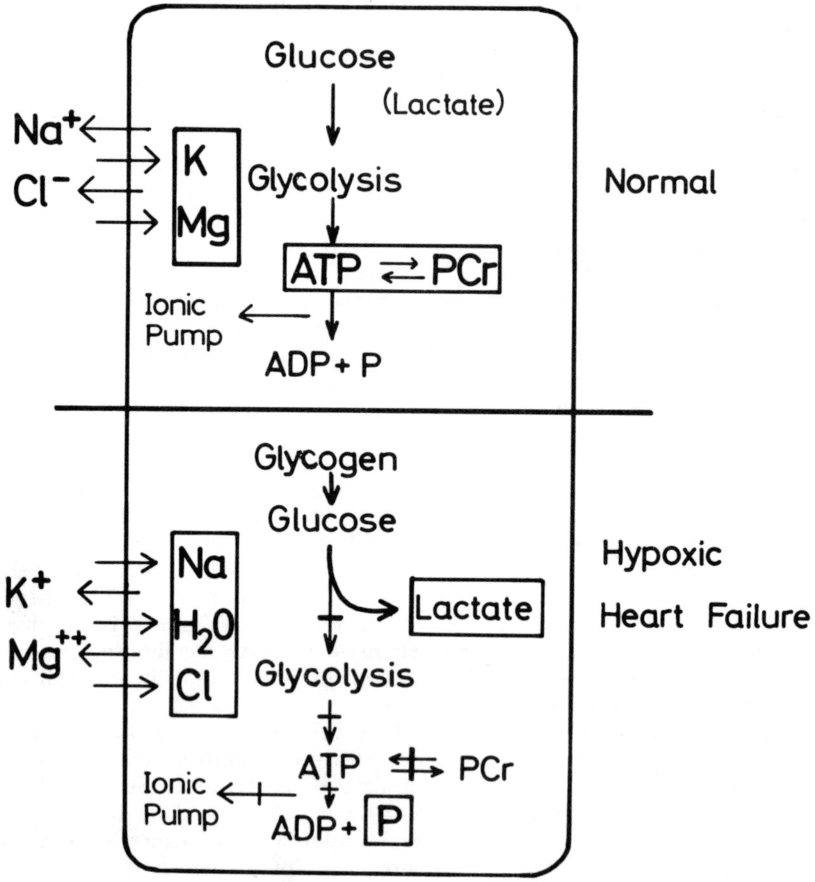

FIGURE 1. Effect of oxygen deficiency on the metabolism of electrolytes in the myocardial cell.

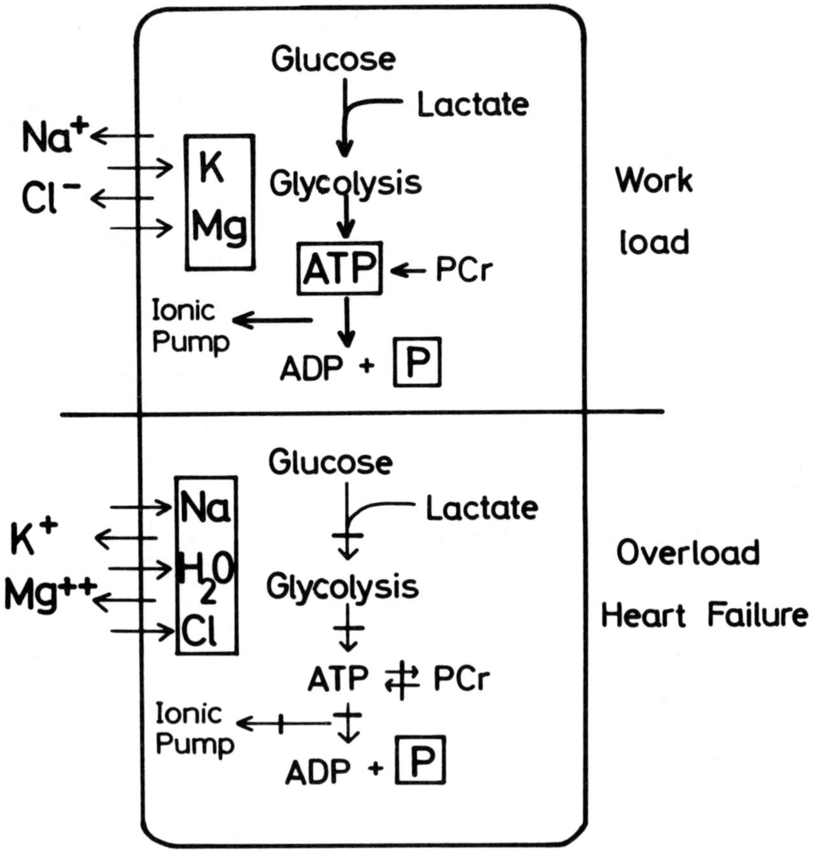

FIGURE 2. Effect of overload on the metabolism of electrolytes in the myocardial cell.

cardiac muscle, there is a complete breakdown of glycolysis—similar to an intoxication with mono-iodine-acetate. The utilization exceeds the production of energy. Therefore, heart failure as a consequence of overload might be expressed as an interruption of the utilization of energy-furnishing substrate.

The intracellular myocardial content of potassium and sodium, measured by flame photometry, shows an identical change in all kinds of heart failure. In all cases—overload, hypoxia, and different intoxications or glucose deficiency—there is an equal loss of potassium in myocardial cells from the normal of 106 mEq/l to 76 mEq/l, on the average. Only in heart failure as a consequence of hypopotassemia does the intracellular potassium content decrease further. The intracellular content of sodium increases proportionately from the normal of 43 mEq/l to 70 or 80 mEq/l (FIGURE 4). Along with these cations, the concentrations of other myocardial electrolytes are also changed in heart failure.[13] Thus, the chloride content, measured by silver-ion titration, increases significantly from 35 to 50 mEq/l, but it probably does so in connection with the increasing sodium concentration, as a passive anion compensation. The myocardial concentration of magnesium decreases, as does the concentration of calcium. Both bivalent cations fulfill an important function in the normal contraction of myocardial muscle. Besides a catalytic effect in different enzymatic actions, the magnesium ion certainly has a direct action on the contractile elements of cardiac muscle fibers. On the average, the intracellular concentration of magnesium is 17 mEq/l, ten times higher than the extracellular concentration, but the intracellular content decreases to 13 mEq/l in heart failure, as noted in spectrofluorometric determinations. Measurements of calcium with the flame photometer, after preparing the cardiac tissue in a vacuum-low temperature asher, showed that the intracellular myocardial calcium content is decreased, possibly as a result of the decreased synthesis of actomyosin, in heart failure as well as in low load.[14] Therefore, changes in calcium, as in chloride, are not specifically dependent on heart failure. Inorganic phosphate increases in the myocardium in an amount proportional to the decrease of energy-rich phosphates, ATP, and creatine phosphate. In this instance, inorganic phosphate performs essentially a buffer function.

Intracellular potassium and sodium concentrations change not only in heart failure, but also in relation to the cardiac load in a normal nonfailing state.

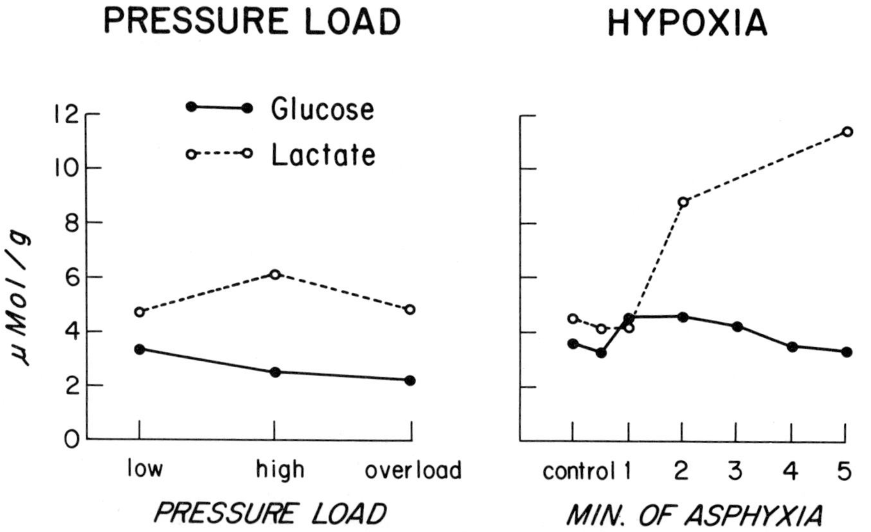

FIGURE 3. Changes of the myocardial glucose and lactate content (expressed in micromoles per gram) during pressure load and in hypoxia of the cardiac muscle.

TABLE 1

GLUCOSE AND LACTATE CONTENT IN THE MYOCARDIUM OF GUINEA PIGS IN HEART FAILURE

	No. of Animals	Glucose*	Lactate*
Control	29	3.72 ± 0.64	4.55 ± 0.85
Overload	14	2.23 ± 0.88	4.91 ± 1.46
Hypoxia (5 minutes of asphyxia)	16	3.55 ± 0.67	11.36 ± 2.68
Mono-iodine-acetate intoxication	12	2.63 ± 0.74	4.69 ± 1.15

* All values with standard deviation, expressed in micromoles per gram.

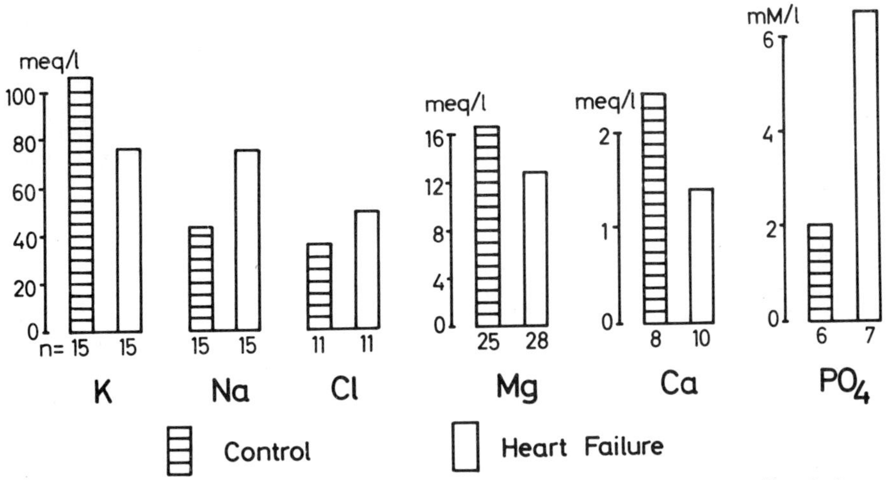

FIGURE 4. Changes of myocardial intracellular electrolytes (expressed in milliequivalents per liter) during experimental heart failure of guinea pig.

With increasing load, intracellular myocardial potassium concentration decreases, and sodium concentration increases correspondingly. These load-conditioned changes of the intracellular metabolism of electrolytes may be a direct cause of insufficient myocardial function, with development of an intracellular edema. If a failing heart is treated with digitalis, causing a positive inotropic effect, the intracellular potassium content increases significantly above the value found in heart failure, but the normal values of a nonfailing heart can never be reached. Sodium reacts in an opposite manner in this therapeutic effect. However, in the myocardium of a heart in shock, values found for potassium are as high and for sodium as low as those found in the myocardium of a low-loaded heart. From a hemodynamic and biochemical point of view, therefore, the heart in shock is a maximally unburdened heart, without any signs of heart failure.

With changing concentrations of extracellular potassium, intracellular myocardial concentrations of electrolytes and, thus, the function of the heart changes, too. In experimental hypopotassemia, with an extracellular potassium concentration of 2.2 mEq/l, only an insignificant decrease in the intracellular potassium concentration is found, with undisturbed normal heart function.[15] Not until an extreme hypopotassemia of 1.2 mEq/l is reached do the myocardial cells lose potassium and take up sodium in a greater amount; then hypopotassemic heart failure develops. Thus, the intracellular metabolism of electrolytes is not controlled directly by changes of the extracellular environment, but is closely connected with the functional state of the heart. In hyperpotassemia, an intracellular loss of potassium also occurs, but not before heart failure develops as a consequence of the high extracellular concentration of potassium. Heart failure first occurs when an extreme level of 11.6 mEq/l extracellular potassium is reached. It is remarkable that intracellular sodium content does not increase as usual under these conditions. In the development of cardiac standstill from hyperpotassemic heart failure—as is the case when an extracellular potassium concentration of 14.8 mEq/l is reached—intracellular potassium content again increases. Possibly, at this stage the mechanism of repolarization of myocardial muscle fibers becomes normal again as a result of an inhibition of the conduction system.

In pretreatment with digitalis, the heart muscle tolerates a higher hyperpotassemia without signs of heart failure. Under the protection of digitalis, heart failure begins at a significantly higher extracellular potassium concentration. Conversely, it is possible to obtain a full recovery from heart failure induced by digitalis intoxication when the extracellular potassium concentration is elevated. With the recovery of digitalis-induced heart failure by elevating the extracellular concentration of potassium to 9.3 mEq/l, an increase of potassium and a decrease of sodium in the myocardial cells was found. Under these circumstances, the favorable therapeutic effect of potassium in digitalis intoxication is as pronounced as the favorable effect of digitalis in hyperpotassemia. In a therapeutic dose (7×10^{-5}g/100 ml), and more significantly in a toxic dose, digitalis causes a loss of potassium from the myocardial cells in a normal nonfailing heart, with an equivalent uptake of sodium. In heart failure, however, a therapeutic dose of digitalis causes an increase of the reduced intracellular content of potassium and a decrease of the elevated sodium content, but the normal values of the nonfailing and untreated heart muscle may never be reached.

Just as potassium acts in digitalis-induced heart failure, the combined solution of potassium-glucose-insulin[16] acts in hypoxic heart failure. Under the influence of this repolarizing solution, in spite of continuous nitrogen breathing of a guinea pig heart-lung preparation, cardiac output and stroke volume increase, pressure in the right atrium decreases, and load capacity of the heart increases.[17] The influence of potassium-glucose-insulin on the hypoxic myocardial cell can be explained as follows: With the help of insulin, the uptake, phosphorylization, and metabolism of glucose in the cardiac cell are improved. In this way, the glycolytic block will be overcome, leading to an increased storage of chemical energy, which intensifies the active transport of cations against the concentration gradient. This means that intracellular potassium concentration in the myocardium increases and sodium concentration decreases. In fact, when potassium-glucose-insulin was given in hypoxic heart failure, intracellular myocardial potassium concentration increased significantly and sodium concentration decreased. The analysis of ten guinea pig hearts treated in this way showed a result quite near the findings of Sodi-Pallares and coworkers.[16]

Another combined solution of electrolytes was examined for its hemodynamic and metabolic effect. Normally, a guinea pig heart *in situ* shows a spontaneous recovery by rebreathing after a maximum asphyxic period of six minutes. This tolerance of asphyxia cannot be improved by potassium, but can be slightly improved by magnesium, and more improved by the combined application of potassium with magnesium. But the application of potassium-magnesium-aspartate, with the same concentrations of potassium and magnesium as above, more than doubles the tolerance of asphyxia. Therefore, the heart muscle is protected against hypoxia by potassium-magnesium-aspartate (FIGURE 5). Furthermore, it was found by metabolic studies, that the outflow of potassium from myocardial cells is less and more retarded when the asphyxic dilating heart is protected by potassium-magnesium-aspartate (FIGURE 6). In regard to the myocardial metabolism of electrolytes, potassium-magnesium-aspartate acts as a protector against hypoxia in the sense of a depolarization inhibitor.[13, 18, 19]

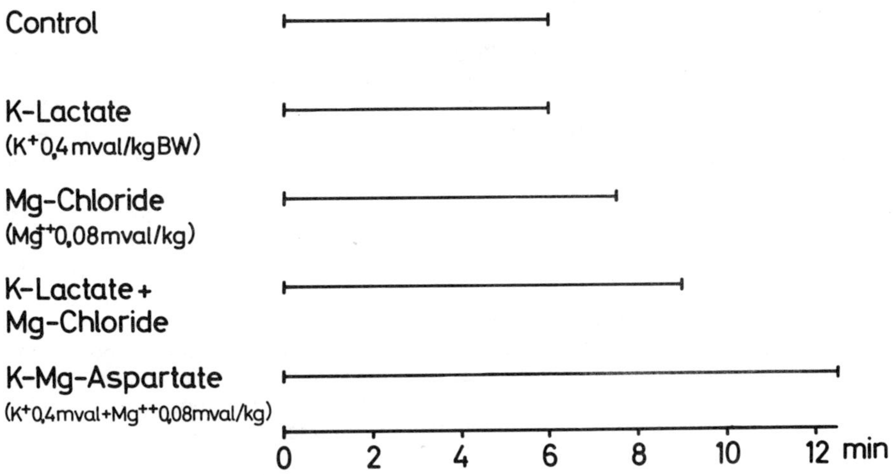

FIGURE 5. Maximal cardiac toleration of asphyxia with spontaneous recovery of respiration in guinea pig heart (*in situ*). mval = milliequivalents per liter.

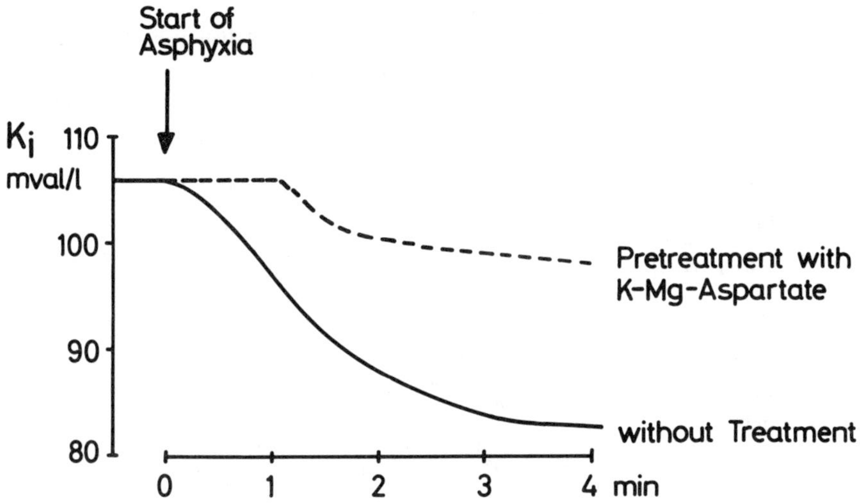

FIGURE 6. Myocardial intracellular potassium concentration during asphyxia. mval = milliequivalents per liter.

In summary, it is clear that there is a close correlation between function of the heart and myocardial metabolism. It has been shown that every positive therapeutic effect is connected with a myocardial loss of sodium and an uptake of potassium. Conversely, every load or damage of the heart leads to an uptake of sodium and a loss of potassium. In connection with this, it is significant that the therapeutic application of certain solutions of electrolytes exerts a favorable influence on the metabolism of electrolytes. This observation may lead to important methods of treatment in the future.

Summary

Experiments were carried out in guinea pigs, whose hearts were examined *in situ* or as heart-lung preparations. It was found that heart failure occurs during myocardial hypoxia because of a reduced energy production. Heart failure as a consequence of overload may be expressed as an interruption of the utilization of energy-furnishing substrate. In all forms of experimentally induced heart failure, myocardial cells lose potassium and take up sodium. With sodium, the intracellular water content increases, and an edema of myocardial cells occurs. The typical changes of other electrolytes in heart failure (chloride, calcium, inorganic phosphate, and magnesium) have been shown. The myocardial metabolism of electrolytes was discussed under the special conditions of shock, changing extracellular potassium concentrations, and digitalis administration. The important therapeutic values of potassium-glucose-insulin and potassium-magnesium-aspartate have been shown. By the use of such electrolyte solutions, the hemodynamic and metabolic consequences of myocardial hypoxia can be prevented or reversed.

References

1. HOCHREIN, H. 1965. Herzinsuffizienz und Myokardstoffwechsel. Editio Cantor. Aulendorf Wurtt.
2. LAMPRECHT, W., G. MICHAL & S. NAEGLE. 1961. Der Stoffwechsel des hypoxischen und anoxischen Herzmuskels. Klin. Wschr. **39:** 358.
3. RUEHL, A. 1934. Ueber die Bedeutung der Milchsaeure fuer den Herzstoffwechsel. Klin. Wschr. **13:** 1529.
4. THORN, W. 1961. Metabolitenkonzentrationen im Herzmuskel unter normalen, hypoxischen und anoxischen Bedingungen. Verh. Deutsch. Ges. Kreislaufforsch. **27:** **76.**
5. ISSELHARD, W. & H. MERGUET. 1962. Metabolite des Glykolyse-Cyclus und des Adenylsaeure-Phosphokreatin-Systems im schlagenden und durchbluteten Warmblueterherzen unter verschiedenen Versuchsbedingungen. Pflueger. Arch. Ges. Physiol. **276:** 211.
6. CORNBLATH, M., P. J. RANDLE, A. PARMEGGIANI & H. E. MORGAN. 1963. Regulation of glycogenolysis in muscle. Effects of glucagon and anoxia on lactate production, glycogen content and phosphorylase activity in the perfused isolated rat heart. J. Biol. Chem. **238:** 1592.
7. FLECKENSTEIN, A. 1955. Der Kalium-Natrium-Austausch als Energieprinzip in Muskel und Nerv. Berlin-Goettingen-Heidelberg.
8. HOCHREIN, H. & P. HECK. 1966. Zur Frage des Glucose- und Lactatverbrauchs bei verschiedenen Belastungszustaenden des Herzens und in Abhaengkeit von der Subtratkonzentration. Arch. Kreislaufforsch. **52:** 175.
9. HOCHREIN, H. & H. J. DOERING. 1960. Die energiereichen Phosphate des Myokards bei Variation der Belastungsbedingungen. Pflueger. Arch. Ges. Physiol. **271:** 548.
10. LOSSNITZER, K. 1966. Herzinsuffizienz und glykolytischer Stoffwechsel. Dissertation. University of Wurzburg, Wurzburg, Germany.
11. HOCHREIN, H. & H. P. HELWING. Intracellular myocardial edema in cardiac failure. VIII Ann. Meet. Internat. Coll. Angiol., Madrid, 1966. Vasc. Dis. In press.
12. KEUL, J., E. DOLL, H. STEIM, U. FLEER & H. REINDELL. 1965. Ueber den Stoffwechsel des menschlichen Herzens. III. Der oxydative Stoffwechsel des menschlichen Herzens unter verschiedenen Arbeitsbelastungen. Pflueger. Arch. Ges. Physiol. **282:** 43.
13. HOCHREIN, H. 1966. Electrolytes in heart failure and myocardial hypoxia. Vasc. Dis. **3:** 196.
14. DAVIES, R. E. 1963. A molecular theory of muscle contraction. Calcium-dependent contractions with hydrogen bond formation plus ATP-dependent extensions of part of the myosin-action crossbridges. Nature **199:** 1068.
15. HOCHREIN, H., Q. ZAQQA, B. PETSCHALLIES & E. WOLLHEIM. 1965. Experimental studies on the hemodynamics and myocardial metabolism of electrolytes in hypo- and hyperpotassemia and under the influence of digitalis. Acta Cardiol. (Brux.) **20:** 148.

16. SODI-PALLARES, D. A. BISTENI, G. A. MEDRANO, A. DEMICHELI, J. PONCE DE LEON, E. CALVA, B. C. FISHLEDER, M. R. TESTELLI & B. C. MILLER. 1966. The polarizing treatment in cardiovascular conditions. *In* Electrolytes and Cardiovascular Diseases. E. Bajusz, Ed. **2:** 198. S. Karger. Basel, Switzerland.
17. HOCHREIN, H., W. HEBERLEIN & K. LOSSNITZER. 1966. Klinische und experimentelle Befunde ueber den repolarisierenden Effekt von Kalium-Glucose-Insulin bei Myokardhypoxie. Verh. Deutsch. Ges. Kreislaufforsch. **32:** 201.
18. LAMARCHE, M., R. ROYER & M. TAPIN. 1961. Action des aspartates sur le coeur isole. C. R. Soc. Biol. (Paris) **155:** 1092.
19. ROSEN, H. J. MCCALLUM, A. BLUMENTHAL & H. P. K. AGERSBORG. 1964. Effects of potassium and magnesium aspartates on the isolated guinea pig heart. Arch. Int. Phamacodyn. **147:** 476.

DISSOCIATION OF FACTORS INFLUENCING MYOCARDIAL DEGENERATION AND GENERALIZED CARDIOCIRCULATORY FAILURE*

E. Bajusz, F. Homburger, J. R. Baker, and P. Bogdonoff
Bio-Research Institute, Cambridge, Mass.

Introduction

"Cardiomyopathy" ("primary myocardial disease" or "heart-muscle disease") is the designation given to an increasingly recognized type of myocardial degeneration which is not caused by coronary artery disease, hypertension, cor pulmonale, or rheumatic and congenital heart diseases. More precisely, the term cardiomyopathy designates a heterogeneous group of diseases that attack primarily the heart muscle and either spare or only minimally involve the endocardium, pericardium, valves, and coronary vessels. The etiology of most cardiomyopathies is unknown, and only the uniformity of the clinical picture they produce warrants their inclusion in a single category.

Experimental studies performed during the past decade have revealed that cardiomyopathies can be induced in laboratory animals by a wide variety of techniques. In fact, the histological findings in the experimentally induced cardiomyopathies are similar to, or often even indistinguishable from, those seen in spontaneous human cases. In both instances there are focal or diffuse lesions consisting of degeneration of muscle fibers, fibroblastic proliferation, fibrosis, and pleomorphic cellular infiltration. However, whereas cardiac enlargement and congestive heart failure are characteristic and constant findings in humans with primary myocardial diseases, these manifestations rarely occur in association with experimentally induced primary heart-muscle lesions.[1, 2] Therefore, the recent successful development, through selective breeding, of a strain of Syrian hamster (BIO 14.6) having a genetically transmitted cardiomyopathy that advances into congestive heart failure should be of great value to workers in various areas of study.

In an earlier paper in this monograph,[3] we noted that three well-defined stages can be distinguished during the spontaneous evolution of the chronic cardiac condition of the BIO 14.6 hamster (FIGURE 1). During the first stage (between the 25th and 65th days of age), myocardial degeneration characterized by focal myolysis occurs in these animals. Structural alterations in the heart muscle are not observed prior to the 25th day of age, but by about the 65th day, the myocardial lesions are severe, comparatively uniform in all animals, and have 100% incidence in both sexes. Thus, although this initial stage of cardiac involvement progresses rapidly, it nevertheless results in negligible mortality. During the second stage (approximately between the 55th and 85th days of age), cardiac enlargement consisting of various degrees of hypertrophy and dilatation develops. These compensatory phenomena are apparently elicited by the extensive muscle damage that occurs during the first stage of the disease; during the second stage, a few new lesions of mild intensity appear, and the older foci of degeneration are already in various stages of healing. In about 10% of the cardiopathic hamster, cardiac dilatation with no appreciable degree

* This work was supported by United States Public Health Service research grant no. HE-09791 (National Heart Institute) and general research support grant no. FR-05525 (Division of Research Facilities and Resources).

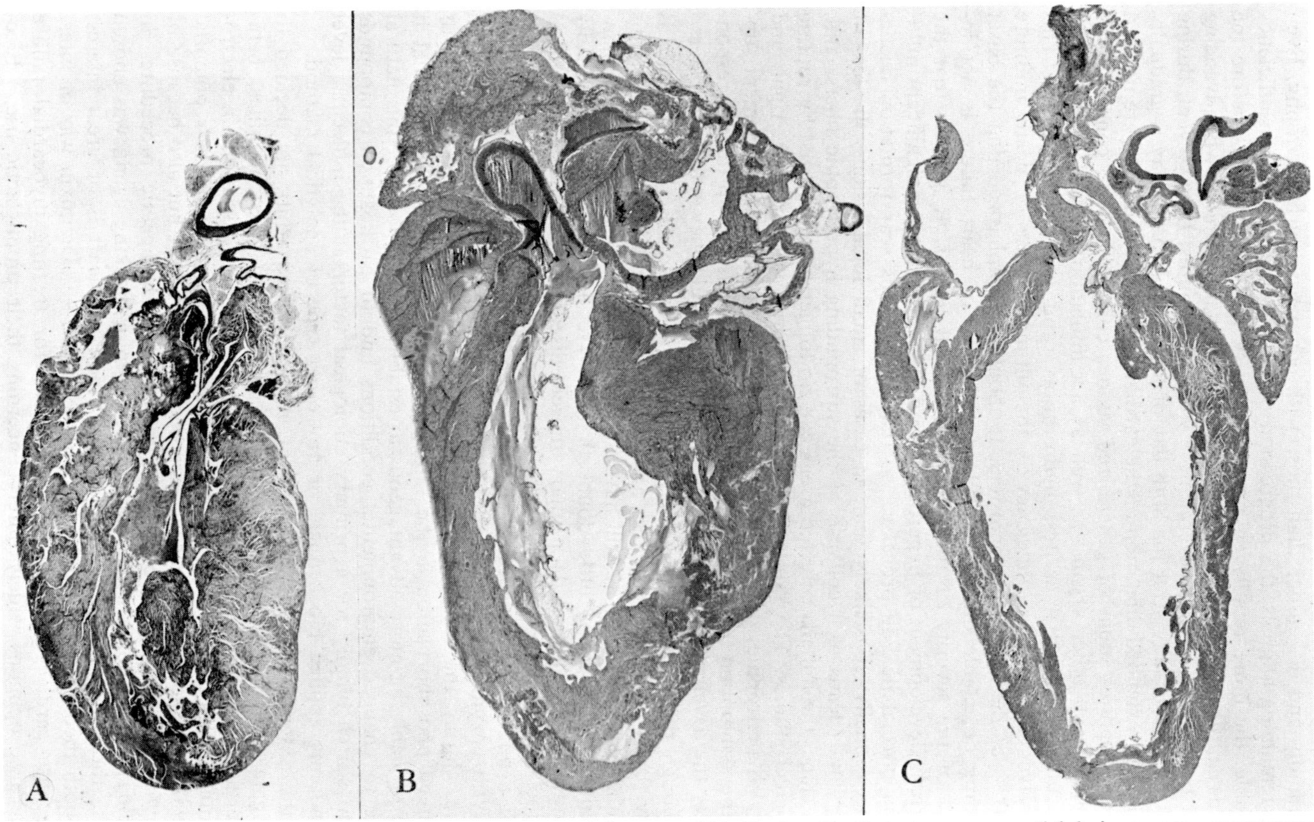

FIGURE 1. Three distinct stages of heart failure in the BIO 14.6 hamster. (A) During the first stage, myocardial lesions occur spontaneously. (B) During the second stage, cardiac hypertrophy and dilatation develop. (C) During the third stage, the hypertrophy is overtaken by extended dilatation. Hearts in photograph are from 62-, 88-, and 105-day old myopathic animals.

of hypertrophy is seen; these animals develop congestive heart failure much more rapidly and die earlier than those with compensatory hypertrophy. Even in the remaining animals, the progression of the cardiocirculatory insufficiency is variable; the more rapidly culminating variety kills the hamsters before the 140th day of age, whereas those showing a more retarded and slowly advancing type of failure may live for several more weeks or months. In any event, during the third stage (usually after the 80th day of age), the hypertrophy is gradually overtaken by extended dilatation of the cardiac chambers, and there are marked peripheral manifestations of generalized venous congestion (i.e., congestion of liver, lungs, and other organs, as well as accumulation of fluids in the form of subcutaneous edema, ascites, hydrothorax, and hydropericardium). This progressive circulatory insufficiency is the ultimate cause of death in more than 92% of the myopathic hamsters. It should be emphasized that the onset of healing detectable during the advanced stages of heart failure is not indicative of the severity of the initial myocardial lesions. It appears that the concurrent development of hypertrophy and dilatation exerts a significant influence on normal healing processes, so that collagenous scar formation occurs only occasionally. It is likely that, in cases of small focal lesions, the loss of muscle bands leads to a collapse of the surrounding hypertrophic fibers, and, at this stage, the initially affected areas can no longer be recognized by routine histological studies. The random occurrence of predominantly left, right, and bilateral hypertrophies during the advanced phases of cardiac involvement supports the assumption that the myocardial degeneration itself is primarily responsible for the development of systemic circulatory insufficiency in these hamsters.[4]

Although these investigations have provided a simple descriptive theory as to how the myocardial pathology and congestive heart failure develop in this particular hamster strain, we still have no knowledge of the underlying mechanisms involved. There is little doubt that we are dealing with a genetically transmitted (or conditioned) primary muscle disease,[5-7] but the histochemical and biochemical studies performed to date have resulted only in the demonstration of a number of nonspecific changes, such as loss of some oxidative and hydrolytic enzymes from degenerating muscle fibers, an elevation of serum enzymes during the active phase of the disease process, or the presence of uncoupled phosphorylation in the failing hearts.[4, 8, 9] We therefore felt that it would probably be more advantageous to establish the response of this natural disease to changed environmental conditions and to cardioactive compounds than to search blindly for a primary etiological factor at the molecular level by randomly applied biochemical or any other type of analytical method.

In the absence of previous pertinent studies, it was arbitrarily decided to investigate the reaction of the myopathic hamster to catecholamines, beta-adrenergic receptor blockade, and digitoxin, as well as to variations in electrolyte intake. Catecholamines were selected not only because of their potential importance in spontaneous cardiac conditions of man,[10, 11] but also because of their wide application to both experimental and therapeutic procedures in cardiology. Propranolol, a beta-adrenergic receptor-blocking agent, was chosen because the effect of this new compound upon the heart is of great interest from both theoretical and practical points of view.[12, 13] Digitoxin was of interest because cardiac glycosides are still basic for treating myocardial failure and because opinions widely differ concerning their prophylactic use.[14] Electrolytes (i.e., K, Mg and Na) were chosen because several recent experimental observations suggest that alterations in the normal ionic balance may play a fundamental role in the genesis of cardiomyopathies,[2] and because electrolytes may profoundly influence the action of cardioactive compounds.[15]

Effect of Various Agents upon the Development of Myocardial Lesions and Congestive Heart Failure in the Myopathic Hamster

Our principal objectives were to determine how the various cardioactive agents influence the development of spontaneous cardiac lesions when given to young myopathic hamsters, and to find out what action the same agents would exert upon the progression of congestive heart failure when given during the advanced stages of the naturally occurring disease.

Methods and Materials

Unless otherwise indicated, each experimental group consisted of ten animals. The myopathic (or dystrophic) hamsters used were those of the BIO 14.6 inbred line. Since myocardial lesions occur earlier in the females than in the males of this strain, and because progression of the subsequent development of congestive heart failure is more rapid in the females than in the males, hamsters of the same sex (i.e., either males, exclusively, or females, exclusively) were included in the groups of a given experimental series. Whenever a comparison between the responses of myopathic and healthy hamsters was deemed necessary, hamsters of an unrelated healthy strain (London School of Hygiene: LSH) served as controls (FIGURE 2). It should be noted that the growth rates of the animals in each of the two different strains (BIO 14.6 and LSH) are significantly different; hence, age and body weight controls were both employed. The animals were kept under identical, controlled-housing conditions in air-conditioned rooms. Guilford hamster chow, supplemented by oats and wheat germ, and tap water were offered *ad libitum*. Distilled water served as drinking fluid in those experiments in which the hamsters were maintained on synthetic (i.e., low-K, low-Mg, and low-Na) diets. The composition of these diets is described in detail elsewhere.[1]

Adrenaline was injected subcutaneously twice daily in doses of 0.2 mg or 0.6 mg/100 g of body weight, depending on the experiment; 0.1 ml of corn oil, was used as a carrier medium in each case, and controls received the same amount of oil by the same route of administration. Propranolol (10 mg/100 g of body weight, per os) and digitoxin (0.06 mg/100 g of body weight, intramuscularly) were also given twice daily. In some experiments, KCl and $MgCl_2$ (of reagent grade degree of purity) were administered at doses of 0.5 millimole/ 100 g of body weight; in others, where the effects of various K- or Mg-salts were compared, each dose contained 100 mg of the cation/100 g of body weight. The electrolytes were always administered twice daily by stomach tube, in 2.0 ml of distilled water, and the controls received the same amount of the solvent. Whenever a possible protective action of some compounds (propranolol, electrolytes) against the adverse effects of other agents (adrenaline, digitoxin) was investigated, a compound of the former group was given one hour prior to the injection of the agent of the latter group.

After death—either spontaneous or by sacrifice—each animal was autopsied, and the gross pathological findings were recorded. Organ weight studies were made on carefully dissected hearts, livers, lungs, and occasionally on other organs (spleen, kidney, and adrenal), and specimens were taken for routine histological study. These specimens always included the heart, liver, diaphragm, and a hind-leg muscle (anterior tibialis). The sections were stained with hematoxylin and eosin. (The myocardial lesions that develop spontaneously in the BIO 14.6 hamster are only occasionally visible by gross inspection or under the dissection microscope, but they can be readily graded on histological preparations because of their focal nature.)

The severity of myocardial lesions was assessed on an arbitrary scale of 0 to 4, with 0 designating no lesions; grade 1, mild lesion; grades 2 and 3, moderate lesions; and grade 4, severe lesions. The following morphological criteria served as the basis for this grading: grade 1, 1 to 3 small focal areas of degeneration, each focus involving not more than 10 adjacent muscle fibers or fiber segments; grade 2, 4 to 6 small foci and/or not more than 2 larger areas; grade 3, 7 to 12 small and/or 3 to 5 large areas; grade 4, more than

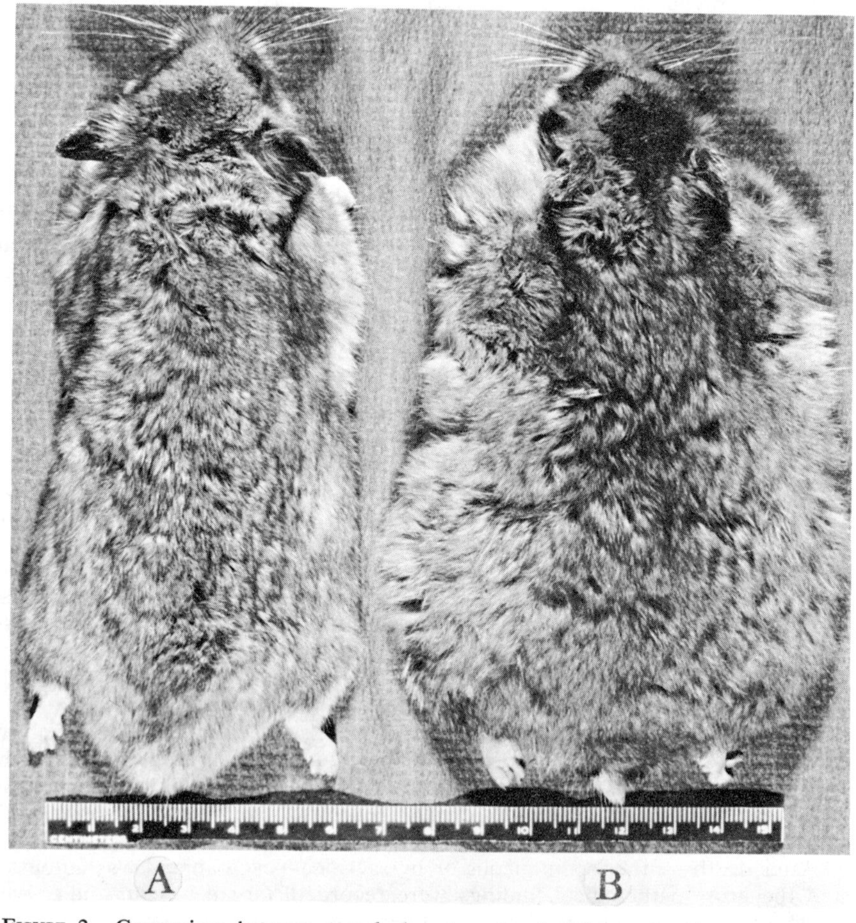

FIGURE 2. Comparison between a male hamster of a healthy strain (A) and a myopathic hamster of the same sex and body length (B). Note that the latter his highly edematous, due to congestive heart failure.

12 small and/or more than 5 larger focal lesions. Confluent and diffuse myocardial involvements were approximated in terms of small focal lesions and graded accordingly.

To estimate the severity of congestive heart failure, the degree of generalized edema was assessed and complemented by histopathological studies of the liver, as well as by observations on the presence of pleural effusion and pulmonary congestion. By means of studies on the progression of various peripheral manifestations of congestive heart failure, the following scale of grading was established and used in the present investigations:

Mild heart failure (grade 1): a moderate degree of subcutaneous edema restricted to the dependent parts; absence of a measurable amount of exudate in the body cavities; liver enlargement accompanied by dilatation of the centrilobular veins and of the sinusoids, but without structural alterations.

Moderate heart failure (grades 2 and 3): diffuse subcutaneous edema; liver pathology consisting of hemorrhages and necroses around the central veins; pleural effusion (grade 2). The additional occurrence of measurable amounts of exudates in the abdominal and chest cavities (not exceeding a total of 2.5 ml) with marked pulmonary congestion was considered to represent a more advanced stage of moderate failure (grade 3). In such cases, the liver pathology was usually diffuse and showed progressive destruction of the parenchymal tissues.

Severe heart failure (grade 4): severe generalized edema involving subcutaneous areas of the entire body (including the facial parts), together with ascites, hydrothorax, and hydropericardium. In such severe cases, the majority of skeletal-muscle groups, especially those of the hind legs and abdominal wall, were markedly swollen. The mesenteries of intestines and the pancreas were highly edematous, and the measurable exudates amounted to well over 2.5 ml. There were diffuse necrotic and fibrotic lesions in the congested liver, and hemosiderin-laden macrophages ("heart-failure cells") were seen in the lungs.

Results and Discussion

Catecholamines

In the first experimental series, adrenaline (0.2 mg/100 g of body weight) was given alone or concurrently with propranolol, KCl, or $MgCl_2$, as indicated in FIGURE 3. Five groups of young BIO 14.6 male hamsters were used to establish the effects of the various treatment combinations upon the development of early myocardial pathology, and five groups of older animals of the same strain and sex were employed to observe the alterations in the disease manifestations (i.e., cardiac lesions, hypertrophy, dilatation, and congestive failure) during the advanced stages of cardiac involvement caused by the same combination of compounds. Groups 1 and 6 served as controls. At the start of the various treatments, the younger animals averaged 25 ($\pm$ 3) days of age, and those in an advanced stage of disease averaged 118 ($\pm$ 9) days. It should be noted that the first myocardial lesions become apparent at about the 45th day of life in male myopathic hamsters; hence, the 25th day represents the "preclinical" (or latent) phase of the genetically determined condition. On the other hand, the older animals were selected from those that had shown only a mild degree of generalized edema by the 118th day of life; these myopathic hamsters were afflicted with the slowly progressing type of the spontaneous cardiac disease and showed cardiac lesions (both fresh and healed) of moderate severity, as well as cardiac enlargement consisting of both hypertrophy and dilatation. All treatments were continued for 20 consecutive days, after which the experiment was terminated by killing the survivors with chloroform. The data in FIGURE 3 indicate the average severity of myocardial lesions, degree of congestive heart failure, and the mortality rate for each experimental group. These results include the clinical and histopathological observations made on all animals, i.e., those that died spontaneously during the experiment and those sacrificed on the 21st day after the initiation of treatments.

When given during the early phase of the disease, adrenaline significantly increased the severity of myocardial lesions from an average degree of 1.9 to 4.0. The difference in the extent of cardiac pathology between untreated group 1 and adrenaline-treated group 2 is statistically quite significant ($p < 0.001$). This aggravating action exerted by adrenaline was completely abolished by the concurrent administration of either propranolol (compare group 2 with group 3) or KCl (compare group 2 with group 4), but these protective compounds apparently did not influence the onset and progression of the spontaneous lesions (compare group 1 with groups 3 and 4). $MgCl_2$ (group 5) proved to be ineffective in counteracting the necrotizing action of the catecholamine. It is important to note that the same duration of treatment wih adrenaline at an identical dose level elicited no histologically demonstrable striated-muscle pathology in the healthy control (LSH) hamsters.

In the adrenaline-injected dystrophic hamsters, the diffuse cardiac-muscle lesions involved the walls of both ventricles and auricles. They were of the mixed type (characterized by both myolysis and necrosis), accompanied by cellular infiltration and proliferation of the sarcolemmal nuclei. These lesions differed only quantitatively from the focal lesions seen normally in the heart muscle of the BIO 14.6 hamsters during the rapidly progressing phase of the hereditary disease. The supersensitivity of these animals to adrenaline was not restricted to the cardiac muscle, since the severity of skeletal-muscle lesions was also enhanced. Unlike propranolol and $MgCl_2$, KCl was again effective (although to a much lesser extent than in the heart) in reducing the adverse action of the hormone. Although noradrenaline exerted a similar aggravating effect, higher doses were necessary than those used for adrenaline to elicit the cardiac pathology in the myopathic hamster during the preclinical stage of the disease. Various catecholamines had different effects on the cardiac and skeletal muscles of the dystrophic animals during the various phases of the genetic disease; these comparative studies, using adrenaline, noradrenaline, and isoproterenol in combination with alpha- and beta-receptor blocking agents, will be published in detail elsewhere.[16]

Further analysis of the data summarized in FIGURE 3 reveals that congestive heart failure did not occur in the untreated young controls (group 1); however, an acute form of often fatal failure was apparent in 60% of the myopathic hamsters treated with adrenaline (group 2). Severe pulmonary congestion with hydrothorax, moderate liver enlargements, and varying degrees of subcutaneous edema were the outstanding findings in these animals. Since the intense myocardial damage elicited by adrenaline is the primary cause of the subsequent development of congestive heart failure, it is hardly surprising that venous congestion was not observed when the myocardial-pathology-eliciting action of the catecholamine was successfully eliminated by propranolol (group 3) or by KCl (group 4). The negative results obtained in the animals treated with adrenaline plus $MgCl_2$ (group 5) should be accepted as an indication that

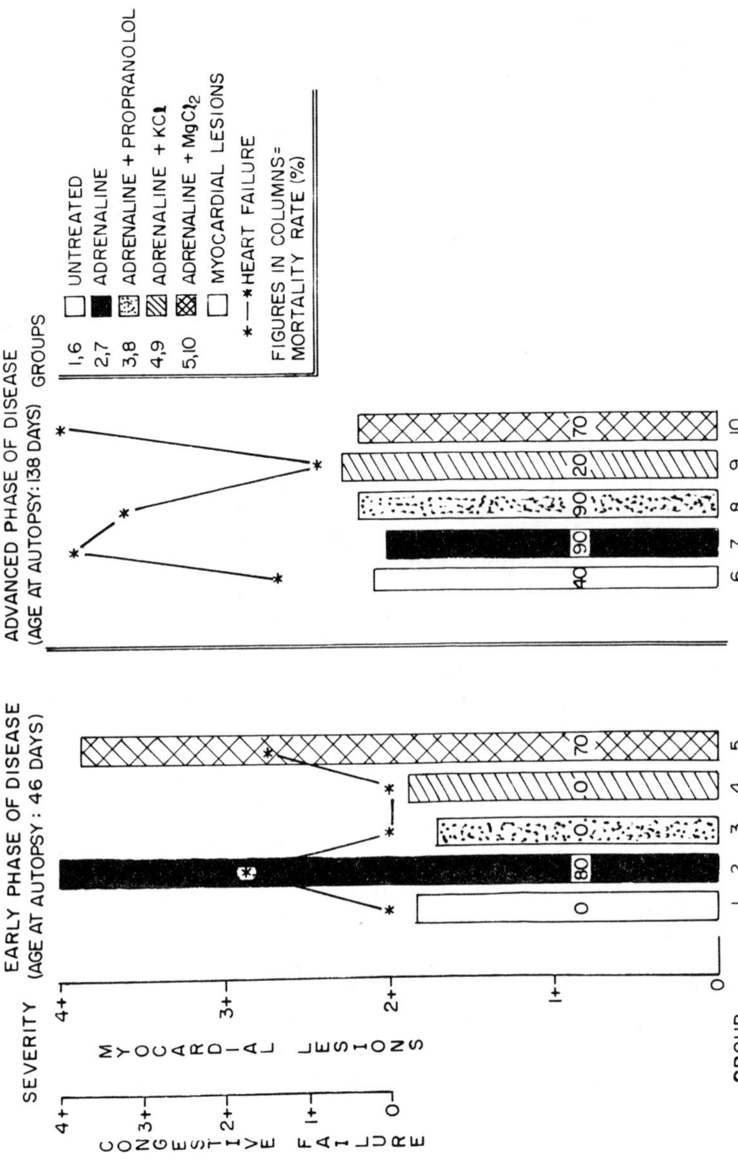

FIGURE 3. Effect of adrenaline upon early and advanced phases of hereditary cardiomyopathy.

this electrolyte exerts no demonstrable effect upon progression of the secondary result of severe myocardial damage.

Interestingly enough, when given during the advanced phase of the disease, adrenaline had no effect on the severity of myocardial degeneration normally present in older BIO 14.6 hamsters (compare group 6 with group 7); in fact, none of the treatment combinations used (groups 8, 9, and 10) exerted influence in this respect. However, the mild-to-moderate degree of failure observed in all of the untreated controls (group 6) was significantly enhanced by the administration of adrenaline (group 7; difference between groups 6 and 7, $p < 0.05$). Propranolol (group 8) and $MgCl_2$ (group 10) proved to be ineffective against the heart-failure-aggravating action of the catecholamine, but concurrent treatment with KCl (group 9) afforded remarkable protection.

There was positive correlation between the mortality rate and the severity of congestive heart failure in all experimental groups. The mortality rates were: group 1, 0%; group 2, 80%; groups 3 and 4, 0%; group 5, 70%; group 6, 40%; group 7, 90%; group 8, 90%; group 9, 20%; and group 10, 70%.

One of the most significant outcomes of these studies is the observation that administration of adrenaline to the dystrophic hamsters greatly enhanced the onset and progression of the spontaneous myocardial lesions when given during the early (preclinical) phase of this hereditary disease; however, the response of the hypertrophied and dilated hearts of animals to adrenaline during a more advanced phase of the spontaneous condition was of a different nature. The muscle fibers of these hearts were apparently no longer sensitive to the necrotizing action of the amine, and the induced sympathetic hyperactivity elicited another type of reaction, which was characterized by an aggravation of the preexisting failure. Whether this aggravation of congestive heart failure was the result of direct action upon the heart muscle or of some other circulatory effects of the amine remains to be established. In any event, it is of interest that beta-adrenergic receptor blockade by propranolol is effective in blocking only the necrotizing action of adrenaline, but KCl is capable of eliminating both types of adverse reaction. Since adrenaline is believed to be equally effective on alpha- and beta-receptors,[17] it appears logical to assume that its adverse effect upon the development of the spontaneous cardiac pathology in the hamster is somehow related to its action on the beta-receptor sites of the heart. On the other hand, the protective action of KCl might be explained by assuming that all effects of adrenaline observed in the present experiments were connected with a depletion of myocardial K. We have no evidence at this time to support the latter theory; future investigations may clarify this point.

The fact that the progression of congestive heart failure is extremely variable within the BIO 14.6 strain hindered the use of this model for serial investigations, e.g. for the testing of new compounds and other therapeutic and prophylactic measures. Therefore, further studies were performed by the injection of adrenaline, and these resulted in the induction of a uniform, subacute form of congestive heart failure in the dystrophic hamsters.

In this second experimental series, adrenaline was injected twice during a single day, in a dose of 0.6 mg/100 g of body weight each time. Two groups of ten female BIO 14.6 hamsters (i.e., one untreated control group and the other injected with adrenaline) served to indicate the extent of myocardial damage. The animals, 25 ($\pm$ 1) days of age at the beginning of the experiment, were killed 72 hours after the last injection. The severity and incidence of skeletal- and cardiac-muscle lesions are given in FIGURE 4. The data reveal a marked aggravation of the striated-muscle pathology induced by the brief period of adrenaline treatment; FIGURES 5–7 show the morphological effects.

In a subsequent experiment, 25 dystrophic hamsters were used in each group. The experimental arrangements were identical with those of the previous study, except that the development of congestive heart failure was observed. Fifteen of the 25 animals injected with adrenaline died within 8 days, and these were eliminated from the experiment. All the survivors of the two groups were killed on the 36th day, and the severity of congestive heart failure was assessed. The data summarized in FIGURE 8 show that a moderate to severe (grades 3 and 4) edema developed in all hamsters injected with the catecholamine, whereas the untreated controls were, on the average, much less edematous and showed a considerable variation in the spontaneous progression of their cardiovascular involvement. The subacute form of congestive heart failure elicited by adrenaline under such experimental conditions was characterized by marked subcutaneous edema, severe pulmonary congestion, moderate liver enlargement, and cardiac dilatation (FIGURE 9).

It is noteworthy that if, under such experimental conditions, 0.5 mM KCl is administered twice daily between the third and tenth days to the myopathic hamsters injected with adrenaline, the otherwise high mortality rate is sig-

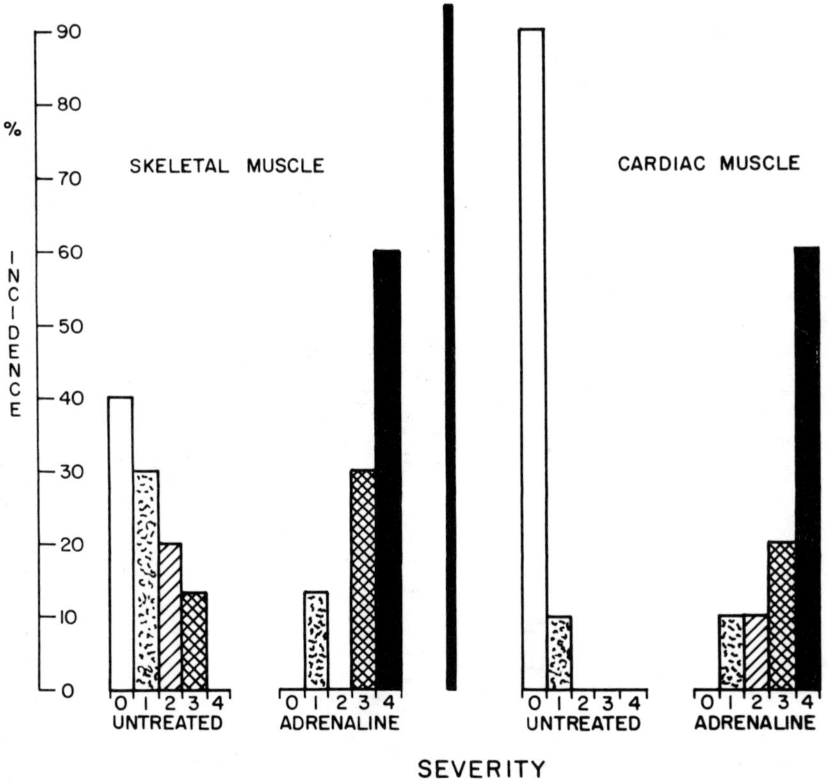

FIGURE 4. Effect of adrenaline on dystrophic hamsters (age, 24-26 days). The numbers under the columns indicate the severity (grade) of skeletal- and cardiac-muscle lesions.

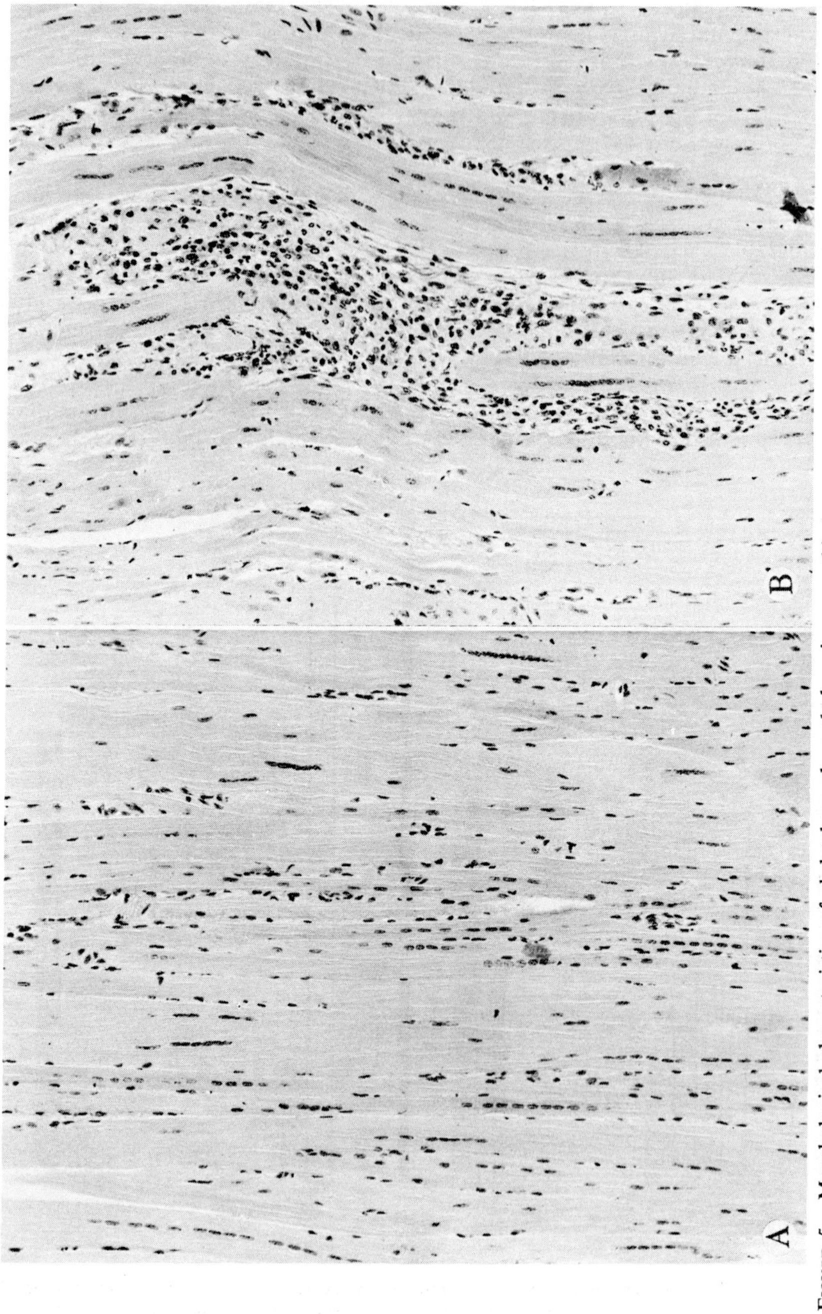

FIGURE 5. Morphological characteristics of skeletal-muscle pathology in myopathic hamsters at 28 days of age. (A) Nuclear rowing. (B) Necrosis of some muscle fibers. Stain: hematoxylin and eosin. × 112 (orig. mag. × 150).

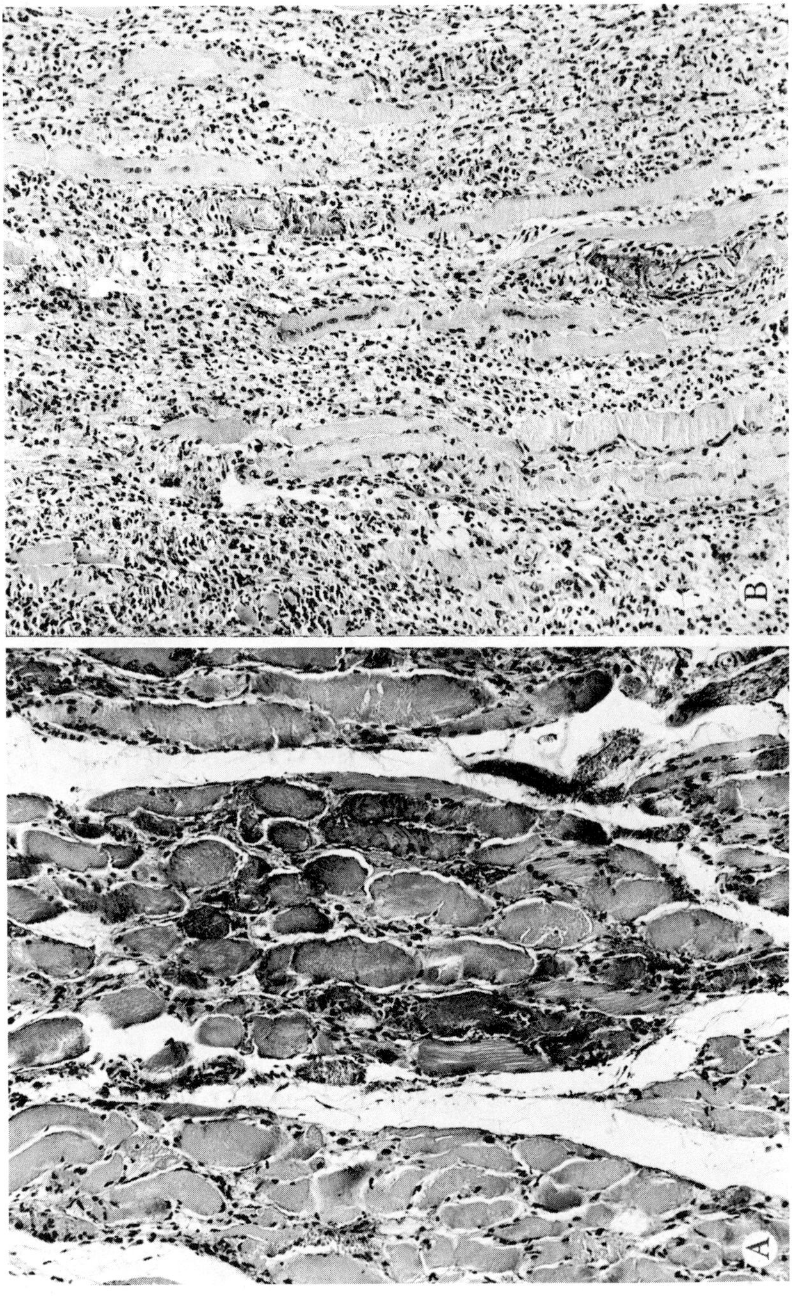

FIGURE 6. Effect of adrenaline (0.6 mg/100 g of body weight, injected twice during a single day into 25-day-old myopathic hamsters) upon the development of skeletal-muscle lesions. (A) Coagulation necrosis 24 hours after last catecholamine injection. (B) Severe, diffuse degeneration 72 hours after last catecholamine injection. Stain: hematoxylin and eosin. × 112 (orig. mag. × 150).

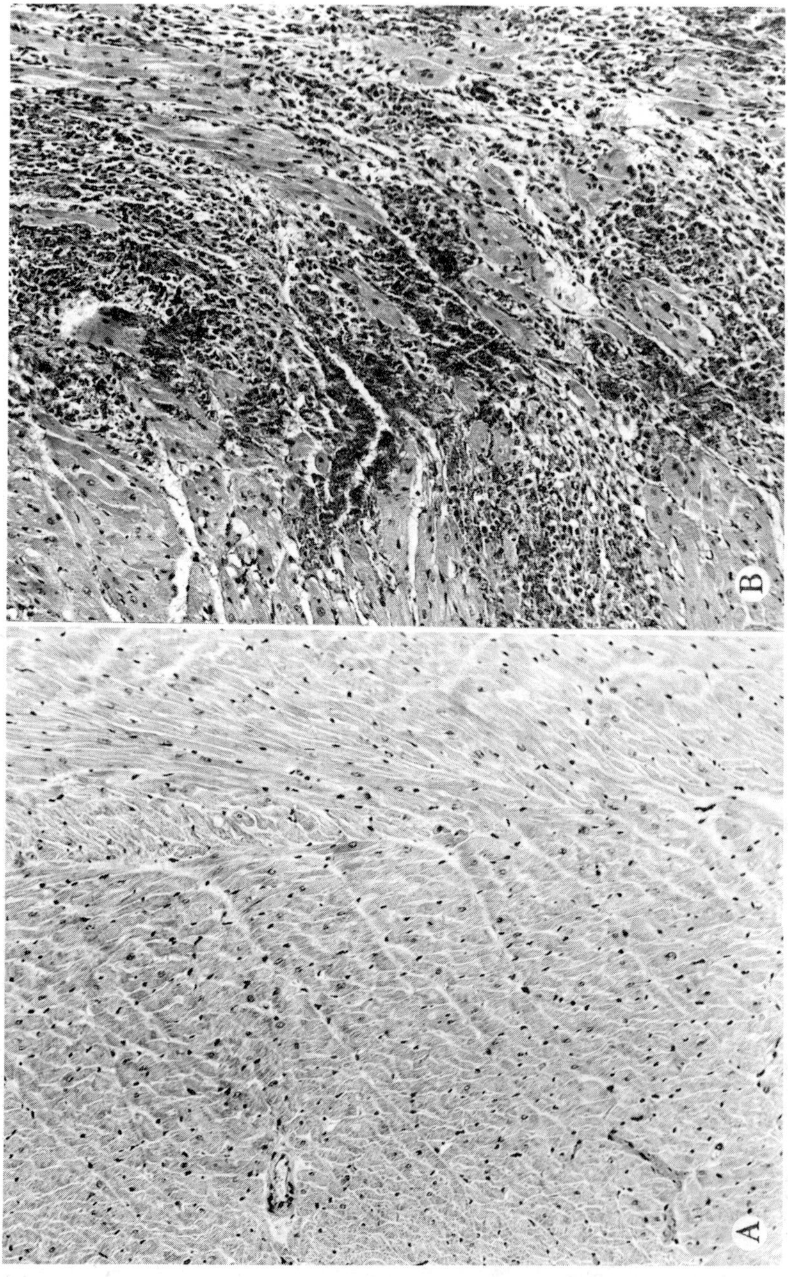

FIGURE 7. Effect of adrenaline (0.6 mg/100 g of body weight, injected twice during a single day) upon development of cardiac-muscle lesions in BIO 14.6 hamsters. (A) No heart lesion is present in the 28-day-old untreated myopathic animal. (B) Severe, diffuse myocardial degeneration is present in the myopathic hamster of same age 72 hours after catecholamine injection. Stain: hematoxylin and eosin. × 112 (orig. mag. × 150).

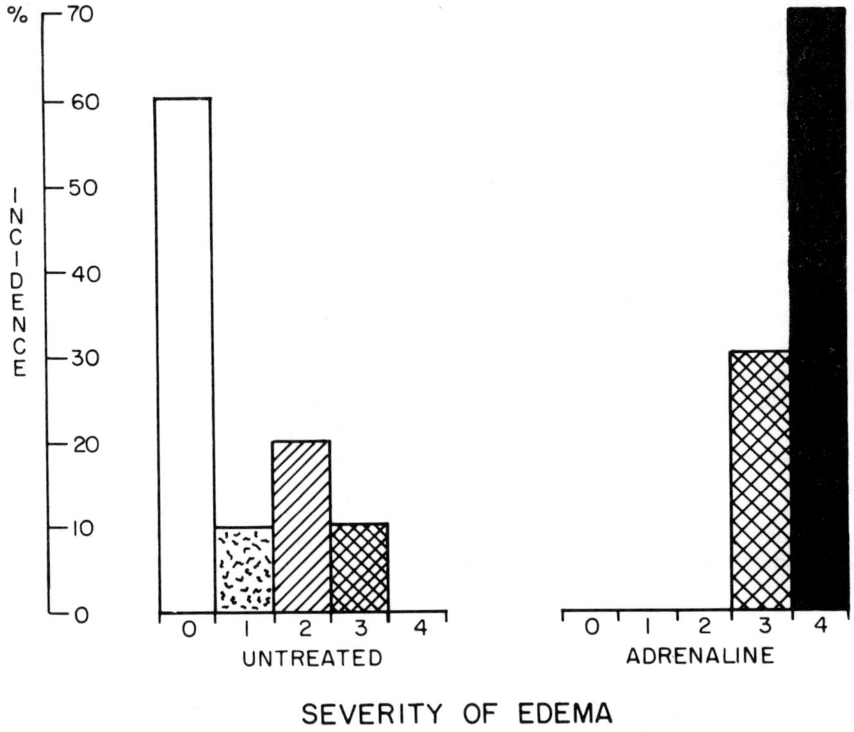

FIGURE 8. Production of congestive heart failure in dystrophic hamsters with adrenaline. The numbers under the columns indicate the severity of generalized edema, including the degree of measurable exudates in body cavities.

nificantly reduced. Congestive heart failure develops uniformly, although somewhat less rapidly, after discontinuation of the electrolyte therapy.

Digitoxin

The edematous BIO 14.6 hamsters react well to digitoxin therapy by a loss of body weight due to increased diuresis, and, unless liver pathology is not too advanced, their life-span may be prolonged considerably. However, the cardiac glycoside elicits an adverse reaction when injected into young myopathic animals. In order to study this phenomenon, the effect of digitoxin was observed during the early phase of the hereditary disease and compared with its action upon the advanced phase of the spontaneous cardiac condition. The young male myopathic animals were, on an average, 27 ($\pm$ 3) days of age at the start of the experiment, whereas the older ones were 109 ($\pm$ 7) days of age. Groups 1 and 6 served as untreated controls. Digitoxin was administered alone (groups 2 and 7), or in combination with propranolol (groups 3 and 8), KCl (groups 4 and 9), and $MgCl_2$ (groups 5 and 10). All treatments were continued for 20 consecutive days, after which the experiment was terminated, and the severity of myocardial degeneration and that of congestive heart failure assessed. The results are summarized in FIGURE 10.

It can be seen that, when given during the early phase of the disease, digitoxin markedly increased the severity of myocardial lesions from an average of 1.6 to 3.7 (difference between groups 1 and 2 is statistically significant at the level of $p < 0.001$). The lesions thus induced were diffuse and closely resembled those seen after administration of adrenaline. However, whereas the adrenaline aggravated the development of both the skeletal- and cardiac-muscle pathology, digitoxin exerted a selective effect on the heart muscle (FIGURE 11). Concurrent treatment with propranolol further increased the toxic action of digitoxin (group 3) and resulted in a high mortality rate. On the other hand, KCl (group 4) and $MgCl_2$ (group 5) were both effective in counteracting the adverse reaction of the heart to the cardiac glycoside. A mild degree of acute cardiocirculatory failure was observed in 40% of the animals treated with digitoxin alone and in 50% of the group that received propranolol in addition to the glycoside.

When given during the advanced phase of the disease, neither digitoxin nor the combined treatments exerted any significant influence upon the heart-muscle pathology (compare group 6 with groups 7–10). Nevertheless, digitoxin somewhat reduced the intensity of both the generalized edema and the morality (group 7), and these beneficial effects were potentiated by the simultaneous administration of KCl (group 9). Propranolol completely eliminated the therapeutic action of the glycoside (group 8), but $MgCl_2$ exerted no influence in any respect (group 10).

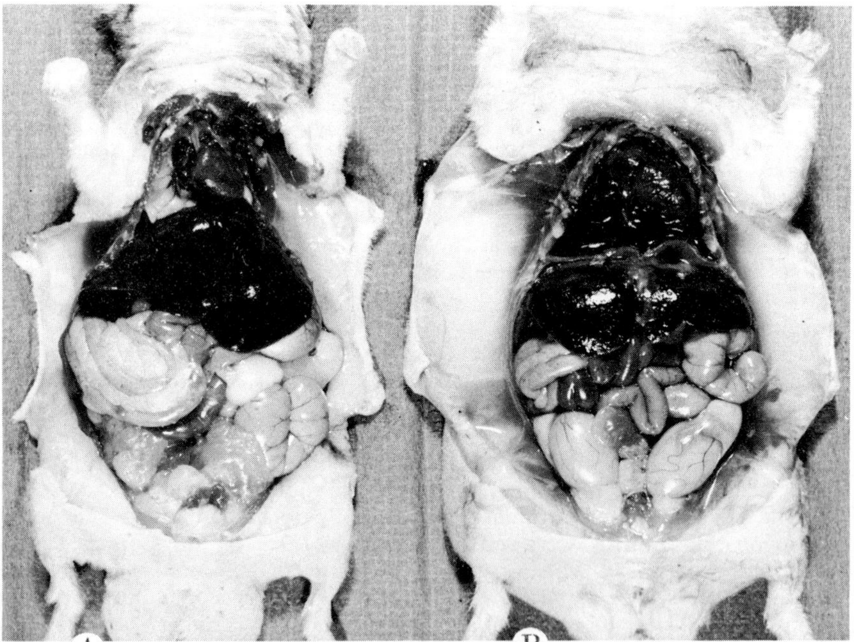

FIGURE 9. Effect of adrenaline (0.6 mg/100 g of body weight, injected twice during a single day) upon development of congestive heart failure in BIO 14.6 hamsters. (A) Congestive heart failure is not apparent in the untreated myopathic animal. (B) Note heart enlargement, pulmonary and hepatic congestion, and severe subcutaneous edema 36 days after adrenaline injection. Both animals were 61 days of age at autopsy.

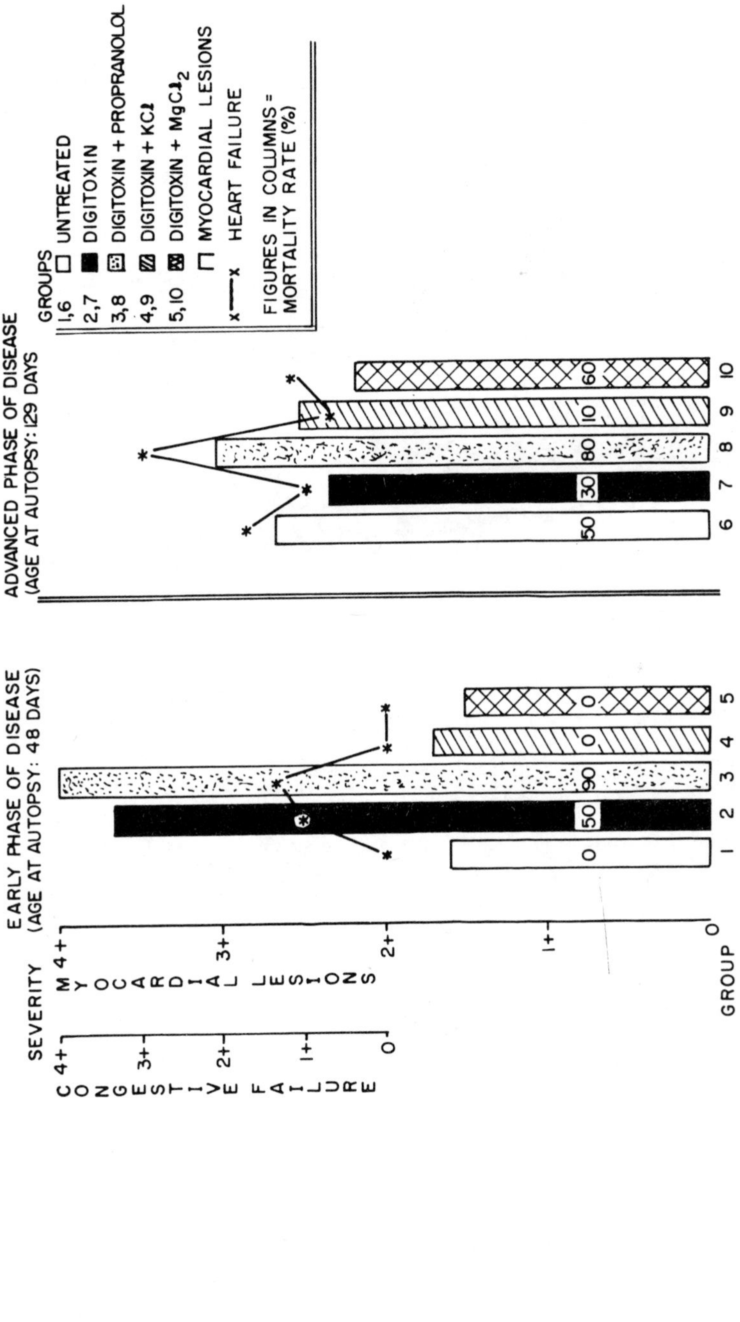

FIGURE 10. Effect of digitoxin upon early and advanced phases of hereditary cardiomyopathy.

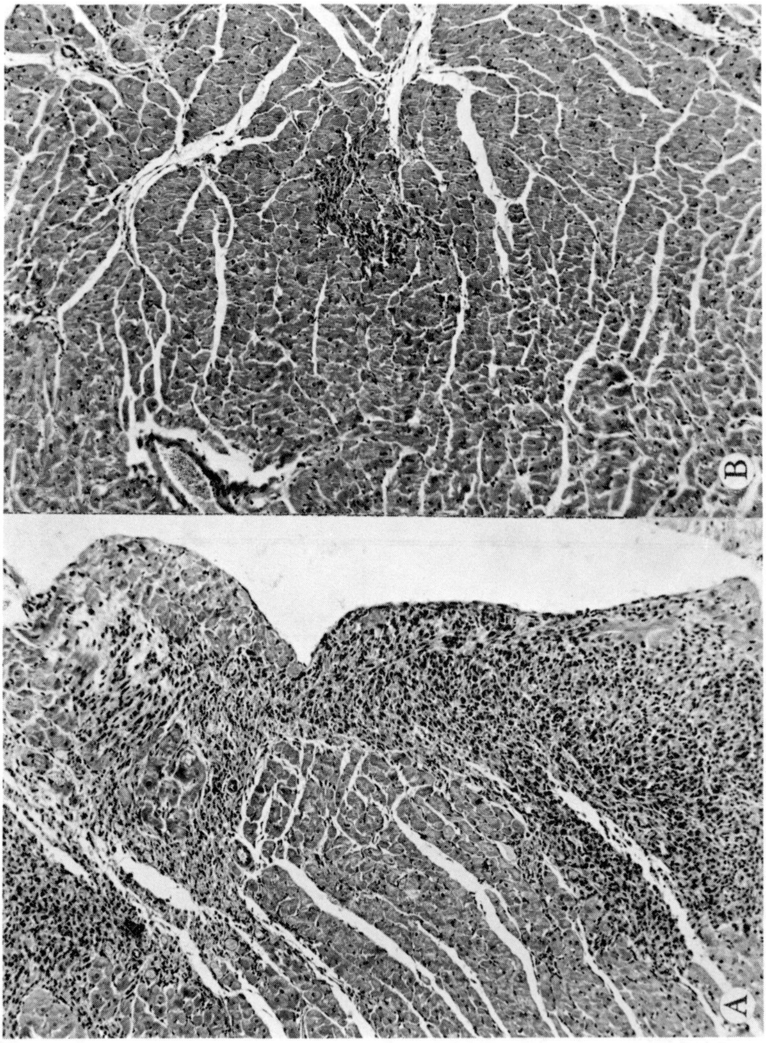

FIGURE 11. Effects of digitoxin alone and in combination with KCl upon the heart-muscle pathology of the myopathic hamster. (A) Diffuse subendocardial lesion in a myopathic hamster treated with digitoxin for 20 consecutive days. (B) Only one small focal lesion is apparent in the heart of another myopathic hamster treated with KCl in addition to digitoxin. Both animals were 48 days of age at autopsy. Stain: hematoxylin and eosin. × 75 (orig. mag. × 100).

It is important to mention that the most effective daily dose of digitoxin in myopathic hamsters with congestive heart failure proved to be around 0.2 mg/100 g of body weight, and this amount could be injected for several months with no toxic manifestations. However, when only about half of the maximally effective dose (i.e., 0.12 mg/100 g of body weight) was administered daily to the young myopathic hamsters, the animals, surprisingly, reacted with marked acceleration of their cardiac pathology. Cardiac glycosides are known to reduce intracellular K and Mg concentrations,[18-20] and the protection afforded by concurrent treatment with KCl or $MgCl_2$ suggests that ionic alterations are probably involved in the mechanism through which digitoxin exerts its aggravating action upon the development of myocardial lesions in young BIO 14.6 hamsters. In fact, all the experimental observations described have pointed to the importance of electrolyte balance; hence, we have studied the effect of various electrolyte deficiencies as well as that of electrolyte administration upon the spontaneous cardiac condition of the myopathic hamster.

Electrolytes

When myopathic hamsters between 25 and 30 days of age were placed on a low-K diet, they died within eight days, invariably showing severe myocardial lesions. Healthy (LSH) hamsters of the same age did not develop histologically demonstrable structural alterations in the heart muscle prior to the 16th day on the same synthetic diet. However, the reaction of the BIO 14.6 animals to K deficiency was different during the various phases of the spontaneous cardiac condition: a fatal enhancement of the cardiac pathology occurred, as a rule, when the usual laboratory diet was replaced by the low-K regimen any time prior to the 50th or 60th day of age; however, in older diseased animals, this dietary treatment exerted little influence on the extent of heart-muscle lesions, but invariably aggravated the progression of the preexisting failure.

The maintenance of young myopathic hamsters on a low-Mg diet resulted in similarly rapid and fatal aggravation of heart-muscle degeneration; however, in animals older than 60 days, this diet had no marked effect on cardiac pathology and congestive heart failure. It should be noted that only a few skeletal-muscle samples were taken from some selected animals for histological studies in these dietary experiments, and these observations do not permit us to draw a final conclusion concerning the influence of dietary electrolyte deficiencies upon skeletal-muscle aspects of the hereditary myopathy. Nevertheless, it seems that the heart muscle of these diseased animals reacts more sensitively to changes in the intake of K and Mg than do the skeletal muscles.

In view of these observations, the working hypothesis has been advanced that K and/or Mg deficiencies play a primary etiological role in the development of the genetically transmitted or conditioned cardiomyopathy in the BIO 14.6 hamster strain. This hypothesis, however, will require further analysis, since the various K and Mg salts administered alone or in combination by different routes (subcutaneously, intraperitoneally, and per os) were completely ineffective in preventing the occurrence and/or in reducing the progression of the spontaneous cardiac lesions. Nevertheless, during these studies it was noted that certain K salts—unlike Mg salts—do exert a decisive influence on the final outcome of the heart disease, despite the fact that equally intense myocardial lesions develop in both the K-treated and untreated animals. More precisely, certain K salts (i.e., K-aspartate and K-orotate), when given during a critical period, are capable of preventing the occurrence of congestive heart

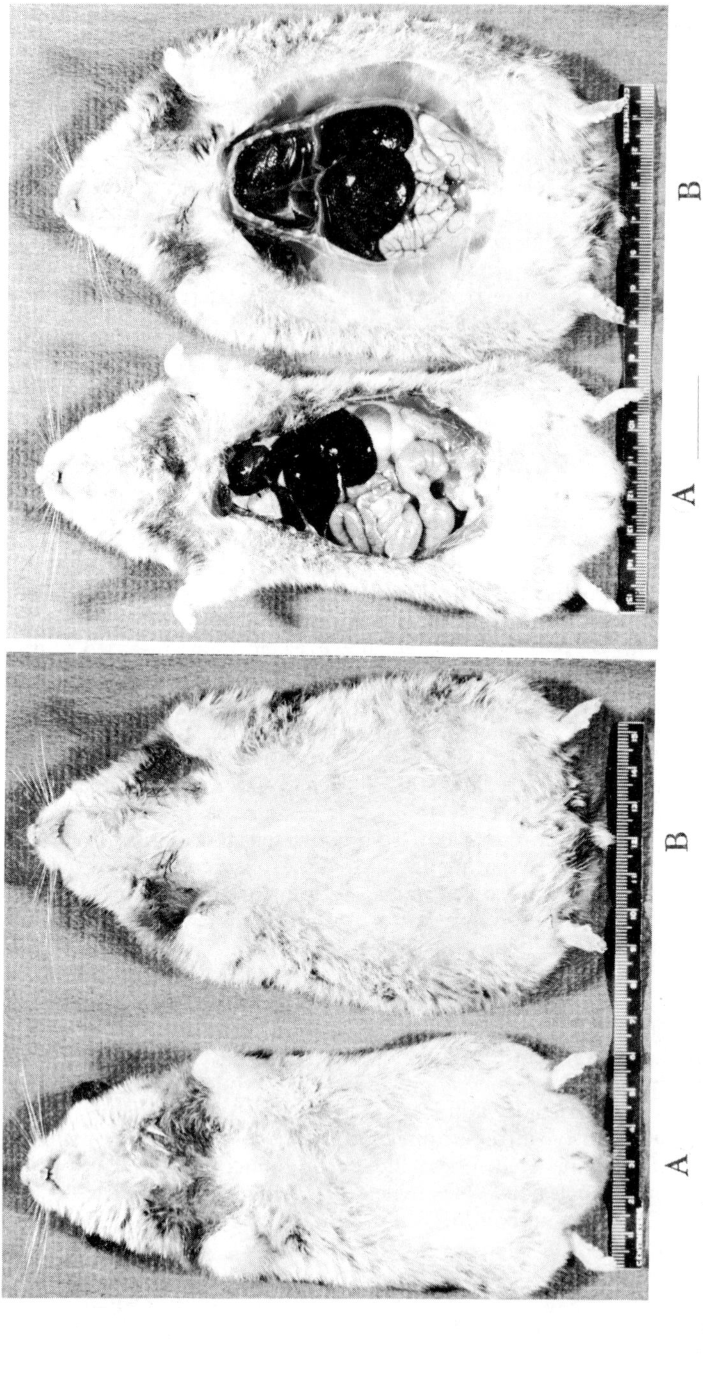

FIGURE 12. Effect of K-aspartate upon development of congestive heart failure in BIO 14.6 hamsters. (A) No edema or gross pathological abnormalities are visible in the animal treated with K-aspartate for 80 days. (B) Marked subcutaneous edema as well as heart and liver enlargement are present in the untreated control. The animals were 109 days of age at autopsy.

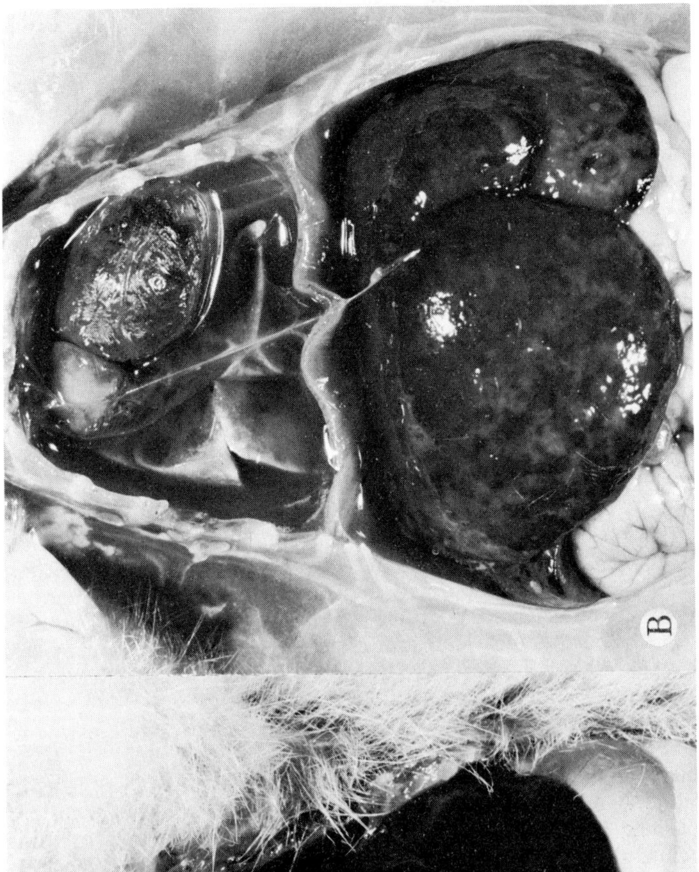

FIGURE 13. Close-up photographs of the hamsters in FIGURE 12. The absence of any pathological alterations in the K-aspartate-treated hamster (A) and heart enlargement with pulmonary congestion and hydrothorax, as well as liver congestion in the untreated control (B) are obvious.

failure, whereas others (i.e., KCl, K-citrate, and K-folate) are less effective or even completely inert in this respect (FIGURES 12 and 13).

In order to analyze this phenomenon more closely the following experiment was performed: 120 female BIO 14.6 hamsters were subdivided into six equal groups and treated as indicated in TABLE 1. The animals were 30 (± 4) days of age at the start of the experiment, and the treatments with the various K salts (as outlined in the section on "Methods and Materials") were continued for 80 days. The experiment was terminated the next day by killing the survivors. The final body weights and the heart and liver weights of the animals that died prior to the 60th day of the experiment are not included in TABLE 1. Only the figures underlined proved to be statistically significant when compared to the untreated group.

Congestive heart failure was found in 85% of the controls, in 70% of the KCl group, in 90% of the K-citrate group, and in 55% of the K-folate group but in only 5% of the K-aspartate group, and in none of the animals receiving K-orotate. The marked protection afforded by K-aspartate and K-orotate is clearly reflected not only by the complete prevention of mortality, but also by the final body and organ weights (FIGURE 14). The difference in body weights between the untreated and protected animals can be attributed to the accumulation of edematous fluids in the untreated groups, whereas the differences observed in heart and liver weights are attributable to the presence of only a mild degree of cardiac hypertrophy and the absence of liver congestion in the protected groups. It should be noted that a considerably larger number of old healed (fibrotic and scarred) cardiac lesions could be seen in the hamsters treated with K-aspartate and K-orotate than in the untreated controls. It is also significant that further studies have shown that the effective K salts must be administered only (approximately) between the 40th and 80th days of age; congestive heart failure no longer develops if the electrolyte treatment is then discontinued.

Experiments were also performed by maintaining the BIO 14.6 hamsters on a low-Na diet. A reduction in dietary Na intake failed to influence the development of cardiac pathology; it was, nevertheless, effective in preventing, or at least reducing, the intensity of congestive heart failure. More precisely, when young myopathic animals were kept on the Na-deficient diet, only about 27%

TABLE 1

EFFECT OF POTASSIUM SALTS UPON THE DEVELOPMENT OF SPONTANEOUS CONGESTIVE HEART FAILURE IN THE HAMSTER*

Group†	Treatment	Final Body Weight (g)	Heart Weight (mg)	Liver Weight (mg)	Mortality (%)
1	None	159 ± 27.8	527 ± 19.7	7,512 ± 478.5	60
2	KCl	152 ± 26.3	502 ± 23.3	7,879 ± 397.1	55
3	K-citrate	157 ± 31.6	511 ± 9.5	6,956 ± 401.0	65
4	K-folate	148 ± 21.4	500 ± 14.8	5,986 ± 458.9	45
5	K-aspartate	108 ± 15.8	409 ± 7.9	4,856 ± 216.0	0
6	K-orotate	101 ± 14.3	353 ± 8.7	5,012‡ ± 324.3	0

* All weight values are means ± standard error.
† Twenty animals in each group.
‡ Six animals showed fatty degeneration.

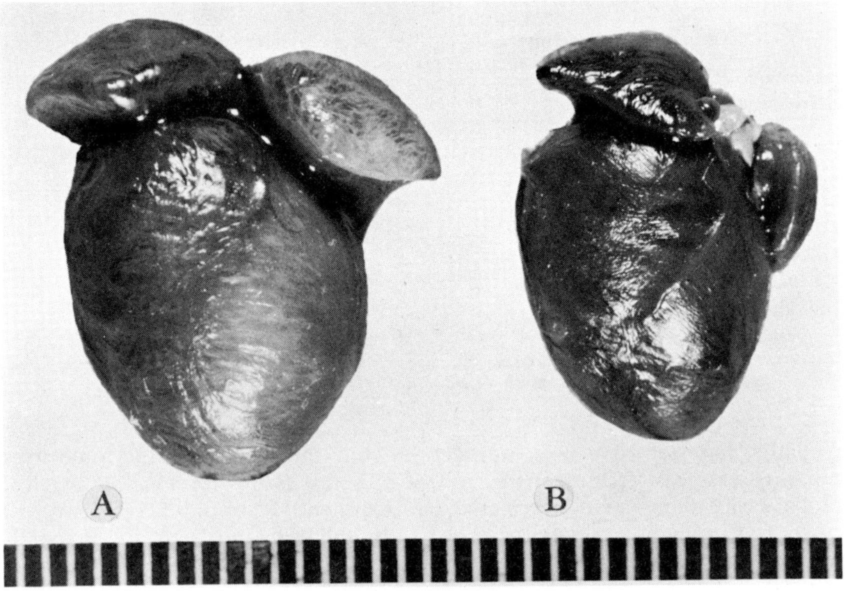

FIGURE 14. Prevention of cardiac enlargement by K-aspartate in the myopathic hamster. (A) Advanced cardiac enlargement consisting of both hypertrophy and dilatation is present in the untreated control. (B) Only a mild degree of hypertrophy (without dilatation) occurred in the hamster treated with K-aspartate. The K-salt was administered from the 40th to the 70th days of age, and the animal was killed 25 days after termination of the K-therapy. Both animals were 95 days of age at autopsy.

developed a moderate degree of generalized edema until the 100th day of life. On the other hand, when older animals, which had already shown signs of venous congestion, were placed on the low-Na diet, an improvement in the clinical condition was observed in the majority, although not all, of the cases. Rapid development of the onset or progression of the peripheral manifestations of congestive heart failure was always observed after discontinuation of the restricted Na intake.

CONCLUSIONS

Congestive heart failure develops regularly in hamsters of the BIO 14.6 strain; the genetically transmitted (or conditioned) spontaneous myocardial degeneration represents the principal lesion responsible for the cardiocirculatory insufficiency. The myocardium of these animals is incapable of maintaining a normal work load because of extensive structural damage. This failure is, thus, somewhat comparable to those occurring clinically in association with acute and chronic degenerative cardiomyopathies, during the progression of primary muscle diseases (e.g. muscular dystrophies), and following myocardial infarction. Nevertheless, it should be kept in mind that, since the fundamental cause of cardiac failure in man is unknown, one cannot be certain that it is being reproduced in the hamster disease.

The experimental observations summarized in TABLE 2 indicate that our attempts to eliminate the principal lesion responsible for cardiac failure in the

TABLE 2

EFFECT OF VARIOUS AGENTS UPON THE DEVELOPMENT OF MYOCARDIAL LESIONS AND CONGESTIVE HEART FAILURE IN THE HAMSTER*

Treatment	Myocardial Lesions	Congestive Heart Failure
Catecholamines	+	+
Digitoxin	+	−
Low-K diet	+	+
Low-Mg diet	+	0
Low-Na diet	0	−
K-salts	0	−
Mg-salts	0	0
Propranolol	0	0

* + = aggravation; − = prevention or beneficial effect; 0 = no effect.

myopathic hamster have been unsuccesful thus far. Just as in the majority of human cases, heart failure in this rodent presents itself with a factor that cannot be easily removed or corrected by treatment. It would be premature at present to formulate any hypothesis as to why the heart muscle of the myopathic hamster is so sensitive to the administration of adrenaline and digitoxin and to a reduction in K or Mg intake. Nevertheless, the fact that such supersensitivity occurs only during the early phase of the spontaneous disease has sparked our search for a reversible factor between the principal myocardial lesion and the subsequent failure. Data showing that the development of congestive heart failure can be prevented despite the presence of myocardial degeneration may be taken to indicate that such factors exist, but are reversible only during a "critical period" of the spontaneous progressive cardiac involvement.

The recognition of a "critical period," i.e., approximately between the 40th and 80th days of age, during the evolution of the cardiac condition in the myopathic hamster makes it possible to distinguish between symptomatically active and therapeutically effective agents in regard to congestive heart failure. If a symptomatically active treatment, such as the administration of digitoxin or restricted Na intake, is interrupted at any time during or after the critical period, congestive heart failure develops rapidly. However, when a therapeutically effective treatment, such as the administration of certain K salts, is maintained during the critical period but is discontinued thereafter, heart failure no longer develops, despite the presence of myocardial degeneration.

It is during this critical period that the myocardial lesions reach their maximal severity; also, healing processes and compensatory phenomena (hypertrophy and dilatation) are initiated in the affected hearts of the diseased hamsters. In animals protected by the administration of certain K salts (or by parabiosis to a healthy partner), the extended cardiac dilatation normally seen in the myopathic animals fails to appear, and only a mild to moderate degree of hypertrophy develops. The reduction in the extent of these compensatory phenomena in turn exerts an influence on the qualitative aspects of the healing of myocardial lesions, as described earlier in this monograph.[3]

Clinical and experimental investigations of the fully developed syndrome of congestive heart failure have provided much important information. It is unlikely, however, that more intensified studies of this end stage of cardiovascular disease, even if more refined methods are placed at the researcher's disposal, will succeed in disclosing the nature and mechanisms of the disorder. Future investigations must be directed toward definition of the physiological and pathological background of the events leading to the congested state, and the hereditary disease model of the hamster appears to be especially suitable for such studies.

Summary

The effects of various cardioactive compounds (adrenaline, digitoxin, and propranolol) and of variations in the intake of electrolytes (K, Mg, and Na) upon the development of a hereditary type of heart disease have been studied in the BIO 14.6 strain of Syrian hamsters. This spontaneous cardiac condition, characterized by the occurrence of focal myolysis in the heart muscle, results in chronic cardiocirculatory failure with generalized subcutaneous edema, ascites, hydrothorax, and hydropericardium, as well as congestion of hepatic and pulmonary tissues and of other organs.

When given during the early stage of the disease, adrenaline greatly accelerated the development of cardiac- and skeletal-muscle lesions, whereas digitoxin intensified only the heart-muscle pathology. The aggravating action of adrenaline—which can be used to induce a uniform, subacute form of heart failure in these myopathic animals—was counteracted by both beta-adrenergic receptor blockade and by the administration of KCl. The adverse action of the digitalis was abolished by concurrent treatment with either KCl or $MgCl_2$.

When given during the advanced stages of the disease, none of the treatments exerted any significant influence upon the extent of fresh and healed lesions normally present in the hypertrophic and dilated hearts. However, the subsequent development of congestive heart failure was enhanced by the induction of sympathetic overactivity, whereas digitoxin proved beneficial in this respect. Propranolol had no influence on the failure-aggravating effect of adrenaline, but it counteracted the beneficial action of digitalis. The latter agent was potentiated by simultaneous treatment with KCl, and the electrolyte abolished the adverse reaction of the myopathic hamster to adrenaline overdosage.

Although the maintenance of young myopathic hamsters on a low-K or low-Mg diet induced a rapidly fatal aggravation of the myocardial pathology, the administration of K and Mg salts, alone or in combination, had no effect on the development of the spontaneous, genetically conditioned heart-muscle lesions. Nevertheless, when given during a "critical period" of the evolution of the chronic cardiac condition, K-aspartate and K-orotate completely prevented the occurrence of generalized venous congestion despite the presence of myocardial degeneration. Other K salts (KCl, K-citrate, and K-folate) were less effective or even completely inert in this respect.

The use of the BIO 14.6 hamster as a disease model makes it possible to distinguish between symptomatically active and therapeutically effective agents. If symptomatically active treatment, such as the administration of digitoxin or restriction in dietary Na intake, is interrupted at any time during or after the critical period, congestive heart failure develops rapidly. However, when a therapeutically effective treatment, such as the administration of certain K salts, is maintained during the critical period but is discontinued thereafter, heart failure no longer occurs in the diseased animals.

References

1. Bajusz, E. 1963. Conditioning Factors for Cardiac Necroses. Intercontinental Medical Book Publ. New York, N. Y.
2. Bajusz, E. 1965. Nutritional Aspects of Cardiovascular Diseases. J. B. Lippincott Co. Philadelphia, Pa.
3. Bajusz, E., J. R. Baker, C. W. Nixon & F. Homberger. 1968. This monograph.
4. Bajusz, E., F. Homburger, J. R. Baker & L. H. Opie. 1966. Ann. N. Y. Acad. Sci. **138**: 213.
5. Homburger, F., J. R. Baker, C. W. Nixon & G. Wilgram. 1962. Arch. Intern. Med. (Chicago) **110**: 660.
6. Homburger, F., J. R. Baker, G. Wilgram, J. B. Caulfield & C. W. Nixon. 1966. Arch. Path. (Chicago) **81**: 302.
7. Homburger, F., C. W. Nixon, M. Eppenberger, J. R. Baker. 1966. Ann. N. Y. Acad. Sci. **138**: 14.
8. Eppenberger, M., C. W. Nixon, J. R. Baker & F. Homburger. 1964. Proc. Soc. Exp. Biol. Med. **117**: 465.
9. Opie, L. H., A. Lochner, A. J. Brink, F. Homburger & C. W. Nixon. 1964. Lancet **i**: 1213.
10. Chidsey, C. A. & E. Braunwald. 1966. Pharmacol. Rev. **18**: 685.
11. Raab, W. (Ed.). 1966. Prevention of Ischemic Heart Disease. Charles C Thomas, Publ. Springfield, Ill.
12. Braunwald, E. 1966. Amer. J. Cardiol. **18**: 303.
13. Shanks, R. G. 1966. Amer. J. Cardiol. **18**: 308.
14. Williams, Jr., J. F. & E. Braunwald. 1965. Amer. J. Cardiol. **16**: 534.
15. Bajusz, E. (Ed.) 1965 & 1966. Electrolytes and Cardiovascular Diseases: Physiology, Pathology, Therapy. **1** & **2**. Williams and Wilkins, Baltimore, Md.
16. Baker, J. R. & E. Bajusz. 1968. Manuscript in preparation.
17. Furchgott, R. F. 1959. Pharmacol. Rev. **11**: 429.
18. Hajdu, S. & E. Leonard. 1959. Pharmacol. Rev. **11**: 173.
19. Hochrein, H., Q. Zaqqa, B. Petschallies & E. Wollheim. 1965. Acta Cardiol. **20**: 148.
20. Kleiger, R. E., K. Seta, J. J. Vitale & B. Lown. 1966. Amer. J. Cardiol. **17**: 520.

ALTERATIONS IN WATER AND ELECTROLYTE DISTRIBUTION IN CONGESTIVE HEART FAILURE AND THEIR SIGNIFICANCE*

C. T. G. Flear

University Department of Clinical Biochemistry
Royal Victoria Infirmary
Newcastle upon Tyne, England

INTRODUCTION

Clinically, the most obvious disturbance of water and electrolyte metabolism in congestive heart failure is a progressive accumulation of edema. It is not, however, the only abnormality. In addition, potassium is lost, and the composition of extracellular fluid is altered. Patients lose potassium partly as a result of the tissue wasting that develops in chronic heart disease, but largely because their cells become depleted of potassium (Flear, 1967). Levels of sodium and chloride in extracellular fluid are often low, whereas that of potassium tends to be high (Flear, 1960a & b). Deterioration in the condition of patients is commonly accompanied by abrupt falls in the levels of sodium and chloride and a rise in the potassium level (Weston *et al.*, 1958; Flear, 1960b, 1966). Moreover, patients in severe congestive heart failure show greater fluctuation from day to day in the serum levels of sodium, potassium, and chloride than do healthy individuals (Flear & Hughes, 1963).

For a number of reasons, I believe that all of these disturbances are directly caused by the progression of heart disease. Throughout the tissues of the body, cells have their own problems of exchange of water and ions with the extracellular fluid. Many lines of evidence indicate that disturbances at the cellular level can provoke net gains or losses from cells, which in turn will, if sufficient cells are involved, determine the balance for the body as a whole, and may also alter the composition of extracellular fluid. Tissue perfusion is progressively impaired in heart failure, which must affect cellular metabolism, and there is indirect (Flear and Domenet, 1961; Flear, 1966, 1967) and some direct (Flear *et al.*, 1961) evidence indicating that cells do, in fact, lose organic solutes, including anions, and gain sodium. Alteration in the amount of solutes contained within cells must cause a net shift of water, whereas change in cellular organic anions will alter the potassium content of cells.

Further support for these conclusions is presented in this paper from an examination of the variability met in the water, sodium, potassium, and chloride contents of replicate samples from a single tissue in a given patient in congestive heart failure. This evidence complements that previously adduced, since the approach involves different assumptions and approximations.

If circulatory inadequacy is responsible for cellular disturbances underlying the alterations of water and electrolyte balance and distribution in congestive heart failure, then one might anticipate some variability in its impact on cells within a tissue. Local factors such as differences in the thickness of the film of extracellular fluid investing cells, differences in the amount of extracellular edema and in the distance of cells from their nearest capillary, and differences in tissue perfusion may well lead to variation in cellular disturbances through-

* The investigations reported in this paper have been supported by the Royal Society, the Dowager Countess Eleanor Peel Fund, the endowment fund of the United Birmingham Hospitals, and the Scientific and Research Committee of the Royal Victoria Infirmary.

out a tissue. The possibility that this is indeed the case, and that it brings about a gain of sodium by cells and loss of organic solutes, including organic anions, may be tested by comparing experimental findings with those predicted on theoretical grounds to follow such variation.

Material and Methods

Variability in water and electrolyte content of samples from within a single tissue (from nine to 60 samples per tissue) has been investigated in 16 patients in congestive heart failure. Three tissues were considered: skeletal muscle, heart muscle, and brain. Findings are strikingly similar in all individuals. Examples presented here are entirely representative. The data will be published elsewhre in full with Irené Florence.

Variability in composition was investigated in a similar fashion in a group of six patients with chronic heart disease who had some symptoms referable to their heart condition but were not in congestive failure. Right ventricle was sampled in four at the time of heart surgery; five skeletal muscles were sampled in each of two subjects.

Over the past five years, Miss Florence and I have investigated the variability within skeletal muscle in more than 200 individuals, including a group of fit subjects admitted to the hospital for cosmetic or minor reparative surgery (e.g. excision of lipoma or repair of inguinal hernia), moderately ill patients admitted for surgery (e.g. peptic ulcer), and patients who were severely ill with acute diseases (e.g. acute pancreatitis, peritonitis, and septicaemia) or chronic conditions (e.g. ulcerative colitis or regional ileitis). These data too, will be presented in full elsewhere. Illustrative examples will be presented in the present paper for comparison with findings in the first two groups.

Tissues were sampled after death from all the patients in congestive heart failure. This was also the case in some of our other severely ill patients. Handling of tissue samples and details of analysis have been described elsewhere (Flear & Florence, 1961). Chloride is currently estimated amperometrically. Each portion of tissue analyzed weighed between 25 and 40 mg. It should be stressed that the water, sodium, potassium, chloride, and fat content is determined for each portion of tissue analyzed.

Variability in the Water and Electrolyte Content of Samples from within a Single Tissue

Considerable variation is met in the composition of samples from patients in congestive heart failure—more, indeed, than in most fit controls. This is a good sign, since differences in the amount of sodium within cells would of course have this effect. But differences in the water and electrolyte content of samples could reflect differences in the relative proportions of cellular and extracellular fluids, either from variation in the volumes of fluid alone or from differences in the relative proportion of entire cellular and extracellular phases, solids as well as fluid.

Were this indeed the case, a piece of muscle with more of the sodium-rich extracellular fluid would of necessity have less of the potassium-rich intracellular fluid than another piece of the same weight but containing a lesser volume of extracellular fluid. The former slice would thus contain more sodium and less potassium than the latter. As pointed out elsewhere, when differences in the relative volumes of cellular and extracellular fluid are caused by variation in relative amounts of entire cellular and extracellular phases, the same negative correlation between sample contents of sodium and potassium is present, whether amounts are expressed per kilogram of fat-free dry weight of tissue or per liter of tissue water (Flear & Florence, 1963; Flear *et al.*, 1965). This situation is almost invariably what we find (FIGURE 1). Variation in the volumes of cellular and/or extracellular fluid alone can therefore be disregarded; in such instances, there is no negative correlation between sample contents of sodium and potassium when 1 kg of fat-free dry weight of tissue is used as the reference base. But the possibility remains that the findings described could arise either from variation in the relative amounts of cellular and extracellular phases or from differences in the average amount of sodium and potassium within the cells of slices if cells containing more sodium contain less potassium and vice versa (Flear & Florence, 1963). It is possible to discriminate between these two alternatives.

Although fluids inside and outside cells have the same osmotic pressure, the concentration of sodium plus potassium in intracellular water ($[Na + K]_i$) exceeds the corresponding concentration in extracellular water ($[Na + K]_o$). Thus,

$$[Na + K]_i > [Na + K]_o \quad (1)$$

and

$$[Na + K]_i > [Na + K]_t > [Na + K]_o \quad (2)$$

where $[Na + K]_t$ is the concentration of the total tissue content of sodium plus potassium, expressed per liter of tissue water. In addition, since samples of skeletal muscle almost invariably contain relatively more intracellular fluid than extracellular:

$$[Na + K]_i - [Na + K]_t < [Na + K]_t - [Na + K]_o \quad (3)$$

It follows, therefore, that, when differences in the sample contents of sodium

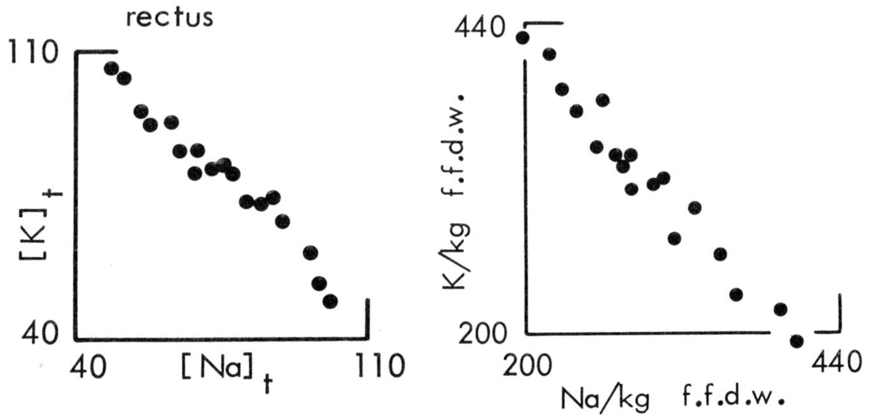

FIGURE 1. Sodium and potassium contents of 18 samples of rectus abdominis muscle taken at the beginning of an operation. (*Left*) Values for sodium and potassium, expressed as milliequivalents per liter (mEq/1) of tissue water ($[Na]_t$ and $[K]_t$, respectively). (*Right*) Values expressed as mEq/kg of fat-free dry weight of tissue (f.f.d.w.).

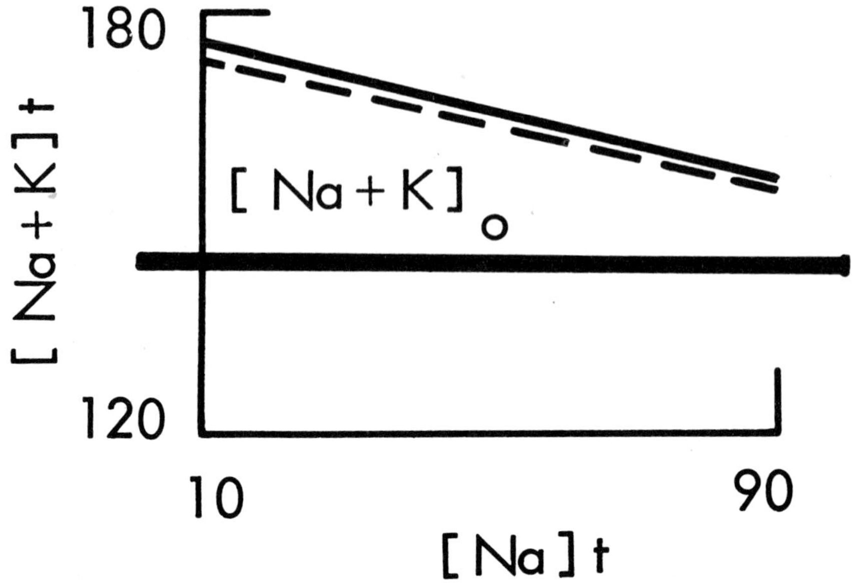

FIGURE 2. Relationship between the combined concentration of tissue sodium and potassium per liter of tissue water ($[Na + K]_t$) and tissue sodium, also expressed as a concentration in tissue water ($[Na]_t$). The differences in tissue sodium are due to variation in relative proportions of cellular and extracellular phases. Solid line, calculated for an intracellular sodium concentration of 10 mEq/1; dashed line, for a concentration of 0 mEq/1. The heavy horizontal line (also seen in FIGURES 3–9 and 11) is drawn through the ordinate at the level corresponding to the value for $[Na + K]_o$ in the patient, or assumed in theoretical examples.

and potassium are *entirely* due to variation in the relative proportions of cellular and extracellular phases, a negative correlation will exist between the concentrations of $[Na + K]_t$ and $[Na]_t$.† The precise relationship is only very slightly influenced by the concentration of sodium in cellular fluid. This is clear from FIGURE 2, which shows the relation resulting when $[Na + K]_o = 145$ mEq/1, $[Na + K]_i = 175$ mEq/1, $[Na]_o = 140$ mEq/1, and $[Na]_i$ is either 10 or 0 mEq/1.

Only once have we encountered such a negative correlation in samples of tissues from patients in congestive heart failure (FIGURE 3, left), and only rarely in samples from other patients (FIGURE 3, right). Superimposed on FIGURE 3 are the theoretical relationships expected, assuming $[Na]_i$ to be 10 mEq/1 (for derivation, see Appendix). It may be concluded, therefore, that variability in water and electrolyte content of samples taken from a single tissue in a particular individual is commonly due to differences in the average composition of their component cells.

† More precisely, the extracellular phase comprises a thin film of extracellular fluid investing the surface of all cells and connective tissue fibers and ground substance, which also contains water and ions. It is legitimate to consider the connective tissue "fluid" and the surface film of fluid collectively as a single fluid, since the value obtained when an ion in connective tissue is expressed as a concentration in connective tissue water closely approximates that of an ultrafiltrate of plasma.

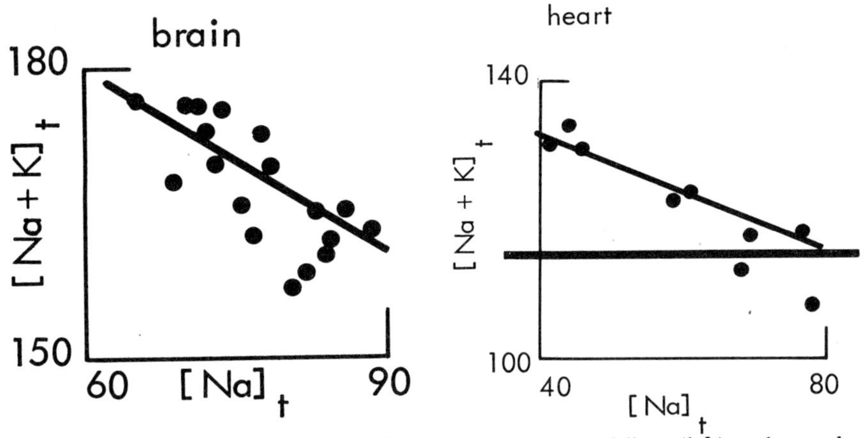

FIGURE 3. Data from a patient who died in congestive heart failure (left) and one who died in diabetic coma (right). (See FIGURE 2.)

PREDICTION OF THE EFFECT OF VARIATION IN THE CELLULAR CONTENT OF SODIUM, NONDIFFUSIBLE SOLUTES, AND THEIR ELECTRICAL CHARGES UPON TISSUE COMPOSITION

Preliminary Remarks

The distribution of water, potassium, and chloride across skeletal muscle cell membranes in what Conway has termed the "balanced state" or state of zero net flux of water and ions (Conway, 1957) is in accord with the requirements of electrical neutrality, osmotic balance, and a double Donnan equilibrium due to the existence of nondiffusible anions within cells and the virtual exclusion of sodium from cells. Accordingly, for electrical neutrality of cellular fluid,

$$[K]_i + [Na]_i = [Cl]_i - (zA/V) \quad \textbf{(4)}$$

for osmotic balance across the cell membrane.

$$[K]_i + [Na]_i + [Cl]_i + (A/V) = C \quad \textbf{(5)}$$

and for a Donnan equilibrium.

$$[K]_i [Cl]_i = [K]_o [Cl]_o \quad \textbf{(6)}$$

where $[K]_i$ and $[Cl]_i$ represent concentrations of potassium and chloride in intracellular water and $[K]_o$ and $[Cl]_o$ their concentrations in extracellular water. In Equations 4 and 5, V represents the volume of cellular water, and is taken as unity in the initial resting circumstance; A represents moles of nondiffusible material in V; and zA represents the sum of the electrical charges on A, represented as milliequivalents of anions (z is the average valence of A); and C represents the total external concentration, less that due to freely diffusible substances such as urea, present in equal concentration on either side of the cell membrane.

Equations 4, 5, and 6 may be combined to give an equation for predicting the outcome of changes in one or more of the terms in Equations 4, 5, and 6:

$$V^2 \{C^2 - (4[K]_o [Cl]_o) + 2[Na]_i C\} + V \{ 2[Na]_i A(1 - z) - 2CA\} + A^2(1 - z^2) = 0 \quad \textbf{(7)}$$

Since $[Na]_i = INa/V$, by substitution in Equation 7:

$$V^2\{C^2 - (4[K]_o[Cl]_o\} - V(2INaC + 2CA) + \{2INaA(1 - z\} + A^2(1 - z^2) = 0 \quad \mathbf{(8)}$$

As defined, INa is the amount of sodium associated with the number of cells which collectively contain 1 kg of cell water.

Equation 8 can be used to predict the effects on cell content and concentration of sodium, potassium, chloride; on A and zA; and on cell content of water relative to (1) gain of sodium by cells, (2) change in A, or (3) change in zA, either singly or jointly. The implications of these effects on total tissue composition are indicated in FIGURE 4, which presents relationships predicted between $[Na + K]_t$ and $[Na]_t$ under the circumstances described in this section.

Assumptions

In deriving the predictions shown in FIGURE 4, it has been assumed that the

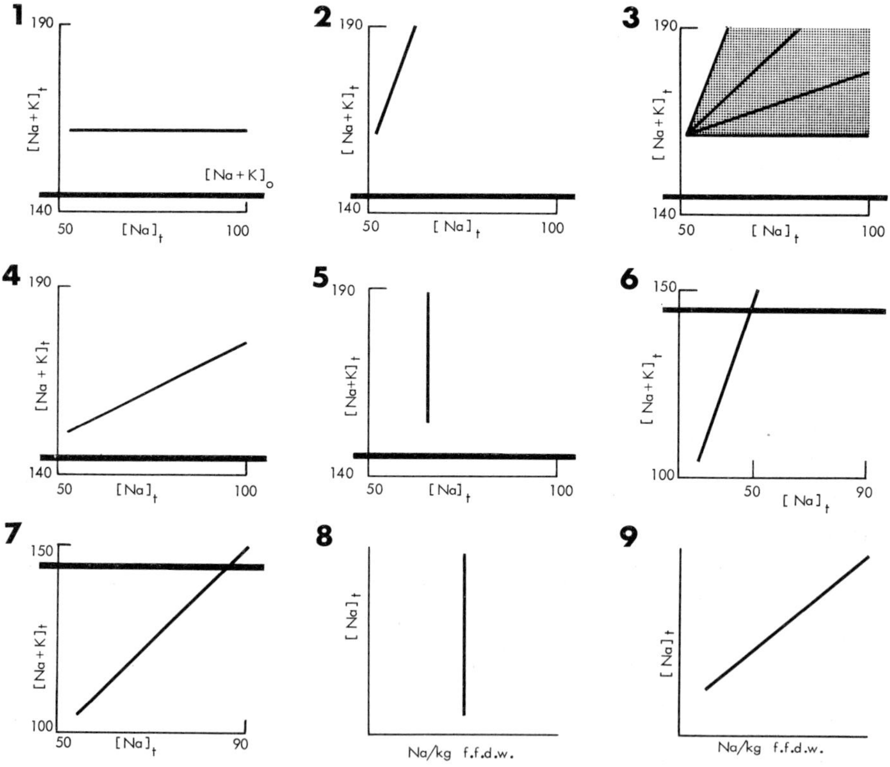

FIGURE 4. (1–7) Relationships predicted between $[Na + K]_t$ and $[Na]_t$ under specified circumstances of variation in cellular contents of sodium, and/or organic solutes within cells, and/or in the sum of the electrical charges on these solutes. (8 and 9) Relationships between $[Na]_t$ and the sodium content of samples expressed per kilogram of fat-free dry weight of tissue (f.f.d.w.). (See FIGURE 2.)

volume of extracellular fluid associated with 1 kg of cell solids is constant, with an initial tissue composition as follows:

$$
\begin{aligned}
[Na]_i &= 10 \text{ mEq/kg of intracellular water}\\
[Na + K]_i &= 170 \text{ mEq/kg of intracellular water}\\
[Na + K]_o &= 140 \text{ mEq/kg of extracellualr water}\\
[K]_o\,[Cl]_o &= 500 \text{ (mEq/kg of extracellular water)}^2\\
C &= 290 \text{ mosm/kg of extracellular water}\\
A &= 117 \text{ mosm/kg of extracellular water}\\
zA &= -\ 167 \text{ mEq/kg of intracellular water}
\end{aligned}
$$

Procedure

Since we are attempting to evaluate variability noted in the composition of a number of slices cut at the same time from one tissue in an individual, the composition of the extracellular fluid (whence C and $[K]_o$ $[Cl]_o$) can be presumed to be constant. Therefore if we substitute the postulated new value for INa, and/or A, and/or z in Equation 8 and solve for V, we can obtain a value for $[Cl]_i$ from Equation 9:

$$2[Cl]_i = C - \{(A/V) \cdot (1 - z)\} \qquad \textbf{(9)}$$

obtained by subtracting Equation 4 from Equation 5. Then $[K]_i$ is obtained from Equation 6, A/V from Equation 5, etc.

Predictions

The consequences of the various postulated changes for the relationship between $[Na + K]_t$ and $[Na]_t$ are shown in FIGURE 4 (1–7).

In the absence of change in zA, gain of sodium by cells causes an equal loss of potassium; thus, when there is also no change in A, the concentration $[Na + K]_i$ is constant. The effect of this sequence is shown in FIGURE 4(1).

Loss of A promotes loss of water from cells and thus gives rise to increases in both $[Na]_i$ and $[Na + K]_i$, as shown in FIGURE 4(2).

A combination of loss of A and gain of sodium results in a positive correlation between $[Na]_i$ and $[Na + K]_i$, with, however, a less steep slope. As shown in FIGURE 4(3), data will give a relationship lying somewhere between the horizontal of FIGURE 4(1) and the steep slope of FIGURE 4(2).

Gain of zA and an associated gain of sodium results, similarly, in a positive correlation between $[Na]_i$ and $[Na + K]_i$. With substantial gain of sodium, the slope will resemble that shown in FIGURE 4(4), but with only slight gain, most of the increase in zA being accommodated by gain of potassium, $[Na + K]_i$ may increase with no change in $[Na]_i$, with the result shown in FIGURE 4(5). A combination of gain of sodium and increase in zA could, therefore, simulate the pattern shown in FIGURE 4(2).

Gain of A promotes gain of water and decreases in both $[Na]_i$ and $[Na + K]_i$, as shown in FIGURE 4(6). Note that values for $[Na + K]_t$ may fall below the value for $[Na + K]_o$. A positive correlation between $[Na]_i$ and $[Na + K]_i$, with values for $[Na + K]_i$, and thus $[Na + K]_t$, below the value $[Na + K]_o$ can arise as a result of gain of sodium associated with loss of A when initial values of A are raised, as shown in FIGURE 4(7).

A correlation similar to that shown in FIGURE 4(7) results from gain of zA coupled with gain of sodium when the initial values for zA are subnormal. Here again, when some of the gain in zA is attended by a gain in potassium, there is a positive correlation between $[Na]_t$ and $[Na + K]_t$, with a slope even steeper than that shown in FIGURE 4(6). In this instance, a change in $[Na]_t$ is brought about by a change in the intracellular water; there is no change in the cell sodium content. A change in $[Na]_t$ will therefore occur without a change in the amount of sodium associated with 1 kg of fat-free dry weight of tissue; this is illustrated in FIGURE 4(8). When a change in $[Na]_t$ is provoked by a change in cell sodium, a positive correlation will be found between $[Na]_t$ and Na/kg of fat-free dry weight tissue, as shown in FIGURE 4(9). In this case, the lowest $[Na]_t$ is most unlikely to be subnormal, whereas in the previous case, this is not at all unlikely.

When the relationship shown in FIGURE 4(2) results from loss of A and a change in water, the pattern shown in FIGURE 4(8) will be found. When the relationship shown in FIGURE 4(2) is associated with a gain of sodium by cells, the pattern shown in FIGURE 4(9) will result.

FINDINGS AND CONCLUSIONS

Congestive Heart Failure

Almost invariably, there is a positive correlation between values for $[Na]_t$ and $[Na + K]_t$ in samples from a single tissue. Usually, data yield a pattern similar to that in FIGURE 4(3), (4), or (7). Findings for skeletal muscle, heart muscle, and brain are essential the same in this respect. Typical findings are presented in FIGURE 5, based on data from four patients. Other data for different tissues in these same patients are similar.

These findings could signify (1) that samples with more sodium in their cells have a greater quantity of organic anions constrained within them (greater values for zA), (2) that samples with more sodium per cell contain fewer nondiffusible solutes (lower values for A), or (3) that samples with more sodium in cells contain both more zA and less A. It is possible to say more than this: When cells that take up sodium and there is no increase in cellular anions, they will lose an equal amount of potassium. Cellular content of cation will remain unchanged, and with it the quantity of (Na + K)/kg of fat-free dry weight of tissue. When cells are also richer in nondiffusible anions, then samples with more sodium in their cells will contain a greater content of (Na + K)/kg of fat-free dry weight. In this latter case, there will be a positive correlation between sample contents of sodium and (Na + K)/kg of fat-free dry weight. In the former case, sodium content will vary without change in (Na + K).

Frequently we find that the sample contents of sodium and (Na + K) are positively correlated, from which we conclude that, of the three possibilities noted above, the first or third may be operative in congestive heart failure. A further finding persuades us that the third possibility is probably the most likely situation in such patients. When cells take up sodium without an increase in their anions, and at the same time lose other solutes normally contained within them, the volume of cellular water will vary with the content of A. The sample content of water/kg of fat-free dry weight will therefore show variation despite constancy of the content of (Na + K)/kg of fat-free dry weight. When the content of A is unchanging but the cellular content of sodium and (Na + K) increases, the water content of cells (and sample) will evidence a striking positive correlation with the cell (and sample) content of (Na + K) (see Rixon & Stevenson, 1956). When the content of A also changes, there will be a positive correlation between the water content and the content of

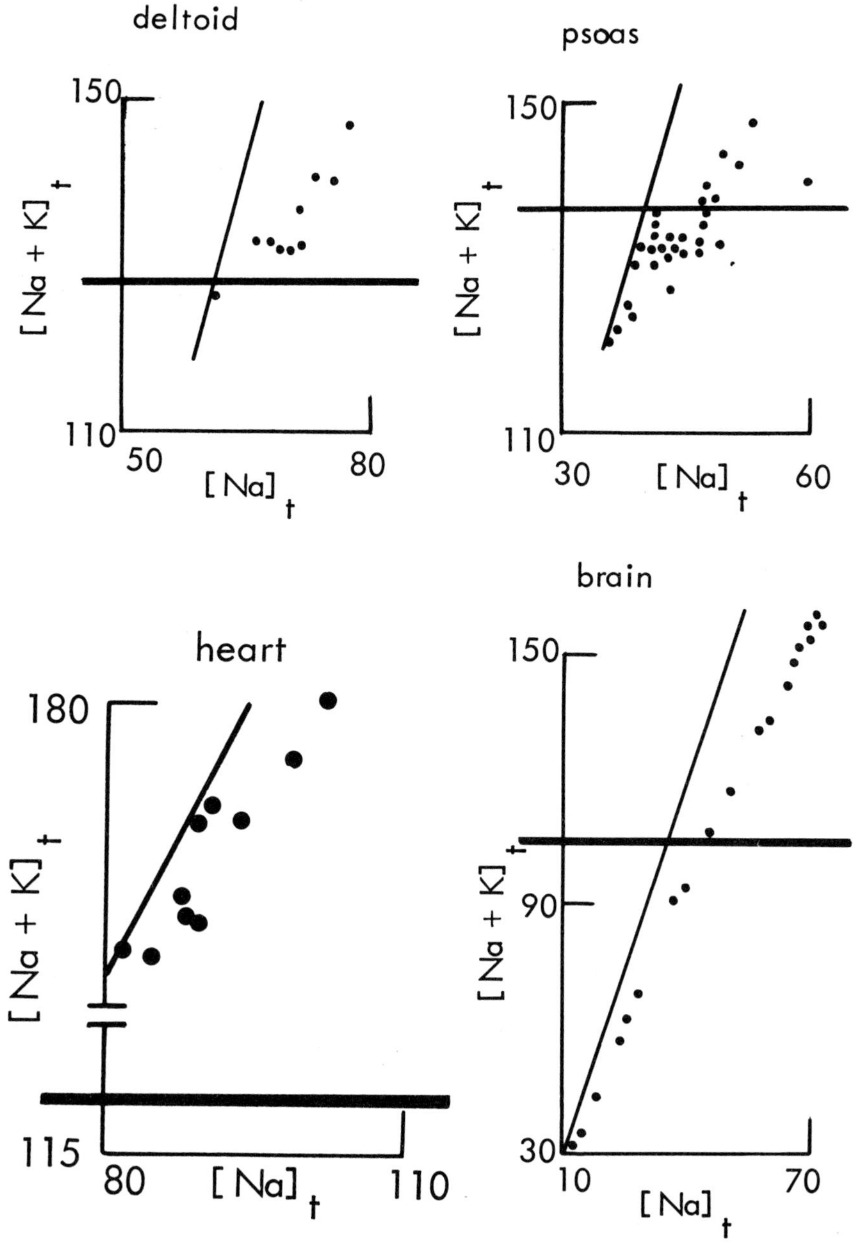

FIGURE 5. Data from four patients who died in congestive heart failure. (See FIGURE 2.)

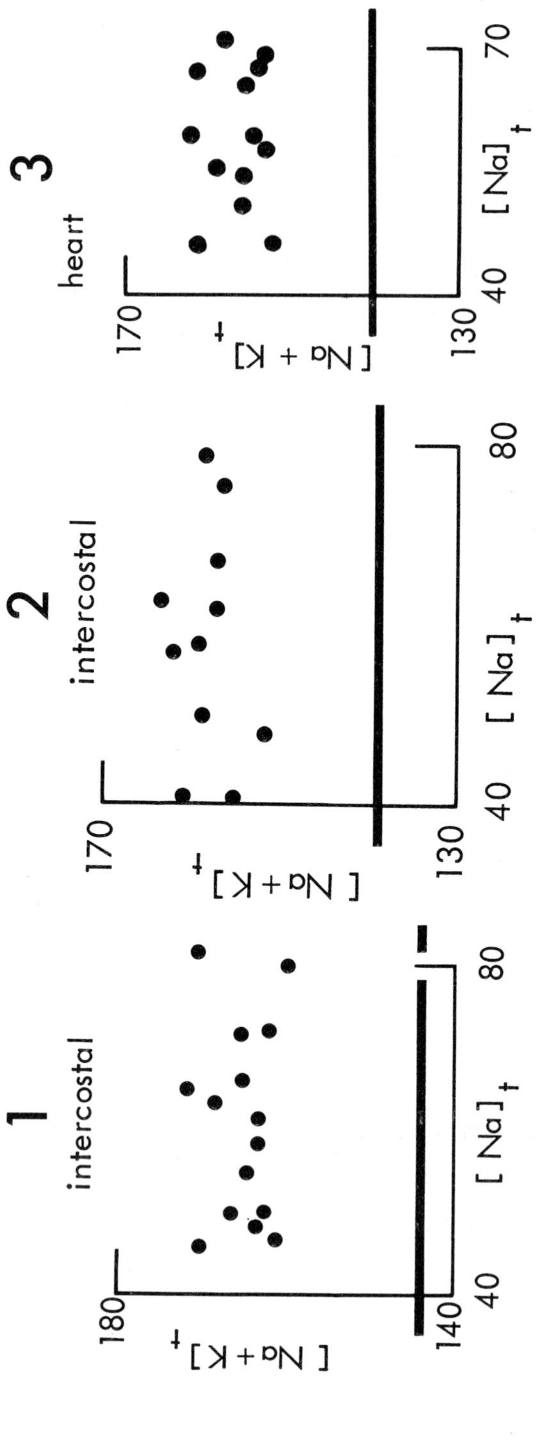

FIGURE 6. Data from three patients with long-standing heart disease. None was in congestive heart failure, but all had some cardiac symptoms. (1 and 2) Patients with rheumatic heart disease and mitral stenosis, undergoing elective commissurotomy. (3) A child with tetralogy of Fallot, undergoing cardiac surgery with bypass of heart and lungs, using a pump oxygenator. (See FIGURE 2.)

(Na + K), but with considerable residual scatter about the regression. This is a frequent observation in congestive heart failure.

The pattern of variability displayed by data from patients in congestive heart failure can be accounted for if one assumes that cells throughout tissues show a variable gain of sodium associated with an increase in organic anions within the cells, and a simultaneous fall in the molar concentration of solutes within the cells. It is inferred that cellular content of sodium is frequently excessive, since almost invariably even the tissue samples with least sodium contain much more than the upper limit of sodium content for samples from fit subjects (some 290 samples from 39 subjects; Flear et al., 1968).

Chronic Heart Disease without Congestive Failure and Edema

Typical findings for this group of patients are presented in FIGURE 6. With one exception, data conform to the pattern shown in FIGURE 4(1), suggesting that, in the absence of frank congestive failure, there is a variation in the amount of sodium within cells in a tissue, without, however, the variation noted in congestive heart failure in either the molar content of nondiffusible solutes or the number of anions within cells. Both heart muscle (right ventricle) and skeletal muscle show these findings.

This conclusion is in accord with other evidence that intracellular sodium is increased in subjects with chronic heart disease who are not yet, or not any longer, in frank congestive failure with edema. Nevertheless, it is not clear from the present data whether the gain of sodium by cells is excessive, since sodium contents of all samples of skeletal muscle (five muscles in each of two subjects) were not greater than those found in samples from the same muscles in control subjects.

It is not possible to comment about the sodium content in samples of heart muscle, since suitable control material is not available. However, samples from one of the four subjects were considerably richer in sodium than those from the other three subjects. This particular patient also had the most symptoms referable to his heart condition. The data from his tissue samples displayed the pattern shown in FIGURE 4(3), the only data that gave this pattern; all other data displayed the pattern shown in FIGURE 4(1). Data from this patient also indicated, for reasons discussed under congestive heart failure, that A fell as cells took up sodium, and that zA rose.

Control Subjects

FIGURE 7 presents findings from one fit 59-year-old male admitted for repair of an inguinal hernia (part 1); from one moderately ill female with chronic peptic ulcer who had lost a considerable amount of weight over the previous two years, was clinically unfit before the operation, and who experienced a protracted and stormy postoperative convalescence (part 2); and from two severely ill patients, both of whom had experienced prolonged ill health (parts 3 and 4). Three skeletal muscles were sampled after death in one of these severely ill patients, and four skeletal muscles were sampled at operation in the other. There was no difference in the pattern displayed by data from tissue taken after death. Indeed, all of the controls presented showed the same pattern, which is the same as that shown by the patients with heart disease but not in failure. This indicates the existence of a variability in the sodium concentration within cells; in contrast to samples from patients in congestive heart failure, cells with more sodium do not show any consistent associated variation in A or zA.

This pattern has been by far the most common one encountered in a wide range of clinical situations. Data obtained from an analysis of heart muscle obtained after death from a patient who died in diabetic coma displayed a different pattern, shown in FIGURE 3, right. In this instance, variation between samples appears to have arisen largely as a consequence of differences in the relative proportions of cellular and extracellular phases in the several samples of tissue.

Conceivably in the fit individual, such as the subject whose data were shown in FIGURE 7(1), variation in the cellular content and concentration of sodium may arise from a variation in the precise permeability characteristics from cell to cell. Influx of sodium will be greater where the membrane is more permeable to it, and this may result in a greater amount within cells. Variation in the permeability of cells within a tissue may arise during the course of normal functioning. On the other hand, it may represent a statistical variation in cell membranes along the lines discussed by Mullins (1959, 1960). In the ill patients, variability in cell sodium may arise as an exaggeration of these

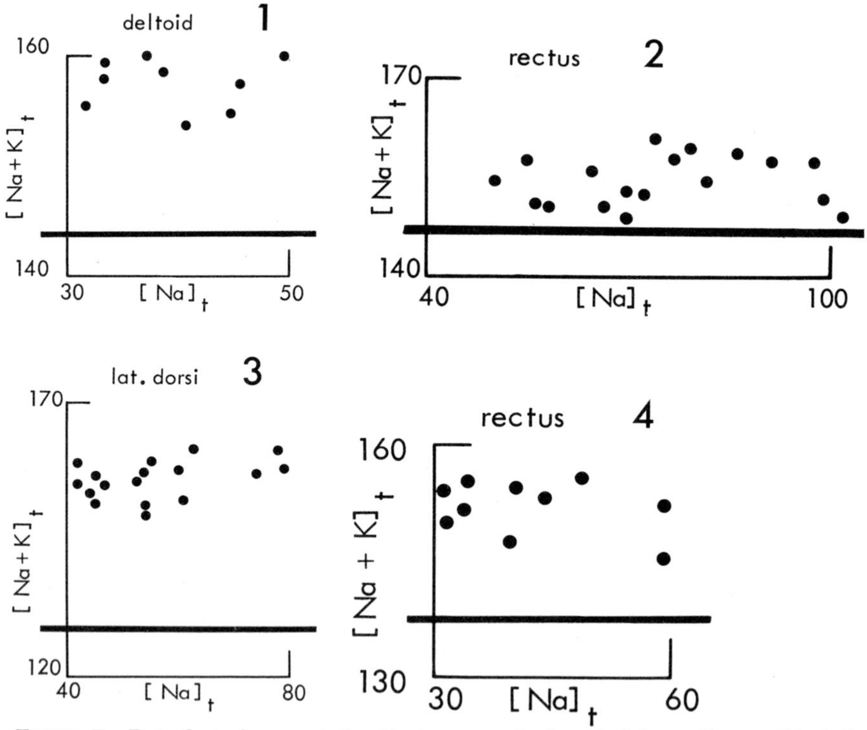

FIGURE 7. Data from four control patients, none of whom had heart disease. (1) A fit male with an inguinal hernia. (2) A moderately ill patient operated upon for peptic ulcer. (Data from this patient is also given in FIGURE 1.) (3) A severely ill patient undergoing thoracic surgery for bronchoplueral fistula following previous peumonectomy. (4) A patient who died in septicemic shock with bronchopneumonia and peritonitis, caused by dehiscence of duodenal stump and anastomosis of polya gastrectomy performed for acute gastric ulcer developing three days after arthroplasty. (See FIGURE 2.)

causes, or as a result of a simple potassium depletion caused by enhanced renal or extrarenal losses.

The possibility that there may be two types of skeletal muscle cell—one rich in potassium and low in sodium, the other poor in potassium but rich in sodium—and that differences between samples from within a given muscle in any one individual reflect differing proportions of the two types of cell in the various samples has been considered briefly elsewhere (Flear, 1967). Evidence against this possibility was also discussed and will be presented in full elsewhere.

How Reliable Are the Conclusions?

Methodology

Perhaps as a prelude I should affirm my belief that the considerable variability noted in our studies results from a genuine variation in composition existing *in situ* and is not introduced by methodological factors. There is considerable evidence in support of this view.

1. Neither general anesthesia (Litchfield & Gaddie, 1958) nor muscle relaxants (Flear *et al.,* 1964) affect composition of samples of skeletal muscle.
2. The water contents of samples taken at operation give an accurate estimate of water content *in situ* with the method we have used for taking and handling samples (Flear *et al.,* 1968).
3. The handling of a tissue involved during its biopsy is unlikely either to introduce systematic bias in its electrolyte content, or to exaggerate the variability in composition between slices subsequently cut from the biopsy. Indeed, electrical stimulation of muscle to repetitive, vigorous contraction for five minutes has been shown to be without effect on its composition, or on the variability between slices cut from biopsies (Flear, 1967; Flear *et al.,* 1968).
4. The small size of samples analyzed ($\simeq$ 25 mg) does not result in variable surface contamination with extracellular fluid, as had been suggested by Johnston (1965; Flear, 1967; Flear *et al.,* 1968).
5. The technique we have employed of lightly freezing the biopsy and slicing the sample while it is still lightly frozen (using a skin grafting blade) does not result in bias or enhanced variability between slices. No correlation has been noted between the order in which slices were cut and their contents of water, sodium, potassium, or chloride (unpublished observations).

Sampling after Death

There can be no doubt about the striking difference between the findings from patients in congestive heart failure and other groups thus far considered. Data from patients in heart failure are all based upon tissue samples taken after death. The possibility that findings in this group are induced by death can be excluded, since similar findings were not seen in controls samples also taken after death (FIGURE 7, part 4); moreover, findings in this group were identical with those seen in comparable controls who were alive (FIGURE 7, part 3). It is also notable that we have found values for $[Na + K]_t$ not infrequently to be lower than values for $[Na + K]_o$ in single biopsies taken from patients in congestive heart failure during life. This is a striking feature of congestive heart failure postmortem findings.

Assumptions Underlying Predictions

How reliable are the assumptions shown in FIGURE 4? Equation 8 is used to predict changes in intracellular amounts and concentrations of sodium, potassium, and chloride.‡ This equation subsumes (1) that sodium is extruded from cells either as an outward current of sodium ions or together with an equal number of anions (see Conway, 1959; Adrian, 1960), and (2) that a balanced state exists. The first assumption, which is implicit in Equation 6, would seem to be a safe one, since Kernan has shown that, when adequate precautions are taken, the resting membrane potential in isolated amphibian (and also mammalian) muscle *in vitro* does not differ from the potassium equilibrium potential (Kernan, 1960, 1963). Equation 6 is based on such an identity. The assumption of a balanced state seems fairly reasonable for the majority of cells in a given muscle. It is possible, however, that some cells, particularly from patients in congestive heart failure, may be in a changing state due to continuing net gains of sodium. Even if this is the case, prediction would remain substantially unchanged, provided, as seems probable, that events during such a period of net gain of sodium could be described by the following equations:

$$\begin{aligned} E_m &= (RT/F)\ \ln\{(P_K[K]_o) + (P_{Na}\,[Na]_o)\ /\ (P_K[K]_i) + (P_{Na}[Na]_i)\} \\ &= (RT/F)\ \ln([Cl]_i\ /\ [Cl]_o) \end{aligned} \qquad \textbf{(10)}$$

and

$$(P_K[K]_o) + (P_{Na}[Na]_o)\ /\ (P_K[K]_i) + (P_{Na}[Na]_i) = [Cl]_i\ /\ [Cl]_o \qquad \textbf{(11)}$$

or

$$[K]_o + b[Na]_o\ /\ [K]_i + b[Na]_i = [Cl]_i\ /\ [Cl]_o \qquad \textbf{(12)}$$

where E_m = resting membrane potential, P_K and P_{Na} represent the permeability factors for potassium and sodium, respectively, and b is the ratio P_K/P_{Na}. Hodgkin and Horowicz (1959) have shown that b is likely to be 0.01 for frog skeletal muscle. It is necessary to consider the consequences of an increase in this ratio caused by an increase in the membrane permeability to sodium. Thus, from Equation 12:

$$[K]_i\ [Cl]_i = [K]_o\ [Cl]_o + b[Na]_o\ [Cl]_o - b[Na]_i\ [Cl]_i \qquad \textbf{(13)}$$

which may be used instead of Equation 6 when deriving an equation for prediction, comparable to Equation 8. The possibility that a changing state might be present from a process of net extrusion can be excluded. All samples were taken from patients who died following progressive deterioration.

Prediction of changes in the total tissue sodium, etc., involves a further assumption regarding the proportion of extracellular fluid present in samples. Relationships shown in FIGURE 4 are based upon an assumed constancy in the volume of extracellular fluid associated with a given quantity of cells. No final decision can be reached about this assumption from observations on muscle or other tissue taking up water *in vitro* as a result of anoxia. Some studies have shown that the quantity of extracellular fluid associated with a given weight of tissue remained constant (Robinson, 1950; Whittam 1956). Others indicated that it fell when cells took up water (Hercus *et al.*, 1955; Rixon & Stevenson, 1956). The fact that our data display certain of the predicted relationships rather well suggests that the assumption made is reasonable. Some stochastic variability is to be expected in the quantity of extracellular fluid associated with

‡ It is not, of course, implied that all of the cells in each sample analyzed show the predicted changes to a precisely equal extent.

a given quantity of cells, and this probably accounts for the scatter noted about the relationships. It is certainly quite clear from the relationships displayed by our data that variation in the quantity of extracellular fluid is not of major significance in the variability met in composition of replicate samples from a given tissue in any one subject. If it is assumed that when cells take up water the volume of extracellular fluid falls, with the total quantity of water associated with a given quantity of cells remaining constant, the relationships shown in FIGURE 4 (3, 4, and 7) could arise as a result of variation in A alone, and without the gain of cellular sodium these relationships have been taken to signify. Whenever our data have displayed these relationships, they have also shown a positive correlation between $[Na]_t$ and the sodium content of samples expressed as milliequivalents per kilogram (mEq/kg) of fat-free dry weight of tissue. This latter correlation would not be evident if the variation in $[Na]_t$ were caused simply by a variation in A (and thus tissue water); its existence, therefore, is evidence of variation in cellular sodium. The conclusions we have reached would thus not be challenged even if this alternate assumption were the correct one.

It should be emphasized that the *patterns* predicted are uninfluenced by the actual value for the volume of extracellular fluid associated with a given weight of cells. It is therefore unnecessary to make any binding assumption about this volume. Of course this means that data from more than one tissue cannot be considered together, even though the different tissues are sampled in the same individual. It is possible that the average value for the volume of extracellular fluid associated with 1 kg of cells would vary in different tissues, which would confound interpretation.

Limitations

Equation 8 enables one to predict the types of pattern likely to exist in variation of tissue composition as a result of specified disturbances. It does not, in the present context, permit quantitative conclusions to be drawn.

It is, for instance, not possible to predict the extent of change in $[Na]_i$ likely to follow a given gain of sodium by cells. Clearly, a given gain of sodium by cells will promote less of a rise in $[Na]_i$ when the average initial volume of water per cell is high than when it is low. The volume of water per cell is likely to vary from individual to individual, as well as from condition (e.g. congestive heart failure) to condition (e.g. regional enteritis). A further reason why quantitative generalization is precluded can be illustrated by the cellular state in congestive heart failure. In this condition, the molar quantity of nondiffusible material contained within cells varies. When a net gain of sodium is associated with an increase in this molar quantity, more water will be gained by cells than if there is a fall in the molar quantity of nondiffusible material. Obviously, a given gain of sodium will promote a greater rise in $[Na]_i$ in the latter circumstance, and an even greater rise should there be a net loss of osmotic material from cells despite the gain of sodium.

Conclusions Are Reliable

I believe that we may reliably conclude that cells in tissues of fit and ill subjects vary in their content of sodium, and consequently also in their potassium content. I believe, too, that one can reasonably infer that differences in cellular sodium in samples from patients in congestive heart failure reflect the variable extent of abnormal net gains by cells throughout tissues; that many tissues, including the heart, participate in such gains of sodium; and that this process of gain begins before the onset of frank congestive heart failure.

We can also conclude that there is an associated variability in cellular content of organic solutes in patients with congestive heart failure, shown by differences in the molar quantity of nondiffusible solutes and their electrical charges. A pattern is distinguishable: Cells with more sodium have more nondiffusible anions and a lesser molar quantity of nondiffusible material. This emphasizes that there is a strong connection between metabolic events and cellular integrity, and the changes in water and electrolyte metabolism which arise in congestive heart failure.

It can also be concluded that the volume of cellular water must vary in congestive heart failure. In its direction and extent, such change is determined by net gains or losses of osmotic material, organic as well as inorganic.

Possible Causes and Wider Implications of Findings in Congestive Heart Failure

Indications from in Vitro Experiments

Findings remarkably similar to those presented for congestive heart failure are shown by tissues, or tissue slices, in saline media and subjected *in vitro* to anoxia, metabolic inhibitors, and factors increasing membrane permeability. Figure 8 presents data from rat right ventricle bathed in Krebs-Ringer phosphate solution and exposed to anoxia for a period, followed by reoxygenation (data of Kopecký and Flear, 1960). The same pattern is shown by data from Heckman and Parsons (1959) for rat liver slices in saline medium at 0.5° C, and by data from Creese and co-workers (1957) for human intercostal muscle before and after soaking, at 38° C, in Krebs-Ringer solution previously equilibrated with 5% CO_2 and 95% O_2.

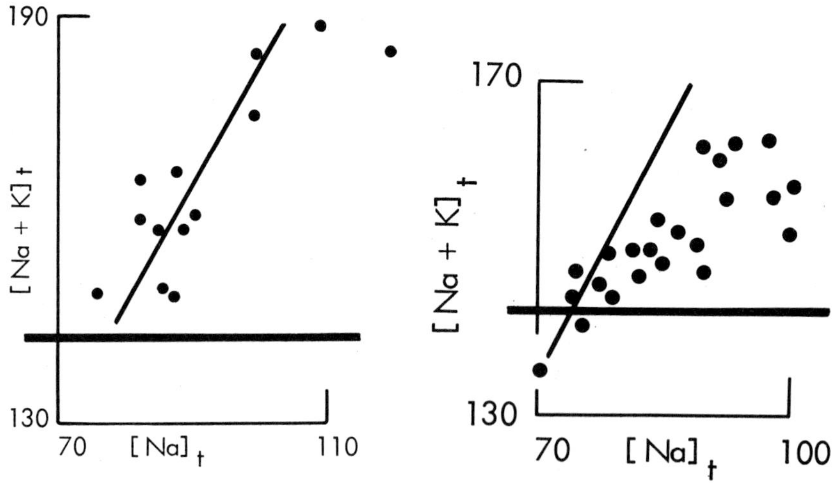

Figure 8. Data from right ventricle of rats *in vitro*, bathed in oxygenated Krebs-Ringer phosphate solution at 33° C and stimulated to contract at a rate of four times per minute. (*Right*) Data from ventricles subjected to a three-minute period of anoxia by bubbling nitrogen through the solution (anoxia preceded by a 75-minute period during which oxygen was bubbled). (*Left*) Data from ventricles reoxygenated after a similar period of anoxia. Experiment previously reported only in brief (Kopeký & Flear, 1960). (See figure 2.)

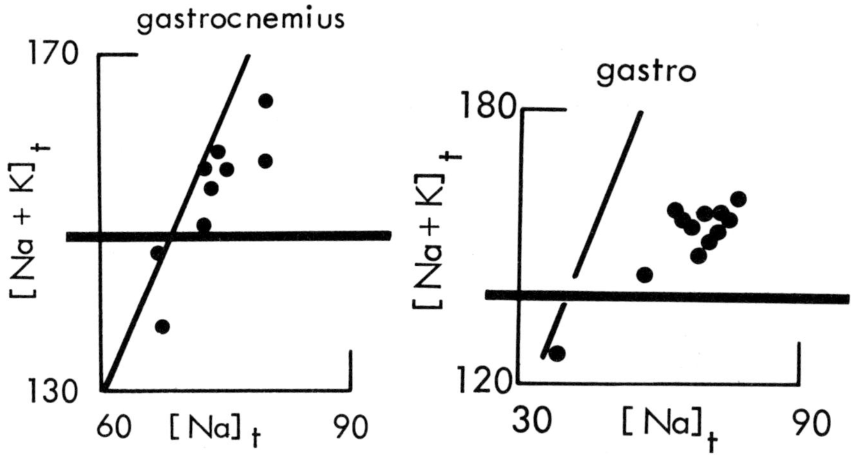

FIGURE 9. Data from two patients undergoing below-knee amputation for ischemia of the lower leg. (See FIGURE 2.)

In a sense, this is not surprising, since several samples from a single tissue bathed by the same extracellular fluid are equivalent to several slices of tissue in the same saline medium. It is also to be expected that the extent of anoxia, inhibition of metabolism, or enhanced permeability induced *in vitro* will vary somewhat from slice to slice, as will similar changes arising *in situ* as a result of impaired tissue perfusion, etc., vary from place to place within the tissue.

Ischemia of the Leg

Similar findings are also seen in ischemia. FIGURE 9 presents findings from two patients with ischemia of the leg. Samples of the gastrocnemius muscle were taken at amputation. In one of these subjects, deltoid muscle was also sampled. Data from the nonischemic muscle were similar to those of the fit individual (FIGURE 7, part 1) and other controls.

For the same reasons enumerated in the discussion of findings from patients in congestive heart failure, data from these patients also indicated an abnormal net gain of sodium and variation in both A and zA.

Possible Causes

Increase in the permeability of cell membranes leads to an increased influx of sodium, which could temporarily swamp sodium extrusion and might lead to the establishment of a different steady state, with cells containing a greater quantity of sodium at a higher concentration. With a great enough increase in permeability, or following damage to cell membranes, there would be a leakage of some solutes previously held within cells by virtue of their size and the normal permeability characteristics of membranes. Consequently, the molar quantity of such substances (A) would fall. This leakage would also affect the balance of electrical charges on residual nondiffusible material. Evidence of an increased permeability in skeletal muscle cell membranes in patients in congestive heart failure is shown in FIGURE 10.

Slices of skeletal muscle bathed at room temperature in 0.9% NaCl gain sodium, chloride, and water. Because of this, their weight may be expected to rise. At the same time, they lose some solids. Therefore, net weight change is

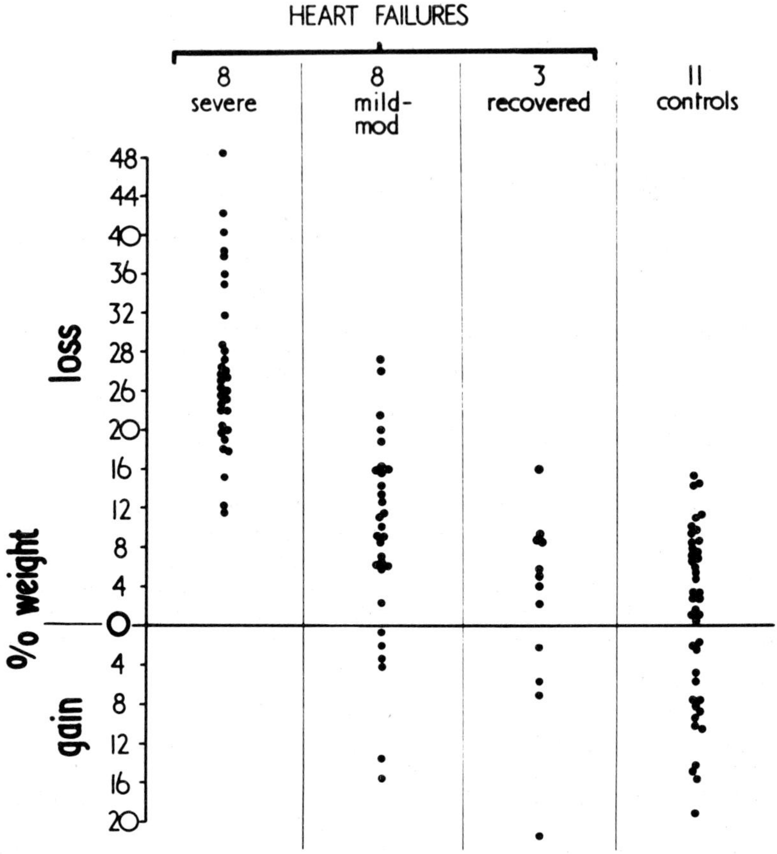

FIGURE 10. Change in weight of slices of skeletal muscle on standing for 45 minutes *in vitro*, in 0.9% saline at room temperature. Muscle obtained by biopsy from eight patients in severe congestive heart failure, eight patients in mild to moderate congestive heart failure, three patients recovering from congestive heart failure, and from 11 control subjects undergoing surgery, none of whom had heart disease.

a result of the two processes, gain of water and loss of solids. It is to be expected that the more permeable cell membranes are, the greater the loss of solids will be. FIGURE 10 shows that slices of skeletal muscle from patients in severe§ congestive heart failure lose weight. Clearly, they lost more solids (and possibly, in consequence, gained less water) than slices from muscle taken after recovery, or from patients without heart disease. Such slices lost less, or gained, weight.

Gain of sodium and changes in the organic substances within cells can also follow metabolic disturbances. Changes in organic substances which may follow anoxia are discussed by Conway and his colleagues (Conway & Geoghegan, 1955; Conway *et al.*, 1955). Extrusion of sodium requires provision of energy.

§ Pragmatic classification: nil or slow response to treatment and/or death during the episode.

It is markedly impaired or, in some tissues, completely abolished by anoxia. Complete inhibition, at least of any bulk of cells, is unlikely *in situ* before death, but impairment is likely for greater or lesser periods of time. In view of the suggestion that lactate dehydrogenase is involved in the anaerobic extrusion of sodium (Conway, 1963), the reported lowering of myocardial lactate dehydrogenase activity in congestive heart failure (Bing *et al.*, 1964) is of considerable interest.

Probably both an increase in membrane permeability and metabolic disturbances arise in congestive heart failure. It is tempting to attribute such changes to tissue anoxia as a result of progressive impairment of tissue perfusion, both during exertion and at rest, which develops with the advance of heart disease. There may, of course, be other factors involved at various stages in the disease, such as an altered release of adrenal stearoids and the presence of polypeptide products released from damaged cells.

Immediate Consequences of Such Events in Situ

Gain of sodium, fall in the molar quantity of nondiffusible material within cells (A), and increase in organic anions (zA) all have consequences not only for the volume and composition of cell fluid, which have already been discussed, but also for extracellular fluid.

Leaf (1959) has directed attention to the importance of sodium pumps in the regulation of the volume of cellular fluid. Conway (1960a) has emphasized the similar importance of the cell membrane, which normally restricts sodium influx. He submits that *in situ* sodium gains only slow entrance into cells (Conway, 1959). Impairment of sodium extrusion, in contrast to its complete inhibition, only results in slight cellular swelling, unless at the same time there is an increase in A or zA, which results in considerable net gain of water. If this gain is abrupt, and a sufficient mass of cells is involved, there must be a shrinkage of extracellular fluid. When a net loss of osmotic material accompanies a gain of sodium, the converse may take place, and hyponatremia (and hypochloremia) will result and persist for as long as the solutes, whose escape through leaky membranes provoked the shift of water, remain in the extracellular fluid. The level of urea in extracellular fluids will not fall, nor, indeed, will potassium. Increase in $[K]_i$, due to a loss of cell water, and in the product of $[K]_i$ $[Cl]_i$, brings about a rise in $[K]_o$ (see Equation 6). Events such as these largely account for the variation in extracellular fluid levels from day to day in severe heart failure (Flear & Hughes, 1963). These matters will receive a more detailed treatment elsewhere.

Clinical Importance

If large enough, changes in volume of extracellular fluid will directly affect the patient's condition. A fall in volume will provoke transient or prolonged circulatory collapse, and will call forth an increased secretion of aldosterone. On the other hand, I believe that alterations in the composition of extracellular fluid often do not have a directly harmful effect. For example, the striking correlation between a fall in the sodium level or a rise in potassium and prognosis (Flear, 1960a & b, 1967) reflects, I believe, a causal relation between prognosis and the cellular events underlying the changes in extracellular composition.

Potassium depletion may provoke myocardial necrosis. Gain of sodium must affect the resting membrane potential of myocardial cells and their excitability; it must also affect their contractile efficiency, since agents that have a positive inotropic action bring about a fall in the intracellular sodium either by lessening the influx of sodium or increasing extrusion. Among the actions of digitalis, for example, is that of lessening membrane permeability. Digitalis will therefore diminish the influx of sodium, as will hyponatremia. Insulin has been shown to increase sodium extrusion (Kernan, 1962). This may explain its therapeutic value in congestive heart failure and myocardial infarction. A low level of sodium in extracellular fluid not only lessens influx, but also lowers the critical energy barrier to extrusion of sodium (Conway, 1960b), and has been shown *in vitro* to exert a greater positive inotropic action after anoxia than does digitalis (Hercus *et al.,* 1955). Similarly, an increased level of potassium lowers the critical energy barrier (Conway, 1960b), and it too has a positive inotropic effect (Hercus *et al.,* 1955).

These considerations urge reflection before treating hyonatremia with fluid restriction or salt. The low value may be beneficial, and may even be the precondition for any steady state at all across cell membranes, for the continued existence of the patient.

Similarly, hyperkalemia may not be directly harmful, as is often supposed. Potassium supplements should not automatically be stopped.

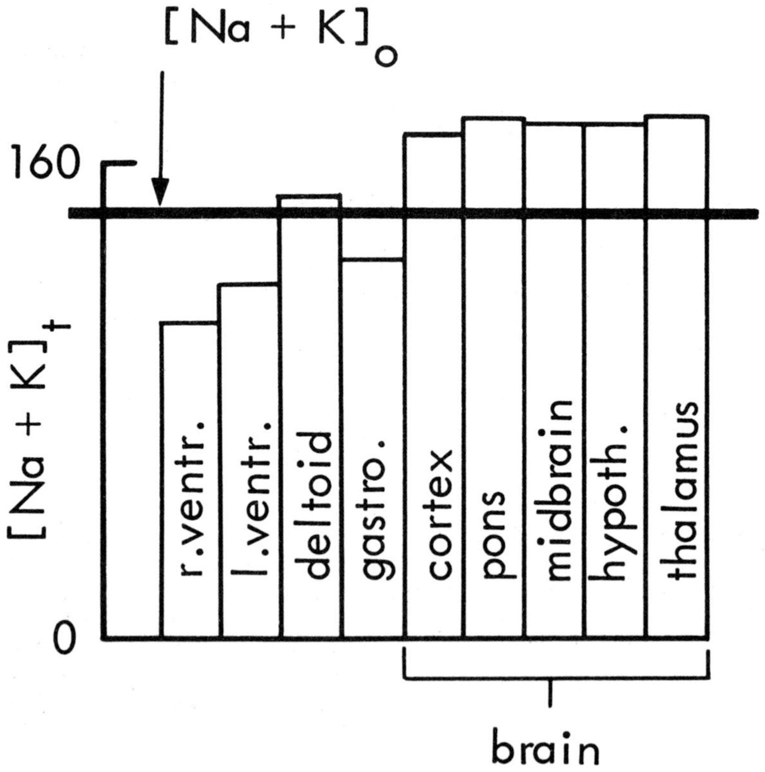

FIGURE 11. Data for five tissues in one patient who died in congestive heart failure; $[Na + K]_o$ is the concentration (Na + K) per liter of extracellular water. (See FIGURE 2.)

SUGGESTED SEQUENCE OF EVENTS IN CONGESTIVE HEART FAILURE

It seems probable that one of the first cellular changes to develop with advancing heart disease is a loss of nondiffusible anions (zA), causing depletion of potassium. In view of the striking correlation between a fall in extracellular sodium level and the extent of potassium depletion (Flear, 1966, 1967), it must be concluded that zA and potassium are lost from cells without water. (Except where hyponatremia is acute, it signifies a fall in the osmotic pressure of extracellular fluid.) By the time a patient is in severe failure, loss of zA and potassium involves many tissues and may be extensive. It commonly causes values for $[Na + K]_t$ to be lower than the value $[Na + K]_o$ (FIGURE 11). This is also apparent in the data of Cort and Matthews (1954).

Increase in membrane permeability leads to a gain of sodium and further loss of potassium unless, as may be the case in severe failure, there is an associated increase of nondiffusible anions. Cells gain water and swell. With still further deterioration, membranes become so leaky that further gain of sodium no longer results in a net gain of osmotic material, and cells do not swell further (FIGURE 12). The progressive cellular gain of sodium may be responsible for its continued retention in the body in the face of a grossly inflated volume of extracellular fluid.

Acute deterioration may be accompanied by further leakage of solutes from cells, provoking a shift of water into extracellular fluid and an abrupt fall in the extracellular sodium level and the development of hyperkalemia. At the same time, there may be an increase in organic anions in cells and a further net gain of sodium.

With improvement, tissue perfusion increases, sodium is extruded from cells, including those of the heart, and potassium is taken up. A more normal cellular metabolism is established, leading to an increase in the molar quantity of mate-

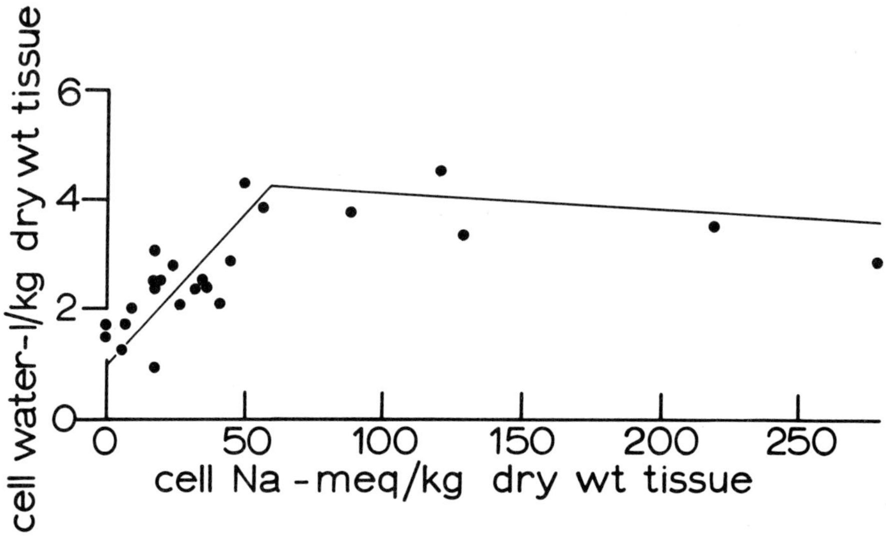

FIGURE 12. Intracellular sodium and intracellular water contents of samples of deltoid muscle taken by biopsy from patients in congestive heart failure with edema. (Flear *et al.*, 1961).

rial within cells, with a resultant secondary increase in the level of sodium throughout the extracellular fluids.

Acknowledgments

Most of these investigations were made with Miss Irené Florence; they have entailed collaboration over a number of years with numerous clinical colleagues at Birmingham and Newcastle whose help I gratefully acknowledge.

I am grateful to Mrs. Lewis and others in the Department of Photography, Newcastle University, for expert assistance with the illustrations. I wish to thank Dr. I. G. Graber (Queens Hospital Center Affiliation, Long Island Jewish Hospital, New Hyde Park, N. Y.) for valued criticism of the manuscript.

References

Adrian, R. H. 1960. Potassium chloride movement and the membrane potential of frog muscle. J. Physiol. **151:** 154.

Bing, R. J., C. Wu & S. Gudbjarnason. 1964. Mechanism of heart failure. Circ. Res. Suppl. 11 (**14 & 15**): 64.

Conway, E. J. 1957. Nature and significance of concentration relations of potassium and sodium ions in skeletal muscle. Physiol. Rev. **37:** 1.

Conway, E. J. 1959. The energetics of ion transport through cell membranes. 21st. Congr. Int. Ciencias Fisiológicas. Fisiol. Farmacol.

Conway, E. J. 1960a. The nature of the differential concentrating of potassium by living cells. Potassium Symp. 1960. : 209. International Potash Institute. Berne, Switzerland.

Conway, E. J. 1960b. Critical energy barriers in the excretion of sodium. Nature **187:** 394.

Conway, E. J. 1963. Significance of various factors including lactic dehydrogenase on the active transport of sodium ions in skeletal muscle. Nature **198:** 760.

Conway, E. J. & H. Geoghegan. 1955. Molecular concentration of kidney cortex slices. J. Physiol. **130:** 438.

Conway, E. J., H. Geoghegan & J. I. McCormack. 1955. Autolytic change at zero centigrade in ground mammalian tissues. J. Physiol. **130:** 427.

Cort, J. H. & H. L. Matthews. 1954. Potassium deficiency in congestive heart failure. Lancet **i:** 1202.

Creese, R., J. B. Dillon, J. Marshall, P. B. Sabawala, D. J. Schneider, D. B. Taylor & D. E. Zinn. 1957. The effect of neuromuscular blocking agents on isolated human intercostal muscles. J. Pharmacol. Exp. Ther. **119:** 485.

Flear, C. T. G. 1960a. Water and electrolyte metabolism in congestive heart failure. Postgrad. Med. J. **36:** 104.

Flear, C. T. G. 1960b. Studies in congestive heart failure: therapeutic and theoretical problems. M.D. Thesis. Birmingham University, England.

Flear, C. T. G. 1966. Disturbance of volume and composition of body fluids in congestive heart failure. *In* Electrolyte and Cardiovascular Diseases. E. Bajusz, Ed. : 357–385. S. Karger. Basel, Switzerland.

Flear, C. T. G. 1967. Significance of potassium and sodium masses in cardiac disease. *In* Compartments, pools, and spaces in medical physiology. P.-E. E. Bergner & C. C. Lushbaugh, Eds. : 53–93 & 126–138. U. S. Atomic Energy Comm., Div. Tech. Info. Symp. No. 11, Conf. 661010.

Flear, C. T. G. & J. Domenet. 1961. Weight changes and sodium balances during deterioration and recovery in patients in congestive heart failure. Clin. Chim. Acta. **6:** 656.

Flear, C. T. G. & I. Florence. 1961. A rapid and micro method for the analysis of skeletal muscle for water, sodium, potassium, chloride, and fat. Clin. Chim. Acta. **6:** 129.

Flear, C. T. G. & I. Florence. 1963. Muscle biopsy in man: an index of cellular potassium? Nature **199:** 156.

Flear, C. T. G. & P. Hughes. 1963. Electrolyte content of extracellular fluid in health and in congestive heart failure. Brit. Heart. J. **25:** 166.

Flear, C. T. G., I. Florence & J. A. Williams. 1964. Muscle relaxants and the water and electrolyte contents of samples of muscle taken at operation. Proc. Ass. Clin. Biochem. **3:** 139.

FLEAR, C. T. G., R. G. CARPENTER & I. FLORENCE. 1965. Variability in the water, sodium, potassium,, and chloride content of human skeletal muscle. J. Clin. Path. **18:** 74.

FLEAR, C. T. G., R. F. CRAMPTON & D. M. MATTHEWS. 1961. Observations on the electrolyte and water composition of skeletal muscle in patients in congestive cardiac failure, using an *in vitro* method for determination of inulin space. Clin. Sci. **21:** 3.

FLEAR, C. T. G., I. FLORENCE & J. A. WILLIAMS. 1968. Water, sodium, potassium and chloride content of skeletal muscle in fit and ill subjects. J. Clin. Path. In press.

HECKMAN, K. D. & D. S. PARSONS. 1959. Changes in the water and electrolyte content of rat—liver slices *in vitro*. Biochim. Biophys. Acta **36:** 203.

HERCUS, V. M., R. J. S. MCDOWALL & D. MENDEL. 1955. Sodium exchanges in cardiac muscle. J. Physiol. **129:** 177.

HODGKIN, A. L. & P. HOROWICZ. 1959. The Influence of K and Cl ions on the membrane potential of single muscle fibres. J. Physiol. **148:** 127.

JOHNSTON, C. I. 1965. Relationship between muscle electrolyte values and varying sample size. Clin. Sci. **28:** 57.

KERNAN, R. P. 1960. Resting potentials in isolated frog sartorius fibres at low external potassium concentrations. Nature **185:** 471.

KERNAN, R. P. 1962. The role of lactate in the active excretion of sodium by frog muscle. J. Physiol. **162:** 129.

KERNAN, R. P. 1963. The resting potentials of isolated rat muscle measured in plasma. Nature **200:** 474.

KOPECKÝ, M. & C. T. G. FLEAR. 1960. Sodium, potassium, and water in isolated anoxic rat myocardium. Cesk. Physiol. **9:** 26.

LEAF, A. 1959. Maintenance of concentration gradients and regulation of cell volume. Ann. N. Y. Acad. Sci. **72:** 396.

LITCHFIELD, J. A. & R. H. GADDIE. 1958. The measurement of the phase distribution of water and electrolytes in skeletal muscle by the analysis of small samples. Clin. Sci. **17:** 483.

MULLINS, L. J. 1959. The penetration of some cations into muscle. J. Gen. Physiol. **42:** 817.

MULLINS, L. J. 1960. An analysis of pore size in excitable membranes. J. Gen. Physiol. **43:** 105.

RIXON, R. H. & J. A. F. STEVENSON. 1956. The water and electrolyte metabolism of rat diaphragm *in vitro*. Canad. J. Biochem. Physiol. **34:** 1069.

ROBINSON, J. R. 1950. Osmoregulation in surviving slices from the kidneys of adult rats. Proc. Roy. Soc. Series B. **137:** 378.

WESTON, R. E., J. GROSSMAN, E. R. BORUN & I. B. HANENSON. 1958. The pathogenesis and treatment of hyponatraemia in congestive heart failure. Amer. J. Med. **25:** 558.

WHITTAM, R. 1956. The permeability of kidney cortex to chloride. J. Physiol. **131:** 542.

APPENDIX

Derivation of Relationship between $[Na + K]_t$ *and* $[Na]_t$ *when the Only Variable in Samples of Tissue is the Relative Volumes of Intracellular and Extracellular Fluid*

Where V_o and V_i are the volumes, in liters, of extracellular and intracellular, respectively:

$$([Na]_o V_o + [Na]_i V_i) \,/\, (V_o + V_i) = [Na]_t \qquad \textbf{(i)}$$

and

$$V_i = \{([Na]_o - [Na]_t) \,/\, ([Na]_t - [Na]_i)\} V_o \qquad \textbf{(ii)}$$

Similarly,

$$\{([Na + K]_o V_o) + ([Na + K]_i V_i)\} \,/\, (V_o + V_i) = [Na + K]_t \qquad \textbf{(iii)}$$

If we substitute the value for V_i defined by Equation ii into Equation iii:

$$\frac{V_o\left([Na+K]_o+[Na+K]_i\{([Na]_o-[Na]_t)/([Na]_t-[Na]_i)\}\right)}{V_o\left(1+\{([Na]_o-[Na]_t)/([Na]_t-[Na]_i)\}\right)} = [Na+K]_t \qquad \textbf{(iv)}$$

Equation iv can be solved for $[Na+K]_i$ after substitution of an assumed value for $[Na]_i$, together with three observed values: $[Na]_o$, the lowest observed value for $[Na]_t$, and the value of $[Na+K]_t$ for that sample.

The value for $[Na+K]_t$ in a sample with identical values for $[Na]_i$ and $[Na+K]_i$ but containing double the volume of extracellular fluid can be derived by appropriate substitution in Equation v:

$$\frac{V_o\left(2[Na+K]_o+[Na+K]_i\{([Na]_o-[Na]_t)/([Na]_t-[Na]_i)\}\right)}{V_o\left(2+\{([Na]_o-[Na]_t)/([Na]_t-[Na]_i)\}\right)} = [Na+K]_t \qquad \textbf{(v)}$$

The corresponding value for $[Na]_t$ (designated $[Na]_{t2}$) is obtained by appropriate substitution in Equation vi:

$$[Na]_{t2} = \frac{V_o\left(2[Na]_o+[Na]_i\{([Na]_o-[Na]_t)/([Na]_t-[Na]_i)\}\right)}{V_o\left(2+\{([Na]_o-[Na]_t)/([Na]_t-[Na]_i)\}\right)} \qquad \textbf{(vi)}$$

The value for $[Na]_t$ entered in Equations v and vi is that already used in Equation iv, i.e., that observed for the sample containing the least sodium.

EXPERIMENTAL CARDIOMEGALIES AND "CARDIOMEGALIES" IN FREE-LIVING ANIMALS

O. Poupa* and B. Ošťádal
Institute of Physiology, Czechoslovak Academy of Sciences
Prague, Czechoslovakia

The heart is capable of extensive adaptive growth in response to its function, since its performance as a pump is directly determined by the mass of its contractile elements. Performance of the heart as a pump, however, must at the same time be precisely adapted to the oxygen consumption of all body tissues. This means that the main factor determining the size of the heart should reflect all influences affecting oxygen consumption of the total active body mass.

In the present report, the following factors are discussed: (1) relationship between size of the heart and various factors determining oxygen consumption with regard to phylogeny; (2) description of changes in the internal heart structure accompanying adaptive growth of the organ; (3) myocardial pathology occurring with these changes during development.

Relationship between Heart and Body Weights in the Animal Kingdom

The size of the heart in different animal species varies considerably. Most authors dealing with this question have attempted to find a relationship between heart weight and body weight. General data, however, concerning the relation between heart weight and "active body mass" are missing. One of the first to draw conclusions from extensive material was Hesse (1921), who collected numerous data after more than ten years of work on the weight of the heart in poikilothermic and homoiothermic animals. His work included the effect of some ecological factors upon changes in heart weight, but his numerical data were not subjected to mathematical analysis. A more general mathematical formulation of the relationship between heart weight and body weight in homoiotherm was attempted by Clark (1927) and later by Brody (1945). In a recent paper, Bartels (1966) stressed the importance of oxygen intake to the size of the heart in a given species.

Mean values of the heart ratio [(heart weight/body weight) × 100] in individual vertebrate classes are given in FIGURE 1. It is apparent that the hearts of poikilotherms represent a much smaller proportion of the total body weight than those of homoiotherms. Thus, it may be concluded that a sharp acceleration of heart growth takes place during evolution, at a time when the metabolic activity of animal tissues has substantially increased. The same conclusion may be drawn from FIGURE 2. A mathematical expression of the heart weight:body weight ratio is illustrated in FIGURE 3:

1. The relationship between log heart weight and log body weight is shown by a straight line regression, the slope of which is always (for poikilotherms, birds, and mammals) smaller than 1. This means that heart growth follows body growth, but with a certain lag.

2. This lag is maximum in poikilotherms (slope = 0.743) and smaller in homoiotherms (birds; slope = 0.892; small mammals, slope = 0.846; large mammals, slope = 0.870).

* Present address: Department of Clinical Physiology, University of Göteborg, Faculty of Medicine, Göteborg, Sweden.

3. Absolute members of regression line equations are different for poikilotherms (− 2.201), birds (− 1.744), and mammals [− 1.970 (small) and − 1.591 (large)]. Thus, the size of animals of the same body weight varies according to whether the animal is a poikilotherm, bird, or mammal.

On the basis of these three points, it is possible to determine three mathematically defined lines expressing the relation between heart and body weights as "poikilothermic," "avian," or "mammalian."

Exceptions and Ecological Factors

Even though it is possible to express the relationship between the heart weight and body weight of vertebrates in simple mathematical terms, it has been found that this expression is not applicable to certain animal species. These exceptions to the rule may be interpreted in connection with the ecology of the animals involved. Such exceptions are readily found among poikilotherms.

When the heart ratios of fish were compared (FIGURE 4) according to their motility, it was found that the hearts of more active fish were larger than those of less active fish. Exceptionally large hearts, however, are to be found in rays with low mobility, apparently because a certain proportion of their musculature is changed into the electric organ, which does not subserve movement but acts rather as ballast. Considerable requirements are laid upon the heart by the work performed in acting against gravity. Thus, it is possible to explain the differences in heart ratios between mammals and birds, or the finding of an avian-type heart ratio (FIGURE 5) in a small-sized flying mammal (bat) and a highly antigravity active mammal (squirrel). The effect of differences in work against gravity seen in various mammals is also observed when the heart weights of amphibians are compared. Frogs permanently living in water (*Rana esculenta*) have a lower heart ratio than frogs predominantly living out of water (*Bufo vulgaris, Hyla*

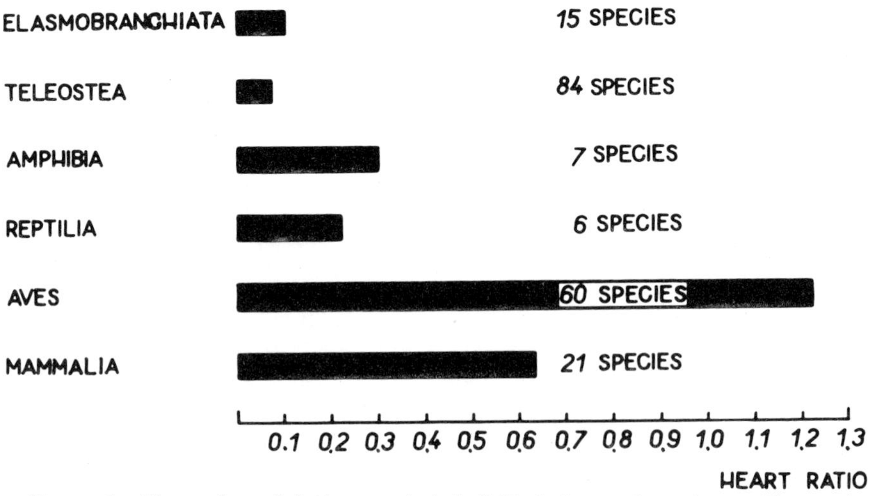

FIGURE 1. Mean values of the heart ratio in individual classes of vertebrates. The number of species from which the mean value was calculated is given in each column. Note the rapid rise in the value of the heart ratio in homoiotherms in comparison with poikilotherms. (Data from Hesse, 1921.)

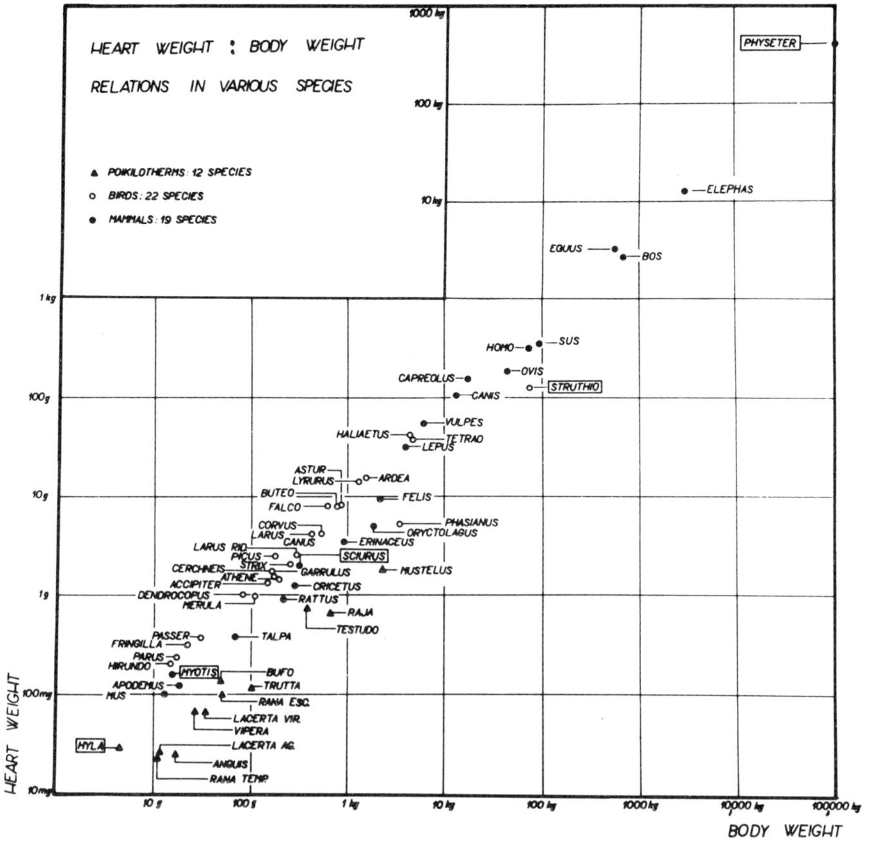

FIGURE 2. Ratios between heart and body weights in various vertebrate species. Values are given in a bilogarithmic scale. Each point represents the mean value for a given species. (Data from Hesse, 1921; Clark, 1927; Oštádal, 1967.)

arborea). It is possible to interpret the findings of a small mammalian-type heart ratio in the ostrich (FIGURE 2) in this manner.

A high work output is also evidently responsible for the fact that the heart ratio in mammals with a large body weight (over 5,000 g) changes into the large-mammalian type (FIGURE 3). The whale is interesting in this respect. Its heart can ensure the metabolic requirements of its huge muscle mass only because its movement is facilitated by the pressure of displaced water. It is a matter of speculation whether the immense body growth of terrestrial animals in prehistoric times did not cause relative insufficiency of the comparatively slowly growing heart muscle and did not thus become the limiting factor of survival of these species (e.g. brontosaurus). It can be concluded from all these facts that one of the main factors determining excessive heart growth in relation to body weight is the amount of work done by muscle, the greater part of which is performed to counteract gravity. Thus, the terms athletic and nonathletic animals, introduced by Clark (1927), may be given a more precise meaning (FIGURES 6 and 7.). It is probable that differences in muscle work may also explain differences in heart ratio in domesticated and wild animal species.

Hesse (1921) pointed out that there are differences in the heart weight:body weight ratio in members of the same animal species living in different geographical latitudes. Poikilotherm animals living in an environment with a low yearly mean temperature have lower heart ratios than animals of the same species living in a warmer climate. For example, toads (*Bufo vulgaris*) living in northern parts of Europe have relatively smaller hearts than toads living in the warmer southern parts of Europe. However, the reverse is true in the case of homoiotherms (FIGURE 8). Heart weight reflects the temperature conditions of the environment which are modified according to whether the animal is homoiothermic or poikilothermic: Overheating, caused by a stay in a hot environment, induces a greater circulatory effort in a poikilotherm than does cooling, which automatically decreases its general metabolic turnover. On the other hand, a homoiotherm exposed to cold is forced to exert considerable circulatory effort associated with physical mechanisms to restrict heat loss. It would seem desirable to obtain much more information about the mechanisms by which environmental temperature and thermoregulation affect the size of the heart and its relation to body weight.

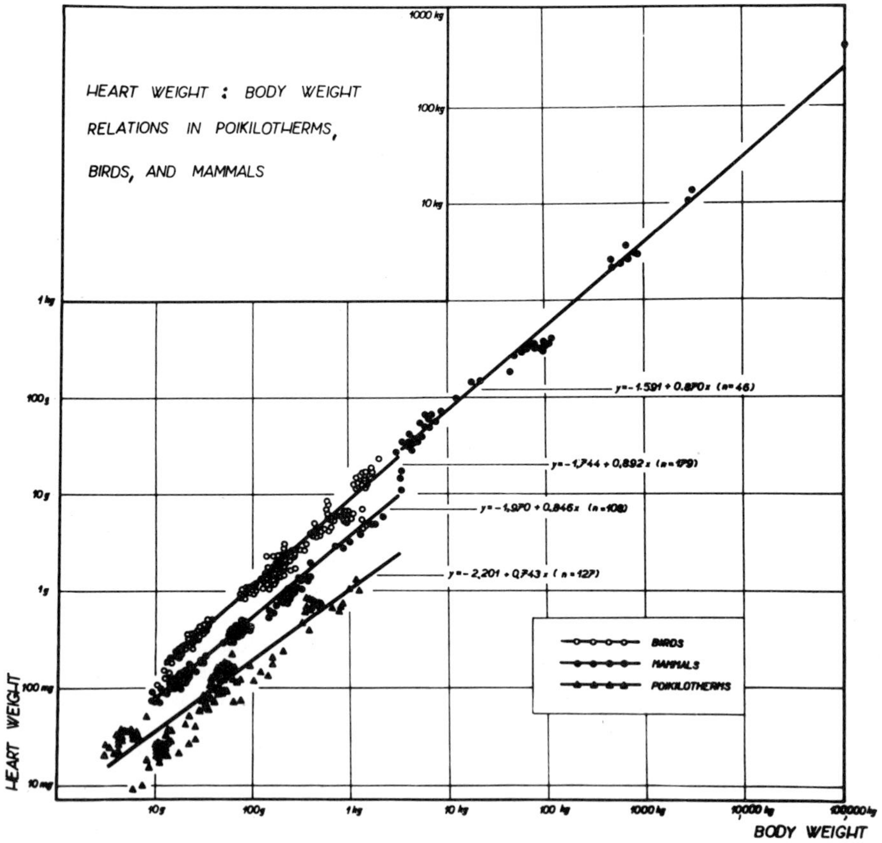

FIGURE 3. Mathematical evaluation of the relation of the heart and body weights in poikilotherms (▲), small (up to 4,000 g) and large mammals (●), and birds (○). Values are given in a bilogarithmic scale. Each point represents the individual value for a given animal. (Data from Hesse, 1921; Clark, 1927; Ošťádal, 1967.)

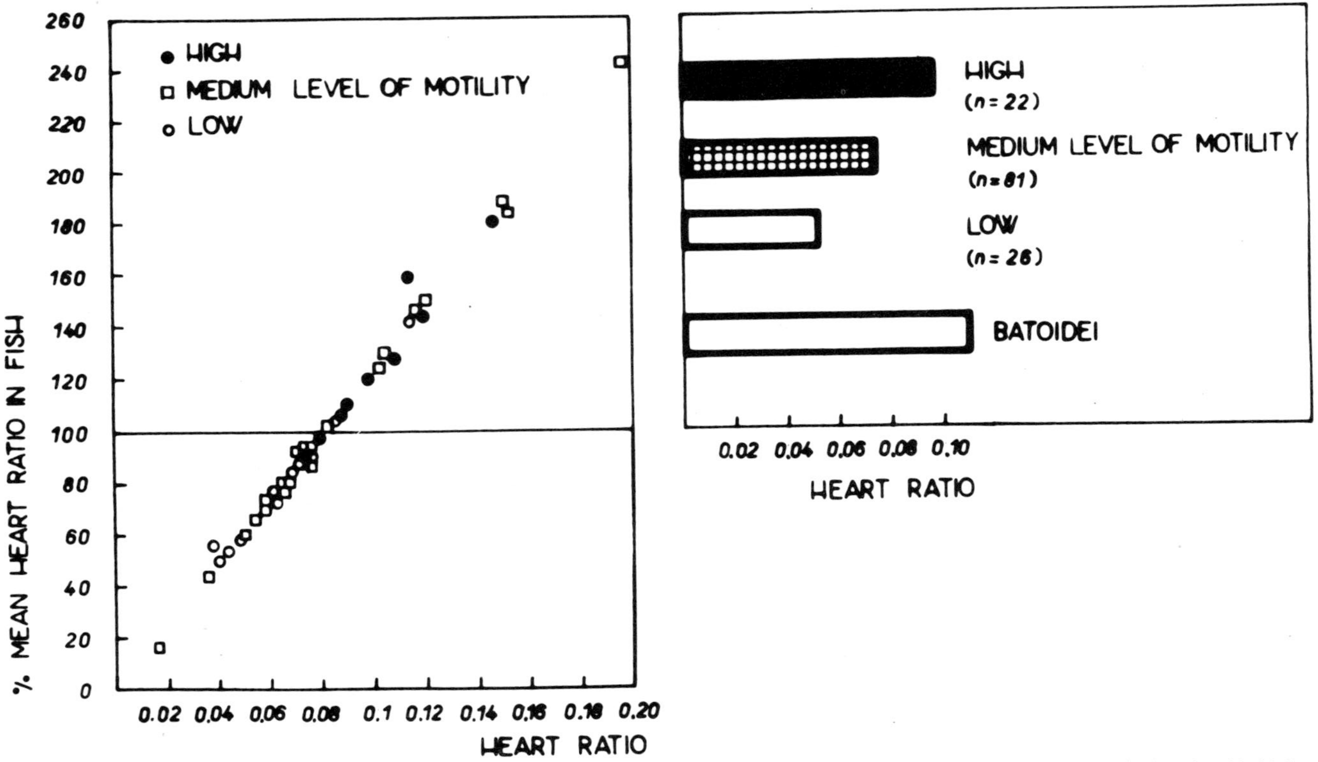

FIGURE 4. (*Left*) Heart ratios in 42 fish species with high, medium, and low motility. (*Right*) Mean values of the heart ratio in fish with high (n = 22), medium (n = 81), and low (n = 26) motility compared with rays (Batoidei). (Data from Hesse, 1921.)

Experimental Cardiomegalies

There are several methods of inducing changes in the heart weight: body weight ratio in laboratory animals. These methods have recently been reviewed elsewhere (Korecký *et al.*, 1967). In principle, three mechanisms are involved: (1) increased peripheral resistance, (2) increased volume work, and (3) unknown factors.

In view of the fact that heart weights in laboratory animals of the same strain, age, sex, and body weight vary within limits of ± 20% (rats), it is necessary to restrict the term "experimental cardiomegaly" only to an increase in heart size

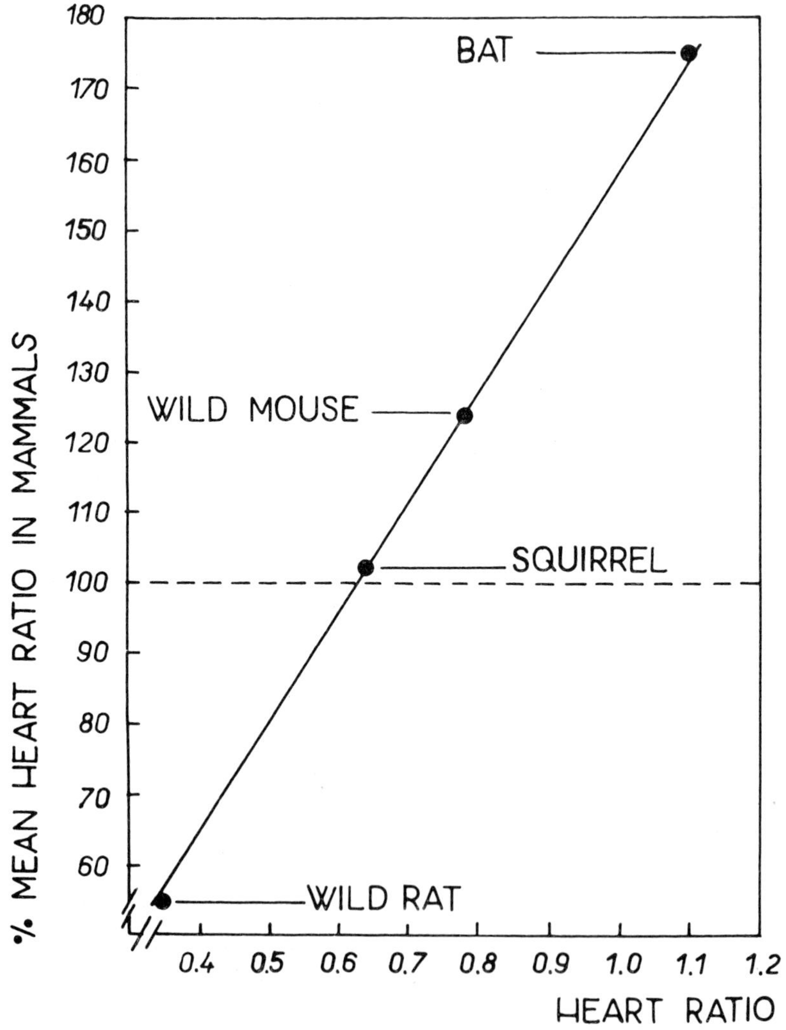

Figure 5. A comparison of heart ratios in mammals of approximately equal weight with different levels of antigravity work (wild rat compared with squirrel, and wild mouse compared with bat). (Data from Hesse, 1921; Ošťádal, 1967.)

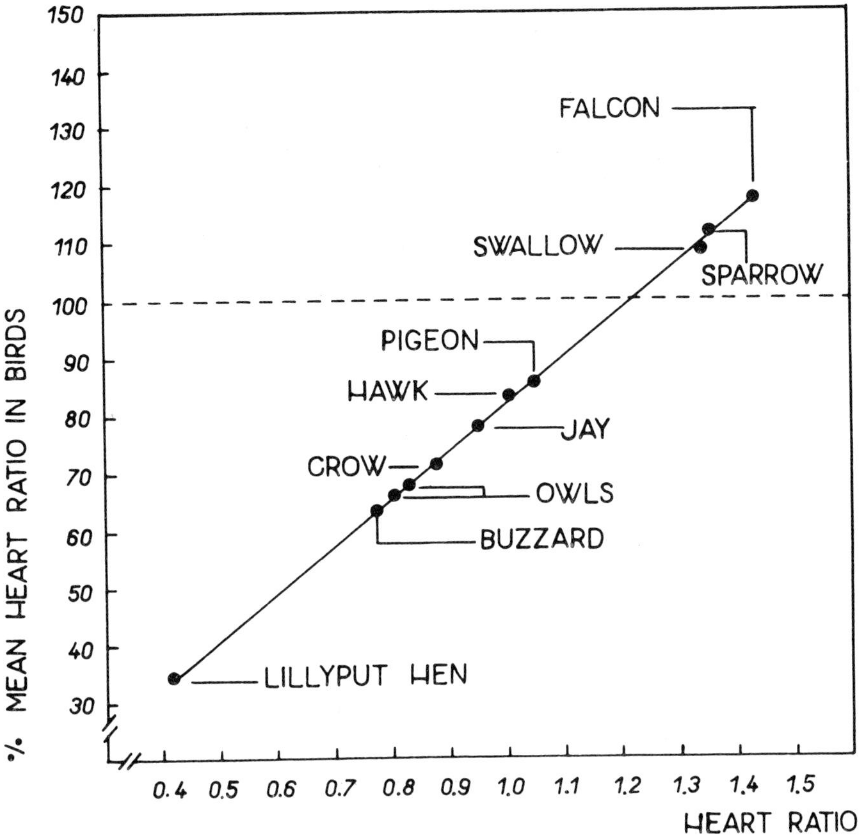

FIGURE 6. Heart ratios in some "athletic" and "nonathletic" birds. (Data from Hesse, 1921; Clark, 1927; Ošťádal, 1967.)

which surpasses this limit. Experimental models of cardiomegaly are usually less marked than "physiological cardiomegaly" and generally exceed normal values only by about 50% (exceptionally by 100%).

Development of Blood Supply of the Heart in Regard to Phylogeny

A functional and anatomical classification of heart structures is given in TABLE 1. In regard to phylogeny, changes in heart size concerning oxygen-consuming structures (muscle cells) are followed by changes in structures supplying the heart with oxygen (blood vessels). To date, however, these relative changes have not drawn sufficient attention. In FIGURE 9, the basic transformation of structures supplying oxygen to the heart is shown in animals representing a critical period of evolution i.e., during transition from poikilothermia to homoiothermia, when maximal acceleration of heart growth occurs (see FIGURE 1). Wide lacunae from which oxygen is brought directly to muscle cells are transformed into an intricate terminal vascular network of coronary circulation. Information about the mode of nutrition of the trabecullar musculature of the heart of poikilotherms from blood lacunae is very sparse. Data dealing with the phylogenetic development of coronary vessels are based on the classical papers of Grant and Reigner (1926), Clark (1927), and, more recently, that of Halpern and May (1958). The branching of the main coronary arteries depends on several phylogenetic factors: (1) Coronary arteries branch off the ventral rather than dorsal aorta, in parallel to the development of pulmonary circulation. (2) At the same time, the heart migrates caudally from the cervical region; in higher vertebrates, it takes up its

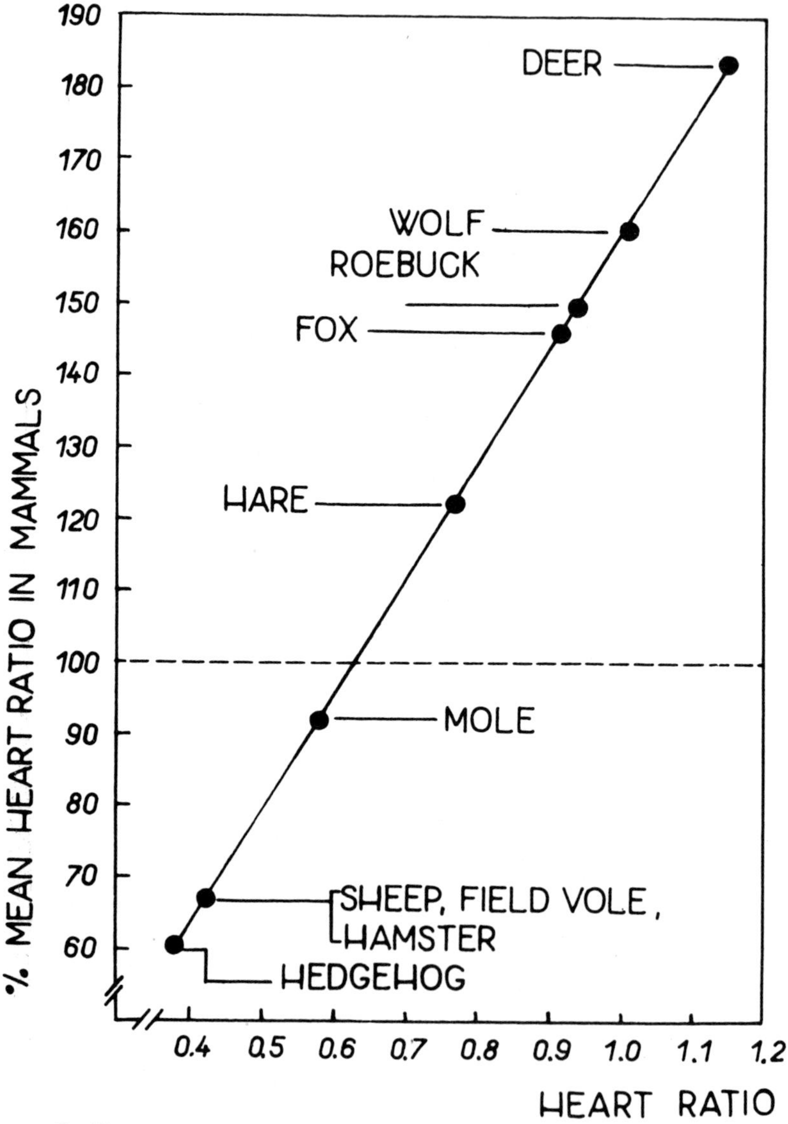

FIGURE 7. Heart ratios in some "athletic" and "nonathletic" mammals. (Data from Hesse, 1921; Clark, 1927.)

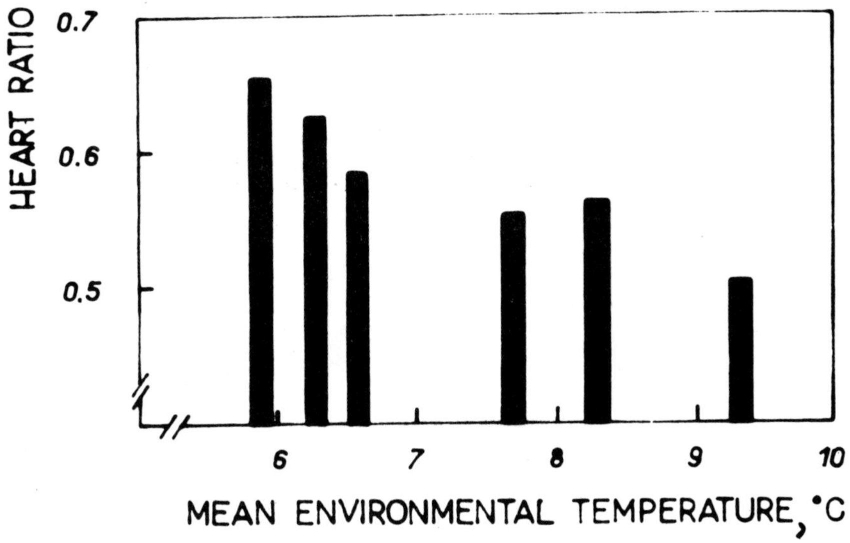

FIGURE 8. Effect of the mean yearly temperature of the environment upon the heart ratio in a homoiothermic species (squirrel). (Data from Hesse, 1921.)

TABLE 1

CLASSIFICATION OF ANATOMICAL AND FUNCTIONAL STRUCTURES OF THE MYOCARDIUM

Functional Structure	Anatomical Structure	Oxygen Consumption
Oxygen-consuming structures		
Contractile proteins	Myofilaments	100
Energy-releasing proteins	Sarcoplasmic organelles (mitochondria, etc.)	
Stromatic proteins	Membranes, fibrocytes, collagen fibers	1
Oxygen-input structures		
Terminal vacular bed	Capillaries	

position in the thorax. During this descent, it is followed by the large vessels, and, for this reason, the coronary arteries leave the aorta nearer to the heart. (3) According to Grant and Reigner (1926), the presence of pericardial connective tissue plays an important role in the development of coronary vessels. This connective tissue is well developed in fish and in some amphibians (e.g. Urodela), whereas it begins to disappear in Anura and reptiles. It is completely missing in mammals. These ligaments contain "coronary" vessels. Where this connective tissue is developed, a twofold arterial supply of the heart is to be found.

Cephalic. The arteries supplying the heart branch off from hypobranchial arteries, and venous blood flows into a sinus venosus. It is from this vascular bed that the future coronary system is derived.

Caudal. Nutritive arteries course along the pericardial connective tissue, and venous blood flows directly into systemic veins.

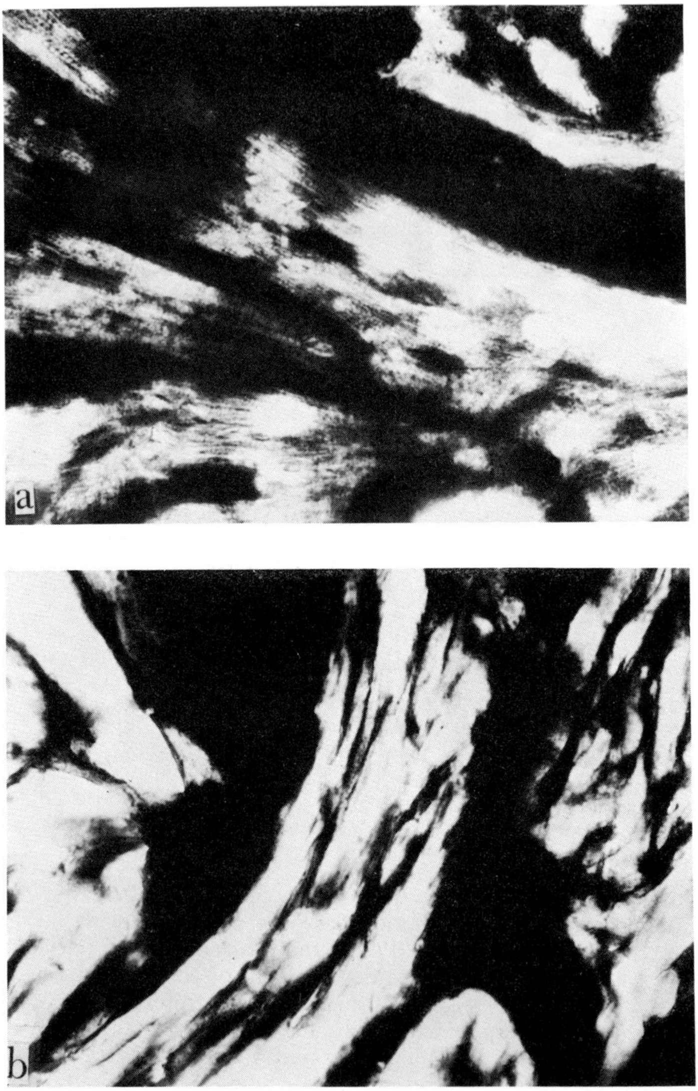

FIGURE 9. A phylogenic comparison of the arrangement of anatomical structures supplying the myocardium with blood. (a) Fish (*Trutta iridea*). (b) Amphibian (*Rana temporaria*). Stain: retrograde injection of India ink with gelatin into aorta. × 250.

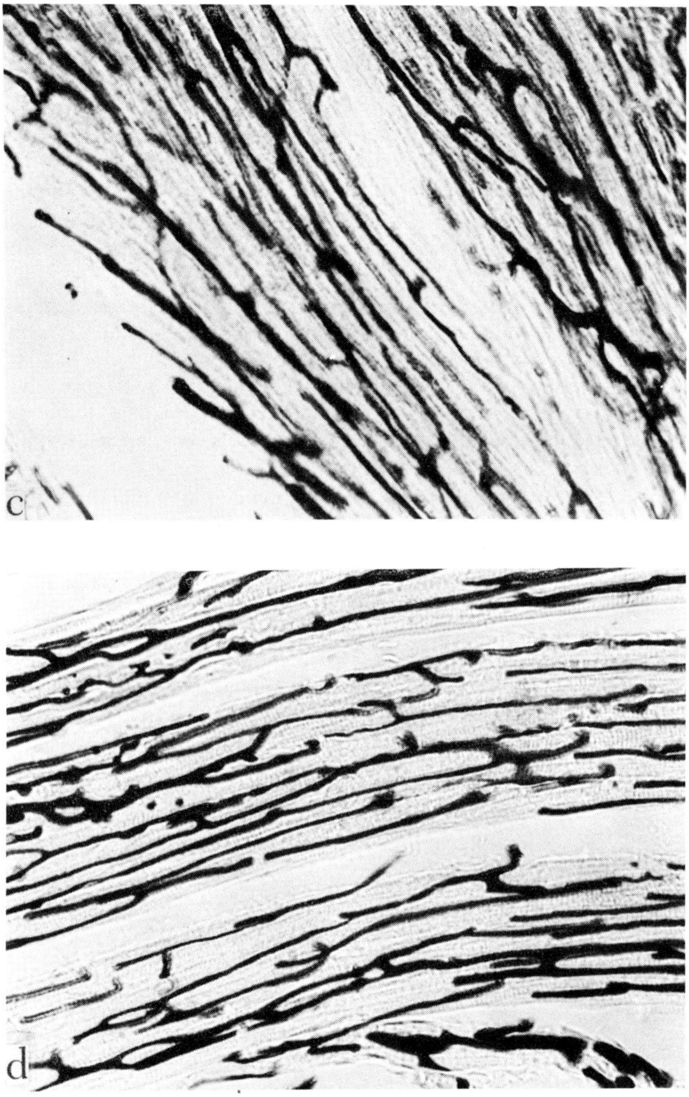

FIGURE 9. (*Continued*) (c) Bird (*Columba livia*). (d) Mammal (*Rattus norvegicus albus*). The change of the lacunar construction in the capillary supply is distinctly visible. Stain: retrograde injection of India ink with gelatin into aorta. × 250. (Data from Oštádal, 1967.)

Over the course of evolution, the caudal heart blood supply disappears, and the cephalic type of supply prevails. The first rudiments of a cephalic blood supply to the heart are encountered in fish.

Thus, nutrition of the myocardium changes over the course of evolution (TABLE 2). Generally, spongious myocardium is supplied by intertrabecullar blood spaces, whereas compact myocardium is supplied by anatomically formed vessels. This means that the heart of cyclostomes and the ventricles of amphibians are supplied by diffusion of blood filling the spongious heart musculature. In fish and reptiles, blood supply of the heart is of the mixed type. In fish, the external subepicardial compact layer of heart musculature is supplied mainly by the so-called caudal arteries, with only a small part supplied by arteries of cephalic origin. The analogous compact layer of the heart muscle in the reptiles is supplied by cephalic (i.e., coronary) arteries (Juhász-Nagy *et al.*, 1963; Brady & Dubkin, 1964).

It is possible to make several general conclusions from these anatomical observations about qualitative changes in nutrition of the heart as it increases in size over the course of evolution:

1. Structures requiring oxygen, represented in the heart by muscle tissue, grow not only quantitatively but also qualitatively, since the spongious arrangement regresses and changes into compact muscle mass.
2. With an increasing proportion of compact musculature, lacunar heart nutrition makes way for vascular nutrition from caudal vessels, as a direct component of the systemic circulation, and from cephalic vessels, as the future specific coronary circulation.
3. The caudal supply is temporary and is present in fish and amphibians.
4. In reptiles, coronary (cephalic) circulation is already formed and becomes dominant in the course of further phylogenetic development, which ensures the most rapid growth of compact cardiac musculature in birds and mammals.

TABLE 2

STRUCTURAL CHANGES OF OXYGEN-CONSUMING AND OXYGEN-INPUT STRUCTURES IN REGARD TO PHYOLOGENY*

Structural Organization	Vertebrate Class					
	Cyclostomes	Fish	Amphibians	Reptiles	Birds	Mammals
Oxygen-consuming structures						
Spongious	+	+	+	+	—	—
Compact	—	±	±	±	+	+
Oxygen-input structures						
Lacunary	+	+	+	+	—	—
Vascular						
Cephalic (coronary)	—	±	±	+	+	+
Caudal (extra-coronary)	—	+	±	±	—	—

* Key: + = present; — = absent; ± = may or may not be present.

Quantitative Data Concerning the Oxygen-Input and Oxygen-Consuming Structures

The oxygen supply of tissues is determined by the blood flow and by the uptake of oxygen from the blood supplying the tissues. In mammals, including man, the coronary arteriovenous oxygen differential is considerable (13–14 vol % according to Rushmer, 1961). The heart is apparently not able to increase its oxygen supply to any appreciable extent by raising the oxygen extraction from the blood. Furthermore it has been shown (Braunwald *et al.*, 1958; Ross *et al.*, 1963) that increased perfusion of the coronary bed (e.g. during work) does not substantially increase oxygen consumption in the heart tissue. If we accept these observations, it can be concluded that the dominant factor affecting the supply of oxygen to cardiac structures is the overall capacity of the terminal vascular bed in the heart, i.e., the density of the capillary network. This conclusion has also been reached by Kety (1957). This assumption may also help to comprehend the transformation of the lacunar blood supply of the heart into the complicated canalicular system of coronary capillaries during the critical period of evolution when the oxygen-consuming cardiac structures are rapidly growing (reptiles → birds).

Although the qualitative characteristics of this transformation are known in rough outline, detailed data are lacking on the quantitative relations between oxygen-supplying and oxygen-consuming systems of the heart at the developmental stages after the main growth of compact cardiac musculature has already been completed (birds and mammals). Even in birds and mammals, however, further transformations may occur, but these concern mainly the quantitative increase of anatomically differentiated structures (cardiac cells and capillaries). According to the classical work of Roberts and Wearn (1941) and some recent work (Rakušan & Poupa, 1963; Brown, 1965), the simple structural relationships between capillaries and muscle cells of avian and mammalian hearts allow the quantitative relations of these two systems to be expressed with the aid of a number of direct measurements; density of muscle cells, density of capillaries or fiber:capillary ratio (Roberts & Wearn, 1941), and diffusion distance (Krogh, 1922; Rakušan & Poupa, 1963). The usefulness of these parameters, of course, depends on the extent to which one is willing to accept the objections of Opitz and Thews (1952) to the older concept of Krogh (1922) concerning eccentric oxygen diffusion in tissues. According to Optiz and Thews (1952), the oxygen supply of the muscles cells is determined specifically by their surface area (concentric diffusion of oxygen in the tissues).

If this basic physical assumption is correct, it is pertinent to ask how the quantitative relations between oxygen-input and oxygen-consuming structures in a heart with canalicular blood supply (coronary vascular bed) are changed when the mass of oxygen-consuming structures is increased. Suitable models for this situation are animals in which the heart ratios are basically different because of ecological reasons (as in the case of mammals with high or low body movement activity, or domesticated or wild forms of near or identical species), and animals in which cardiomegaly is induced by experimental conditions (experimental cardiomegaly).

"Physiological Cardiomegaly" in the Hearts of Animals with High and Low Activity Level

Figure 10 shows a comparison of the quantitative differences between oxygen-input and oxygen-consuming structures in the heart of the hare (*Lepus europeus*) and rabbit (*Oryctolagus domesticus*) (Wachtlová *et al.*, 1965). Although the

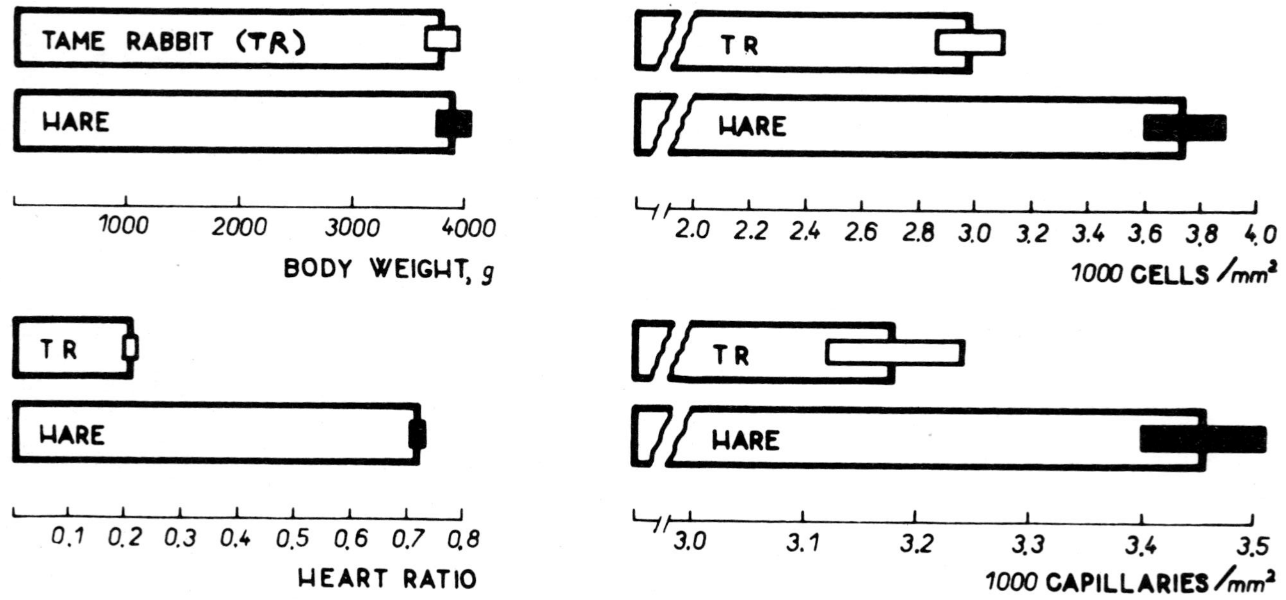

FIGURE 10. A comparison of quantitative relations (mean values, with standard deviations) in the internal structure of the hearts of "athletic" (*Lepus europus*, $n = 11$) and "nonathletic" (*Oryctolagus domesticus*, $n = 10$) mammals. Although the body weights are equal, the heart ratio is three times greater in the wild form ($p < 0.01$). Statistical significance of difference in cell density, $p < 0.01$; difference in capillary density, $p < 0.02$. (Data from Wachtlová *et al.*, 1965.)

body weights of the experimental animals were the same, the heart ratio of the hare was more than three times as great as that of the tame rabbit. A greater cell density was found in the heart of the hare, as well as a greater density of capillaries. The same result was found when the hearts of the wild and domesticated forms of the Norwegian rat were compared (Poupa & Rakušan, 1966). Although the difference between the heart ratios was not as marked as it was between the rabbit and hare (owing to the different form of movement in the wild rat, which is more of a sprinter than a long-distance runner), a higher density of cells and capillaries was noted in the heart of the wild form of rat than in the domesticated form. Each capillary supplies oxygen to a smaller muscle mass and the diffusion distance is shorter in the heart of the wild form than in the domesticated form (FIGURE 11).

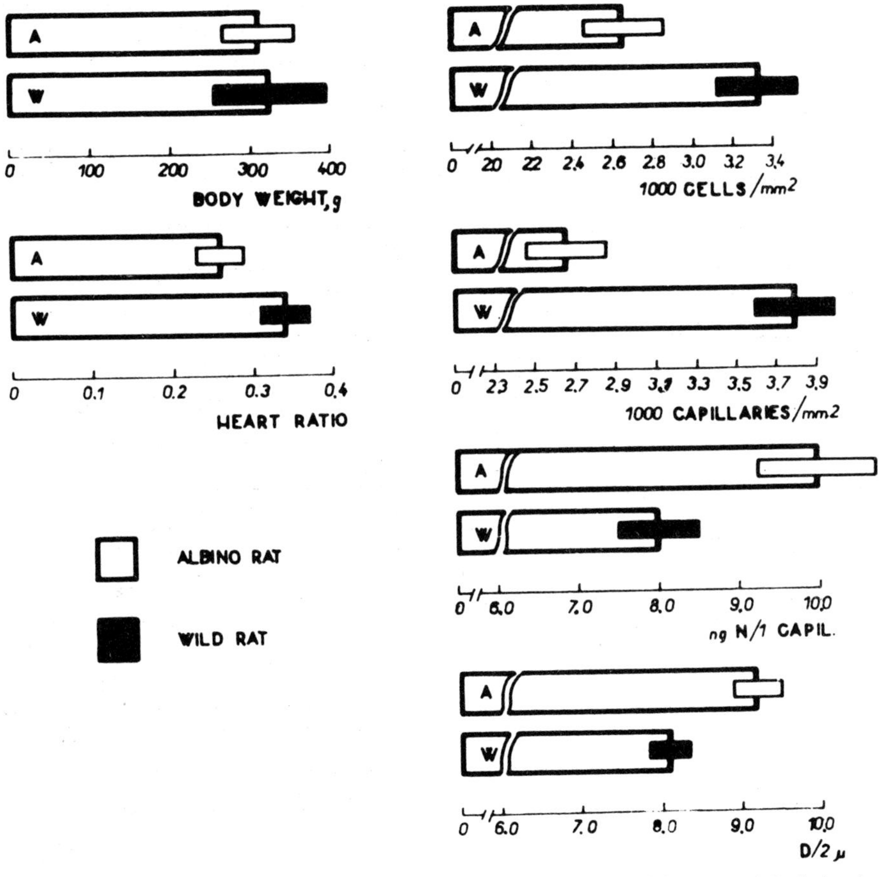

FIGURE 11. A comparison of quantitative relations (mean values, with standard deviations) in the internal structure of the hearts of wild (W, n = 7) and domesticated (A, n = 18) rats (*Rattus novegicus*). Statistical significance of difference in heart ratio, $p < 0.01$; cell density, $p < 0.01$; capillary density, $p < 0.01$; ng N/capillary, $p < 0.01$; D/2, $p < 0.01$.

Experimental Cardiomegaly

Analogous parameters were measured in the hearts of animals after the muscle mass had been increased experimentally by one of two methods: (1) by fitting a loose ring around the aorta of growing animals, so that growth of the aorta gradually caused an increased resistance and subsequent cardiomegaly (FIGURE 12), which took 150 days to develop (Rakušan & Poupa, 1966); or (2) by inducing sideropenic anemia at the time of weaning and maintaining it for 100 days (FIGURE 13), so that the heart was overstrained by hypercirculation due to a chronically lower supply of oxygen to the tissues.

In both cases, cardiomegaly of varying extent was obtained. It was found by an analysis of quantitative relations between capilaries and heart cells that the muscle mass became greater in cardiomegaly due to constriction of the aorta, i.e., growth of oxygen-consuming structures occurred, but this was not followed by a proportional growth of oxygen-input structures. The cell density in experimental animals was lower than in control animals, as was capillary density. The reverse was found in cardiomegaly due to anemia, in which heart growth was accompanied by an increased number of cells and capillaries, so that a heart hypertrophied by 100% ultimately exhibited the same capillary density as that of normal animals.

Comparison of "Physiological" and Experimental Cardiomegaly

FIGURES 14 and 15 illustrate the differences in the internal structure of hypertrophied hearts of two very closely related animal species (wild rat and albino

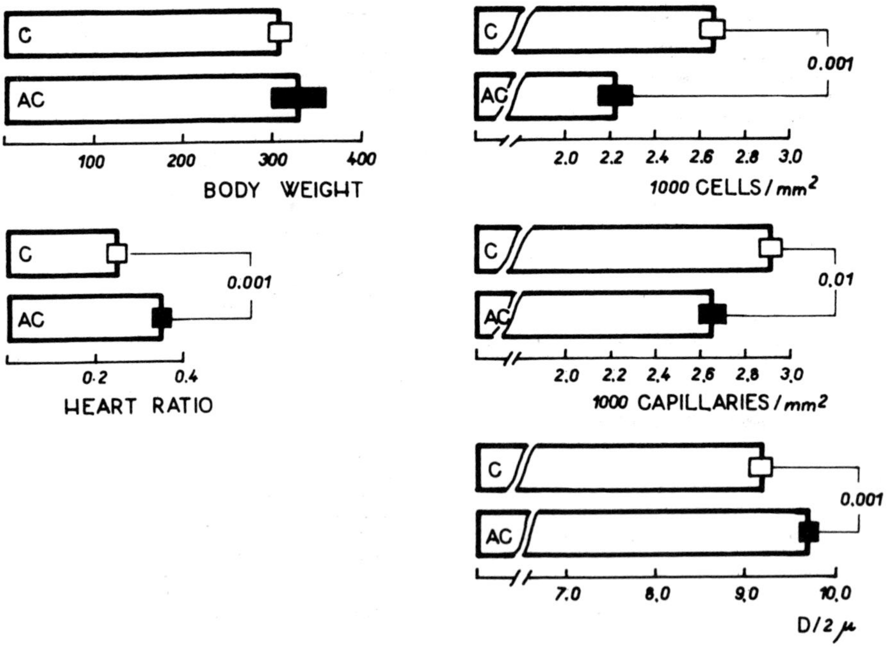

FIGURE 12. A comparison of quantitative relations (mean values, with standard deviations) in the internal structure of the hearts of normal rats (C, n = 18) and rats with experimental cardiomegaly due to aortic constriction for 150 days (AC. n = 10). Note the statistical significance in each case. (Data from Rakušan & Poupa, 1966.)

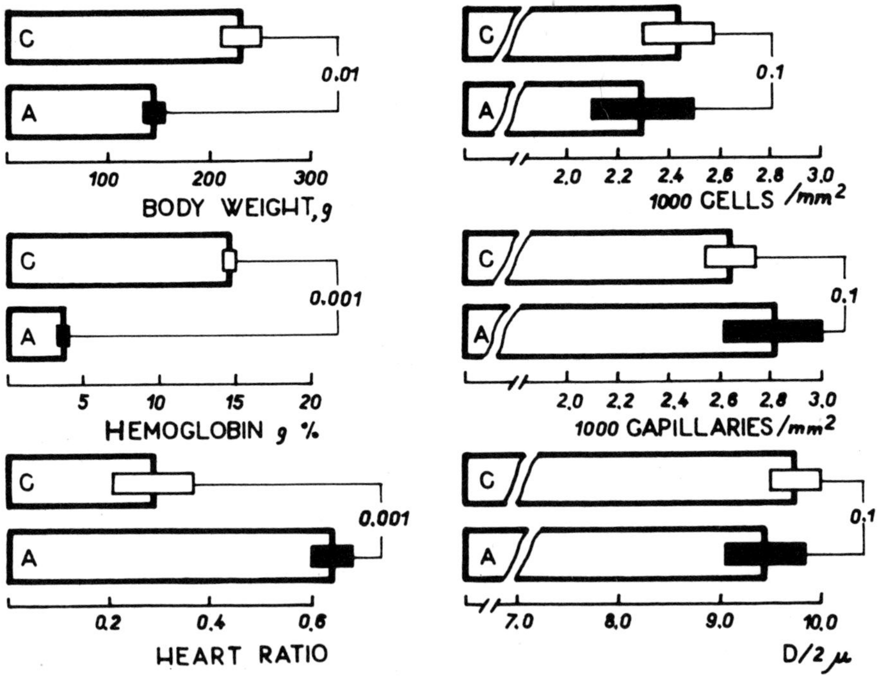

FIGURE 13. A comparison of quantitative relations (mean values, with standard deviations) in the internal structure of the hearts of normal rats (C, n = 14) and rats with experimental cardiomegaly due to volume load on the heart as a result of sideropenic anemia induced by a milk diet for 100 days after weaning (A, n = 15). Note the statistical significance in each case. (Data from Poupa *et al.*, 1964.)

rat), in which cardiomegaly was induced by two different mechanisms. "Physiological" cardiomegaly in wild rats is probably evoked by greater general motor activity. Experimental cardiomegaly was induced in albino rats by aortic constriction with a silver ring. For a meaningful comparison, animals were chosen with "physiological" and experimental cardiomegaly of the same extent, approximately 35% greater than the mean heart ratio in controls (normal albino rats). It is evident from FIGURE 14 that the cell density was greatest in wild rats and lowest in rats with experimental cardiomegaly; similarly, capillary density was highest in wild rats and lowest in rats with experimental cardiomegaly. Oxygen-consuming structures were supplied by the smallest number of capillaries in the hearts of animals with experimental cardiomegaly, and each capillary supplied the smallest muscle mass in the hearts of wild animals. A measurement of the sizes of heart cells in these three groups of animals showed that the smallest cells were in the hearts of the wild animals, and the largest were in the hearts of animals with aortic constriction (FIGURE 15). If the theory of Opitz and Thews (1952) concerning the concentric diffusion of oxygen in cardiac tissues is taken into account, it is obvious that the most suitable structural conditions for supplying oxygen to cardiac tissues are present in the large heart of a wild animal with its considerable internal surface, due to the smaller cell dimensions, from which oxygen brought in by the dense capillary network diffuse concentrically. Structural conditions in a heart with resistance cardiomegaly due to aortic construction are the reverse of those found in "physiological" cardiomegaly in the wild animal, even though the extent of cardiomegaly may be the same.

ACUTE "METABOLIC" MYOCARDIAL NECROSIS IN REGARD TO PHYLOGENY

The basis of acute myocardial necrosis, which can be induced in mammals by administering high doses of isoproterenol, has not been explained satisfactorily to date. Two explanations of its mechanism appear to be the most relevant:

Vascular Theory. It is assumed that the pressure relations in the vascular bed are changed after isoproterenol administration to such an extent that the oxygen supply of the heart is transiently decreased. Thus, isoproterenol-induced necrosis would be ischemic (Handforth, 1962).

Metabolic Theory. In view of the fact that some authors have proved the absence of vascular changes following isoproterenol administration in some animal species (Rosenblum *et al.*, 1965), and since histological examinations have shown necrotic foci in the heart following low doses of isoproterenol, which do not cause circulatory changes either in the coronary or systemic vascular bed, it has been concluded that this type of acute cardiac necrosis is metabolic in character. This explanation has been accepted by Rona and his colleagues (1963), who believe that myocardial necrosis following isoproterenol administration is due to an imbalance between the supply of oxygen and the high demand for it.

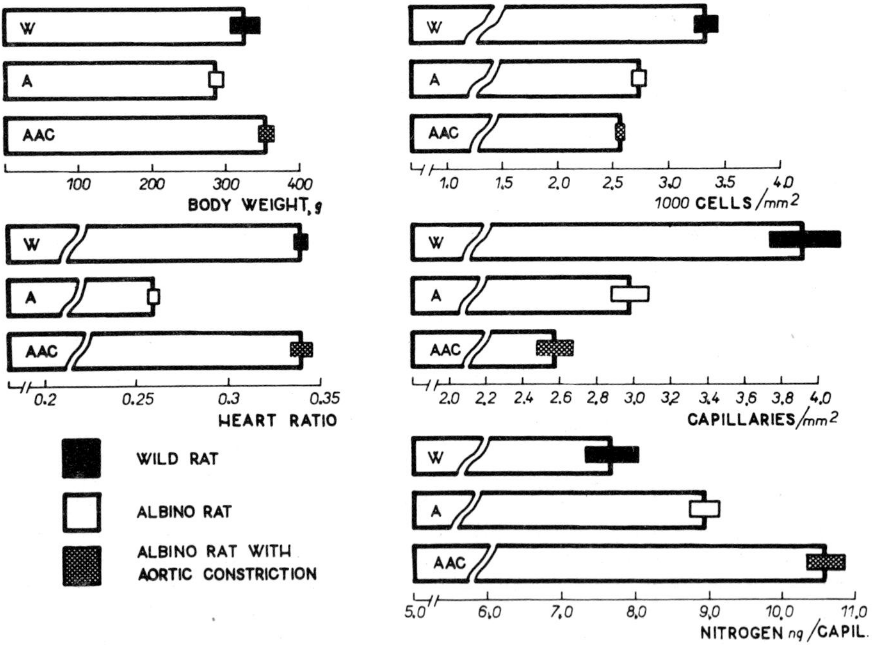

FIGURE 14. A comparison of quantitative relations (mean values, with standard deviations) in the internal structure of the hearts of wild rats (*Rattus norvegicus*) with "physiological" cardiomegaly (W, n = 3), albino rats with cardiomegaly due to aortic constriction (AAC, n = 4), and control albino rats (A, n = 6). Statistical significance of differences between AAC and W: body weight, no significance; heart ratio, $p < 0.01$; cell density, $p < 0.01$; capillary density, $p < 0.01$; ng N/capillary, $p < 0.01$. (Data from Poupa and Rakušan, 1966.)

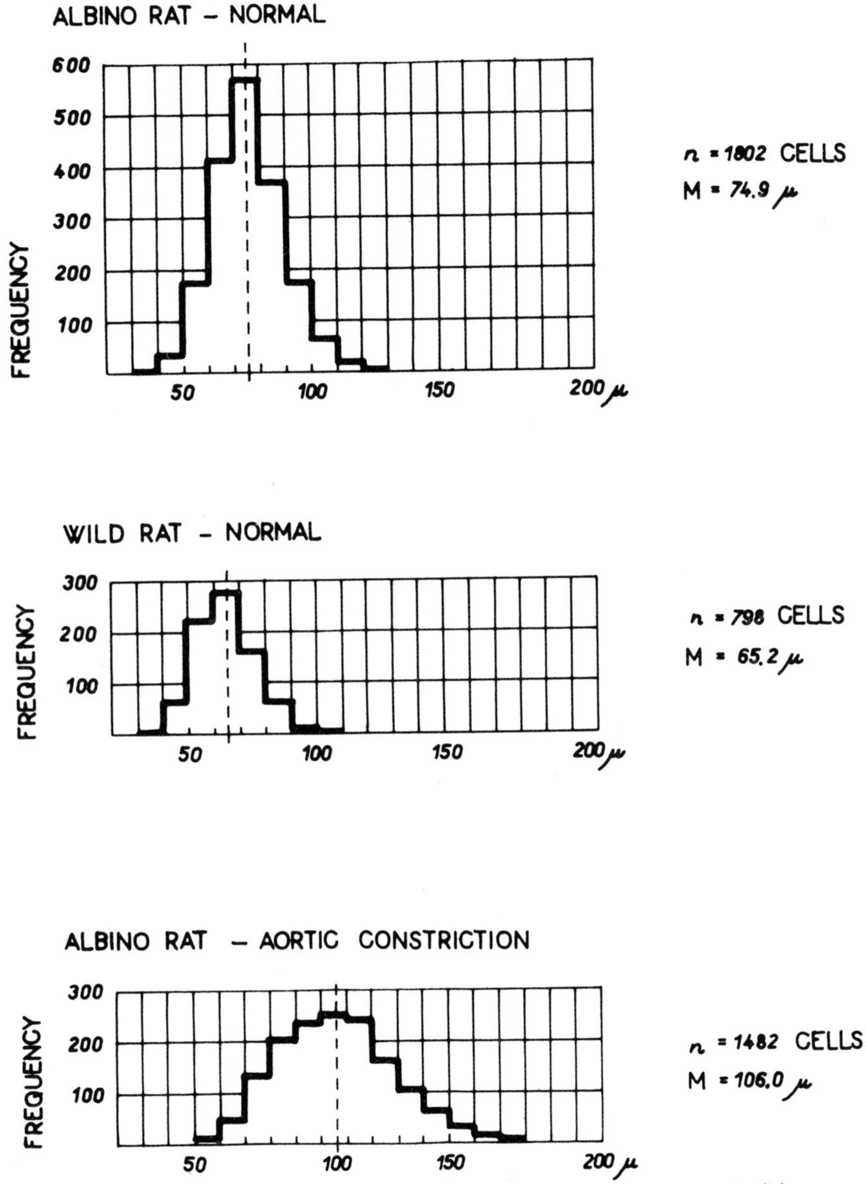

FIGURE 15. Occurrence of cells of various sizes in the hearts of a normal albino rat, a normal wild rat, and an albino rat with aortic constriction. M = mean values; n = number of cells evaluated. (Data from Poupa & Rakušan, 1966.)

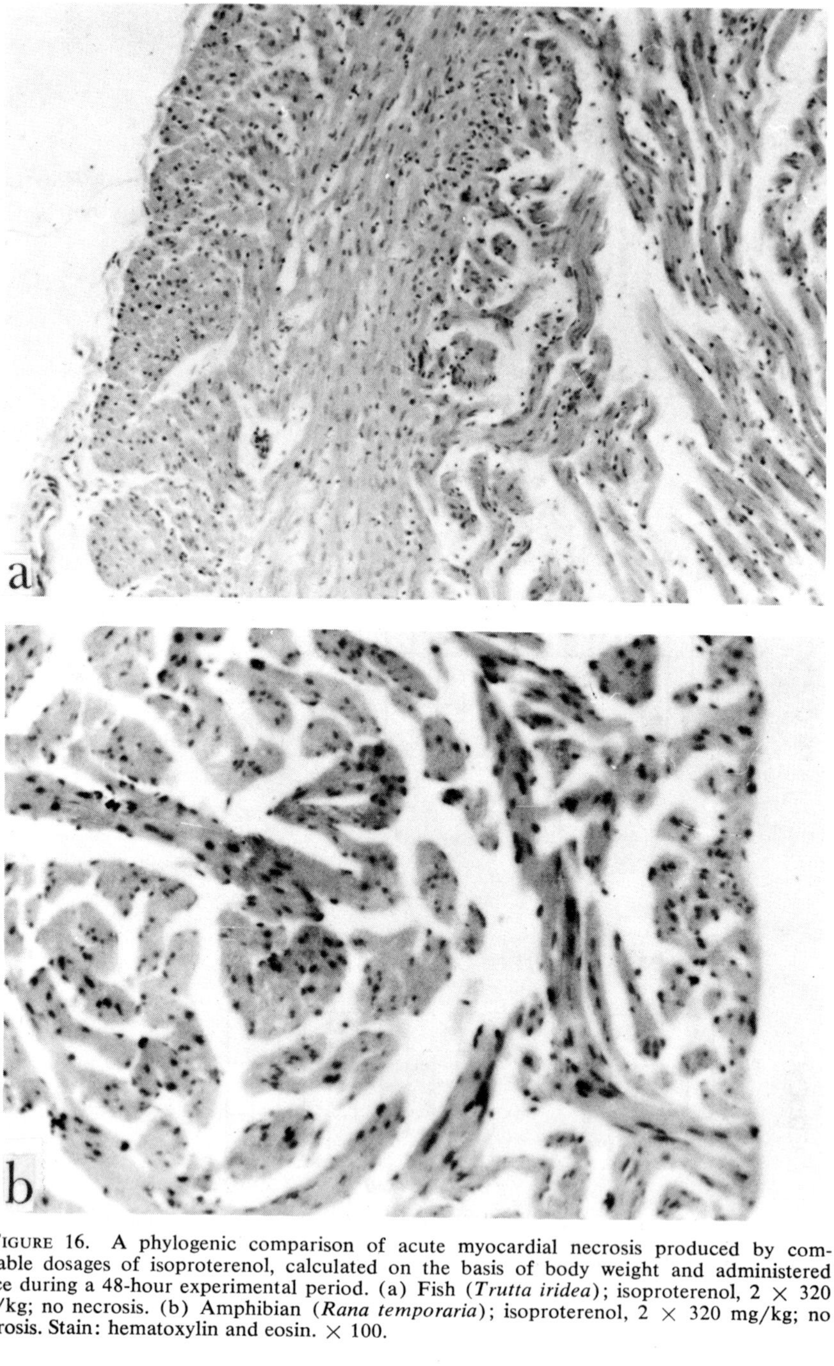

FIGURE 16. A phylogenic comparison of acute myocardial necrosis produced by comparable dosages of isoproterenol, calculated on the basis of body weight and administered twice during a 48-hour experimental period. (a) Fish (*Trutta iridea*); isoproterenol, 2 × 320 mg/kg; no necrosis. (b) Amphibian (*Rana temporaria*); isoproterenol, 2 × 320 mg/kg; no necrosis. Stain: hematoxylin and eosin. × 100.

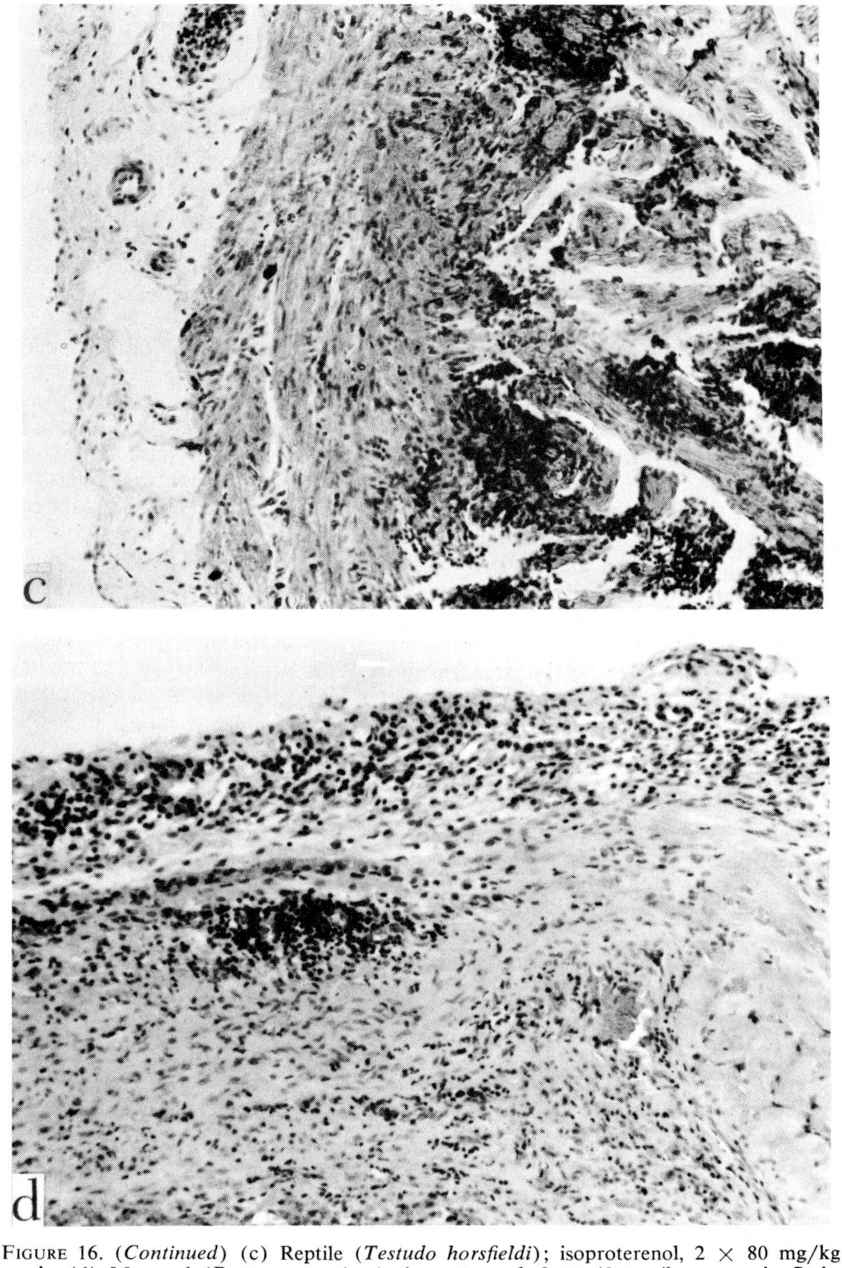

FIGURE 16. (*Continued*) (c) Reptile (*Testudo horsfieldi*); isoproterenol, 2 × 80 mg/kg; necrosis. (d) Mammal (*Rattus norvegicus*); isoproterenol, 2 × 40 mg/kg; necrosis. Stain: hematoxylin and eosin. × 100. (Data from Oštádal, 1967.)

The increase in size of the heart over the course of phylogeny and the accompanying transformation of the heart blood supply (lacunary to coronary) and of the internal microcirculatory coronary vascular bed offer a number of anatomical and functional models for analyzing the mechanism of the origin of acute myocardial necrosis following isoproterenol administration. To date, little attention has been paid to this field, and the main effort has been concentrated studying the morphology of myocardial necrosis following isoproterenol administration in common laboratory mammals. Recently, we administered isoproterenol to a variety of animals under identical conditions (two doses in 48 hours) in comparable amounts (calculated on the basis of individual body weight) so that a comparative study could be made concerning the occurrence of myocardial necrosis in relation to the position of the given species in the phyogenic scale, with regard to the known facts about the blood supply of the myocardium at that developmental level (Oštádal, 1967).

As shown in FIGURE 16 and TABLE 3, it was not possible to induce necrotic changes in the myocardium in two classes of poikilothermic vertebrates (fish and amphibians), even though isoproterenol was administered in doses four to eight times greater than those sufficient to induce myocardial necrosis in mammals (rats). Lesions of the myocardium which were similar in character to those found in homoiotherms were observed in reptiles (*Testudo horsfieldi*). Interpretation of this finding is not simple. It must be borne in mind that the resorption of an injected substance in homoiotherms is faster than in poikilotherms. This would seem to be disproved by the fact that necrosis-like lesions of the myocardium were induced by isoproterenol in reptiles but not in fish or amphibians, although all three classes are poikilothermic. A further consideration is that necrosis in fish and amphibians might have developed later, in view of the slow general metabolic rate in these animals and the slower transport of the necrogenic agent in the body. However, the finding of myocardial necrosis in reptiles seems to rule out this possibility. The external layer of the heart, which is more compact in fish and reptiles and to a lesser extent in frogs (bulbus arteriosus), exhibits differences in vascularization in both classes resistent to necrosis (fish and amphibians) compared with that of reptiles. The main supply of the reptilian heart is cephalic, i.e., a coronary vascular bed proper, whereas the hearts of the lower poikilotherms are supplied predominantly by caudal blood vessels (extracoronary). Furthermore,

TABLE 3

PRODUCTION OF EXPERIMENTAL MYOCARDIAL NECROSIS WITH ISOPROTERENOL IN REGARD TO PHYLOGENY*

Class	Species	n	Isoproterenol Dose (mg/kg)	Score
Fish	*Trutta iridea*	8	2 × 80	0
		6	2 × 320	0
Amphibians	*Rana temporaria*	8	2 × 80	0
		5	2 × 320	0
Reptiles	*Testudo horsfieldi*	8	2 × 80	0.85
Birds	*Columba livia*	7	2 × 80	2.6
Mammals	*Rattus norvegicus* (*albus*)	20	2 × 80	2.1

* n = number of animals investigated in each case. The specified dose of isoproterenol was injected twice during the 48-hour evxperimental period. The effect was observed macroscopically and microscopically 24 hours after the second injection. An explanation of the score is given by Poupa *et al.* (1966). (Data from Oštádal, 1967.)

it is not possible to exclude metabolic differences in the cardiac tissue itself, especially insofar as water and ion metabolism is concerned, due to the transition from an aquatic to a terrestrial form of life. It is interesting that necrosis-like lesions appear first at that stage of evolution when the myocardium undergoes the most rapid outburst of its anatomical development (Oštádal *et al.*, 1968).

Summary

1. The size of the heart in normal animals is adapted to its work output. Since the heart ensures the tissue oxygen supply, it can be assumed that there is a relationship between the size of the heart and factors determining overall oxygen consumption, including: (1) size of the lean body mass, (2) muscle activity, and (3) maintenance of body temperature.

Size of the heart in different animals (fish, amphibians, reptiles, birds, and mammals) is discussed in relation to these factors. The type of relationship between the size of the heart and the body weight of vertebrates is characterized as "poikilothermic," "avian," or "mammalian." The designation of individual animal species as one of these three types may be interpreted in terms of the factors determining oxygen consumption in the given species.

2. Heart tissue mass increases over the course of evolution, and there is a distinct difference in size between poikilothermic and homoiothermic animals. At this stage of the phylogenic scale, a change in the blood supply of the heart also occurs. In reptiles, the heart increases in size when "lacunar" nutrition is supplemented by "coronary" nutritional circulation.

3. Changes in the internal structure of the heart (cells and capillaries) associated with increased heart muscle mass in homoiotherms are manifested differently, depending on whether cardiomegaly is experimentally induced or caused by ecological adaptation to higher oxygen requirements (e.g. athletic and non-athletic free-living animals).

4. There is a marked difference in the resistance or susceptibility of the heart muscle to acute heart necrosis in vertebrates. In reptiles, necrosis of the myocardium has been produced. On the other hand, it has not been possible to evoke acute heart necrosis with isoproterenol in fish and amphibians with the same procedure used in reptiles.

References

Bartels, H. 1966. Some aspects of circulatory and respiratory functions in mammals. Amer. Heart J. **72:** 1.

Brady, A. J. & C. Dubkin. 1964. Coronary circulation in the turtle ventricle. Comp. Biochem. Physiol. **13:** 119.

Braunwald, E., S. J. Sarnoff, R. B. Case, W. N. Stainsby & G. H. Welch. 1958. Haemodynamic determinants of coronary flow: Effect of changes in aortic pressure and cardiac output on the relationship between myocardial oxygen consumption and coronary flow. Amer. J. Physiol. **192:** 157.

Brody, S. 1945. Bioenergetics and Growth. Hafner Publishing Co. New York, N. Y.

Brown, R. E. 1965. The pattern of the microcirculatory bed in the ventricular myocardium of domestic mammals. Amer. J. Anat. **116:** 355.

Clark, A. J. 1927. Comparative Physiology of the Heart. Cambridge University Press.

Grant, R. T. & M. Reigner. 1926. The comparative anatomy of the cardiac coronary vessels. Heart **13:** 283.

Halpern, M. H. & M. M. May. 1958. Phylogenetic study of the extracardiac arteries to the heart. Amer. J. Anat. **102:** 469.

Handforth, C. P. 1962. Isoproterenol-induced myocardial infarction in animals. Arch. Path. (Chicago) **73:** 161.

Hesse, R. 1921. Das Herzgewicht der Wirbeltiere. Zool. Jahrb. Abt. Allg. Zool. Physiol. **38:** 243.

JUHÁSZ-NAGY, A., M. SZENTIVÁNYI, M. SZABO & S. VAMOSI. 1963. Coronary circulation of the tortoise heart. Acta Physiol. Acad. Sci. Hung. **23:** 33.

KETY, S. S. 1957. Determinants of tissue oxygen tension. Fed. Proc. **16:** 666.

KORECKÝ, B., K. RAKUŠAN & O. POUPA. 1967. Experimental cardiomegaly. *In* Methods and Achievements in Experimental Pathology. E. Bajusz, Ed. **2:** 158–171. S. Karger. Basel, Switzerland.

KROGH, A. 1922. Anatomy and Physiology of Capillaries. London.

OPITZ, E. & G. THEWS. 1952. Eifluss von Frequenz und Fasserdichte auf die Sauerstoff-versorgung des menschlichen Herzmuskels. Arch. Kreislaufforsch. **18:** 137.

OŠŤÁDAL, B. 1967. The phylogenetic and ontogenetic development of the terminal vascular coronary bed and its influence on experimental heart necrosis. Ph.D. Thesis.

OŠŤÁDAL, B., V. RYCHTEROVA & O. POUPA. 1968. Isoproterenol-induced acute experimental cardiac necrosis in the turtle (*Testudo horsfieldi*). Amer. Heart J. In press.

POUPA, O., B. KORECKÝ, K. KROFTA, K. RAKUŠAN & J. PROCHÁZKA. 1964. The effect of anaemia during the early postnatal period of vascularisation of the myocardium and its resistance to anoxia. Physiol. Bohemoslov. **13:** 281.

POUPA, O., K. KROFTA, J. PROCHÁZKA & Z. TUREK. 1966. Acclimation to simulated high altitude and acute cardiac necrosis. Fed. Proc. **25:** 1243.

POUPA, O. & K. RAKUŠAN. 1966. The terminal microcirculatory bed in the heart of athletic and non-athletic animals. *In* Physical Activity in Health and Disease. : 18–29. Universitets-forlaget. Oslo, Norway.

RAKUŠAN, K. & O. POUPA. 1963. Changes in the diffusion distance in the rat heart muscle during development. Physiol. Bohemoslov. **12:** 220.

RAKUŠAN, K. & O. POUPA. 1966. Differences in capillary supply of hypertrophic and hyper-plastic hearts. Cardiologia **49:** 293.

ROBERTS, J. T. & J. T. WAERN. 1941. Quantitative changes in the capillary muscle relation-ship in human hearts during normal growth and hypertrophy. Amer. Heart J. **21:** 617.

RONA, G., D. S. KAHN, C. I. CHAPPEL. 1963. Studies on infarct-like myocardial necrosis produced by isoproterenol. A review. Rev. Canad. Biol. **22:** 241.

ROSENBLUM, I., A. WOHL & A. A. STEIN. 1965. Studies in cardiac necrosis. III. Metabolic effects of sympathomimetic amines producing cardiac lesions. Toxic. Appl. Pharmacol. **7:** 344.

ROSS, I., F. KLOCKE, G. G. KEISER & E. BRAUNWALD. 1963. Effect of alterations of coronary blood flow on the oxygen consumption of the working heart. Circ. Res. **13:** 510.

RUSHMER, R. F. 1961. Cardiovascular Dynamics. W. B. Saunders Co. Philadelphia, Pa.

WACHTLOVÁ, M., K. RAKUŠAN & O. POUPA. 1965. The coronary terminal vascular bed in the heart of the hare (*Lepus europeus*) and the rabbit (*Oryctolagus domesticus*). Physiol. Bohemoslov. **14:** 328.

A QUANTITATIVE STUDY OF MYOCARDIAL MITOCHONDRIA IN EXPERIMENTAL CARDIAC HYPERTROPHY*†

Ben D. McCallister‡ and Arnold L. Brown, Jr.
Sections of Medicine and Experimental and Anatomic Pathology
Mayo Clinic and Mayo Foundation
Rochester, Minn.

In the hypertrophic heart there is a twofold demand for an increase in available energy: to meet the added work load[1-3] that initiated the hypertrophy and to support the increase in protein synthesis that produced the hypertrophy.[4,5] The production of this energy, in the form of adenosine triphosphate, occurs only within the mitochondrion.[6,7]

The present study was undertaken to determine whether an increased demand for energy is reflected in an alteration of the fine structure in the mitochondrion of the myocardial muscle cell. The newborn heart and the adult hypertrophic heart, which represent conditions of accelerated cardiac growth, were used as the experimental models.

Methods

Unilateral perinephritis and subsequent renal hypertension were produced in 20 rats by wrapping the left kidney in Saran Wrap§ after removing the right kidney. The rats were killed six weeks later, and the hearts were weighed after the auriclular appendages and great vessels had been clipped off and the heart emptied of blood. The ten rats with the most extensive cardiac hypertrophy were chosen as the experimental group. The percentage of hypertrophy was calculated from the mean heart weight expected for a normal animal of the same body weight. The expected heart weights were obtained from a log-log regression based on the heart and body weights of 100 normal rats of various sizes. The weights of the hypertrophic hearts all were well above the 95th percentile (FIGURE 1). The weights of the hypertrophic hearts varied from 29 to 65% above the expected weights, with a mean hypertrophy of 48% (TABLE 1).

Sections from the left ventricle of each animal were fixed in Dalton's solution, embedded in an aliphatic epoxy resin (Epon 812), and stained with uranyl acetate for study with the RCA-EMU 3E electron microscope. Identical techniques were carried out on a control group of ten normal rats of similar age and body weights and on four newborn rats. Individual sections of left ventricular myocardium were selected for definitive study only if the heart muscle appeared to be maximally contracted. In order to standardize the fixation and preparatory techniques, the tissues were fixed and processed in the following order: five normal rat hearts, ten hypertrophied hearts, five normal hearts, and four newborn rat hearts.

There are a number of problems in a quantitative electron microscopical investigation. These include day-to-day differences in the environment and calibration of the microscope, differences in the degree of muscle fiber shortening, differences in fixation and dehydration of tissue specimens, variation in the compression of tissue by the ultratome knife, and difficulties in working with fetal tissue. All of these factors were taken into consideration and minimized as much as possible.

† This investigation was supported in part by United States Public Health Service research grant no. H-4856 from the National Institutes of Health.
‡ Recipient of United States Public Health Service fellowship no. HE-15623.
§ The Dow Chemical Co., Midland, Mich.

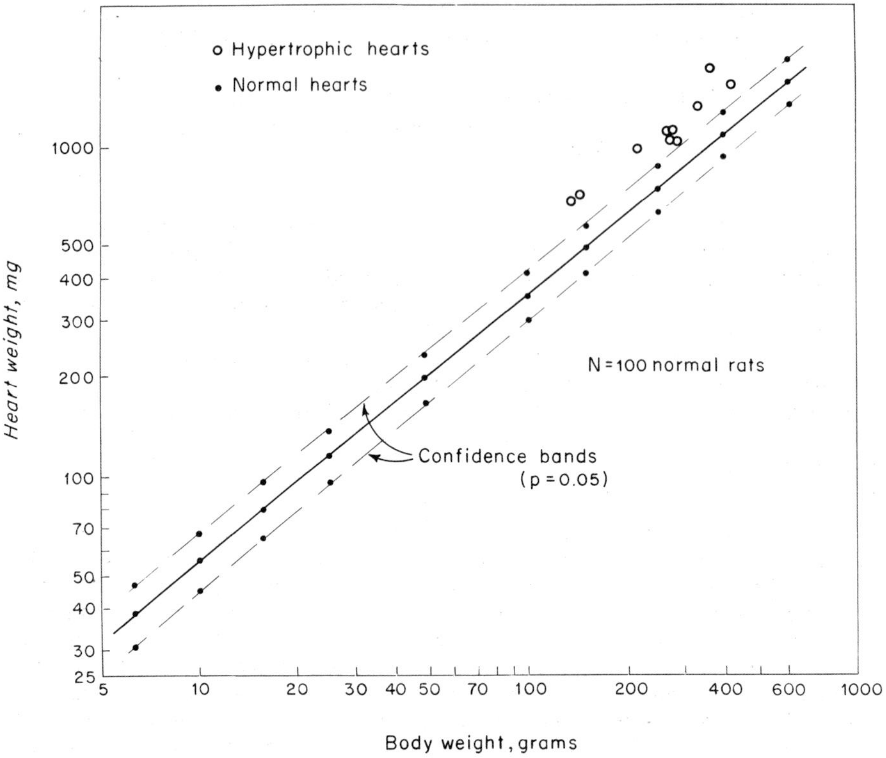

FIGURE 1. Log-log regression of heart weight:body weight in normal rats. The 95th percentile confidence limits were calculated from the heart and body weights of 100 normal rats.

The first part of this study was concerned with an evaluation of the number and area of the mitochondria in the myocardial muscle cell and the percentage of the cytoplasm of the muscle cell that is occupied by the mitochondria. Twenty random fields were photographed in sections from each of five of the control rat hearts, five of the hypertrophic rat hearts, and four of the newborn rat hearts at a magnification of approximately × 8,000. The prints were further enlarged four times, resulting in a final magnification of approximately × 32,000. A planimeter was used to determine the area of the individual mitochondrion and the percentage of cytoplasm occupied by the mitochondria. The number of mitochondria in each picture also was counted at the same magnification. Approximately 2,000 mitochondria were measured in each of the hypertrophic and normal hearts for these determinations and were related to an area of 35 μ^2 of the cytoplasm (FIGURE 2).

For all measurements in the hypertrophic and normal rat hearts, the cell was divided into two arbitrary areas: the perinuclear zone and the rest of the cell. The perinuclear zone included only those mitochondria that were nestled adjacent to the nuclear poles. The zone designated as the rest of the cell refers to fields of cytoplasm that were greater than 12μ from the nuclear membranes. In the newborn rat hearts, the percentage of cytoplasm occupied by the mitochondria and the number of mitochondria per field were not determined.

TABLE 1

HEART WEIGHTS AND BODY WEIGHTS OF NEWBORN RATS AND RATS WITH HYPERTROPHIC HEARTS

Rat No.	Body weight (g)	Heart Weight (mg)		Hypertrophy* (%)
		Mean Expected Normal	Actual	
Hypertrophic				
1	272	775	1160	50
2	422	1110	1510	36
3	286	810	1198	48
4	332	910	1434	57
5	220	660	850	29
6	145	460	719	56
7	391	1040	1719	65
8	275	790	1114	41
9	136	440	681	54
10	267	760	1093	44
Newborn				
1	8	—	39†	—
2	8	—	39†	—
3	16	—	53†	—
4	13	—	58†	—

* Calculated from the mean predicted heart weight.
† In newborn rats, the term "heart weight" applies only to left ventricular weight.

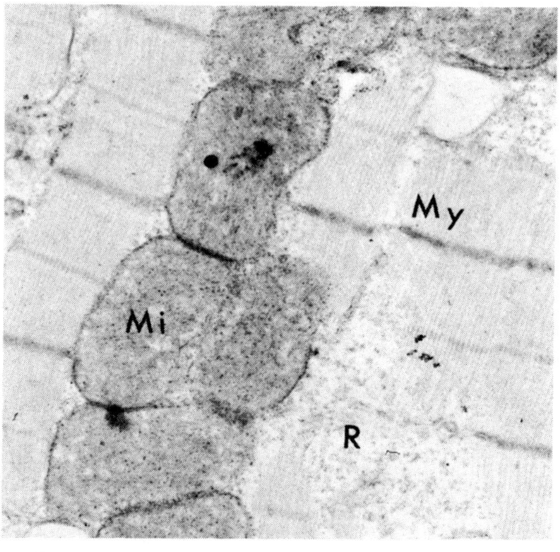

FIGURE 2. Myocardium of rat, showing mitochondrion (Mi), myofibril (My), and ribosomes (R). × 32,400.

The second part of the study was concerned with an evaluation of the inner structure of the mitochondrion. Ten photographs of mitochondria were taken in each of ten control, ten hypertrophied, and four newborn rat hearts at a magnification of approximately × 19,000. The prints were then enlarged four times to a total magnification of approximately × 76,000.

Calipers were used to measure the widths of the outer membranes of the mitochondria, the widths of the cristae mitochondriales, the sizes of the intercristal spaces, and the widths of the cristal membranes (FIGURE 3). Approximately 100 measurements were made of each of these inner structures in each of the 24 rats. Appropriate conversions of the measurements were made to Ångström units (Å), utilizing the magnification of the electron microscope, as determined by periodic calibrations with a grating replica. The mean value of the measurement, the standard deviation, and the standard error of the mean were computed for each individual rat as well as for the entire control, newborn, and hypertrophied groups.

The t-test was used to determine the statistical difference between the means, and 0.001 was chosen as the level of significance. Each group of measurements was compared among individual animals, as was the perinuclear zone to the rest of the cell among individuals. All of the intragroup measurements were then pooled, and the three main groups were compared. These individual measurements were also compared with the heart weight and the percentage of hypertrophy by a correlation and regression analysis.

Results

There was no significant difference between the normal and hypertrophic groups in regard to the mean values of the number of mitochondria per field or in the percentage of cytoplasm of the myocardial muscle cell occupied by the mito-

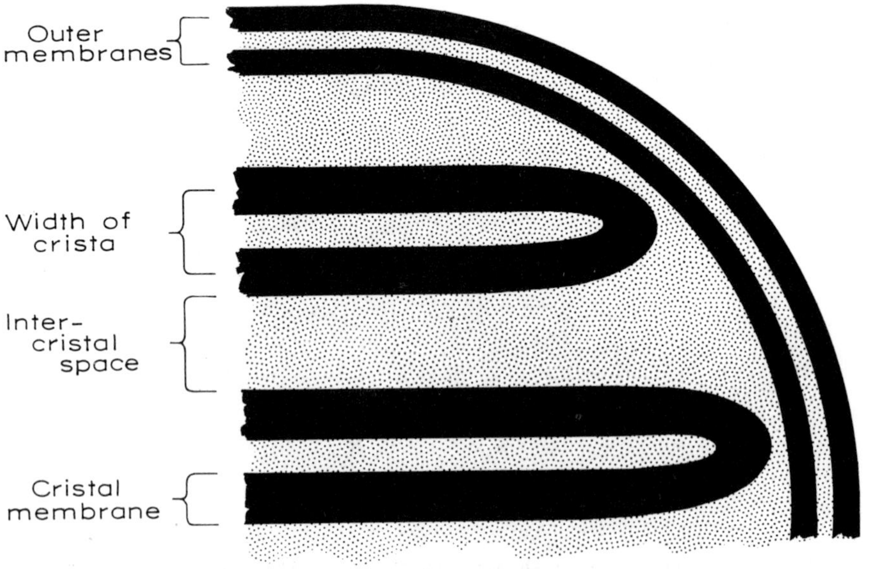

FIGURE 3. Schematic illustration of the inner structure of a mitochondrion.

chondria (TABLE 2). However, the mean area of the individual mitochondria in the hypertrophic hearts (0.581 μ^2) and in the newborn group (0.261 μ^2) is significantly different from the mean area of the control (0.517 μ^2). It should be pointed out that the statistical conclusions concerning the mean area that were published in preliminary abstract form were in error.[8] The difference in the means between the number of total mitochondria per field (35 μ^2) in the hypertrophic heart (mean, 8.7) and in the normal heart (mean, 9.9) is small and is not statistically significant. However, there are significantly fewer mitochondria in the nuclear zone of the hypertrophied cardiac muscle cell (mean, 7.9) than in the nuclear zone of the normal cell (mean, 11.0).

All of the inner structures of the mitochondria in the hypertrophic hearts were significantly larger than those in the normal hearts (TABLE 3 and FIGURES 4 and 5). There is a tendency for the differences in the inner structures to be greater in the peripheral portions of the cell than in the perinuclear zone. The inner structures in the newborn group were also significantly different from those of the normal group and were larger even than those of the hypertrophic group (TABLE 3 and FIGURE 6). The only exception to this was the width of the cristae mitochondriales, in which there was no significant difference between the newborn and the normal group (TABLE 3). One representative photograph from each group of rat hearts is shown in order to illustrate the main differences noted. For the purposes of publication, smaller magnifications are shown than those actually used in the study, as described under "Methods." As can be noted, it was not always possible to make all four of the measurements illustrated in FIGURE 3 on each individual mitochondrion.

The areas of the mitochondria as well as the widths of their inner structures varied little with changes in heart weight in both the hypertrophic and normal groups (slope, 0.001 to 0.02; range, +0.03 to +0.23) throughout the ranges of heart weights that were studied. These relationships were not studied in the newborn group, since the range in heart weights in this group was too limited.

No definite difference could be seen in the density of the apparently structureless internal matrix of the mitochondria among the groups studied. However, in general, the cristae of the hypertrophic rat mitochondrion appeared subjectively

TABLE 2

MITOCHONDRIAL MEASUREMENTS IN NORMAL, NEWBORN, AND HYPERTROPHIC HEARTS OF RATS

Measurement*	Normal Adult	Hypertrophic	Newborn
Area			
Mean (μ^2) ± S.E.	0.517 ± 0.12	0.581 ± 0.13†	0.261 ± 0.02†
No. of observations	770	784	84
S.D.	0.33	0.37	0.19
No. per field (35 μ^2)			
Mean ± S.E.	9.86 ± 0.53	8.66 ± 0.38	
No. of observations	78	98	
S.D.	4.7	3.6	
Percentage of cytoplasm			
Mean ± S.E.	31.5 ± 1.44	29.4 ± 0.99	
No. of observations	78	91	
S.D.	12.7	9.4	

* S.E. = standard error; S.D. = standard deviation.
† Statistically significant from normal beyond the 0.001 level.

TABLE 3

MEASUREMENTS OF INNER STRUCTURE OF MYOCARDIAL MITOCHONDRIA IN NORMAL, NEWBORN, AND HYPERTROPHIC HEARTS OF RATS

Measurement*	Normal Adult	Hypertrophic	Newborn
Width of outer membranes			
Mean (Å) ± S.E.	143 ± 1.5	149 ± 1.3†	153 ± 2.4†
No. of observations	526	716	133
S.D.	35	36	28
Width of cristae mitochondriales			
Mean (Å) ± S.E.	101 ± 0.71	106 ± 0.22†	101 ± 0.97
No. of observations	939	987	160
S.D.	22	17	12
Width of cristal membranes			
Mean (Å) ± S.E.	168 ± 1.13	179 ± 0.84†	185 ± 1.96†
No. of observations	998	1034	210
S.D.	36	27	28
Width of intercristal spaces			
Mean (Å) ± S.E.	174 ± 1.7	208 ± 1.5†	243 ± 3.8†
No. of observations	1033	1028	238
S.D.	55	48	59

* S.E. = standard error; S.D. = standard deviation.
† Statistically significant from normal beyond the 0.001 level.

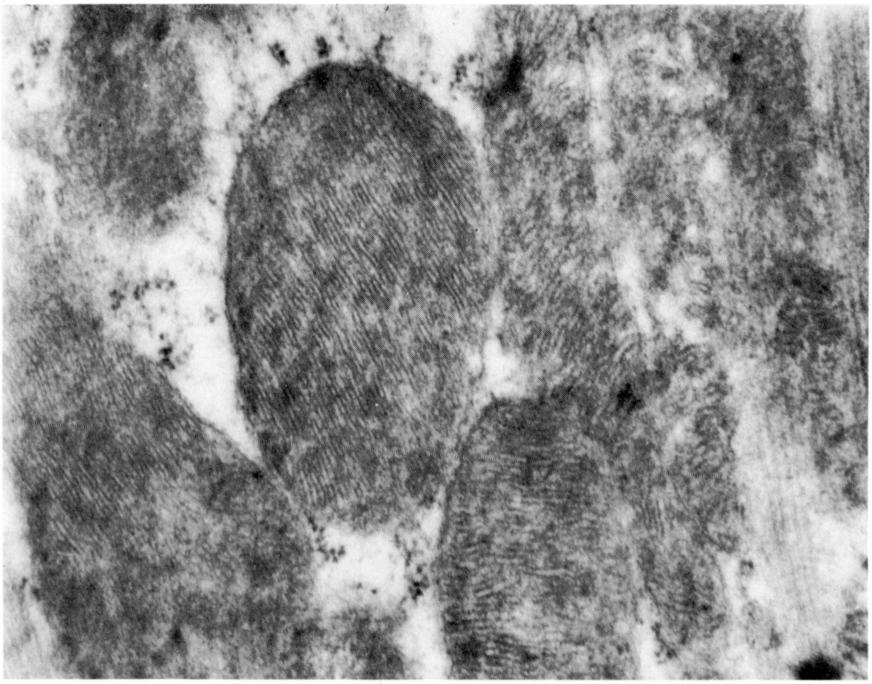

FIGURE 4. Mitochondrion from normal rat myocardium. × 49,200.

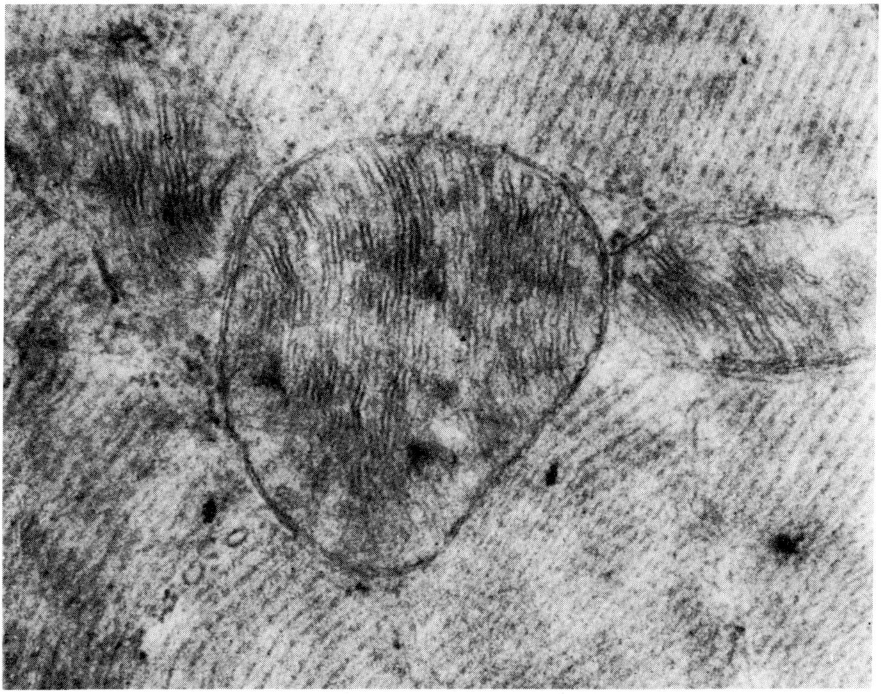

FIGURE 5. Mitochondrion from hypertrophic rat myocardium. × 48,200.

to be more osmiophilic, as evidenced by the greater ease of focusing on these cristae as compared with those of the normal rat mitochondrion.

When renal hypertension and subsequent cardiac hypertrophy were produced, by the technique described previously under "Methods," significant cardiac hypertrophy developed in about 50% of the operated animals. None of the rats in the hypertrophic group gave any clinical or pathological evidence of heart failure.

Discussion

In the present study, a quantitative analysis of the inner structure of the mitochondria of the rat myocardium revealed that the mitochondria of hypertrophic and newborn hearts are similar. These mitochondria differ from those of the normal adult rat heart in that there is a decreased concentration of the cristae mitochondriales and an increased width of the cristal membranes. In addition, the mitochondria of the hypertrophic heart are slightly larger than those of the normal rat heart, and the mean area of the newborn mitochondrion measures about one-half that of either form of the adult mitochondrion.

The differences in the measurements of the inner structures are, indeed, small, and the most striking differences are noted in the widths of the intercristal spaces. In support of the latter observation, Mölbert and Iijima[9] and Wollenberger and his associates[10–12] have previously noticed a decrease in the concentration of cristae in the mitochondria of hypertrophic rat and dog hearts, respectively. Wollenberger and his co-workers[10] also stated recently that Schwartz and Lee[13] noted a decrease in the concentration of the cristae in the mitochondria of failing guinea pig hearts. Edwards and Challice[14] have observed further that the cristae mitochondriales of the newborn mouse myocardium are unusually thin and lacking in alignment. In none of these previous studies, however, were mensuration data presented.

It is likely that some of the mitochondria seen in the rapidly growing hearts of the present study represent newly formed mitochondria. Mitochondria of other newly formed structures, such as spermatocytes, have also been described as containing few cristae.[15]

In the present study, mitochondria that resembled each other were found in all of the three groups. Nevertheless, in the hypertrophic group, the majority of mitochondria appeared abnormal. In no instance was there 50% "disappearance of cristae," as described by Wollenberger and Schulze.[11] Also, abnormal elongated forms of mitochondria with irregular cristae, such as were described in the failing dog heart,[11] were not seen.

Wollenberger and Schulze[12] also noted a ratio of myofibrillar to mitochondrial area of 3.57:1 in the hypertrophic heart and one of 2.23:1 in the normal heart. They concluded that the relative amount of contractile matter that the mitochondria must supply with energy is increased in cardiac hypertrophy. However, these conclusions are not supported by the present study, in which the portion of the cellular space occupied by the mitochondria was essentially the same in both the normal and the hypertrophic heart. In support of our findings are studies of other cell types which show an equilibrium between the total amount of cytoplasm

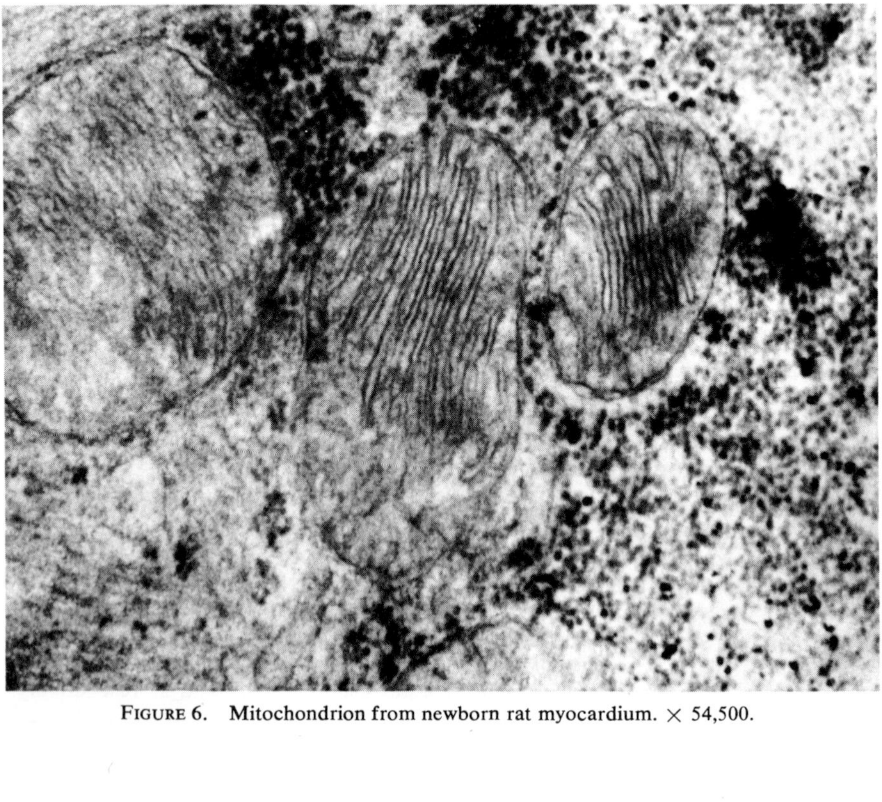

FIGURE 6. Mitochondrion from newborn rat myocardium. × 54,500.

and the mitochondrial mass, at least as noted in spermiogenesis and cell regeneration.[15]

It is known that the enzymes of the Krebs cycle and the fatty acid cycle are situated within the mitochondrial matrix.[16,17] However, histochemical and biochemical evidence has shown that the respiratory enzymes, that is, the dehydrogenase and cytochrome complexes, are attached directly to the membranes of the mitochondrion.[6,18–23] Recently, using negative staining techniques, Parsons,[24] Smith,[25] Stoeckenius,[26] and Fernández-Moran[27,28] demonstrated projecting subunits that measure 80–100 Å in diameter and are attached by stalks to the cristal membranes. Chance and Parsons[29] also have shown a relationship between the number of these projecting spheres and the cytochrome c content of the mitochondria. The slight increase in thickness of the cristal membranes that was noted in the hypertrophic hearts in this study, therefore, might be due to a change in the size or distribution of these subunits.

A relationship exists between metabolic activity, as measured by oxygen consumption, and the concentration of cristae within the mitochondria.[15,30–32] The concentration of the cristae has further been related directly to the concentration of the respiratory pigments, that is, the cytochromes and flavoproteins.[30] As an example, the highly active mitochondria of cardiac tissue have been shown to have greater amounts of the respiratory enzymes than do the mitochondria of liver tissue,[30,33] in which the cristae are less densely concentrated.

The hypertrophied myocardium is able to reach a higher level of cardiac work than is the normal heart.[1–3] Observations that show an increase in succinic dehydrogenase[34] and cytochrome c[35] in the hearts of animals with cardiac hypertrophy would seem to confirm the expected physiological result of cardiac hypertrophy, that is, an increased ability to do work. Nevertheless, the decrease in concentration of the cristae mitochondriales which was noted in the present study might be expected to be associated with a decrease in enzyme content and activity.[6,19,30] To support this hypothesis, a decrease in malic dehydrogenase activity in the hypertrophic heart has been noted by Wollenberger and his co-workers.[10] In addition, they reported a study on isolated mitochondria from hypertrophic dog hearts in which they found a decrease in oxidation and phosphorylation to 54% and 64%, respectively, below normal rates.

Besides their function in the production of energy for the contractile apparatus, the mitochondria are known to play a double role in protein synthesis: in the manufacture of protein[36,37] and in the elaboration of the energy required for protein synthesis.[37,38] Thus far, biochemical studies have shown that mitochondria synthesize only their own proteins, yet Ward[39] has reported morphological studies that show the location and apparent formation of yolk protein within the mitochondria of the frog oocyte. This raises the possibilities that the mitochondria may be able to synthesize extramitochondrial protein and that the mitochondria of the heart may synthesize myofibrillar as well as mitochondrial proteins. Mitochondrial synthesis of myofibrils has been suggested by Edwards and Challice,[14] who observed that the incomplete myofibrils of the newborn mouse are closely associated with Palade granules and mitochondria.

It is possible that the requirements for an increase in protein synthesis, such as occurs in the newborn and hypertrophic heart, may result in a decrease in the concentration of the cristae mitochondriales.[4,5,40] Biochemical data of Wollenberger and his associates[10] seem to support the concept that a decrease in the concentration of the cristae may subsequently compromise the oxidative capacity of these mitochondria.

A priori, since the hypertrophic heart requires more energy, the myocardial muscle cells would be expected to have either more mitochondria or a greater concentration of cristae, or both. However, this is not the case, because the energy-producing apparatus of the hypertrophic heart seems to respond with an alteration in structure that would not appear to enhance the oxidative capacity of the cell.

In the healthy, growing, newborn heart coping with only physiological demands, the level of oxidative capacity associated with the protein synthesis of rapid growth conceivably might not be detrimental to the function of the contractile apparatus. However, in the hypertrophic heart a decrease in the energy-producing ability of the myocardial cell could possibly lead to the development of heart failure, as well as to a decreased ability to synthesize protein.[5] This could further limit the extent of myocardial growth, which is a primary requirement of the myocardium in adjusting to an increasing work load.

Summary

The mitochondria of the hypertrophic rat heart have been observed to have distinct morphological characteristics. These characteristics have been quantitatively studied; they differ significantly from those of the mitochondria of the normal rat heart. The mitochondria of the hypertrophic rat heart are distinguished from those of the normal rat heart by increases in the width of the cristae mitochondriales, in the width of the intercristal space, in the width of the cristal membranes, and in the width of the outer membranes, as well as by an increase in the size of the mitochondrion itself.

References

1. BEZNAK, M. 1958. Cardiac output in rats during the development of cardiac hypertrophy. Circ. Res. **6:** 207–212.
2. KERR, JR., A., A. R. WINTERBERGER & M. GIAMBATTISTA. 1961. Tension developed by papillary muscles from hypertrophied rat hearts. Circ. Res. **9:** 103–105.
3. NOVACK, P. 1962. Hemodynamic alterations accompanying diastolic hypertension. Amer. J. Cardiol. **9:** 659–662.
4. GUDBJARNASON, S., TELERMAN & R. J. BING. 1963. Protein synthesis in myocardial hypertrophy and experimental heart failure (abstr.). Fed. Proc. **22:** 345.
5. MEERSON, F. Z. & T. L. ZAYATS. 1960. Changes in the intensity of protein synthesis in the myocardium during compensatory hyperfunction of the heart. Bull. Exp. Biol. Med. **50:** 678–680.
6. GREEN, D. E. & Y. HATEFI. 1961. The mitochondrion and biochemical machines. Science **133:** 13–19.
7. LEHNINGER, A. L. 1961. How cells transform energy. Sci. Amer. **205:** 63–73.
8. MCCALLISTER, B. D. & A. L. BROWN. 1963. A quantitative morphologic study of the mitochondria in experimental cardiac hypertrophy (abstr.). Fed. Proc. **22:** 194.
9. MÖLBERT, E. & S. IIJIMA. 1958. Beitrag zur experimentellen Hypertrophie und Insuffizienz des Herzmuskels im elektronenmikroskopischen Bild. Naturwissenschaften **45:** 322–323.
10. WOLLENBERGER, A., B. KLEITKE & G. RAABE. 1963. Some metabolic characteristics of mitochondria from chronically overloaded hypertrophied hearts. Exp. Molec. Path. **2:** 251–260.
11. WOLLENBERGER, A. & W. SCHULZE. 1961. Mitochondrial alterations in the myocardium of dogs with aortic stenosis. J. Biophys. Biochem. Cytol. **10:** 285–288.
12. WOLLENBERGER, A. & W. SCHULZE. 1962. Über das Volumenverhältnis von Mitochondrien zu Myofibrillen im chronisch überlasteten, hypertrophierten Hertzen. Naturwissenschaften **49:** 161–162.
13. SCHWARTZ, A. & K. S. LEE. Cited by Wollenberger, Kleitke & Raabe.[10]
14. EDWARDS, G. A. & C. E. CHALLICE. 1958. The fine structure of cardiac muscle cells of newborn and suckling mice. Exp. Cell Res. **15:** 247–250.
15. NOVIKOFF, A. B. 1961. Mitochondria. *In* The Cell. J. Brachet & A. E. Mirsky, Eds. **2:** 299–404. Academic Press, Inc. New York, N. Y.

16. Green, D. E. 1960. Structure and function in the mitochondrial electron-transport system. Radiat. Res. Suppl. **2:** 504–526.
17. Lehninger, A. L. 1959. Relation of oxidation, phosphorylation, and active transport to the structure of mitochondria. *In* Symposium on Molecular Biology. R. E. Zerkle, Ed. : 122. University of Chicago Press. Chicago, Ill.
18. Ball, E. G. & R. J. Barrnett. 1957. An integrated morphological and biochemical study of a purified preparation of the succinate and DPNH oxidase system. J. Biophys. Biochem. Cytol. **3:** 1023–1035.
19. Estabrook, R. W. & A. Holowinsky. 1961. Studies on the content and organization of the respiratory enzymes of mitochondria. J. Biophys. Biochem. Cytol. **9:** 19–28.
20. Green, D. E. 1964. The mitochondrion. Sci. Amer. **210:** 63–79.
21. Green, D. E., P. V. Blair & T. Oda. 1963. Isolation and characterization of the unit of electron transfer in heart mitochondria. Science **140:** 382.
22. Scarpelli, D. G., E. L. Craig & C. G. Rosa. 1962. Submicroscopic localization of two dehydrogenase systems. *In* Proc. Fifth Int. Cong. for Electron Microscopy, Philadelphia, 1962. **2:** L–6. Academic Press, Inc. New York, N. Y.
23. Sedar, A. W., C. G. Rosa & K.-C. Tsou. 1962. Tetranitro-blue tetrazolium and the electron histochemistry of succinic dehydrogenase. J. Histochem. Cytochem. **10:** 506–508.
24. Parsons, D. F. 1963. Mitochondrial structure: Two types of subunits on negatively stained mitochondrial membranes. Science **140:** 985–987.
25. Smith, D. S. 1963. The structure of flight muscle sarcosomes in the blowfly *Calliphora erythrocephalia* (*Diptera*). J. Cell Biol. **19:** 115–138.
26. Stoeckinius, W. 19634. Some observations on negatively stained mitochondria. J. Cell Biol. **17:** 443–454.
27. Fernández-Morán, H. 1962. Cell mebrane ultrastructure: Low-temperature electron microscopy and x-ray diffraction studies of lipoprotein components in lamellar systems. Circulation **26:** 1039–1065.
28. Fernández-Morán, H. 1963. Subunit organization of mitochrondrial membranes. Science **140:** 381.
29. Chance, B. & D. F. Parsons. 1963. Cytochrome function in relation to inner membrane structure of mitochondria. Science **142:** 1176–1179.
30. Mattisson, A. G. & A. Birch-Andersen. 1962. On the fine structure of the mitochondria and its relation to oxidative capacity in muscles in various invertebrates. J. Ultrastruct. Res. **6:** 205–228.
31. Pringle, H. Cited by Smith.[32]
32. Smith, D. S. 1961. The structure of insect fibrillar flight muscle: A study made with special reference to the membrane systems of the fiber. J. Biophys. Biochem. Cytol. **10**(Suppl. 4): 123–158.
33. Hulsmans, H. A. 1961. "Microsomes" in heart-muscle homogenates. Biochim. Biophys. Acta **54:** 1–14.
34. Kerr, Jr., A. & E. J. Kollar. 1958. Histochemical study of hypertrophied heart muscle (abstr). Clin. Res. **6:** 212.
35. Harnischfeger, E. & E. Opitz. 1950. Über den Cytochromgehalt verschiedener Kaninchenorgane nach Höhenanpassung. Arch. Ges. Physiol. **252:** 627–635.
36. McLean, J. R., G. L. Cohn, I. K. Brandt & M. V. Simpson. 1958. Incorporation of labeled amino acids into the protein of muscle and liver mitochondria. J. Biol. Chem. **233:** 657–663.
37. Truman, D. E. & A. Korner. 1962. Incorporation of amino acids into the protein of isolated mitochondria: A search for optimum conditions and a relationship to oxidative phosphorylation. Biochem. J. **83:** 588–596.
38. Borsook, H. 1950. Protein turnover and incorporation of labeled amino acids into tissue proteins in vivo and in vitro. Physiol. Rev. **30:** 206–219.
39. Ward, R. T. 1962. The origin of protein and fatty yolk in *Rana pipiens*. II. Electron microscopical and cytochemical observations of young and mature oocytes. J. Cell Biol. **14:** 309–341.
40. Sobel, H. & F. M. Cohen. 1958. Proteins of heart in experimental cardiac hypertrophy in the rat. Proc. Soc. Exp. Biol. Med. **99:** 656–658.

INTERSTITIAL EDEMA IN VALVULAR ENDOCARDITIS

A. Angrist, M. Oka, and K. Nakao
Department of Pathology, Albert Einstein College of Medicine, Bronx, N. Y.

The cardiac valve and chordae tendinae are composed of unique tissues, and resemble the connective tissue of the sex skin in their propensity to edema and sensitivity to certain hormones. This tissue is very susceptible to stress, infection, and local stimulation, as well as to the administration of certain hormones, and yields edema initially. The valvular edema (FIGURE 1) is encountered so often in autopsy material that its significance is apt to be neglected. It is not a postmortem change, for it is seen in freshly killed experimental animals. Such edema is also an initial and common, if not a universal, response to nonspecific stress in the experimental animals (FIGURE 2). The reactivity of valves depends upon the constituent components of valvular tissue per se and varies with age and probably other factors.

Deiss and Leon[1] and Meyer and his colleagues,[2] using bovine and pig heart valves, respectively, reported that the mucopolysaccharides in the heart valves are mainly chondroitin sulfate A/C and B, with minimal hyaluronic acid. Boström and his co-workers[3,4] found a higher incorporation of ^{35}S into the heart valves of the calf than into any other tissues of the heart; they advanced the possibility of a continuous mucopolysaccharide synthesis in the heart valves. Moretti and Whitehouse[5] reported that chondroitin sulfate A/C was the main acid mucopolysaccharide in bovine heart valves and that there was less hyaluronic acid in valves of old animals than in those of the young. A change in acid mucopolysaccharides with aging in human heart valves[6] has also been noted.

Torii and co-workers[7] studied the mucopolysaccharides in human valves and found variations with age and in different valves. In contrast to the results of Deiss and Leon[1] and those of Meyer and co-workers[2] in bovine and pig heart valves, they found a higher amount of hyaluronic acid in human heart valves. These results may represent a characteristic of the species. In both humans and animals, the valves are generally more edematous and have more cellular elements in younger than in older subjects. Bashey and his colleagues[8] found that the collagen content also varied with age and in different valves in the human heart.

Various workers[9–12] have found an increased soluble collagen in chicken following a lathyritic diet. Our data[33] with β-aminopropionitrile (BAPN) also showed a more active uptake, and possibly synthesis, in the heart valves of rats, as judged by utilization of tritiated L-proline. A higher uptake was found in rats on a BAPN diet in the heart valves with severe lesions, including marked edema.

This paper deals with the development and effects of the interstitial valvular edema of heart valves, with its implications in the development of nonbacterial and bacterial endocarditis.

Methods and Materials

In addition to human autopsy material, Holzman strain rats were used as test animals. For the study of uptake in normal rats, tritiated L-proline (proline-^{3}H) was given to 77 rats of various ages. A dose of 4 μc/g of body weight of proline-^{3}H was administered intraperitoneally (i.p.), and the rats were sacrificed four, 24, 48, and 96 hours later. The uptake was measured by scintillation counting in a Packard Tricarb and also evaluated *in situ* by autoradiographic studies.

Similar uptake studies were done in a group of 16 rats maintained on a high salt diet and also in 14 rats on a 0.2% BAPN diet.

For the experiments on the incorporation of ^{35}S, labeled sulfate was administered to normal rats and rats on a high salt diet (12 rats), BAPN diet (24 rats), and to each of six rats subjected to the administration of adrenocorticotropic hormone (ACTH) alone and a combination of ACTH and deoxycorticosterone acetate (DOCA). A dose of 2 $\mu c/g$ of body weight of ^{35}S was given i.p., and rats were sacrificed 24, 48, and 96 hours later. *In vitro* experiments were also done with thin slices of fresh heart valves from human autopsies and rats with and without vegetations; fresh thin slices were incubated in 5 cc of balanced salt solution (described by Curran[14]) with ^{35}S (50 μc) for two hours at 37° C. The

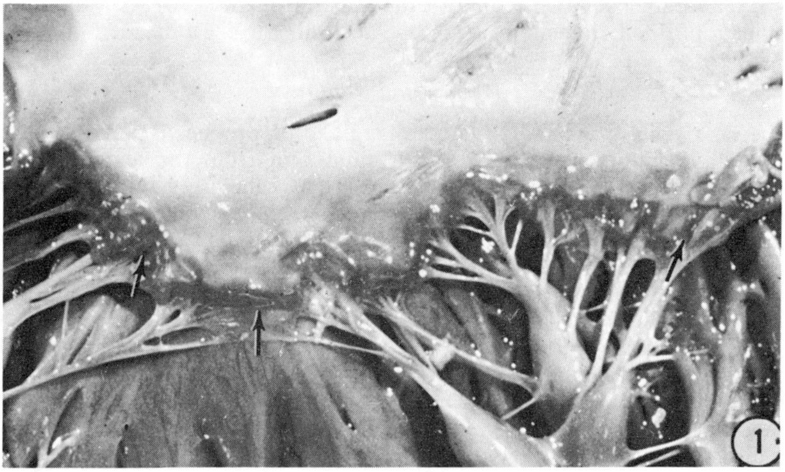

FIGURE 1. Mitral valve from a 24-year-old male who died of uremia. The edge of the valve is edematous and is a bit darker (arrows) because of mild hemoglobin staining.

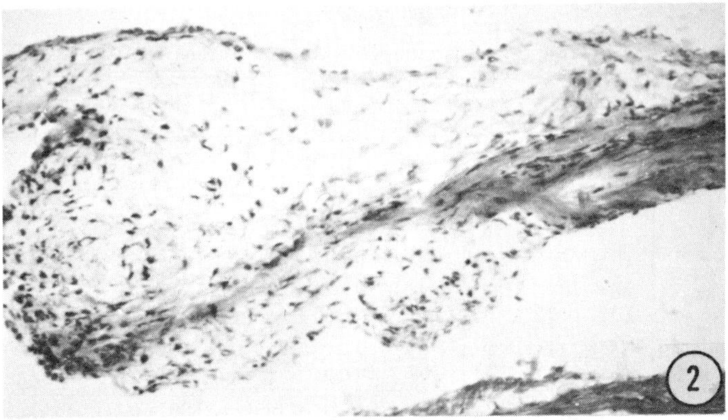

FIGURE 2. Mitral valve from a five-month-old male rat who had undergone arteriovenous shunt procedure two weeks previously. The valve shows marked edema and some cellular reaction. Stain: hematoxylin-eosin. × 120.

tissue slices were fixed in buffered formalin overnight and washed in tap water for four hours. Paraffin sections for microscopy and autoradiography were prepared in the usual manner.

For histoenzymatic reactions, cryostat sections were used after fixation for 20 minutes in cold buffered calcium formalin. The following reactions were performed; alkaline phosphatase, as described by Gomori; adenosinetriphosphatase (ATPase), adenosinediphosphatase (ADPase), and adenosinemonophosphatase (AMPase) by Wachstein-Meisel's methods; and DPNH diaphorase reaction with Nitro-Bt, as described by Novikoff.

For routine staining techniques, hematoxylin-eosin, combined periodic acid-Schiff (PAS) and alcian blue, phosphotungstic acid hematoxylin (PTAH), and oil-red-O stains were used. For electron microscopical studies, tissues were prepared in standard manner, using 2% osmium tetroxide, as described by Palade, or 4% glutaraldehyde, according to the Sabatini method, with or without post-osmification. Epon embedding was done according to the Luft method.

Results and Comment

The heart valves showed the highest uptake of proline-^{3}H among all tissues examined, including heart valve, aorta, and skin from the abdominal region (TABLE 1). The results revealed that growing rats generally have a higher uptake than older rats. The uptake decreased with time (biological half-life), except that the highest uptake was found at 24 hours in the older rats. Although the number of animals studied is small, young rats (four to seven weeks old showed the highest uptake after 96 hours of proline-^{3}H administration. There was considerable individual variation, which was more prominent in older rats (over 18 months). Older rats with valves distorted by edema, cellular reaction, and increased thickness showed a higher uptake than did young rats with normal valves, which may account for the variation noted. These findings indicate that there may be a continuing collagen synthesis in the heart valve throughout life and that it may vary with different conditions, including basic diseases, sex, and nonspecific stress. In the valves with edema only, without any increase of cells, the cytoplasmic proline may be ruled out in accounting for the increased uptake. The uptake of L-proline-

TABLE 1

TIMED UPTAKE OF PROLINE-^{3}H IN RATS OF DIFFERENT AGES*

Age of Rat	4 Hours			24 Hours			48 Hours			96 Hours		
	Valve	Aorta	Skin	Valve	Aorta	Skin	Valve	Aorta	Skin	Valve	Aorta	Skin
4–7 weeks	—	—	—	34	8	—	20	4	—	39†	4	—
	—	—	—	(4)	(4)	—	(2)	(2)	—	(3)	(3)	—
9–15 weeks	31†	14	19	29	11	13	18	3	4	17	16	20
	(9)	(9)	(3)	(10)	(10)	(7)	(4)	(4)	(2)	(5)	(5)	(4)
17–28 weeks	46†	10	9	34	9	—	29	9	—	20	7	—
	(9)	(9)	(5)	(5)	(5)	—	(3)	(3)	—	(5)	(5)	—
Over 18 months	35	11	9	46†	17	20	21	2	—	14	7	—
	(6)	(6)	(4)	(6)	(6)	(3)	(3)	(3)	—	(3)	(3)	—

* Proline-^{3}H was administered at a dose of 4 μc/g of body weight, i.p. Time is given in hours after administration of proline-^{3}H. All values given in μc/g. Number of rats used in each experiment given in parentheses below each value.

† Highest uptake in a given age group.

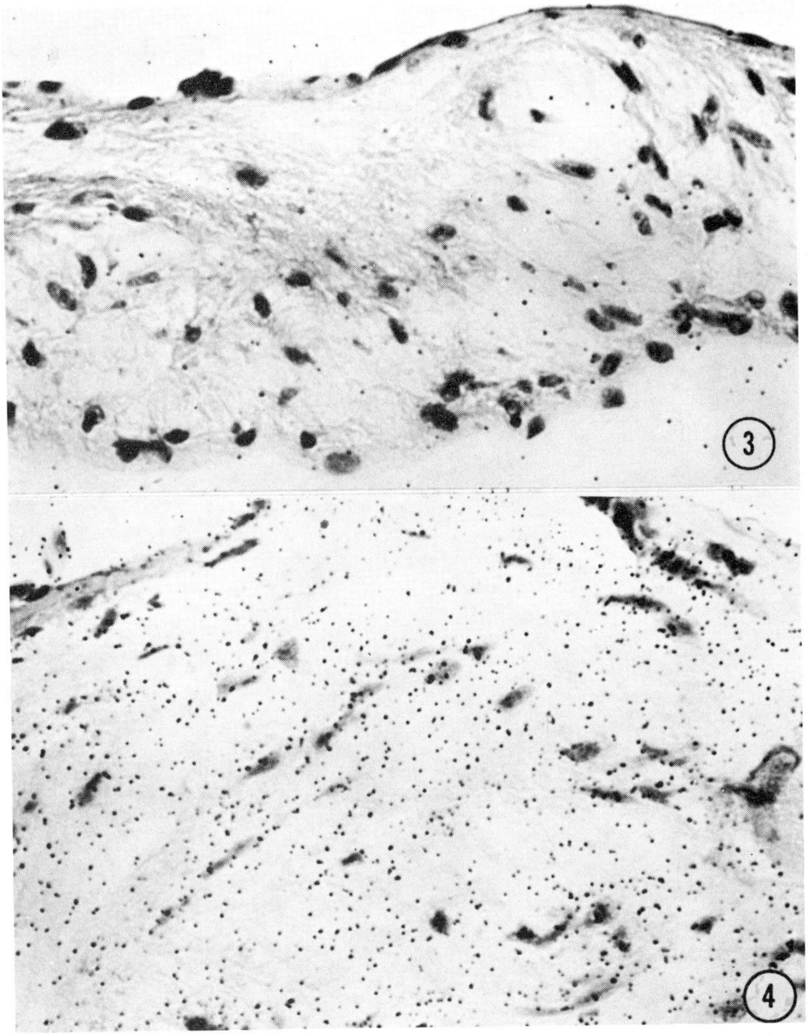

FIGURES 3 and 4. Range of biological variation in uptake of tritiated L-proline in tricuspid valves from rats of similar age, embedded side by side for sectioning and autoradiographic preparations. Proline-^{3}H was given at a dose of 4 $\mu c/g$ of body weight, i.p., and the rats were sacrificed 4 hours later. NTB-3 emulsion (Kodak) was used and exposed for 25 days. FIGURE 3 shows a valve from a 23-month-old female rat, with minimal thickening in the valve; only a few reduced silver grains are seen. × 420. FIGURE 4 shows a valve from a 25-month-old male rat, with swelling and edema in the valves. Numerous reduced silver grains are present all over the valve. × 420.

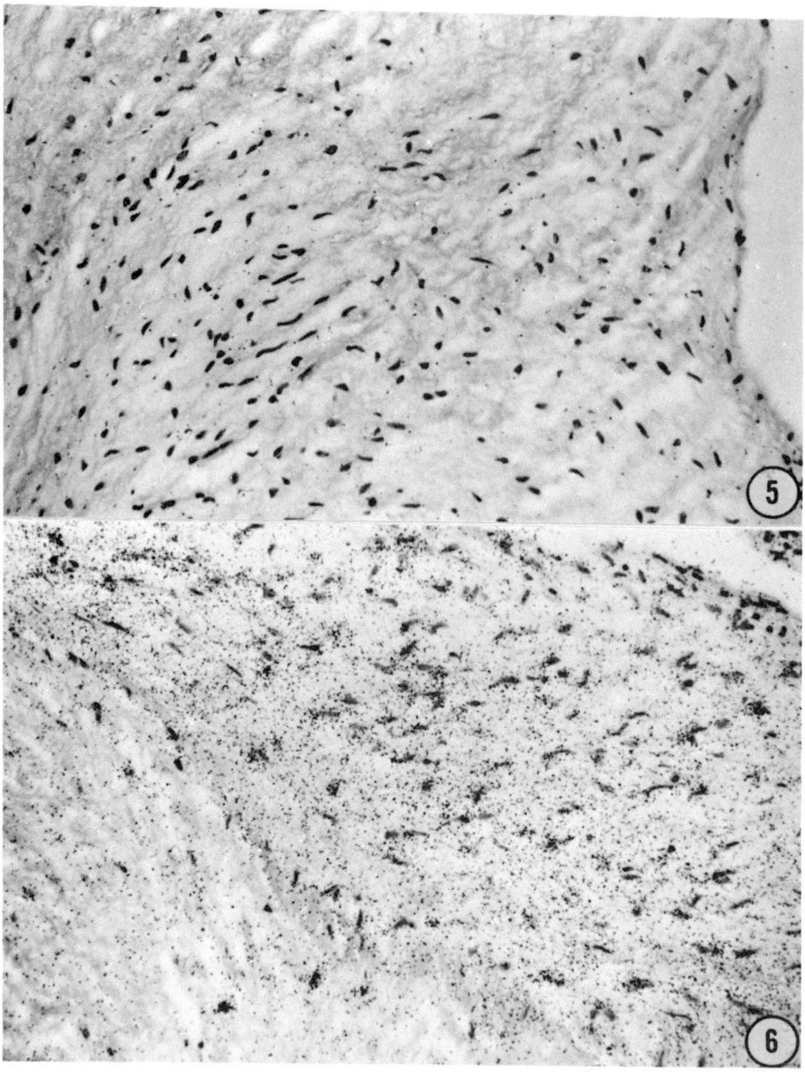

FIGURES 5 and 6. *In vitro* experiments of thin slices of fresh valves incubated in 5 ml of balanced salt solution (Curran[14]) containing 50 μc of ^{35}S for two hours. The exposure time was 15 days. FIGURE 5 shows a fibrotic thickened mitral valve from a 68-year-old female who died with pneumonia and cirrhosis. Only a few reduced silver grains are found in this fibrotic valve. $\times$ 170. FIGURE 6 shows a mitral valve taken from a 74-year-old male who died with cerebral infarction. This edematous valve showed a prominent incorporation of ^{35}S compared with FIGURE 5. $\times$ 170.

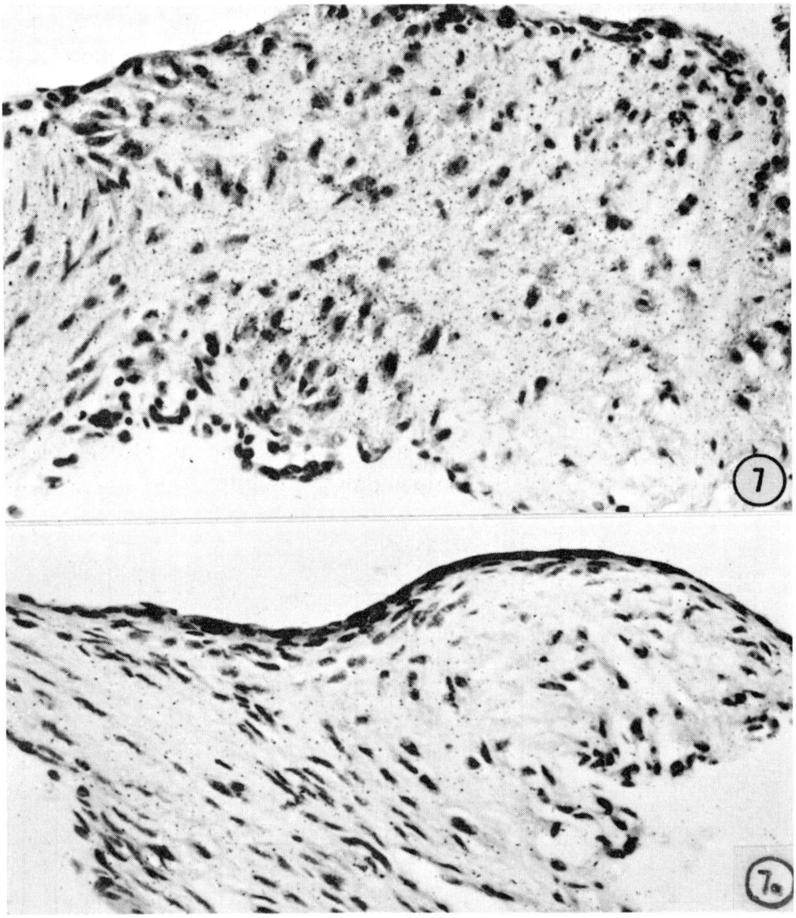

FIGURES 7 and 7a. Autoradiographs from two-month-old rats given ^{35}S at a dose of 2 $\mu c/g$ of body weight, i.p. and sacrificed two days later. The exposure period was 14 days. FIGURE 7 shows a mitral valve from a rat on a 0.2% BAPN diet for 34 days. A fair amount of reduced silver grains is present in the valve, corresponding to the incorporated ^{35}S × 200. FIGURE 7a shows a mitral valve of a control rat fed with regular Purina chow. Note that there are far fewer reduced silver grains than in FIGURE 7. × 200.

^{3}H depended not only upon the age and growth status, but also upon the nature of the valvular distortion. FIGURES 3 and 4 are autoradiographs from a 25-month-old male and a 23-month-old female rat, sacrificed four hours after administration of proline-^{3}H. Tricuspid valves of both rats were embedded side by side for sectioning and autoradiographic preparation. The valve of the male rat showed a higher uptake than did that of the female, and the uptake in the 25-month-old-male was higher in this instance than in most growing rats.

With combined PAS-alcian blue staining, the edematous area showed an early alcian blue staining, but staining with PAS was weak in the early stage of edema; the alcian blue reaction increased in prolonged edema. In the longer experiments, the thickened valve showed an increase in the PAS-positive fibers, presumably collagen, and then the alcian blue-positive material diminished. This coincides with Dahman's results[1] that mucopolysaccharides decrease as collagen increases in maturation of connective tissues. In edematous regions of valves, the incorporation of ^{35}S was high, in both *in vitro* and *in vivo* experiments (FIGURES 5 and 6). Such an increased incorporation of ^{35}S was observed in the edematous regions of valves in older subjects as well as in the young. An increased uptake of ^{35}S was seen in the rats fed on the BAPN diet; such valves showed edema and cellular reaction (FIGURES 7 and 7a).

Edema in the valve also seemed to be associated with alteration in enzymatic reactions.[13,16] The AMPase reaction was usually pronounced in the valvular tissue proper of very young rats, and was found to be decreased in older rats. However, in the young rat and even in the older rat with visible distortion of the valve, including edema and cellular reaction, the AMPase reaction was found to be increased in the valvular tissue proper, whereas the ATPase reaction was positive only in the surface endothelial lining of the valve, in both young and older atherosclerosis relationship may exist in the vascular system, but such a relationship of AMPase to arteriosclerosis is still speculative in the heart valve, at least acincreased in the older rats, particularly in those with distorted valves.

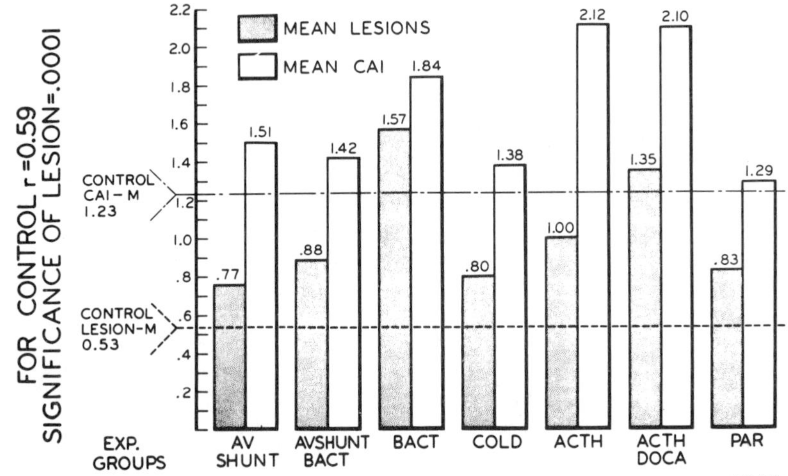

EXP. GROUPS	AV SHUNT	AVSHUNT BACT	BACT	COLD	ACTH	ACTH DOCA	PAR
r	.54	.69	.30	.84	.06	.29	.50 (R) .90 (L)
t TEST FOR LESIONS	.10	N.S.	.0005	.87	.01	.0005	.03
t TEST FOR CAI	.01	N.S.	.001	.07	.0005	.0005	N.S.

FIGURE 8. Comparison of enlargement of adrenals with severity of valvular lesions under various experimental conditions. Enlargement of adrenals by weight includes factors of hypertrophy, hyperplasia, congestion, and edema. The comparative adrenal index (CAI) is the index of enlargement, using the normal values in the tables of Gray and Addis for rats of the same weight and sex as a reference. Experimental conditions: AV SHUNT refers to an experimental opening of about 2 mm in size between the aorta and vena cava below the renal vessels; BACT refers to an intravenous injection of 0.5 cc of a 24-hour culture of *Streptococcus fecalis*; COLD refers to repeated exposure at 4° C for varying periods; ACTH refers to adrenocorticotropic hormone administration for varying periods at varying dosage; DOCA refers to deoxycorticosterone acetate administration for varying periods at varying dosage; PAR refers to the parabiotic joining of two rats by the technique of Bunster and Meyer. N.S. = not significant.

Riss[17,18] suggested a relationship between 5-nucleotidase and atherosclerosis in the aorta. Kirk[19,20] was in accord with this suggestion, based on the results of his extensive biochemical studies of the vascular tree. The 5-nucleotidase-atherosclerosis relationship may exist in the vascular system, but such a relationship of AMPase to arteriosclerosis is still speculative in the heart valve, at least according to our histoenzymatic preparations.

Hormonal effects on the connective tissue and ground substances are well known (Dorfman & Schiller,[21] Asboe-Hansen,[22] Boström *et al.*[3]). The heart

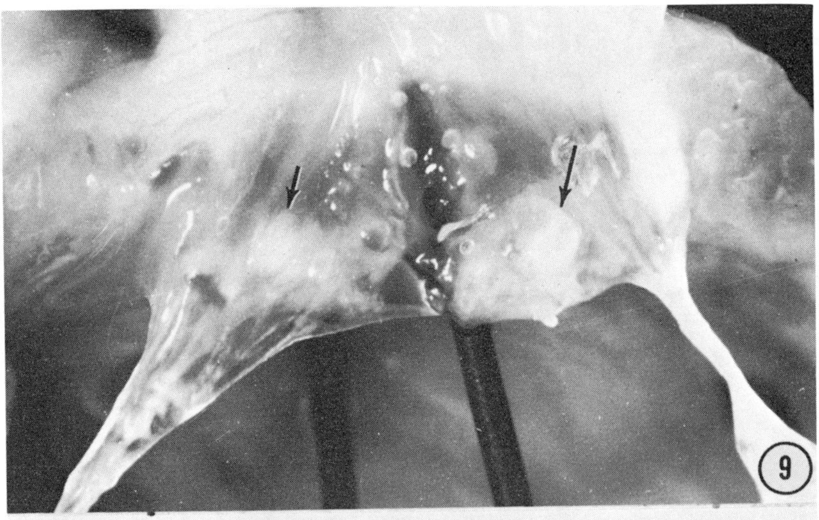

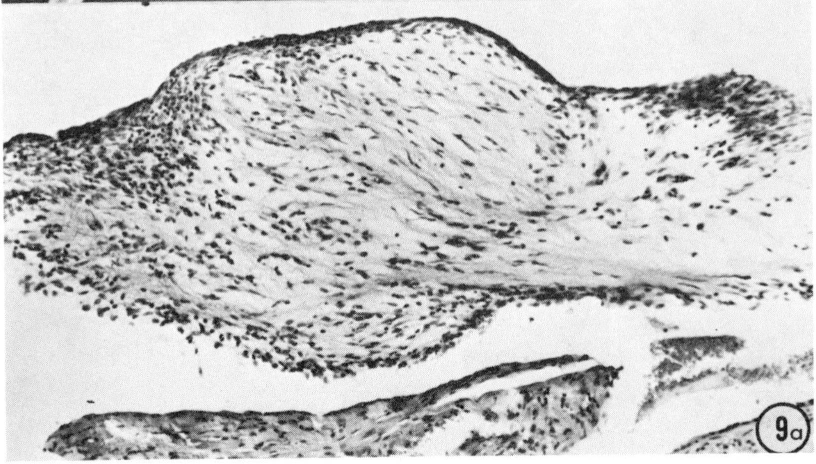

FIGURE 9. Tricuspid valve from a four-month-old male rat given a combination of ACTH (8 units) and DOCA (5 mg) daily, five times per week for five weeks. Focal edema and thickening (arrows) are noted. × 12.

FIGURE 9a. A microphotograph of the valve in FIGURE 9 through the thickened area (FIGURE 9, right arrow). Marked edema and cellular reaction are present. Stain: hematoxylin-eosin. × 90.

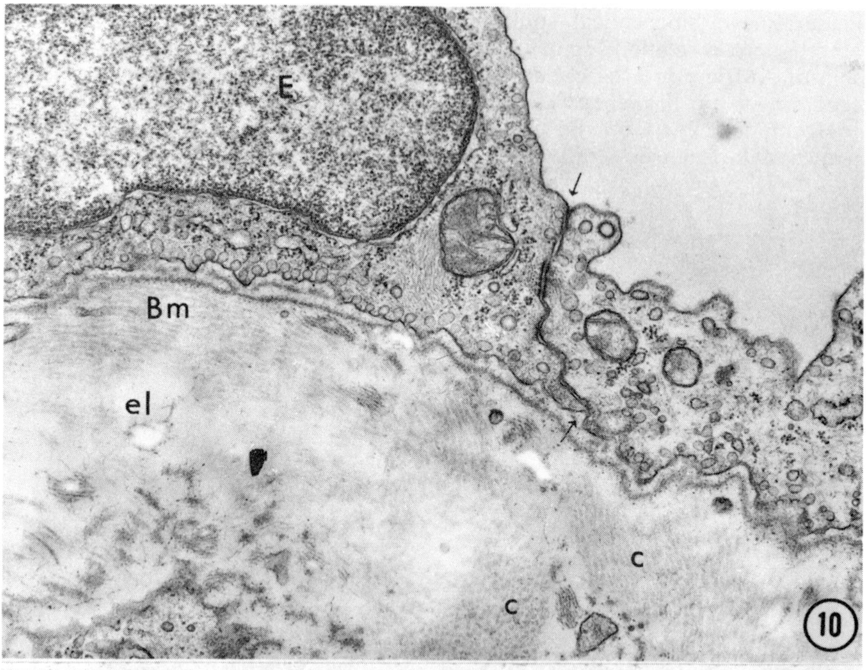
E
Bm
el
c
c
10

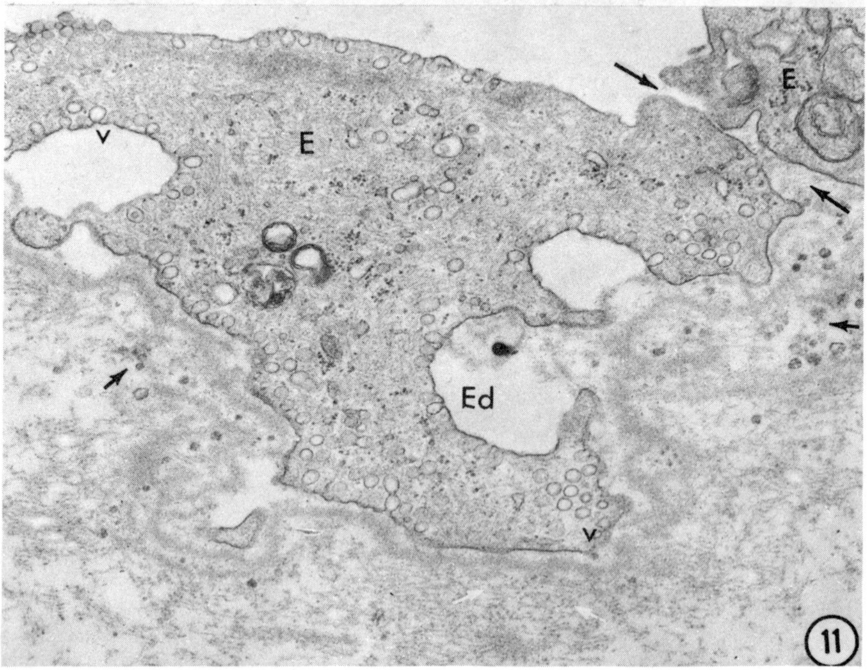
E
E
v
Ed
v
11

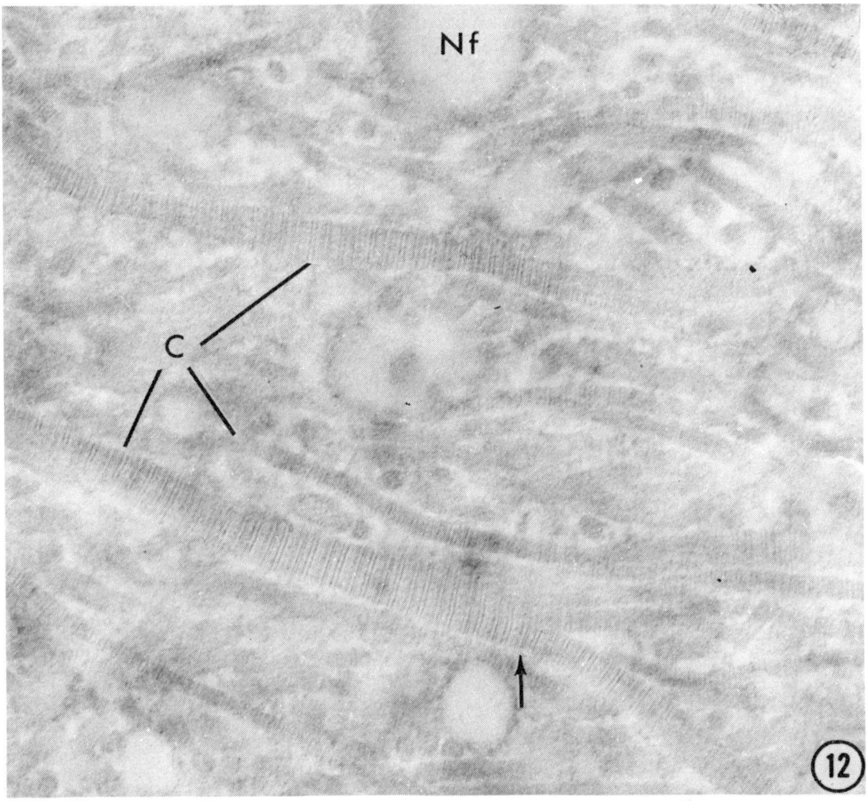

FIGURE 12. Micrograph of a human heart valve, showing variation and atypical morphology of collagen fibrils (C) in chronic edema. There is branching (arrow) and irregularity in width of each collagen fibril. Nf = neutral fat droplet. × 69,000.

valve is also affected by hormones, and to some extent rather selectively. Our studies[16,23,24] revealed that adrenal hypertrophy was correlated with the valvular lesions in experimental rats (FIGURE 8).

Edema is not only an initial and transient change in many forms of nonspecific stress, but edema may last for a long period and be followed by cellular reaction and/or collagen changes and fibrous thickening (Dahme *et al.*[25]). It was found that ACTH administration yielded adrenal hypertrophy, and the heart valves showed edema with little cellular reaction, whereas DOCA yielded a more

FIGURE 10. A portion of the auricular endothelial surface of an intact rat heart valve. The intercellular junctional complexes are neat and regular (between arrows). The basement membrane (Bm) is closely apposed to the cell membrane of the endothelial cells. The underlying connective tissue shows parallel-arranged unit collagen fibrils, mostly in form of collagen bundles (C). The elastic fibers appear electron-light (el). E = endothelial cell. × 20,000.

FIGURE 11. Subendothelial edema following *Streptococcus fecalis* injection. The endothelial cell (E) shows an increase of pinocytotic vesicles along the cell membrane (v). Intercellular space appears widened and without junctional complexes (long arrows). Focal subjacent edema (Ed) above the basement membrane is striking. The basement membrane appears prominent and mixed with granular and vesicular structures (short arrows) and microfibrils (white arrows). × 24,000.

prominent cellular response with the edema. Combined ACTH and DOCA gave both edema and cellular reaction, with thickening and other alterations in the valvular tissue proper (FIGURES 8, 9, and 9a). Our experimental data also indicated that endogenous ACTH seemed to be more effective in yielding severe valvular lesions.[26]

Several workers[27-29] have demonstrated that arteriovenous fistula (AV shunt) resulted in susceptibility of the heart valves to bacterial infection. Our results also showed an increased bacterial susceptibility with AV shunts in the rat, even though with AV shunt alone the incidence of severe valvular alterations was not significant, as judged by gross and macroscopical studies, although changes were seen with the electron microscope. The incidence of severe valvular lesions increased significantly (from 5 to 15%) when the procedure of adrenalectomy was

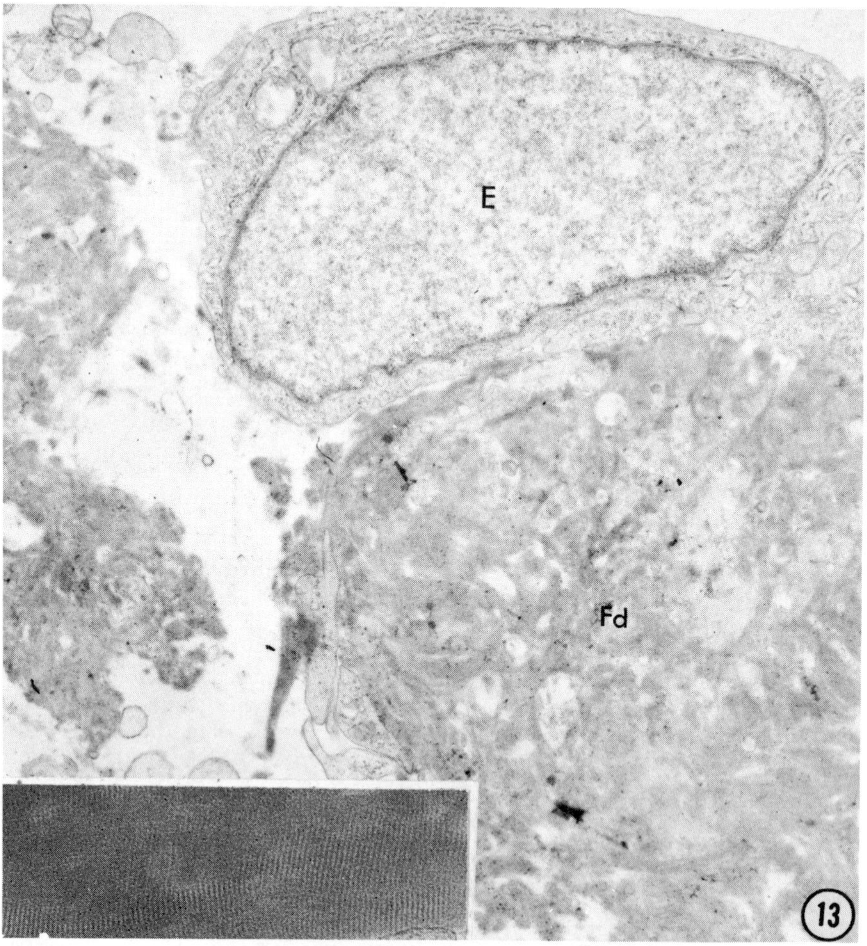

FIGURE 13. Electron micrograph showing subendothelial accumulation of fibrinoid material (Fd). E = endothelial cell. × 23,000. The inset shows the periodicity of 220 Å, typical for fibrin. × 37,500.

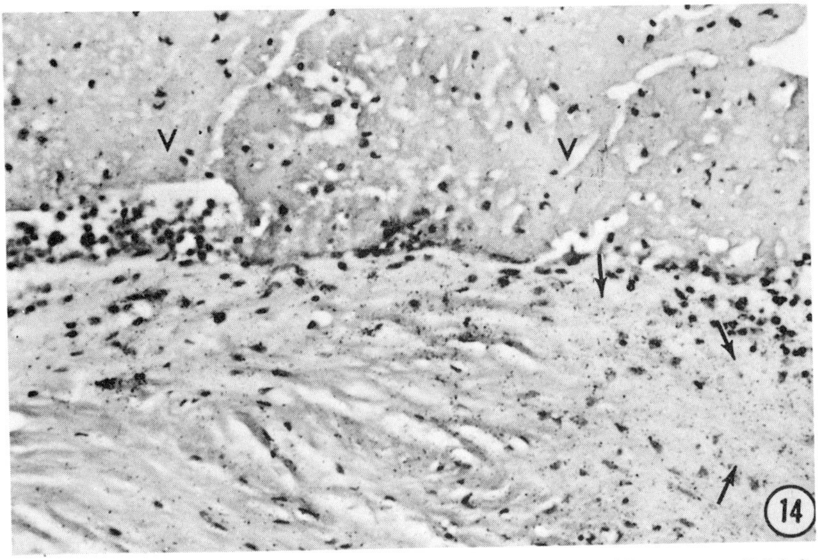

FIGURE 14. Mitral valve from a 76-year-old female who died with a myocardial infarct. A fresh slice of valve, including attached vegetation, was incubated in 5 ml of buffered salt solution (Crane) with 50 μc of ^{35}S for two hours. Uptake of ^{35}S was prominent in the valve at the base of the vegetation (V), particularly in the edematous region (arrows). Some cell infiltration is also present. × 170.

added to the AV shunt procedure in the rat.[26] Adrenalectomy alone yielded edematous valves with some cellular reaction.[23]

How edema is related to the valvular lesions, or what role edema may play in the production of valvular lesions, is the main topic of this paper. Interstitial edema is fluid related to mucopolysaccharides and other ground substances. This retention of edema causes an alteration in the fibrillar components, basement membrane, cellular elements, and endothelium, as has been observed with the electron microscope by Nakao and Angrist[30] (FIGURES 10–13).

During the study of nonbacterial thrombotic endocarditis (NBTE) in human material, an association was also found between edema and fresh NBTE formation. Fresh NBTE was found frequently on the surface of the altered edematous or scarred valve. When the valvular tissue was fibrotic, the collagen often showed fatty degeneration. Alcian blue-positive material was present toward the valvular surface at the base of the fresh NBTE. An incorporation of ^{35}S was also evident *in vitro* (FIGURE 14) in this location in the valve.

Various authors[31–34] have demonstrated that platelets tend to adhere to collagen. Others[35–39] have clarified the significant role of ADP in the platelet agglutination. When edema appeared in the valve proper, particularly if it lasted for a certain period, it distorted the endothelial lining at the surface of the valve, which led to an exposure of underlying ground substance of the valve proper and of collagen fibers directly to the bloodstream. Under such conditions, platelets adhere to the valve surface, and NBTE formation occurs. This phenomenon has been observed by Nakao and co-workers[40] at the electron microscope level (FIGURES 15–17).

Increments of fresh platelets tend to superimpose (FIGURE 18), possibly as the result of release of ADP from the agglutinated platelets already caught and

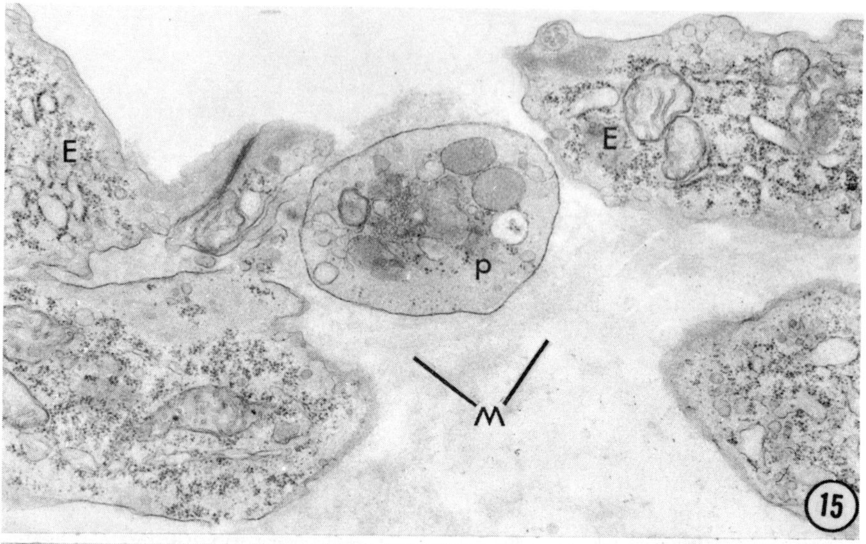

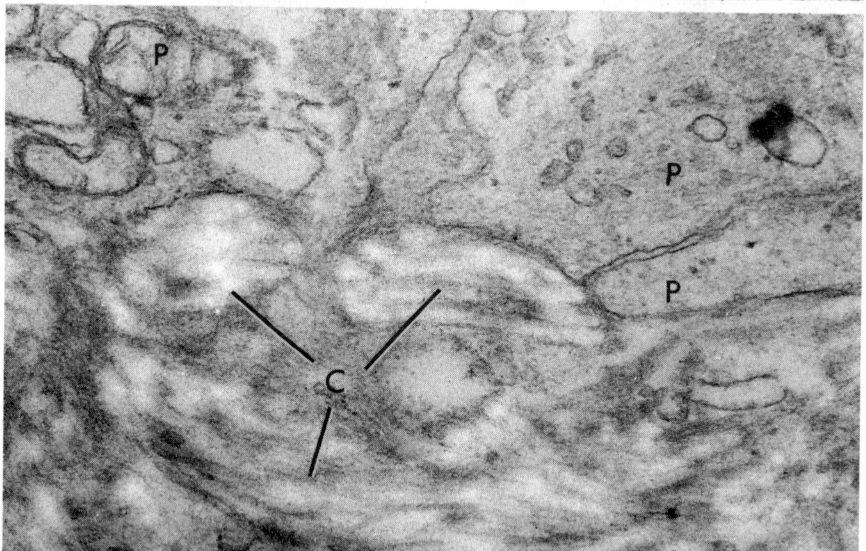

FIGURE 15. Platelet (P) is seen in contact with fine fibrils of the subendothelial stroma. This platelet indicates normal morphology without much alteration. E = endothelial cell; M = microfibrils. Stained: lead citrate. × 20,000.

FIGURE 16. Micrograph showing platelet (P) very closely adherent to bundles of unit collagen fibrils (C). × 37,500.

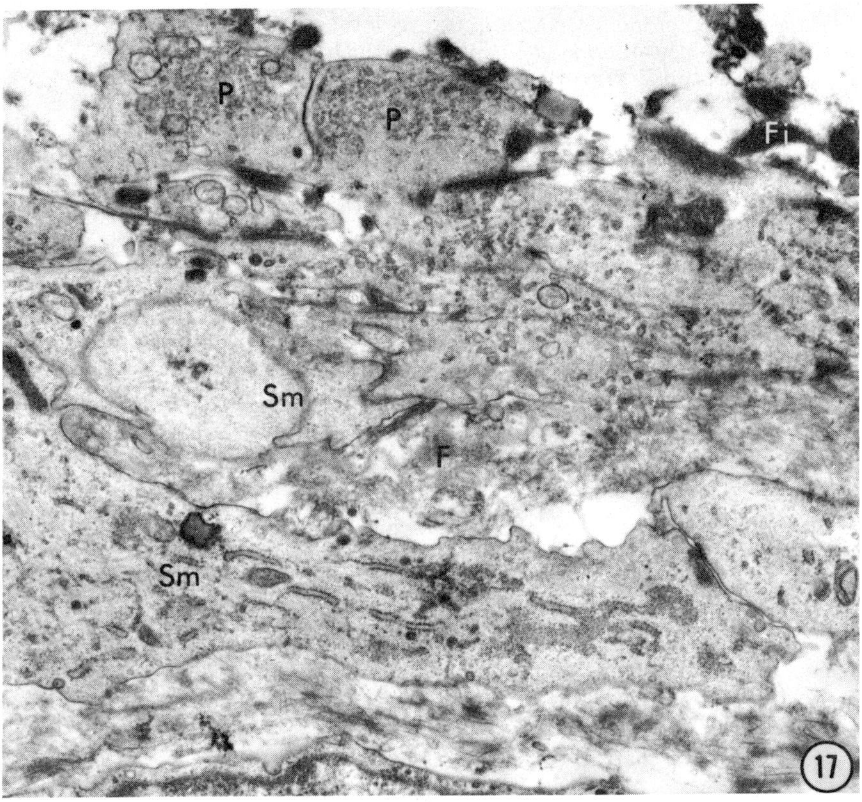

FIGURE 17. Miniature platelet (P) vegetation located on the auricular surface of a human heart valve. Altered smooth muscle cells (Sm) are seen surrounded by fiber elements (F). Dark strands at the surface are fibrin (Fi). × 10,000.

clustered at such valve sites. Endothelialization and organization of platelet vegetations can also cause valvular thickening (Duguid,[41] Tweedy,[42] Margarey[43]). With sepsis or even passive bacteremia, bacterial contamination can occur with infection of the platelet deposits and of the vegetation, and then bacterial endocarditis follows.[44] Leary[45] and Nedzel[46] have shown that mechanical or chemical traumatic injury to the valve yields *initial* local platelet accretion as a nidus for the *subsequent* contamination that follows with a later bacterial injection.

The ebb and flow of enzymatic activities in the NBTE or bacterial formation is of interest. The DPNH diaphorase reaction readily demonstrates the platelets and the aging of the platelets after the vegetation forms (FIGURE 18). This reaction has been helpful in understanding the mechanisms of NBTE formation, and in clarifying the relationship of NBTE to other enzymatic activities in their time sequence with regard to the age of the vegetation.[47,48] The AMPase reaction appeared earlier than did the ATPase reaction in the valve at the base of fresh NBTE. The AMPase reaction became weaker or disappeared, and the ATPase reaction was positive when the NBTE became older.

With very fresh NBTE obtained experimentally, the enzymatic reactions, including alkaline phosphatase, AMPase (FIGURE 19), ADPase (FIGURE 20), and ATPase, were all pronounced on the surface of the valve at the base of vegetation. The endothelium was often desquamated, which is best seen with the DPNH diaphorase reaction. With early edema, the DPNH diaphorase reaction was rather weak in the fibroblasts in the valve proper. However, after NBTE was well established, the enzymatic activities diminished or disappeared quickly at the base of the vegetation. The AMPase reaction was retained longer than the others. The ATPase and ADPase reactions increased with the decrease of AMPase reaction. The enzymatic activities in the valve behaved differently in NBTE as compared with bacterial vegetations; the alkaline phosphatase reaction was positive at the base of bacterial vegetations but not with NBTE.[49] The enzymatic activities at the base of vegetations also varied according to the site. When NBTE formed in relation to an edematous region of the valve, the enzymes disappeared sooner than when NBTE formed on a fibrotic site. Cellular reaction occurred frequently in the edematous background of the valve. This phenomenon and the alteration in the enzymatic activities suggest that edema plays a role in the evolution of cardiac valvular lesions.

Summary and Conclusion

Interstitial edema is a common initial change of valves, occurring with nonspecific or specific stress. This edema often initiates other valvular distortions, such as swelling, separation of endothelium, and exposure of collagen and other stromal elements, plus morphological changes in collagen and adherence and further agglutination of platelets and fibrin. These distortions may lead to other

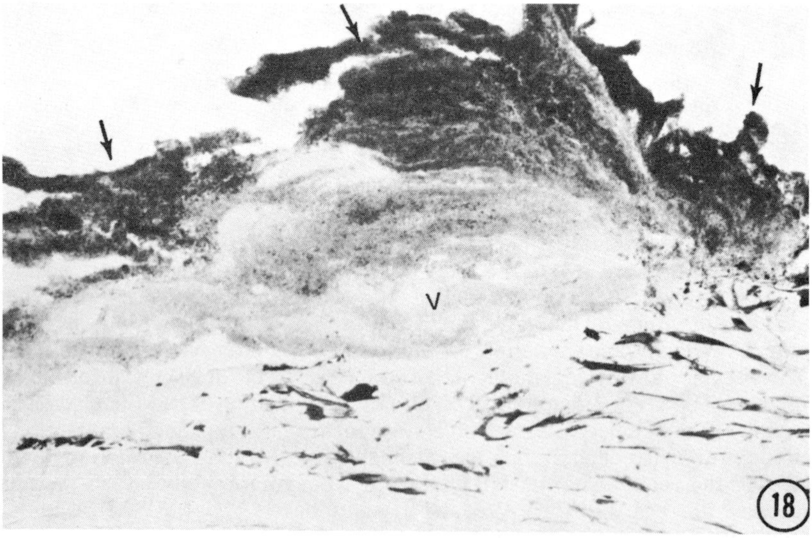

FIGURE 18. Mitral valve from a 77-year-old female who died two days after colostomy for colon carcinoma. The DPNH diaphorase reaction reveals superimposed fresh platelet vegetation (arrows) on an older platelet vegetation (V), which is lighter with little or no formazan precipitation. There is some cell reaction present in the valve at the base of vegetation. × 120.

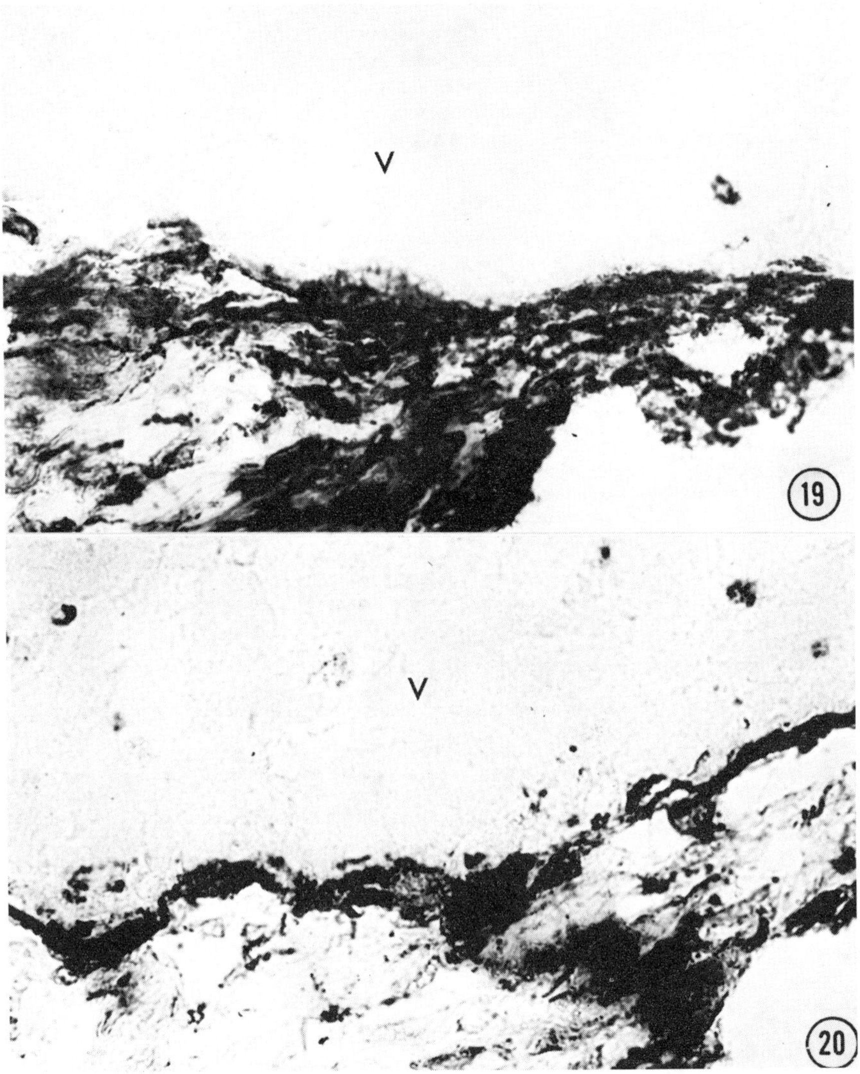

FIGURES 19 and 20. Consecutive sections of the mitral valve from a 17-week-old male rat fed with high salt diet for ten weeks. FIGURE 19 shows the abundant AMPase reaction in the depths of the valve proper, as well as at the base of the vegetation (V). The vegetation shows no reaction product. × 620. FIGURE 20 shows a positive ADPase reaction at the surface of valve at the base of the vegetation. × 620.

consequences, such as vegetation formation, valvular thickening, insufficiency, stenosis, calcification, and bacterial endocarditis.

The significance of interestial valvular edema in experimental endocarditis and in human autopsy material was discussed. Evidence is suggestive that mucopolysaccharide and collagen, whose synthesis seems to continue through life in heart valves, may be altered in the edematous area. The connective tissue may be modified by many factors and cause the valvular distortion. Enzymatic activities were found to vary, and may also be important in the valvular alterations, in particular as related to early vegetation formation.

References

1. DEISS, W. P. & A. S. LEON. 1955. Mucopolysaccharides of heart valve mucoprotein. J. Biol. Chem. **215:** 685.
2. MEYER, K., E. DAVIDSON, A. LINKER & P. HOFFMAN. 1956. The acid mucopolysaccharides of connective tissue. Biochim. Biophys. Acta **21:** 506.
3. BOSTRÖM, H., A. MORETTI & M. H. WHITEHOUSE. 1963. Studies on the biochemistry of heart valves. I. On the biosynthesis of mucopolysaccharides in bovine heart valves. Biochim. Biophys. Acta **74:** 213.:
4. JACOBSON, B. & H. BOSTRÖM. 1964. Studies on the biochemistry of heart valves. II. The effect of aging and anti-inflammatory drugs on the synthesis of glucosamine 6-phosphate and phosphoadenosine phosphosulfate by bovine heart valves. Biochim. Biophys. Acta **83:** 152.
5. MORETTI, A. & M. H. WHITEHOUSE. 1963. Changes in the mucopolysaccharide composition of bovine heart valves with age. Biochem. J. **87:** 396.
6. MORETTI, A. & V. ZAMBOTTI. 1964. Mucopolysaccharide composition of human heart valves. 6th Int. Congr. Biochem., New York. Pt. **6:** 519 (Abstr.).
7. TORII, S., R. I. BASHEY & K. NAKAO. 1965. Acid mucopolysaccharide composition of human-heart valve. Biochim. Biophys. Acta **101:** 285.
8. BASHEY, R. I., S. TORIE & A. ANGRIST. 1965. Connective tissue compositions of human-heart valves. Fed. Proc. **24:** Part I.
9. LEVENE, C. I. & J. GROSS. 1959. Alterations in the state of molecular aggregation of collagen induced in chick embryos by β-aminopropionitrile (lathyrus factor). J. Exp. Med. **110:** 771.
10. LEVENE, C. I. 1962. Studies on the mode of action of lathyrogenic compounds. J. Exp. Med. **116:** 119.
11. GROSS, J., C. I. LEVENE & S. ORLOFF. 1960. Fragility and extractable collagen in the lathyritic chick embryo: an assay for lathyrogenic agents. Proc. Soc. Exp. Biol. Med. **105:** 148.
12. GROSS, J. 1963. An intermolecular defect of collagen in experimental lathyrism. Biochim. Biophys. Acta **71:** 250.
13. OKA, M., S. GERERD, S. BRODIE & A. ANGRIST. 1966. Cardiac valve and aortic lesions in beta-aminopropionitrile (BAPN) fed rats with and without high salt. Amer. J. Path. **48:** 45.
14. CURRAN, R. C. 1960. The effects of x-ray on the uptake of radioactive sulphate. Proc. Roy. Soc. Biol. **152:** 410.
15. DAHMAN, G. 1965. Beobachtungen bei der Reifeing des Bindesgewebes Z. Rheumaforsh. **24:** 332.
16. ANGRIST, A. & M. OKA. 1967. Experimental endocarditis. *In* Methods and Achievements in Experimental Pathology. E. Bajusz & G. S. Jasmin, Eds. S. Karger. Basel, Switzerland. In press.
17. REIS, J. L. 1950. Studies on 5-nucleotidase and its distribution in human tissues. Biochem. J. **46:** 21.
18. REIS, J. L. 1951. The specificity of phosphomonoesterase in human tissues. Biochem. J. **48:** 548.
19. KIRK, J. E. 1959. The 5-nucleotidase activity of human arterial tissue in individuals of various ages. J. Geront. **14:** 288.
20. KIRK, J. E. 1963. Enzyme chemistry of the vascular wall. *In* Fundamentals of Vascular Grafting. S. A. Weschowski & C. Dennis, Eds. : 32–62. McGraw-Hill Book Co. New York, N. Y.
21. DORFMAN, A. & S. SCHILLER. 1958. Effects of hormones on the metabolism of acid mucopolysaccharides of connective tissue. Recent Progr. Hormone Res. **14:** 427.

22. Asboe-Hansen, G. 1958. Hormonal effects on connective tissue. Physiol. Rev. **38:** 446.
23. Oka, M. & A. Angrist. 1963. Experimental endocarditis. Rev. Canad. Biol. **22:** 297.
24. Angrist, A., M. Oka, K. Nakao & J. Marquiss. 1960. Studies in experimental endocarditis: 1. Production of valvular lesions by mechanisms not involving infection or sensitivity factors. Amer. J. Path. **36:** 181.
25. Dahme, E., P. Dorn & F. M. Eletreby. 1965. Zur Endocarditisfrage beim Huhn. 1. Formen der Endocarditis und ibre Häufigkeit. Berlin. Munchen. Tieraerz. Wschr. **78:** 222.
26. Oka, M., A. Shirota & A. Angrist. 1966. Experimental endocarditis: Endocrine factors in valve lesions on AV shunt rats. Arch. Path. (Chicago) **82:** 85.
27. Lillehei, C. W., J. R. R. Bobb & M. B. Visscher. 1950. The occurrence of endocarditis with vascular deformities in dogs with arteriovenous fistulas. Ann. Surg. **132:** 577.
28. Lee, S. H., B. Fisher, E. R. Fisher & A. Little. 1962. Arteriovenous fistula and bacterial endocarditis. Surgery **52:** 463.
29. Davis, R. L., J. A. Brunson & P. E. Fehr. 1957. Cardiac fibrinoid lesion produced by cross circulation on temporary A-V shunt. Circ. Res. **5:** 11.
30. Nakao, K. & A. Angrist. 1967. Electron microscopy of nonbacterial valvular vegetations in rats with arteriovenous shunt. Brit. J. Exp. Path. **48:** 294.
31. Zucker, M. B. & J. Borrelli. 1962. Platelet clumping produced by connective tissue suspensions and by collagen. Proc. Soc. Exp. Biol. Med. **109:** 779.
32. Hovig, T. 1963. Aggregation of rabbit blood platelets produced *in vitro* by saline "extract" of tendons. Thromb. Diath. Haemorrh. **9:** 248.
33. Glynn, M. F., H. F. Movat, E. A. Murphy & J. F. Mustard. 1965. Study of platelet adhesiveness and aggregation with latex particles. J. Lab. Clin. Med. **65:** 179.
34. Hughes, A. & R. S. Tonks. 1962. Intravascular platelet clumping in rabbits. J. Path. Bact. **84:** 379.
35. Born, G. V. R. & M. J. Gross. 1963. The effects of inorganic ions on the aggregation of platelets by adenosine phosphatase. J. Physiol. (London) **168:** 41.
36. Born, G. V. R. 1965. Uptake of adenosine and of adenosine diphosphatase by human blood platelet. Nature **206:** 1121.
37. Honour, A. J. & J. R. A. Mitchell. 1963. Platelet clumping in injured vessels. Brit. J. Exp. Path. **45:** 75.
38. Haslam, A. J., A. E. Odegaard & B. A. Skalhegy. 1963. Investigations on adenosine diaphosphate (ADP) induced platelet adhesiveness *in vitro*. Part I. The ADP-platelet reaction in various experimental conditions. Thromb. Diath. Haemorrh. **10:** 61.
39. Mitchell, J. & A. Sharp. 1964. Platelet clumping *in vitro*. Brit. J. Haemat. **10:** 78.
40. Nakao, K., A. Angrist & P. Mao. 1967. Collagen and platelet interaction in experimental vegetative cardiac valvular lesions. Exp. Molec. Path. **6:** 213.
41. Duguid, J. B. 1959. The role of the connective tissue in arterial disease. *In* Connective Tissue, Thrombosis, and Atherosclerosis. I. H. Page, Ed. : 13. Academic Press Inc. New York, N. Y.
42. Tweedy, P. S. 1956. The pathogenesis of valvular thickening in rheumatic heart disease. Brit. Heart J. **18:** 173.
43. Magarey, F. R. 1949. On the mode of formation of Lambl's excrescences and their relation to chronic thickening of the mitral valve. J. Path. Bact. **61:** 203.
44. Angrist, A. & M. Oka. 1963. Pathogenesis of bacterial endocarditis. J.A.M.A. **183:** 249.
45. Leary, T. 1932. Early lesions of rheumatic endocarditis. Arch. Path. (Chicago) **13:** 1.
46. Nedzel, A. J. 1937. Experimental endocarditis. Arch. Path. (Chicago) **24:** 143.
47. Oka, M. & A. Angrist. 1964. Histochemical studies of thrombotic nonbacterial endocarditis. Lab. Invest. **13:** 1504.
48. Angrist, A., M. Oka & K. Nakao. 1967. Vegetative endocarditis in pathology. Annal. S. Sommers, Ed. Appleton-Century-Crofts. New York, N. Y.
49. Oka, M. & A. Angrist. 1965. Comparative histochemical studies of nonbacterial and bacterial valvular vegetations. Lab. Invest. **14:** 48.

PART VI. PRIMARY CARDIOMYOPATHIES AND CONGESTIVE HEART FAILURE IN CLINICAL MEDICINE

THE AFRICAN CARDIOMYOPATHIES*

J. N. P. Davies
Department of Pathology, Albany Medical College
Albany, New York

It seems unfortunate that an old-fashioned morbid anatomist should open the section of the monograph dealing with human implications, because it might imply that we take a dim view of the prognosis in human cases of cardiomyopathy. This is by no means the case, but, until our clinical diagnostic methods in this field are more advanced, the ultimate diagnosis of a case will be made at autopsy. This diagnosis, however, will usually be in terms of the lesions found rather than in terms of etiology; if the clinician has failed in attempts to elucidate the etiological factors, it is unlikely that these can be specified by the autopsy findings. In many cases, definite lesions can be found, but the specificity and significance of these lesions are in doubt. Whereas I agree with Dr. Wartman's statement in his opening remarks on the limited range of reactions of the myocardium to disease processes, I still do not think that this is as limiting a factor as might be supposed. Even if tissue reactions are limited in the overall sense, there is still a sufficient interplay of factors, of cell reactions, of tissue reactions, of cell infiltrates, of vascular, nervous, endocardial, and epicardial reactions, of infiltrations and "degenerations," that in conjunction with the factors of time, of intensity, of concurrent lesions elsewhere and with the clinical findings, the chemical and functional findings, and with the armamentarium we now have for studying morphological changes, we can hope, with time and careful study, to determine much more specificity in lesions than we recognize at present. There is, however, one danger that should be warned against, and that is of premature identification and of using terms that imply specific etiological factors when, in fact, we have no evidence pointing to these factors.

The common cardiomyopathies of the African continent can at present be distinguished only by the lesions they produce in the heart, as studied in autopsied patients, that is, usually in those with advanced disease. Since to date we have no clear ideas as to etiology, and we have as yet no closely comparable lesions in either wild or experimental animals, we can only describe the lesions as accurately as possible to note the features that any etiological explanation will have to account for and to which any experimental model must conform. Before considering the specific lesions, however, some attention must be given to the populations in which these diseases occur with particular frequency. The African continent is very large, and the trans-Saharan part is not only large but also inhabited by an astonishing variety of peoples with a remarkable degree of variation in habits, customs, diets, and ways of life. It includes some of the tallest and the shortest of human beings, but, insofar as it is safe to generalize, these negroid peoples tend to be of small stature and low body weight. They are often poorly nourished, if not malnourished, and consume a high carbohydrate diet, often based on a single staple, with resulting periods of feast or famine. The diets are often low in protein and fat, and many of the people are no doubt in marginal

* This work was supported by United States Public Health Service research grant no HE–09417 from the National Heart Institute.

deficiency states, although frank outbreaks of vitamin deficiency diseases are usually seen only under rather unnatural conditions.

The basic factors in the cardiovascular system of these peoples have been little studied, and there has been a tendency to take over concepts established in other countries and apply these, rather uncritically, to the African peoples. This is unhappily a risky procedure. In Uganda, we have found that there is no correlation of body height with heart weight, but that body weight and heart weight are linearly related between body weights of 35–55 kg.[1] Below 35 kg, there is no proportional diminution of heart weight with lower body weight; above 55 kg, there is no proportionate increase in heart weight with greater body weight. A degree of aortic hypoplasia is also commonly seen.[2] Blood pressure does not seem to rise with age, and heart weight falls with increasing age once adulthood is achieved, the heaviest normal hearts being found in young adults. Thus, the average normal heart weight in Africans is appreciably less than in caucasoid peoples, and the limits of normality and the point where hypertrophy is recognizable are uncertain. Against this uncertainty, there are some favorable factors. In Uganda, it has been clearly established that disease of the major coronary arteries is, for practical purposes, nonexistent and that coronary artery thrombosis, myocardial infarction, and systemic thromoboembolic disease are extremely uncommon and clinically of negligible importance.[3,4]

At the moment, no classification of the African cardiomyopathies can be more than tentative, but we can discern certain broad groupings, and it is convenient to distinguish those in which there is no constant concomitant endocardial changes, other than intracavitary thrombi in the ventricles, from those in which there is a marked endocardial component.

Cardiomyopathies without an Endocardial Lesion

In the first group of diseases, those without significant endocardial changes, we have many cases that cannot be classified at this time because of the lack of specific features revealed by the light microscope. Common to nearly all of these diseases is the presence of vacuolation of myofibers, often initially marked in the perinuclear region and extending to marked hydropic degeneration; severe interfibrially edema; loss of sarcoplasm or its degeneration into a smudgy amorphous mass; evidence of loss of myofiber; the development of patchy fibrosis, especially in the trabeculae; some obliterative changes in small coronary arterial vessels; and a slight degree of cellular infiltration, often with lymphocytes or monocytes. These changes may be seen with or without evidence of cardiac hypertrophy. There is often an apparent increase in nuclear size, and hyperchromatic or eccentric nuclei with blunt ends. Because we cannot discern any specificity in these lesions, we tend to classify these cases according to some social, geographic, nutritional, or other factor or with some concomitant disease process.

Firstly, it is worth considering the frequency of hypertensive disease in these peoples, since hypertensive heart disease is one of the most common causes of heart failure in Uganda.[5] These patients pass into severe decompensation and die without any evidence of coronary artery disease, and some without any notable cardiac hypertrophy, although there is always some increase in the heart weight above normal. Some or all of the changes mentioned may be found in the hearts at autopsy, and it seems that the hearts of many Africans for some reason cannot stand up to sustained hypertension. Thus, there is good reason to put hypertension high on the list of African cardiomyopathies.

Since the specificity of the changes in the heart is not yet recognized, we find somewhat similar changes in the heart in other conditions. Common to many areas, notably Nigeria, is the so-called "heart-muscle disease" described by Edington and Jackson,[6] although cardiomegaly is evident in these cases. This is probably the same type of disease as that which Stuart and Hayes[7] described as common in Jamaica in which the histological changes are also slight and lack specificity. Somewhat similar changes are seen in the hearts of palm-wine tappers who consume vast quantities of concentrated fermenting carbohydrate-rich juice and develop a congestive failure that has been described as cardiac beriberi.[8] However, it seems that the response to thiamine is often poor in contrast to the response seen in acute fulminant cardiac beriberi in other areas. Similar cases of unexplained congestive cardiac failure have been described in South Africa[9] and in Ceylon;[10] these cases are unresponsive to thiamine or, indeed, to any specific nutriment, but they respond to a generally good diet, only to relapse upon return to the patient's own normal diet.

There is a vague aura of malnutrition about many of these cases, as about so many in this country, and there is great difficulty, both clinically and pathologically, in the separation of possible thiamine deficiency and alcoholism. It seems of the highest importance that methods be devised by which the effects of ethanol and of thiamine deficiency on the heart may be separated, if they are separable. In my own laboratory, using a multidisciplinary approach in the experimental rat, an attempt has been made to separate the effects of ethanol from those of thiamine deficiency; it is our impression that there are clearly definable differences which will in time, we hope, provide a solution to this problem.

True cardiac beriberi, especially in its acute fulminant form, is a rare disease of African adults or infants, certainly much less common than it was in the Far East. There has been so much confusion about beriberi, both from the clinical and pathological aspects, that there were, it seemed, only two fixed points of agreement: first that it is preventable and second that, save when patients are *in extremis,* acute cardiac beriberi is rapidly responsive to the administration of thiamine.[11] The pathology of cardiac beriberi is not well described; existing descriptions are confusing, often contradictory and inadequate, and of course notoriously at variance with the lesions produced by thiamine deficiency in experimental animals.[12] Recently, Dr. Bishop and I have been able, thanks to the curators of various medical museums, to reexamine several hearts on exhibit as cases of acute beriberi. We have found that some show evidence of cardiac hypertrophy alone, but others show various degrees of myofiber vacuolation and myocardial edema without fibrosis, fatty droplets, or cell infiltrates. I have never, even in the Far East, been able to find an authenticated case of chronic cardiac beriberi. I doubt if such a condition exists, and, if it does, I would not care to speculate on what the histological changes might be.

At present, therefore, this group of cardiomyopathies defiies classification or explanation, but clearly central to this problem is the nature and causation and effects of the watery vacuolation of the myofibers. We do not know if these diseases are the same, are variants within a spectrum of disease, or if the lesions represent some common final pathway of myofiber damage entered on by a multiplicity of routes. A subsidiary problem is whether such watery vacuolation can lead to myofiber dissolution without the production of an inflammatory cell response.

Cardiomyopathies with an Endocardial Lesion

With the cardiomyopathic diseases in which there is an endocardial component, we are on firmer grounds, first because there is a higher degree of specificity to these lesions, and second because we can distinguish between primary and secondary lesions[13] and can see something of the pathogenetic mechanisms by which these lesions are produced.[14] Thus, we can distinguish between those conditions in which the endocardial lesion is a reactive one and those in which the endocardium has been destroyed and replaced by scar tissue. Indeed, this is the justification for including these conditions in the cardiomyopathies, since a severe degree of endocardial destruction seems only to be brought about by disease "or destruction" of the adjacent subendocardial myocardium.[14] In the United States, the underlying disease is usually a myocardial infarction due to coronary artery disease, an uncommon condition in Africans.

In Africa, there are two cardiomyopathies in which the myocardial destruction is associated with an arteritis that is not confined to the heart, although the brunt of the damage falls on this organ. The best recognized is Loffler's disease, in which there is an eosinophilic arteritis, usually with a marked eosinophilia in the blood and arteritic lesions in many organs; to the damage produced by the arteritis, there may be added frequent embolic accidents.[15,16] In the heart, there is frequently a valvulitis, with vegetations and destruction of the myocardium which often extends to its full thickness and which, if the patient survives long enough, will exhibit organization and fibrosis. The original endocardium is swept away and replaced by scar tissue covered by extensive mural thrombi which commonly detach. The myocardial destruction, and hence the endocardial scarring, seems haphazardly distributed, without special involvement of any particular area of the myocardium. In Africa, there is a subvariant of this condition; described by Brink and Weber,[15] in which the predominant cell is not an eosinophilic but a neutrophilic polymorphonuclear cell. Loffler's disease is a recognizable clinical and pathological entity.

Another clinical entity is the condition described by Becker[17] as common in South Africa but which exists in other countries.[18] Clinically a relapsing form of congestive cardiac failure with increasing resistance to treatment in each episode, the course is marked by pyrexia, leukocytosis, and evidence of microinfarcts of a bland type. The cardiac lesions consist of a mucinous edema of the endocardium, with small polypoidal hemorrhagic masses on the endocardial surface. Areas of the damaged endocardium go on to develop small fibroelastotic patches, with evidence of smooth muscle hypertrophy. Associated with these lesions is a curious verrucose angitis affecting only the small subendocardial blood vessels and manifesting initially as small areas of fibrinofibrinoid deposition on the walls which change into a nexus of capillary tissue and fibrous tissue being organized into eccentric cushions of fibrous tissue. Occasionally, small polypoid masses are seen, and sometimes the lesions are so extensive as to occlude the vessels. The distribution of these lesions is haphazard, affecting all areas of the endocardium, but multiple blocks may be necessary to reveal them. On the whole, the myofibers show little change other than edema with separation of the muscle bundles. This disease thus presents both clinical features and specific pathological lesions which enable it to be distinguished, but its cause is quite unknown.

Distinct from all these conditions is endomyocardial fibrosis, as my colleagues and I reported in Uganda.[16,19] It is clear that this disease exists in many countries, and I have seen typical instances of it in United States residents who have never left this country. The pathology exhibits some highly specific features. First, it is a disease of the inflow tract endocardium, with fibrosis in severe cases extending in a massive sheet from the atria, over the posterior cusp of the atrioventricular (AV) valve, to the apex of the ventricle, ending in a sharply defined rough ridge at the region where the differences between inflow and outflow types of endocardium become distinct. Fibrosis is very evident in the left ventricle, where the septal and anterior walls are largely spared, although there may be patches of reactive elastomyofibrosis on the septum. The posterior cusps of the AV valve are bound down at an early stage to the mural endocardium behind and may ultimately completely disappear in the mass of fibrous tissue. The valves show no evidence of vegetations or valvulitis, and the semilunar valves are always spared. The endocardium in the affected areas of the inflow tract is swept away by a destructive process, and all features of it are lost. It is replaced by fibrous tissue, more densely scarred toward the cavitary aspect, but more loosely meshed and softer on the myocardial side, from which it is separated by a thin layer of granulation tissue with a sparse cell infiltrate. The cavitary aspect is covered by a variable amount of thrombus, but embolic accidents are curiously uncommon. On the myocardial side, tongues of fibrous tissue run down into about the middle of the myocardium and surround large dilated thin-walled blood vessels, probably obstructed Thebesian veins, and arterioluminal vessels. The myocardial fibers show watery vacuolation varying in degree from slight to very severe.

Gross changes on the right side are modified only by the ease with which the right ventricular cavity becomes filled with organized fibrous tissue and the cavity becomes obliterated and reduced to a small saucer beneath a monstrously dilated right atrium. This obliterated right ventricle is conveniently recognized by a marked recession of the right ventricular apex when viewed externally.

My clinical colleagues in Uganda[20] and Nigeria[21,22] have demonstrated elegantly how the clinical features of this disease, and the radiological and angiographic features, correlate beautifully with the gross anatomical changes according to the involvement of one or other ventricle, or both ventricles, and to the extent of the disease, particularly the extent of the involvement of the posterior cusps of the AV valves. Although in many cases it can be diagnosed accurately in life, with the diagnosis confirmed at autopsy, we have not made any great advances in our knowledge of its etiology. I do not propose to review or add to the etiological explanations, but I would like to discuss certain features which any etioiogical suggestion must explain. On the clinical side, there is the infrequency of embolic phenomena; this is not a racial factor, since it is noted in non-African cases. Also, there is the anatomical factor to be explained: Why is the inflow tract endocardium involved and the outflow tract spared. This is of course secondary, in that an early lesion must be the destruction of the endocardium from disease of the underlying muscle of the inflow tract region. There must be some specific factor to cause this localization, because the myofiber vacuolation is as evident in the uninvolved septum as it is in the affected areas.

Some of the difficulties may be partially resolved through some recent work by Drs. D. H. Connor and W. Mannion of the Armed Forces Institute of Pathology in Washington and their co-workers in Uganda[23] which they have been kind enough to draw to my attention prior to publication. They have found that the lesions contain very large amounts of acid mucopolysaccharide and exhibit a series of reactions that seem to be unique to this disease. Much of what has been considered thrombus apparently may be this acid mucopolysaccharide, which may explain the infrequency of embolic accidents. Just what this discovery will mean in a larger context must await their full report, but I think their paper will constitute a considerable advance in our knowledge of this disease.

One can only conclude this review of African cardiomyopathies with the remark that none of them, and this includes the frequent submitral aneurysms recorded in Nigeria,[24] are confined to the African continent. They occur in all parts of the world where cardiovascular disease is carefully evaluated clinically and at autopsy. Years ago, it was possible to explain any odd disease of the tropics as malarious because everyone has malaria. Coronary atherosclerosis is so common in the United States that it is almost always possible to find some at autopsy in a human heart. How many cases of cardiomyopathy are missed in this country because of the prevalence of coronary atherosclerosis is an open question.

References

1. DAVIES, J. N. P. & R. M. COLES. 1959. The normal heart weight of Uganda Africans. E. Afr. Med. J. **36:** 76–84.
2. DICK, G. W. A. 1947. Aortic size in East African natives. Ann. Trop. Med. Parasit. **41:** 48–54.
3. THOMAS, W. A., J. N. P. DAVIES, R. M. O'NEAL & A. A. DIMAKULANGAN. 1960. Incidence of myocardial infarction correlated with venous and pulmonary thrombosis and embolism. Amer. J. Cardiol. **5:** 41–47.
4. LEE, K. T., J. N. P. DAVIES & R. A. FLORENTIN. 1966. Geographic studies in atherosclerosis. Geriatrics **21:** 160–182.
5. DAVIES, J. N. P. 1961. The heart of Africa. Lab. Invest. **10:** 205–215.
6. EDINGTON, G. M. & J. G. JACKSON. 1963. The pathology of heart muscle disease and endomycardial fibrosis in Nigeria. J. Path. Bact. **86:** 333–344.
7. STUART, K. L. & J. A. HAYES. 1963. A cardiac disorder of unknown aetiology in Jamaica. Quart. J. Med. **32:** 97–114.
8. HARLING, D. S., P. D. MARSDEN & D. S. RIDLEY. 1965. Some observations on the pattern of heart disease in the Gambia. Trans. Roy. Soc. Trop. Med. Hyg. **59:** 628–641.
9. GILLANDERS, A. D. 1951. Nutritional heart disease. Brit. Heart J. **13:** 177–196.
10. OBEYESEKERE, I. 1966. Nutritional heart disease in Ceylon. Paper to the 5th World Cong. Cardiol., New Delhi, India.
11. BLEGEN, S. D. 1965. Post-partum congestive heart failure. Beri beri heart disease. Acta Med. Scand. **178:** 515–524.
12. FOLLIS, R. D. 1958. Deficiency disease. Charles C Thomas, Publ. Springfield, Ill.
13. OKADA, R. 1961. Clinicopathologic study on the thickening of the parietal endocardium. Jap. Heart J. **2:** 220–255.
14. DAVIES, J. N. P. 1962. Pathology and pathogenesis of endocardial disease. Cardiologia (Basel) **42:** 161–175.
15. BRINK, A. J. & H. W. WEBER. 1963. Fibroplastic parietal endocarditis with eosinophilia. Amer. J. Med. **34:** 52–70.
16. DAVIES, J. N. P. & R. M. COLES. 1960. Some considerations regarding obscure diseases affecting the mural endocardium. Amer. Heart J. **59:** 600–631.
17. BECKER, B. J. P. 1963. Idiopathic mural endocardial disease in South Africa. Med. Proc. **9:** 124–128; 147–158.
18. DAVIES, J. N. P. & A. HOLLMAN. 1965. Becker type cardiomyopathy in a West Indian woman. Amer. Heart J. **70:** 225–232.
19. DAVIES, J. N. P. & J. D. BALL. 1955. The pathology of endomyocardial fibrosis in Uganda. Brit. Heart J. **17:** 337–359.
20. BALL, J. D., A. W. WILLIAMS & J. N. P. DAVIES. 1954. Endomyocardial fibrosis. Lancet **i:** 1049–1053.
21. ABRAHAMS, D. G. 1962. Endomyocardial fibrosis of the right ventricle. Quart. J. Med. **31:** 1–20.
22. PARRY, E. H. O. & D. G. ABRAHAMS. 1965. The natural history of endomyocardial fibrosis. Quart. J. Med. **34:** 383–408.
23. CONNOR, D. H., W. MANNION, M. S. R. HUTT & K. SOMERS. Personal communication about a manuscript in press.
24. ABRAHAMS, D. G., C. J. BARTON, W. P. COCKSHOTT, G. M. EDINGTON & E. J. M. WEAVER. 1962. Annular subvalvular left ventricular aneurysms. Quart. J. Med. **31:** 345–360.

LACK OF CORRELATION BETWEEN CORONARY THROMBOSIS AND MYOCARDIAL INFARCTION OR SUDDEN "CORONARY" HEART DEATH*

Giorgio Baroldi

Istituto Anatomia e Istologia Patologica, Universita di Milano, Milan, Italy and Cardiovascular Branch, Armed Forces Institute of Pathology, Washington, D. C.

Since 1881, the etiopathogenetic interpretation of myocardial infarction in man has been based on Cohnheim's concept[1] that physiologically the coronary arteries are end arteries. In one of the most recent textbooks on cardiovascular pathology, the chapter "Ischemic Heart Disease and Myocardial Infarction" is introduced by the following statement: "Functionally the coronary arteries are 'end arteries' and obstruction anywhere in the arterial tree almost certainly will cause infarction somewhere in the heart."[2] Such a statement is justified on the basis of Cohnheim's experiences and by numerous experimental studies of myocardial infarction, with or without associated ventricular fibrillation followed acute coronary occlusion. Assuming that this conclusion is correct within the limits of pertinent experimental pathology, it seems especially worthy of discussion in relation to human pathology in general, and to coronary thrombosis in particular, since the latter is considered to be the main cause of acute occlusion in the coronary diseases. Human cases of myocardial infarction in which no occlusion or acute occlusion has been detected have been regarded as relatively rare, and have been labeled with the questionable, if not contradictory, term "myocardial infarction without occlusion or acute occlusion." It should be noted that there is a good deal of confusion insofar as terminology is concerned.

Definitions

"Myocardial infarction," "coronary thrombosis," "coronary occlusion," "ischemic heart disease," and "coronary insufficiency" are terms frequently used synonimously without regard to the specific nature of a given lesion, its chronological evaluation, or consideration of the total pathological background in which the lesion evolves. Thus, the correlation between myocardial and vascular damage seems to be based more on preconceived ideas than on any objective data. A brief review of the current meaning of the terms used in the present discussion may be helpful.

Myocardial Infarct. A myocardial infarct is a "coagulation necrosis" of the myocardium which is generally believed to be secondary to an acute occlusion of the coronary arteries or branches. It should be emphasized that this coagulation necrosis is a basic pathological finding, which undergoes a relatively well-known repair process. It is, however, only during the acute or recent phase that we are able to differentiate this lesion from other necrotic damage. For instance, myocytolysis or necrotic changes secondary to inflammatory processes show a divergent morphological pattern and evolution. In the final stages, however, it becomes impossible to differentiate between them, since the necrosis ends in a dense scar, the extent of which cannot be considered distinctive enough for the etiopathogenesis of the different necrotic lesions. Finally, myocardial coagulation necrosis begins by involving a single fiber or a few scattered fibers.[3,4] It may remain focal, or it may become focal-confluent or massive. Other characteristics

* This study was in part supported by a Postdoctoral Research Fellowship, grant no. FF-485, from the National Institutes of Health, United States Public Health Service.

seem superfluous in the present discussion (i.e., laminar, subendocardial, transmural, and subepicardial).

Acute Coronary Occlusion. Different causes or mechanisms are involved in an acute coronary occlusion. The lesion occurs frequently at the level of the extramural coronary arteries or branches, but only rarely at the level of the intramural arterial ramifications. Among the major causes that have been thought capable of producing a mechanical obstruction of the vessels are, first, thrombosis, and, less frequently, hemorrhage into an atherosclerotic plaque per se or, by secondary thrombosis or vascular spasm, rupture of an atheromatous plaque, vascular spasm, acute intimal edema, settling of blood masses, embolization, and dissecting aneurysm.

Acute Coronary Insufficiency or Ischemia. In the absence of an acute mechanical coronary occlusion, an acute coronary insufficiency or ischemia, in the sense of a critical coronary flow reduction (as in shock), has also been considered cause of myocardial coagulation necrosis. Acute coronary insufficiency, even if possible in normal coronary vessels, is considered more likely when chronic stenosing-obstructive vascular damage and/or cardiac hypertrophy are present (i.e., cases of so-called chronic coronary insufficiency or ischemia).

Sudden "Coronary" Heart Death. Sudden "coronary" heart death defines those cases of sudden death in which the main pathological finding at autopsy is a coronary disease, with or without myocardial involvement. The inability to detect myocardial damage by routine histological methods may be due to the short period of time between the onset of the attack and the demise of the patient, too short a period to allow the lesion to become manifest. It is well known that several hours pass before the first signs of coagulation necrosis appear by light microscopical methods. Therefore, uncertainty exists as to whether or not these are true cases of myocardial infarction.

On the basis of such definitions, and using our present knowledge, the following basic criteria should be essential to any human study on the so-called myocardial infarct and its relationship to vascular impairment. (1) Selection of the material must be limited to cases with acute or recent coagulation necrosis. In this way, it is possible to identify the lesion with certainty and evaluate its approximate age. (2) In these cases, a careful gross and microscopical examination of the arterial coronary tree must be made at the level of both the extramural and intramural systems. (3) The frequency, nature, and location of the acute or recent occlusion must be calculated. (4) The previous sclerotic lumen reduction at the site of the resultant acute or recent occlusion must be calculated. (5) The relationship of the anastomotic circulation to the sclerotic lumen reduction (previous to the acute or recent occlusion) must be considered. (6) An attempt must be made to correlate the age of the acute or recent occlusion to the age of the myocardial necrosis.

During the past 14 years, a similar study comprising cases of so-called "sudden coronary heart death" was completed. An extensive report of the methods and materials employed has been published.[5–10] Hence, only a brief summary will be given here.

Methods and Materials

Plastic Injection Method

The arterial and venous circulation was studied after the injection of plastic substances (Geon Latex 576 and Neoprene 842A) in 522 normal and pathological human hearts.† The arterial coronary tree in particular was examined by

† Taken from the files of the Institute of Morbid Anatomy and the Institute of Forensic Medicine, Medical School, University of Milan, Milan, Italy.

aortic injection in 79 selected normal hearts, in 48 "pure" (without vascular damage) hypertrophic hearts, in 25 pure atrophic hearts, in 18 normal hearts from patients dying from chronic hypoxic disease, and in 217 hearts with coronary stenosing-occlusive disease, in most instances arterio-atherosclerosis. Of the last group, 147 were hospitalized patients, and 70 were sudden unexpected coronary heart death cases. After a hermetic closure of the aortic valve below the coronary ostia, the plastic substances were injected at a pressure of 130–200 mm Hg. The penetration of the latex as far as the precapillary vessels (30–10 μ) was enhanced by artificial pulsation determined by rhythmical compression of the aortic bulb. Solidification of the latex fluid at room temperature was accomplished by placing the heart in 10% formalin at 40–50° C. Prior to hydrochloric acid corrosion, several samples of the myocardium were taken for histological study. Since the plastic material employed in this study underwent minimal, if any, shrinkage during the solidification process, the resulting vascular cast reproduced an accurate mold, making it possible to calculate the vasal diameter and its eventual pathological reduction.

By this method, a tridimensional and complete view of the arterial anastomotic intracardiac circulation in normal and pathological conditions was reached, and a definitive correlation between the grade of the obstructive vascular lesion, the enlargement of the anastomotic channels, and the myocardial damage was possible. This method was devised and chosen for this particular study since numerous other suggested methods have given only a partial view of the anastomotic circulation (i.e., injection of radiopaque material with or without "unrolling" the heart, mixed dye with dissection, or injection of calibrated spheres).

According to their location, the arterial anastomoses were designated as "intercoronary" when there were connecting branches of the two or, if a third coronary artery was present, three coronary arteries, or as "homocoronary," when there were joining branches of the same coronary artery. The collaterals‡ were so numerous that it was impossible to estimate their exact number. Thus, in order to compare the behavior of the anastomotic channels in the different groups examined, the following "anastomotic index" (AI) was formulated for each heart: $AI = [max. \phi + (av. \phi \times freq.)]/100$, in which the "maximum diameter" in microns of the largest anastomosis found (max. ϕ), the "average diameter" of the anastomoses having a diameter larger than 100 μ (av. ϕ), and the "frequency" (freq.) of the anastomoses with a diameter greater than 100 μ were considered. The "frequency" refers to the normal heart, which has been arbitrarily regarded as 1.

Histological Study

A histological study was done in 499 selected cases from the files of the Armed Forces Institute of Pathology (AFIP), Washington, D.C., which includes case material from military, Veterans Administration, and civilian sources. The following three distinct groups were included: (1) 208 hospitalized patients (180 men and 28 women) in whom an acute or recent coagulation necrosis of the heart was substantiated at autopsy; (2) 116 subjects (112 men and four women) whose demise was attributed to sudden unexpected "coronary" death, without clinical history of previous cardiac symptoms and signs; and (3) 125 subjects (112 men and 13 women) who died from sudden but not unexpected "coronary" heart death (they had had previous clinical histories of heart attacks).

‡ In the present study, the term "collateral" has been used synonymously with "anastomosis."

The extramural coronary arteries and branches were sectioned by serial transverse incisions, and any severe stenosis or occlusion was histologically examined. The type of occlusion was recorded, and the preexisting sclerotic luman reduction of the acutely or recently occluded vessel was measured by a micrometer. The percentage of lumen reduction was then noted, based on the normal diameter of the involved vessels. This normal diameter was derived from the plastic casts of normal hearts and, according to the method used, the diameter corresponds to the diameter of the vessel in maximum dilatation. In all of the hearts, several specimens of the myocardium were taken. An attempt was then made to correlate the age of the myocardial coagulation necrosis with the age of the acute or recent occlusion, using the criteria of Mallory and co-workers[11] and Irniger.[12]

In 205 additional cases (129 men and 76 women) with varying degrees of extramural coronary athero-arteriosclerosis, a systematic histological study of the intramural branches was done on several specimens taken from damaged and undamaged areas of the same heart.

Finally, 39 cases (24 men and 15 women) of Moschcowitz disease (so-called thrombotic thrombocytopenic purpura) from the files of AFIP, including case material from military, Veterans Administration, and civilian sources, were studied. This disease exhibits a peculiar, generally widespread, stenotic-occlusive involvement of the intramural cardiac arterioles. In human pathology, therefore, it represents a unique, almost "experimental," opportunity for a select study of the relationship between intramural arterial obstructive lesions and myocardial necrosis.

Synthesis of the Results of This Study

A summary of the conclusive results follows. Only those results pertinent to the present discussion are reported.

Intracardiac Arterial Anastomotic Circulation in Relation to Coronary Occlusion and Myocardial Coagulation Necrosis (Plastic Injection Study)

The coronary arteries, anatomically speaking, are not end arteries, since all vascular areas communicate with adjacent vascular areas by way of anastomotic channels. In fact, a well-developed, extensive collateral circulation is present in all normal hearts, connecting branches of the same coronary artery (homocoronary anastomoses) and branches of the two (or, when present, three) coronary arteries (intercoronary anastomoses). The differentiation between homo- and intercoronary anastomoses must also account for the different patterns of the coronary arterial distribution. For example, when the posterior descending branch is supplied by the right coronary artery, the septal anastomoses will be intercoronary; however, when the posterior descending branch arises from the circumflex branch of the left coronary artery, they will be homocoronary. The anastomotic arterial vessels are generally parallel or oblique to the muscular planes, and they frequently show a characteristic "corkscrew" appearance. Their disposition, however, assumes a definite pattern in some cardiac regions; for example, in the interventricular septum, the collaterals are arranged in bundles of parallel branches. In the atria, they form a large mesh-like vascular structure, but beneath the ventricular endocardium, they are dispersed as a fine net-like reticulum, parallel to the endocardial surface. In general, in the normal human heart, with the exception of the immediate subepicardial layer, a fine anastomotic reticulum is distributed throughout the entire thickness of the cardiac walls, making it impossible to recognize a true subepicardial and/or subendocardial plexus.[13-15] In the normal adult heart, the homocoronary and intercoronary anastomoses show diameters of 20–250 μ and 20–350 μ, respectively. The maximum diameter found in newborn hearts was about 50 μ.

According to the methods applied in this study, "diameter" must be considered the diameter of the vessel in maximum dilatation. Anastomoses having a diameter of less than 20 μ probably exist, but, because of the multitude of small injected ramifications, they were not demonstrated with certainty despite microscopical examination of the casts.

In order to compare the frequency of the collaterals in the normal and pathological hearts, an "average diameter" for each heart was calculated by measuring only those grossly visible anastomoses with a diameter greater than 100 μ. From 15 to 30 intercoronary collaterals of this type were counted in the interventricular septum, and an equal number were noted in the cardiac walls; the homocoronary collaterals, however, averaged in the hundreds. The average diameter was 150–280 μ, with an average of 200 μ for the total number of normal adult hearts studied. The frequency of the larger anastomoses in the right ventricle was proportionally less, in accordance with the relative reduction in vascularization of the right ventricle compared with the left. No differences were noted in respect to sex and age. The anastomotic intracardiac arterial circulation is already present at birth, and its growth is parallel to that of the whole coronary tree. No further modifications in relation to age were noted following the attainment of adulthood.

In the pathological hearts examined in this study, i.e., pure atrophic and hypertrophic hearts, normal hearts in chronic hypoxia, and hearts with stenotic-occlusive coronary diseases, the following variations of the arterial anastomotic circulation was detected: In pure atrophy, subnormal values of the caliber and length of the anastomoses were found, concurrent with the general involution of the coronary intramural arterial system occurring in this condition. The opposite was observed in pure hypertrophy, in which a proportional enlargement of the collateral circulation exists together with an increase in the diameter and length of both extramural and intramural branches, giving the false impression of an apparent increase in number. A more salient "phanerosis" of the anastomoses also occurs in chronic hypoxia, and particularly in the presence of severe stenotic-occlusive coronary damage (FIGURE 1).

In FIGURE 2 and TABLE 1, the mean values of the "anastomotic index" are shown. Although in hypertrophy and hypoxia the vascular enlargement is diffuse throughout the entire anastomotic system, in stenotic-occlusive coronary disease the increase in size and length of the anastomoses coming from any adjacent vessels is strictly related to the severe stenosis (60–70% of lumen reduction) or occlusion ("satellite anastomotic circulation"). Due to the presence of numerous normal collaterals in all cardiac regions, the "anastomotic reserve" appears to be capable of compensating for multiple severe stenoses and/or occlusions. In fact, the increase of the collateral compensation was found proportional to the severity of the coronary disease, and was maximum when multiple severe stenoses and occlusions were present.

FIGURE 2 and TABLE 2 show that the anastomotic increase is not only proportional to the number of occlusions, but also to the degree of lumen reduction in other main branches, if those cases with only one occlusion are considered. Arterio-atherosclerosis is the most frequently encountered coronary disease; it is a slow, chronic, progressive process that generally involves the various extramural arteries and branches at different times and on different levels. Thus, it is understandable how anastomotic compensation occurs. A potential, diffuse col-

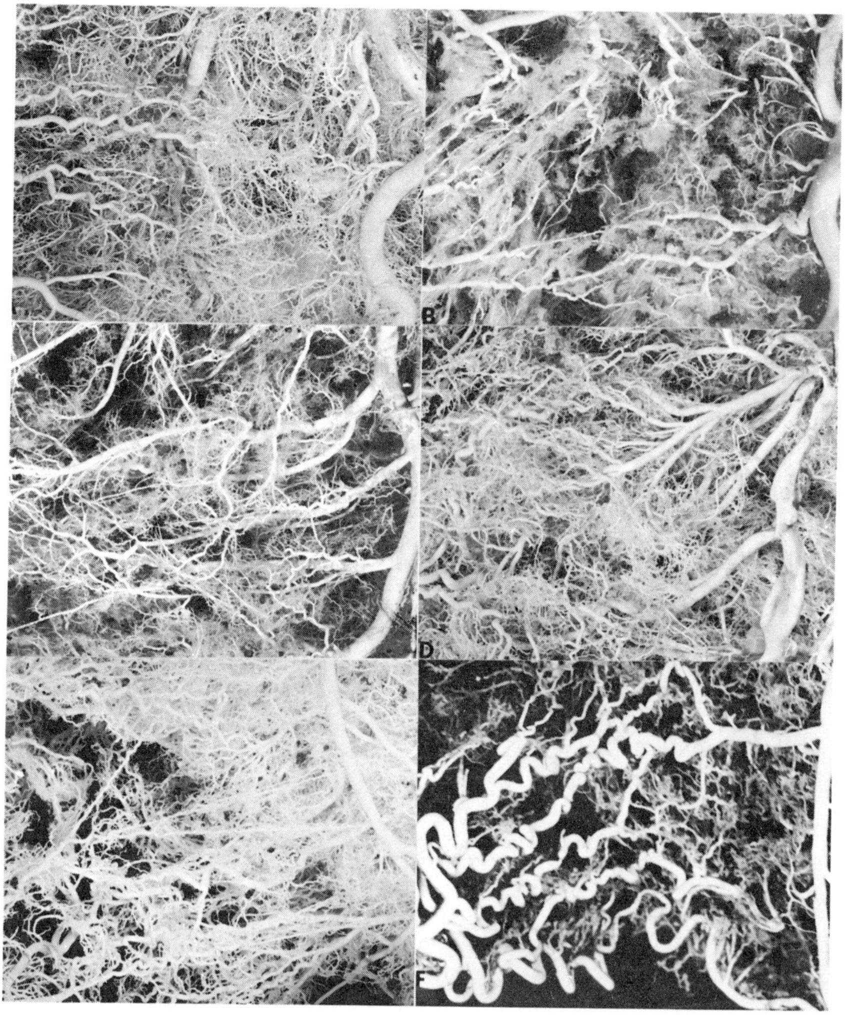

FIGURE 1. Intracardiac arterial anastomoses in normal and pathological conditions. Intercoronary anastomoses between the anterior descending branch of the left coronary artery (main vessel on the right) and the right anterior branches of the right coronary artery. (A) Normal heart. (B) Right cardiac hypertrophy. (C) Normal heart in chronic hypoxic condition. (D) Coronary stenosis, $>$ 60–70%. (E, F) Occlusion of the anterior descending branch. Two different patterns of collateral compensation.

lateral source is present everywhere, easily adaptable to any further compensatory demands. This is a protective function and has been well demonstrated in experimental studies with "chronic" coronary occlusion. It has also been clearly shown in the high frequency of human cases with single or multiple coronary occlusions without myocardial damage (occurring in 20.5% of the 112 cases in our material) or with minimal focal sclerotic damage (24.1% of the cases).

Moreover, the collateral increase does not seem to correspond to the myo-

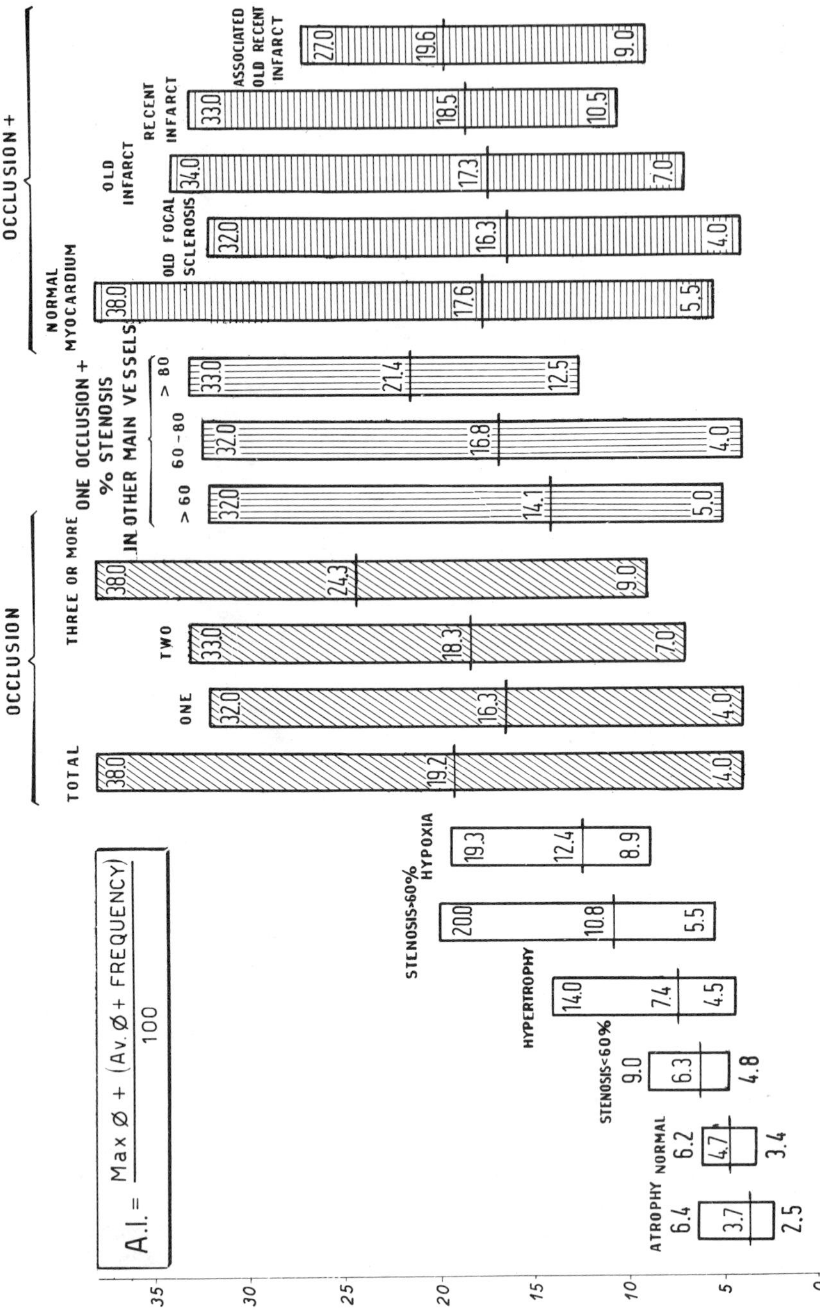

FIGURE 2. Mean values of anastomotic index in normal and pathological conditions.

TABLE 1

MEAN VALUES OF ANASTOMOTIC INDEX IN NORMAL HEARTS AND IN PATHOLOGICAL CONDITIONS

	Anastomotic Index		
Conditions	Minimum	Maximum	Average
Atrophy	2.5	6.4	3.7
Normal	3.4	6.2	4.7
Stenosis < 60%	4.8	9.0	6.3
Hypertrophy	4.5	14.0	7.4
Stenosis > 60%	5.5	20.0	10.8
Hypoxia	8.9	19.3	12.4
Occlusion	4.0	38.0	19.2

TABLE 2

MEAN VALUES OF ANASTOMOTIC INDEX IN RELATION TO THE NUMBER OF CORONARY OCCLUSIONS AND STENOSES

	Anastomotic Index		
Condition	Minimum	Maximum	Average
One occlusion	4.0	32.0	16.3
Two occlusions	7.0	33.0	18.3
Three or more occlusions	9.0	38.0	24.0
One occlusion plus			
< 60% stenosis in other main branches	5.0	32.0	14.1
60–80% stenosis	4.0	32.0	16.8
> 80% stenosis	12.5	33.0	21.4

TABLE 3

ANASTOMOTIC INDEX IN CORONARY OCCLUSION IN RELATION TO MYOCARDIAL DAMAGE

		No. of Occlusions*			Anastomotic Index		
Myocardial Damage	No. of Cases	1	2	3	Minimum	Maximum	Average
Without damage	23	73.9	21.7	4.3	5.5	38.0	17.6
Old focal sclerosis	27	74.0	22.2	3.7	4.0	32.0	16.3
Old infarct	15	53.3	33.3	13.3	7.0	34.0	17.3
Recent infarct	27	66.6	25.9	7.4	10.5	33.0	18.5
Associated infarct (old and recent)	20	30.0	50.0	10.0	9.0	27.0	19.6

* Values in percentage distribution.

cardial damage. As shown in TABLE 3 and FIGURE 2, approximately the same values of anastomotic index were found in hearts with occlusive coronary disease and a normal myocardium as in those with a focal sclerotic myocardial lesion, with an old infarct, acute-recent infarct, or associated (old and recent) infarcts; the higher values were found when recent damage was present. This would indicate that coagulation necrosis occurs even in the presence of an apparently well-functioning anastomotic circulation in human pathology, and, therefore, that function cannot be judged by the status of the myocardium. On the other hand, myocardial coagulation necrosis may occur in the presence of normal or non-functionally damaged coronary arteries (in this study, 10.8% of 46 cases with a lumen reduction below 60%). If we consider only the 47 cases of acute-recent infarct with coronary occlusion: in 95.8% (45 cases), a highly elevated collateral circulation was found, and in the remaining two cases (4.2%), it was moderately increased. It was concluded that myocardial coagulative necrosis occurred in all the examined "occlusive" cases where there was an anastomic circulation greater than normal, and that in most of these cases, the collateral compensation was markedly elevated.

In the heart with stenotic-occlusive coronary disease, the satellite collateral circulation may show two different patterns. It may be composed of numerous relatively smaller anastomotic channels or a relatively small number of greatly enlarged vessels. The explanation for this odd behavior becomes evident if we bear in mind the vascular changes that take place in and around the area of coagulation necrosis.[7,8] The intramural vascular structure, and the anastomoses, undergo secondary necrotic changes and disappear, whereas the arteriolar structures at the periphery show an obliterating arteritis that follows the necrosis and its repair process. The result is a more or less "avascular," or "hypovascular," area, according to the extent of the necrotic lesion. By plastic casting, this avascular or hypovascular area is clearly demonstrable as a region in which the intramural vessels are diminished or have disappeared, whereas the extramural branches are always demonstrable after injection, the distal portion of the occluded branch being injected via the surviving peripheral anastomoses (FIGURE 3). When such a loss of anastomoses occurs, a further enlargement of the surviving collaterals is expected. It must be emphasized that this vascular disappearance and the finding of sclerotic, stenosed, or occluded vessels within an old infarcted area must be considered secondary to the necrotic process, and not the primary cause, as is frequently believed. Moreover, with respect to the degree of the anastomotic compensation in the acute-recent infarct, it must be noted that its evaluation must take into account this secondary disappearance of the anastomoses. In other words, before the occurrence of the infarct, a more extensive anastomotic circulation, greater than that found in the postmortem postinfarct study, has to be present.

The angiomatous-like pattern in and around the myocardial scar, as well as in the subendocardial region (so-called "subendocardial plexus"), has been interpreted by us[8] as due mainly to the vascular changes in the necrotic areas. The enlargement of the preexisting precapillaries or surviving structures of the capillaries, especially the collaterals, is understandable because of the new hemodynamic conditions imposed on these vessels in this condition. The angiomatous or plexus-like findings were interpreted as more of a consequence of these changes than as new vascular formation,[16] or as a consequence of the questionable "ebb and flow" subendocardial mechanism, which is thought to increase in the "ischemic" heart.[14] Finally, on the basis of our findings, the concept of coronary insufficiency following progressive atherosclerosis involvement of the anastomoses or of the branches from which they originate[17] was not substantiated, nor was the mechanism of the so-called "infarct at a distance."[18] In regard to the behavior of the arterial anastomotic coronary circulation, no differences were found in relation to age or sex, or between hospitalized patients and those subjects dying from sudden coronary heart death. Nor do the different types of anatomical distribution of the coronary arteries or the presence or absence of the third coronary artery have any significance in relation to the anastomotic compensation or myocardial necrotic damage.

In addition, because of the preexisting enlarged competing intracardiac anastomoses, neither recanalization of occluded vessels nor the eventual new formation

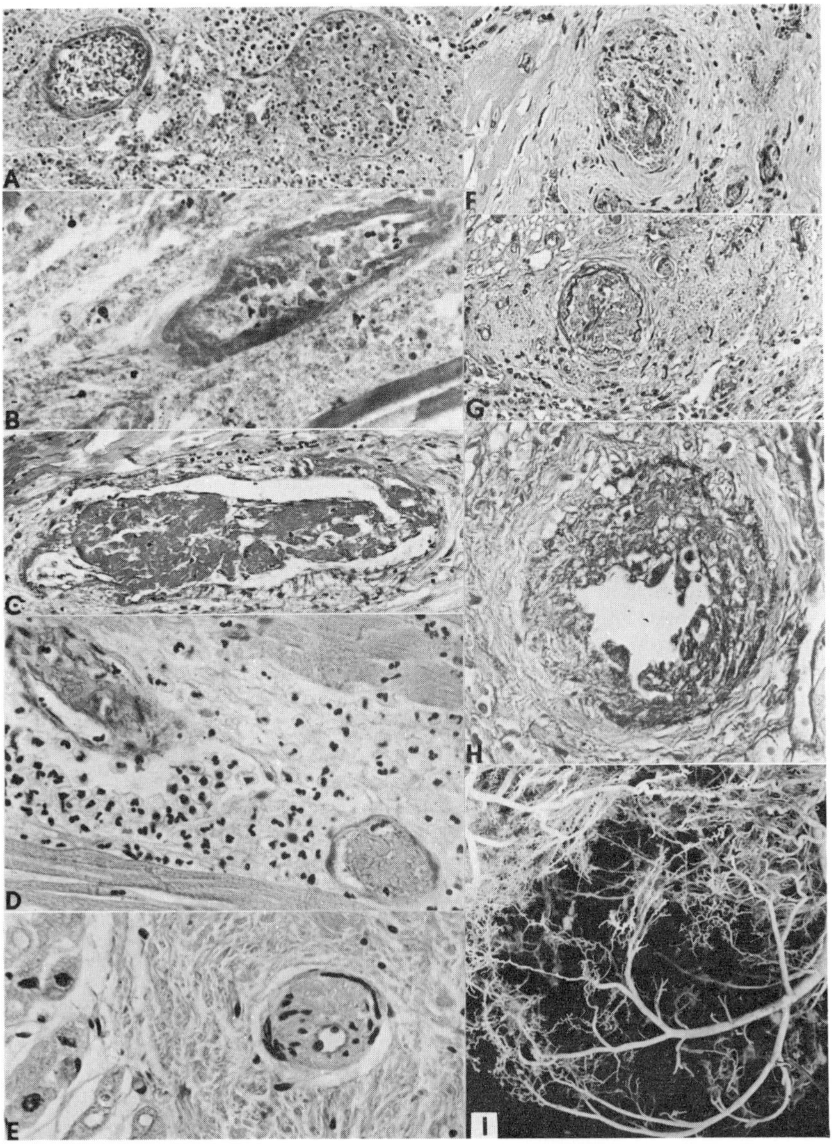

FIGURE 3. Intramural vascular changes secondary to myocardial coagulation necrosis. (A) Stain: hematoxylin and eosin. × 110 (orig. mag. × 180). (B) Stain: hematoxylin and eosin. × 270 (orig. mag. × 450). (C) Stain: periodic acid-Schiff. × 95 (orig. mag. × 160). (D) Stain: hematoxylin and eosin. × 270 (orig. mag. × 450). (E) Stain: hematoxylin and eosin. × 330 (orig. mag. × 550. (F) Stain: hematoxylin and eosin. × 110 (orig. mag. × 180. (G) Stain: Movat. × 110 (orig. mag. × 180). (H) Stain: Movat. × 270 (orig. mag. × 450). (I) "Avascular area" shown by plastic cast in a case of acute myocardial infarction of the apex. The main vessel on the right is the anterior descending branch of the left coronary artery.

of an anastomotic vessel at the site of a repair process or surgical procedure have much, if any, significance in human stenotic-occlusive coronary disease. This is also true for the extracardiac anastomotic circulation and arterioluminal as well as Thebesian vessels. Only in those rare cases of bilateral occlusion or subocclusion of the coronary ostia secondary to aortitis do the extracardiac collaterals probably have a compensatory function.[8,19] In the present study, coronary arterovenous anastomoses were not demonstrated.

Acute-Recent Occlusion of the Coronary Artery in Acute-Recent Coagulation Necrosis and in Sudden "Coronary" Heart Death (Histological Study)

Using the plastic and corrosion method, it was possible in our studies to fill the distal portion of all occluded vessels, in most cases (91% of the cases with occlusion and 95.8% of the cases with occlusion and acute-recent coagulation necrosis) through an anastomotic circulation of an "occlusive type." However, it was not possible to histologically determine whether the occlusion was acute or old. Therefore, a histological study was undertaken.

In 449 examined cases, the thrombosis was found as the only cause of acute occlusion, when present. Among the other proposed pathological causes of acute occlusion were eight cases of rupture of atheromatous "abscesses" and one hundred instances of intimal hemorrhage into an atherosclerotic plaque, generally detected at the site of severe stenosis or occlusion. In fact, in only six cases did intimal hemorrhage associated with an acute thrombosis occur in vessels with a lumen reduction below 65%. Referring to the total case material of the three groups examined, 53% of the 208 hospitalized patients, 53% of the 116 sudden unexpected "coronary" heart death patients, and 54% of the 125 sudden but not unexpected "coronary" death cases failed to demonstrate an acute or recent occlusion.

In regard to the approximate age of the acute or recent thrombosis and the age of the myocardial lesion, in only 23%, 22%, and 19% of the three groups, respectively, was a coeval relationship considered possible. Because it is difficult to arrive at an exact chronological evaluation for these lesions, a rough estimation was made according to the following classification: (1) early thrombus without an associated reaction to early coagulation necrosis and a leukocyitc infiltration stage of the myocardial necrosis, or both; (2) thrombus with early endothelial proliferation and capillary growth associated with an early phase of organization and a granulomatous stage, or both; (3) thrombus with early formation of collagen fibrils associated with a granulomatous stage of the myocardial necrosis; (4) recent organization of thrombus associated with recent myocardial fibrosis; (5) in the cases of sudden death, blood clot or early thrombus without reaction associated with normal-appearing myocardium or myocardial fibrosis without acute necrosis. According to this evaluation, in 77%, 78%, and 81% of the respective groups there were no objective findings of an acute occlusion which might explain the myocardial coagulative necrosis or sudden death.

The third factor taken into consideration was the degree of the sclerotic lumen reduction at the level of the acute occlusion. In only 8% of the total group of hospitalized patients, 4% of the sudden unexpected death group, and 2% of the sudden but not unexpected death group was an acute occlusive thrombosis associated with a lumen reduction below 65% found. If we consider the coeval cases only, an acute thrombosis combined with less than 65% lumen reduction was shown in 4%, 3%, and 0% in the three groups, respectively. In conclusion, as shown in FIGURE 4, this means that in 96%, 97%, and 100% of the groups

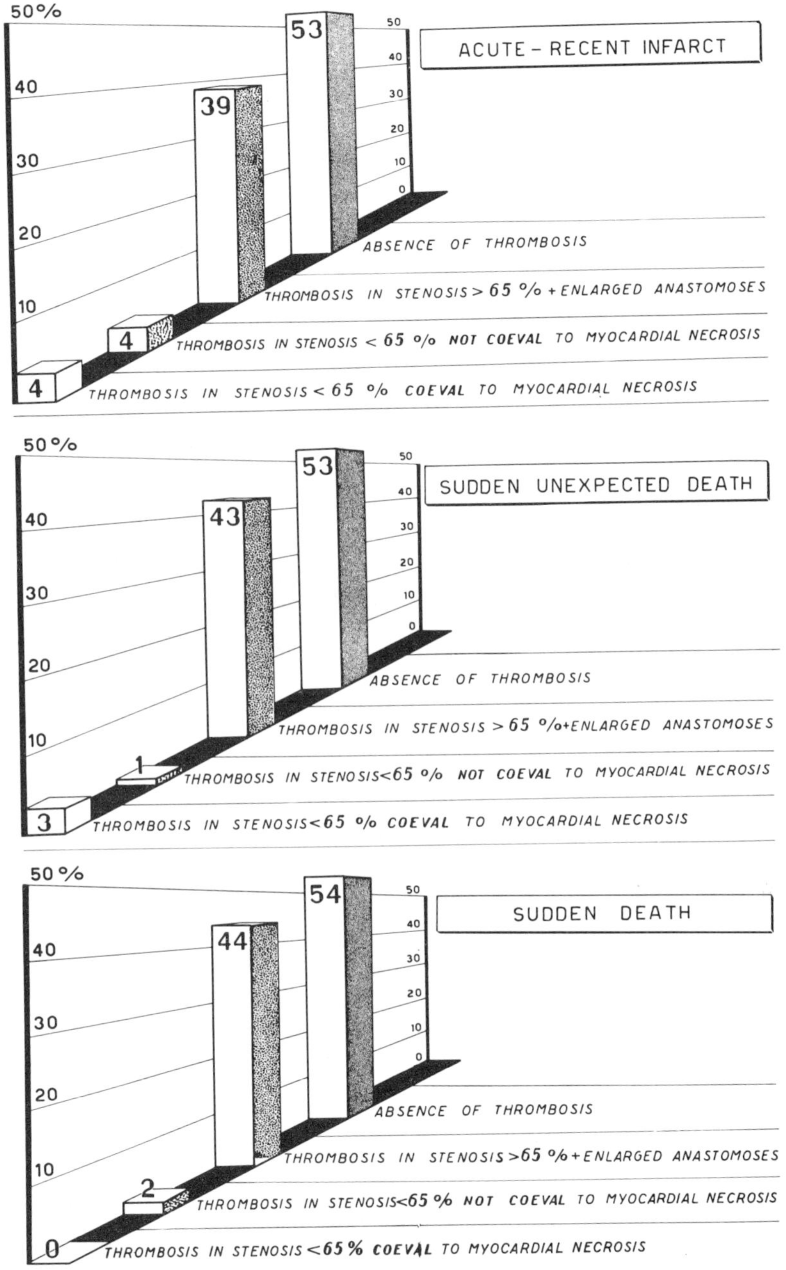

FIGURE 4. Frequency of coronary thrombosis in relation to previous lumen reduction and age of myocardial coagulative necrosis.

examined, an acute occlusion was: (1) not detected in 53%, 53%, and 54% respectively; (2) found in the presence of a highly developed anastomotic compensation in 39%, 43%, and 44%, respectively, and (3) not chronologically correlated to the myocardial coagulative necrosis or sudden death in 4%, 1%, and 2%, respectively.

Incidence of Stenosing-Occlusive Vascular Changes of the Intramural Arterial System in Coronary Arterio-Atherosclerosis

Coronary arterio-atherosclerosis involves the extramural arterial branches and particularly the main vessels, but not the intramural ramifications. In all the examined hearts of arterio-atherosclerotic heart disease without myocardial infarction, and in the normal areas of those hearts with infarct damage, the intramural arteriolar system only occasionally showed a moderate sclerotic thickening of the arteriolar wall of some isolated vessels. It must also be emphasized that intramural involvement was never observed in the cases of so-called myocardial infarction without occlusion, with a mild or relatively mild degree of extramural arterio-atherosclerosis. To suggest that intramural coronary sclerosis is the cause of myocardial damage, one must take into account the previously mentioned vascular reaction that follows any repair process. In fact, it is only within and around the infarcted areas that the surviving intramural branches undergo an obliterative arteritis secondary to the necrosis and its repair changes, and this may result in a sclerosis of the vascular wall of the residual vessels. Such an arteritis has been considered secondary to the necrosis because it begins afterward, showing a pattern of evolution parallel to that of the myocardial damage, but arteritis was never detected in the normal areas of the infarcted heart. Therefore, apart from the frequently forgotten block apparatuses,[20,21] which are interpreted as pathological findings, the regressive and reactive or sclerotic vascular changes in the presence of a similar myocardial lesion do not permit the conclusion that intramural ischemia is the cause of the myocardial damage.

Thrombotic Thrombocytopenic Purpura

The typical obstructive vascular lesion present in the Moschcowitz syndrome (so-called thrombotic thrombocytopenic purpura) has its maximum frequency in the intramural myocardial branches. In many instances, it is a widespread lesion involving most of the vessels of the same section (FIGURE 5). The nature of the lesion is debated, despite the fact that it is usually defined as "thrombotic." What is of interest in the present discussion is its severe and widespread stenotic-occlusive character. Moreover, due to the generally rapid and progressive course of the disease, this lesion may be considered as an acute-recent lesion (82% out of 159 cases reported in the literature and 90% of the AFIP cases died within 35 days, 21% and 20%, respectively, within the first week). In relation to the frequency of the myocardial coagulative necrosis, in only 33.3% of the 159 literature cases and in 10.2% of the 39 AFIP cases were there rare, isolated, small foci of an early coagulative necrosis, without any apparent relationship to the occluded arterioles. This was further shown by a serial section study. Finally, it must be remembered that the hemolytic anemia present in these patients, even in the early phase of the disease, results in an extremely marked anemia. An evaluation of the percentage of hemoglobin in these subjects had the following results: In the 159 cases from the literature, 86.2% showed a hemoglobin value below 60% (69.2% below Hb 50%); of the 39 AFIP cases, 82.6% had a hemoglobin value below 60% (71.2% below Hb 50%).

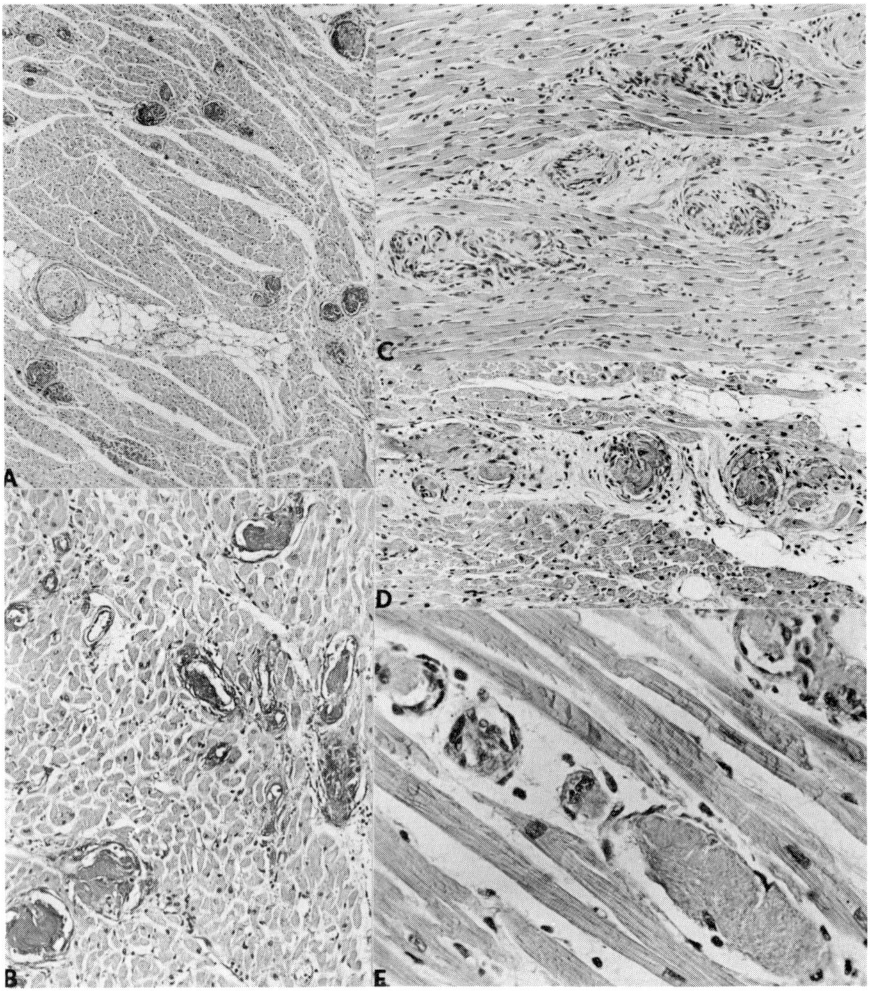

FIGURE 5. Lack of myocardial damage in widespread obstructive lesions of intramural arterioles. Moschcowitz's syndrome (so-called thrombotic thrombocytopenic purpura). (A) AFIP acc. no. 204944. Stain: periodic acid-Schiff. × 30 (orig. mag. × 50). (B) AFIP acc. no. 1088461. Stain: periodic acid-Schiff. × 110 (orig. mag. × 180). (C) AFIP acc. no. 268893. Stain: hematoxylin and eosin. × 110 (orig. mag. × 180). (D) AFIP acc. no. 1105110. Stain: hematoxylin and eosin. × 110 (orig. mag. × 180). (E) AFIP acc. no. 316098. Stain: hematoxylin and eosin. × 330 (orig. mag. × 550).

Discussion

An infarct is defined as "an area of coagulation necrosis in a tissue due to local anemia resulting from obstruction of circulation to the area."[22] The following findings in our study led to the conclusion that only in a few instances could the term "infarct" be accepted in human pathology: (1) the absence of a coronary thrombosis in more than 50% of the cases of acute or recent "infarct" and sudden "coronary" death; (2) sclerotic lumen reduction up to 65% at the site of the thrombosis in most of the remaining cases in which an acute or recent thrombosis was detected; (3) marked enlargement of the normally existing anastomoses, parallel and proportional to progressive, severe obstructive coronary disease; (4) the low incidence of a chronological relation between the thrombosis and the myocardial lesion in the acute-recent "infarct" cases with thrombosis and with a previous lumen reduction of less than 65%. As a rule, in the so-called human myocardial infarct as well as in the so-called sudden "coronary" death, there is no morphological basis consistent with an acute "functioning" occlusion; therefore, the human infarct cannot be compared with an experimental acute occlusion of a normal coronary artery. In fact, either there is no acute occlusion, or the acute occlusion is not coeval with the myocardial lesion, or the acute occlusion cannot be effective since it takes place in a severely stenosed vessel in the presence of a collateral circulation many times greater than the normal condition. The compensatory ability of these anastomotic channels is well demonstrated, not only by numerous experimental studies,§ but generally in the human cases with severe, occlusive coronary disease, with or without minimal, but not proportional, myocardial damage (44% of the "occlusive" cases in the plastic injection study).

As shown in FIGURE 6, when a 60–70% stenosis occurs, a particular hemodynamic situation exists in the rigid, stenosed vessels, characterized by a slowing or blockage of the blood flow due to the reduction of the normal proximal flow and the competing anastomotic distal backflow. Such a hemodynamic condition may explain, at least in part, the occurrence of the thrombosis in these tube-like stenosed vessels, especially when an increase of the peripheral resistance occurs secondary to the stretching of the cardiac wall, as in cardiac insufficiency or extensive necrosis with consequent stasis, edema, and occlusion of the intramural vessels ("avascular area"). Other conditions may aggravate the critical flow in the stenosed vessels, such as a fall in the systemic blood pressure (as in shock), and other cofactors may act with the altered hemodynamic factor in the genesis of the thrombosis in damaging the endothelium of these pathological vessels[23] or in altering the local or general "hemostatic balance"[24,25] between fibrinolytic and thromboplastic substances. An increase of the coagulant activity has been demonstrated when a tissue necrosis in the heart or in other organs takes place[26–28] or in the so-called "emergency reaction."[29] It would seem reasonable, therefore, to consider the eventual thrombosis as secondary to the infarct, bearing in mind that it occurs generally when an extensive, massive coagulative necrosis is present.[9] On the other hand, it may occur in the absence of documented myocardial necrosis by the same mechanism mentioned previously.

In conclusion, the coronary thrombosis, at any level of the coronary tree, does not seem to be responsible for myocardial coagulation necrosis, and sudden "coronary" death. The same conclusion may be drawn with respect to other suggested mechanical obstructions, such as intimal hemorrhage, "rupture" of an

§ Khouri and Gregg demonstrated a rapid collateral response after experimental coronary stenosis (40% flow reduction) which was effective in compensating a further occlusion (personal communication).

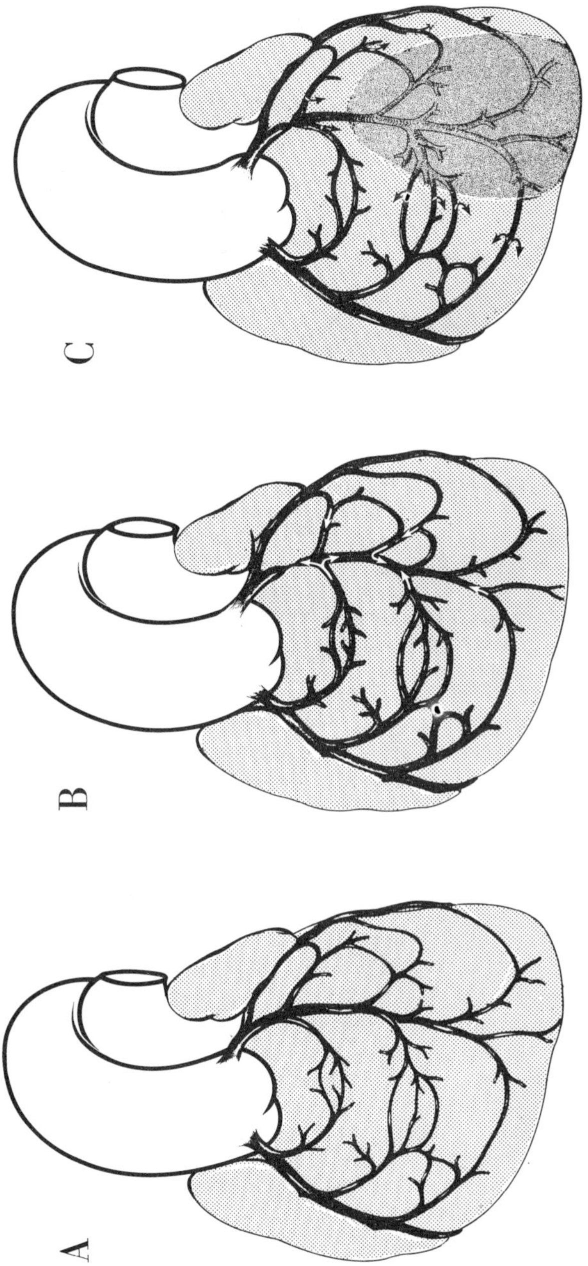

FIGURE 6. Hemodynamic changes in increased peripheral resistance. (A) Normal heart. (B) > 60–70% stenosis. (C) > 60–70% stenosis, and infarct.

atheromatous plaque, and acute edema of the intima. Other causes, such as coronary embolization and coronary dissecting aneurysm, are rare exceptions, and without significance where their incidence in cardiac pathology is concerned. They may, therefore, be overlooked in the present discussion.

In short, at the present stage of our knowledge of human pathology, the term "infarct" will remain incorrect until we are able to prove rather than merely speculate a true occlusive cause. In order to avoid the improper definition of "infarct without occlusion or without acute *'functioning'* occlusion" the human infarct may be classified on a morphological basis, as "idiopathic coagulation necrosis." This definition stresses the obscurity of its pathogenesis, despite the many proposed theories, and emphasizes the typical myocardial lesion, thereby segregating it from other types of cardiac necrosis.

A review of the pertinent literature of the past 60 years reveals general agreement on the finding of myocardial infarct in association with coronary arterio-atherosclerosis. Even recently, a significant correlation between these two patterns has been claimed.[30–34] The presence of a moderate to severe coronary arteriosclerosis in 95.5% of the cases of recent infarct with recent occlusion, and in 93.6% of the cases of recent infarct without occlusion, led to the following statement: "From this finding, it seems inescapable that the problem of myocardial infarction is the problem of coronary arteriosclerosis. . . . The importance of thrombosis as a cause of infarction may seem of less magnitude than has usually been supposed. This would be so, were it not for the evidence . . . that thrombosis is a factor in the inception and progression of the arteriosclerotic lesions and, therefore, a major cause of 95 per cent of the cases of myocardial infarction."[30] This conclusion refers to Rokitansky's encrustation theory of arterio-atherosclerosis. Even in our study, independent of the presence of absence of an acute or recent occlusive thrombosis, in about 90% of both acute-recent myocardial infarct and sudden coronary death cases, a severe stenosing (greater than 65%) or old occlusive coronary arterio-atherosclerosis was found. However, the "inescapability" of a correlation between myocardial infarct and coronary arterio-atherosclerosis is worthy of discussion. In fact, although it may be possible to state that most of the infarct and sudden death heart cases show severe coronary involvement, the reverse is certainly not true: in a high percentage (44%) of cases with severe occlusive coronary arterio-atherosclerosis and 88% of cases with severe stenosis greater than 60%, no proportional myocardial damage was detected, and, in most instances, the cases did not terminate in sudden death. Furthermore, in spite of this relatively low frequency (10%), cardiac infarct and sudden "coronary" death do occur, with or without minimal, but not functionally, stenosing damage to the coronary arteries.

In some geographic pathological studies (e.g. the Roseto community[35] and other racial groups[36,37]), the significant low incidence of the myocardial infarct was concurrent with a nearly equal incidence of arteriosclerotic heart disease when compared with the control groups. Finally, if we accept Rokitansky's theory as the pathogenetic mechanism in the "inception and progression of the arteriosclerotic lesion," it is difficult to accept thrombosis as the major cause of infarction, since the slow progressive thrombotic encrustation is neutralized or counterbalanced by a parallel increase in anastomotic compensation. Bearing in mind this phenomenon and the particular hemodynamic condition leading to it, it seems likely that the high incidence of occlusions in the recurrent infarct (see TABLE 3) is due to the infarct itself, especially in the old plus recent infarct cases. In other words, the infarct can apparently aggravate the coronary damage.

All these considerations seem to justify questions such as whether or not the "cardiac infarct/coronary arterio-atherosclerosis" combination is only a possible association or a true correlation, and, if so, how and at what level does this correlation occur. The reasons mentioned previously at least in part oppose the widespread opinion that the arterio-atherosclerotic heart is characterized by chronic coronary insufficiency as is maintained by those who believe in the complete lack of, or at least disproportionate, anastomotic compensation. On this subject, the lack of significant differences between the occlusive coronary cases in the anastomotic index with and without different myocardial involvement, but with slightly higher values in the recent infarct cases, is worthy of mention.

This and the finding of the myocardial infarct without significant coronary lesions support the concept that the cardiac coagulation necrosis may occur independent, or almost so, of the coronary status. The same conclusion may be drawn in sudden "coronary" heart death, in which both the lack of an effective coronary occlusion and the collateral compensation speak against the "oxygen differential theory,"[38] which is, furthermore, not supported by experimental study.[39]

The ability of the myocardium to resist ischemia or hypoxic conditions, both acute and chronic, is well documented by experimental studies.[40,41] This has also been demonstrated in some human cardiopathies. In addition to occlusive atherosclerotic heart disease without corresponding myocardial damage, cases of bilateral occlusion or severe stenosis of the coronary ostia due to aortitis, generally with marked cardiac hypertrophy,[42,43] and so-called thrombotic thrombocytopenic purpura cases should be recalled. The latter is an impressive example of widespread, severe acute-recent involvement of the intramural coronary arterial tree, combined with a very severe anemia and only relatively few instances[10] of exceptionally rare microfoci of a terminal, early coagulation necrosis of the myocardium. From this point of view, the distinction between "noncoronarogenic" or "primary necroses" and "coronarogenic" necrosis[33] needs further elucidation. "Noncoronarogenic" or "primary necrosis" indicates a process that is secondary to anoxia, anemia, mechanical stress, shock, a metabolic process, hormone action, toxic conditions, or an allergic infectious status. The first four are akin to the coronarogenic necrosis. "Coronarogenic" necrosis, on the other hand, indicates a process in which atherosclerosis is the main predisposing factor on which (a) a functional overstrain of the heart muscle may act; (b) a supervening coronary spasm may act; or (c) a supervening thrombosis may act.[33] Moreover, any classification of cardiac necrosis should take into consideration the different morphological types of myocardial necrosis.[44–55] Certainly it seems reasonable that a different etiopathogenesis or, at least, a different pathogenesis may explain the different morphology.

In conclusion, if we exclude thrombosis as the cause of cardiac infarct and sudden "coronary" death, and consider the arterio-atherosclerotic heart less "ischemic" than generally believed, the roles of a metabolic disturbances at the myocardial level,[54–62] e.g. electrolyte-steroid toxic action or cathecolamine "oxygen-wasting effect," (b) the too often advocated vascular spasm, and (c) the "settling of the blood cell masses"[63,64] or an abnormal hemoglobin-oxygen affinity[65] appear, at present, to be among the most interesting subjects of future investigation with respect to the coronarogenic or noncoronarogenic pathogenesis of the human cardiac infarct.

Summary

The coronary circulation in general and the anastomotic intracardiac coronary circulation in particular have been studied by plastic casts plus myocardial histological examination in 522 normal and pathological hearts. This material includes arterio-atherosclerotic hearts from hospitalized patients and subjects dying from sudden "coronary" heart death. In another 208 cases of acute-recent cardiac infarct in hospitalized patients, and in 241 sudden "coronary" death cases, the frequency of the acute-recent coronary thrombosis in relation to the previous sclerotic lumen reduction and to the age of the myocardial lesion was investigated by histological methods. Finally, in 208 cases of arterio-atherosclerotic coronary disease and in 39 cases of Moschcowitz's syndrome (so-called thrombotic thrombocytopenic purpura), the relationship between the arterial lesions of the intramural coronary branches and the myocardial damage was studied. The following are the main findings:

1. An extensive anastomotic arterial circulation exists in every area of the normal heart.

2. Its enlargement is proportional to the severity of the coronary disease, being maximum in the presence of multiple occlusions and severe stenoses.

3. The "anastomotic reserve" appears capable of compensating for the progressive evolution of the arterio-atherosclerotic coronary disease.

4. The adequate function of this enlarged collateral circulation is demonstrated by the relatively high frequency (44%) of cases with one or more coronary occlusions and stenoses with normal myocardium or with minimal, not proportional, myocardial damage.

5. The myocardial damage is independent of the degree of enlargement of the collateral circulation.

6. No difference exists in the behavior of the anastomotic channels in the two sexes or in "hospitalized" or "sudden death" subjects of different age.

7. In more than 50% of the examined acute-recent infarct and sudden coronary heart death cases, an acute-recent occlusion was not detected.

8. In most of the remaining cases, the acute-recent thrombosis had little if any effect either because it took place in highly stenotic vessels (more than 65%) with enlarged anastomotic circulation, or because the acute-recent thrombosis was not coeval with the myocardial damage.

The high resistance of the heart to ischemia and hypoxic conditions, as shown by experiments and by different patterns of human cardiac pathology (such as in so-called thrombotic thrombocytopenic purpura), has been emphasized, and the association of "coronary arterio-atherosclerosis and myocardial infarct" has been discussed. In 96% of the acute-recent infarct cases and in 98% of the sudden unexpected "coronary" death cases, as well as in 100% of the sudden but not unexpected "coronary" death cases, there is no morphological proof of either an acute occlusion or an acute functioning occlusion. Therefore, not only does the term "infarct" appear incorrect, but the human cardiac infarct cannot be compared to the experimental infarct following acute ligature of a coronary artery. The particular hemodynamic condition existing at the level of the severe stenosis (i.e., slowing or hindrance of the blood flow due to a decrease of the normal proximal flow and an increase in the anastomotic distal flow), either alone or combined with other cofactors, supports the concept that the thrombosis, when present, may be secondary to the infarct. At the present stage of our knowledge, "metabolic disturbances" on the myocardial level, spasm of the coronary vessel, and "settling or aggregation of blood cell masses" seem among those mechanisms worthy of greater discussion in the pathogenesis of the human infarct.

References

1. Cohnheim, J. & A. von Schulthess-Rechberg. 1881. Ueber die Folgen der Kranzarterienverschliessung für das Herz. Virchow. Arch. Path. Anat. **85:** 503–537.
2. Hudson, R. E. B. 1965. Cardiovascular Pathology : 649. Edward Arnold Publ. London, England.
3. Caulfield, J. & B. Klionsky. 1959. Myocardial ischemia and early infarction: an electron microscopy study. Amer. Heart J. **35:** 489–524.
4. Mölbert, E. 1957. Die Herzmuskelzelle nach akuter Oxydationshemmung im elektronenmikroskopischen Bild. Beitr. Path. Anat. **118:** 421–435.
5. Baroldi, G., O. Mantero & G. Scomazzoni. 1954. Su di una nuova metodica di studio del circolo coronarico mediante sostanze plastiche. Policlinico [Prat.] **61:** 745–749.
6. Baroldi, G., O. Mantero & G. Scomazzoni. 1956. The collaterals of the coronary arteries in normal and pathologic hearts. Circ. Res. **4:** 223–229.
7. Baroldi, G. 1962. Histopathological study of the intramural artery vessels in relation to the pathology of extramural coronary arteries and myocardial damage. Cardiologia **41:** 364–380.
8. Baroldi, G. & G. Scomazzoni. 1967. Coronary circulation in the normal and the pathologic heart. U. S. Govt. Printing Office. Washington, D. C.
9. Baroldi, G. 1965. Acute coronary occlusion as a cause of myocardial infarct and sudden coronary heart death. Amer. J. Cardiol. **16:** 859–880.
10. Baroldi, G. & W. C. Manion. 1967. Microcirculatory disturbance and human myocardial infarction. Amer. Heart J. **74:** 173–178.
11. Mallory, G. K., P. D. White & J. Salcedo-Salgar. 1939. The speed of healing of myocardial infarction. A study of the pathologic anatomy in seventy-two cases. Amer. Heart J. **18:** 647–671.
12. Irniger, W. 1963. Histologische Altersbestimmung von Thrombosen und Embolien. Virchow. Arch. Path. Anat. **336:** 220–237.
13. Spalteholz, W. 1924. Die Arterien der Herzwand. Anatomische Untersuchungen an Menschen und Tieren. S. Hirzel. Leipzig, Germany.
14. Fulton, W. F. M. 1964. The dynamic factor in enlargement of coronary arterial anastomoses, and paradoxical changes in the subendocardial plexus. Brit. Heart J. **26:** 39–50.
15. Estes, H. E., M. L. Entman, H. B. Dixon & D. B. Hackel. 1966. The vascular supply of the left ventricular wall. Anatomic observations, plus a hypothesis regarding acute events in coronary artery disease. Amer. Heart J. **71:** 58–67.
16. Mitchell, J. R. A. & C. J. Schwartz. 1963. The relation between myocardial lesions and coronary artery disease. II. A selected group of patients with massive cardiac necrosis or scarring. Brit. Heart J. **25:** 1–24.
17. Anitschkow, N. N., K. G. Wolkoff, E. E. Kikaion & K. M. Pozharisski. 1964. Compensatory adjustments in the structure of coronary arteries of the heart with stenotic atherosclerosis. Circulation **29:** 447–455.
18. Blumgart, H. L., M. J. Schlesinger & D. Davis. 1940. Studies on the relation of the clinical manifestations of angina pectoris, coronary thrombosis and myocardial infarction to the pathologic findings with particular reference to the significance of the collateral circulation. Amer. Heart J. **19:** 1–91.
19. Bloor, C. M. & A. A. Liebow. 1965. Coronary collateral circulation. Amer. J. Cardiol. **16:** 238–252.
20. Zinck, K. H. 1940. Sondervorrichtungen an Kranzgefässen und ihre Beziehungen zu Coronarinfarkt und miliaren Nekrosen. Virchow. Arch. Path. Anat. **305:** 288–297.
21. Bucher, O. 1947. Ueber den Bau der Blutgefässe des menschlichen Herzens. Acta Anat. **3:** 162–189.
22. Dorland, W. A. N. 1954. The American Illustrated Medical Dictionary. : 737. W. B. Saunders Co. Philadelphia, Pa.
23. Engelberg, H. & H. Tanney. 1965. Effects of scarring of the wall on the thrombosis of human blood in vitro. Circulation **32** (Suppl. II, Abstr.)**:** 11.
24. Astrup, T. 1958. The hemostatic balance. Thromb. Diath. Haemorrh. **2:** 347–357.
25. Alexander, B. 1962. Blood coagulation and thrombotic disease. Circulation **25:** 872–884.
26. Myasnikow, A. L., N. N. Kipschidze & E. I. Tchazov. 1961. The experimental induction of myocardial infarction. Amer. Heart J. **61:** 76–80.
27. Brinkhous, K. M. & D. Geratz. 1961. 'Paradoxical' thrombosis and hemorrhage (Penick's syndrome). Some intermediary sequence in its pathogenesis. R. L. MacMillan & J. F. Mustard, Eds. Int. Symp. "Anticoagulants and fibrinolysins' : 28–34. Toronto, Canada.

28. EISENBERG, S. 1966. Blood viscosity and fibrinogen concentration following cerebral infarction. Circulation **33–34** (Suppl. II) : 10–14.
29. SHIMAMOTO, T. 1963. The 'emergency reaction' in thrombogenesis and in atherogenesis. Amer. Heart J. **66:** 572–573.
30. MORE, R. H. & M. D. HAUST. 1961. The role of thrombosis in occlusive disease of coronary arteries. R. L. MacMillan & J. F. Mustard, Eds. Int. Symp. 'Anticoagulants and Fibrinolysins' : 143–153. Toronto, Canada.
31. STRONG, J. P. & H. C. McGILL. 1962. The natural history of coronary atherosclerosis. Amer. J. Path. **40:** 37–49.
32. DAOUD, A. S., R. A. FLORENTIN & F. GOODALE. 1964. Diffuse coronary arteriosclerosis versus isolated plaques in the etiology of myocardial infarction. Amer. J. Cardiol. **14:** 69–74.
33. MYASNIKOV, A. L. 1964. Myocardial necroses of coronary and non coronary genesis. Amer. J. Cardiol. **13:** 435–440.
34. LIEBOW, I. M., G. E. BARTSCH & W. J. INSULL. 1965. Diffuse coronary arteriosclerosis infarction to severity of coronary atherosclerosis in the young male. Amer. Heart J. **70:** 54–58.
35. STOUT, C., J. MORROW, E. N. BRANDT & S. WOLF. 1964. Unusually low incidence of death from myocardial infarction. J.A.M.A. **188:** 845–849.
36. GILLMAN, J., C. GILBERT & M. D. PRATES. 1960. Patterns of reaction in the coronary artery of the Portuguese East African with special reference to age. S. Afr. J. Med. Sci. **25:** 47–58.
37. LEE, K. T., F. GOODALE, R. F. SCOTT & E. S. SNELL. 1964. Geographic pathology of myocardial infarction. III. Myocardial infarction in Africans in Africa and Negroes and White in United States. Amer. J. Cardiol. **13:** 30–40.
38. BECK, C. S. 1958. Coronary heart disease. An evaluation and criticism of present day concepts. Amer. J. Cardiol. **1:** 547–552.
39. BADEER, H. S. 1966. Present status of the concept of oxygen differential in the etiology of ventricular fibrillation after coronary occlusion. Amer. Heart J. **72:** 238–241.
40. COFFMAN, J. D., F. B. LEWIS & D. E. GREGG. 1960. Effect of prolonged periods of anoxia on atrioventricular conduction and cardiac muscle. Circ. Res. **8:** 649–659.
41. CORDAY, E., H. C. BERGMAN, L. L. SCHWARTZ, R. J. SPRITZLER & M. PRINZMETAL. 1949. Studies on the coronary circulation. IV. The effect of shock on the heart and its treatment. Amer. Heart J. **37:** 560–581.
42. REDWITZ, E. 1909. Der Einfluss der Erkrankungen der Koronararterien auf die Herzmuskulatur mit besonderer Berücksichtigung der chronischen Aortitis. Virchow. Arch. Path. Anat. **197:** 433–472.
43. SCHARFMAN, W. B., J. B. WALLACH & A. ANGRIST. 1950. Myocardial infarction due to syphilitic coronary ostial stenosis. Amer. Heart J. **40:** 603–613.
44. SCHLESINGER, M. J. & L. REINER. 1955. Focal myocytolysis of the heart. Amer. J. Path. **31:** 443–459.
45. SARAM, M. 1957. Ueber die azelluläre Entstehung von Narben bei Durchblutungstörungen im Herzmuskel. Beitr. Path. Anat. **118:** 275–291.
46. BAJUSZ, E. & G. JASMIN. 1965. Observations on histochemical differential diagnosis between primary and secondary cardiomyopathies. Amer. Heart J. **69:** 83–92.
47. RONA, G., D. S. KAHN & C. I. CHAPEL. 1961. Study on the healing of cardiac necrosis in the rat. Amer. J. Path. **39:** 473–489.
48. MARTIN, A. M., D. B. HACKEL & S. M. KURTZ. 1964. The ultrastructure of zonal lesions of the myocardium in hemorrhagic shock. Amer. J. Path. **44:** 127–140.
49. FERRANS, V. J., R. G. HIBBS, W. C. BLACK & D. G. WEILBAECHER. 1964. Isoproterenol-induced myocardial necrosis. A histochemical and electron microscopic study. Amer. Heart J. **68:** 11–90.
50. MOLNAR, Z., K. LARSEN & B. SPARGO. 1962. Cardiac changes in the potassium-depleted rat. Arch. Path. (Chicago) **74:** 339–347.
51. KORB, G. & V. TOTOVIC. 1963. Licht- und fluorescenzmikroskopische Befunde am Herzmuskel nach einer akuten, kurzfrüstigen Koronarinsuffizienz. Virchow. Arch. Path. Anat. **336:** 475–484.
52. CORREA, P., C. RESTREPO, C. GARCIA & A. QUIROZ. 1963. Pathology of heart diseases of undetermined etiology which occur in Cali, California. Amer. Heart J. **66:** 584–596.
53. JENNINGS, R. B., J. P. KALTENBACH & G. W. SMETTERS. 1957. Enzymatic changes in acute myocardial ischemic injury. Arch. Path. (Chicago) **64:** 10–16.
54. SELYE, H. 1958. The Chemical Prevention of Cardiac Necrosis. The Ronald Press Co. New York, N. Y.

55. RONA, G., C. I. CHAPPEL, T. BALZARS & R. GAUDRY. 1959. An infarct-like myocardial lesion and other toxic manifestations produced by isoproterenol in the rat. Arch. Path. (Chicago) **67:** 443–455.
56. RONA, G., D. S. KAHN & C. I. CHAPPEL. 1963. Studies on infarct-like myocardial necrosis produced by isoproterenol: A review. Rev. Canad. Biol. **22:** 241–255.
57. RAAB, W. 1960. Key position of catecholamines in functional and degenerative cardiovascular pathology. Amer. J. Cardiol. **5:** 571–578.
58. RAAB, W. 1963. Neurogenic multifocal destruction of myocardial tissue. (Pathogenic mechanism and its prevention). Rev. Canad. Biol. **22:** 217–239.
59. RAAB, W., J. P. CHAPLIN & E. BAJUSZ. 1964. Myocardial necroses produced in domesticated rats in wild rats by sensory and emotional stresses. Proc. Soc. Exp. Biol. Med. **116:** 665–669.
60. BAJUSZ, E. & G. JASMIN. 1963. Comparative morphogenesis and enzyme histogenesis of some occlusive and metabolic cardiac necroses. Rev. Canad. Biol. **22:** 181–199.
61. SHIMAMOTO, T., T. FUJITA, H. SHIMURA, H. YAMAZAKI, S. IWAHARA & G. YAJIMA. 1959. Myocardial infarct-like lesions and arteriosclerosis induced by high molecular substances and prevention by magnesium salt. Amer. Heart J. **57:** 273–288.
62. HANDFORTH, C. P. 1962. Isoproterenol-induced myocardial infarction in animals. Arch. Path. (Chicago) **73:** 161–165.
63. KNISELY, M. H. 1963. The settling of blood cell masses to the lower sides of vessels during life and the probable significance. *In* The Etiology of Myocardial Infarction. : 557–585. Little, Brown & Co. Boston, Mass.
64. LONG, D. M., M. W. MYER, E. B. BROWN & C. W. LILLEHEI. 1962. Myocardial necrosis and electrocardiographic changes related to microcirculatory abnormalities. Amer. J. Cardiol. **10:** 695–705.
65. ELIOT, R. S. & H. MIZUKAMI. 1966. Oxygen affinity of hemoglobin in persons with acute myocardial infarction and in smokers. Circulation **34:** 331–336.

A DISTINCTIVE MYOCARDIOPATHY OCCURRING IN OMAHA, NEBRASKA: CLINICAL ASPECTS

James F. Sullivan, John D. Egan, and Ralph P. George

Department of Medicine of Creighton University School of Medicine and Medical Service of the Veterans Administration Hospital Omaha, Neb.

During a 20-month period, extending from December, 1964, to July, 1966, 64 patients with primary myocardial disease of uncertain etiology were seen in three hospitals in the city of Omaha. The only recognized factor of possible pathogenetic significance common to all was the excessive ingestion of alcoholic beverages, particularly beer. Of the 64, 30 died; autopsy was performed on 26 and revealed similar myocardial pathology in each case.

An epidemic of cardiac decompensation, also associated with beer drinking, was recently described in Québec, Canada. The Omaha and Ouébec patients appear to be quite similar in clinical aspects and pathology.[1] This report is concerned primarily with the epidemiological and clinical features of the entity observed.

Epidemiological Factors

Hospitals. All patients were seen in one of three hospitals. The number in each and other statistics pertinent to the hospital are shown in TABLE 1. In 1963, in the same three hospitals, only eight cases of primary myocardial disease were observed in which alcohol ingestion could be incriminated. The predominance of involvement in caucasians is in striking contradistinction to most series of alcoholic myocardopathy described in the United States.[2-4] It is also noteworthy that the Douglas County Hospital (DCH), which receives the majority of skid row alcoholics, had few cases of myocardial disease.

Observers. When the diagnosis rested on clinical grounds alone, with relatively few exceptions, the patients were seen by one or both of the senior investigators. It is of intreest that recognition at autopsy occurred at St. Joseph's Hospital (SJH) prior to clinical recognition. The simultaneous occurrence of the entity in the Veterans Administration Hospital (VAH) and SJH was initially unknown to either pathologists or clinicians. The specific combination of clinical, laboratory, and pathological findings to be described were not recognized by the same clinicians or pathologists working in the same hospitals prior to December, 1964.

Geographical Location. Of the 64 patients, 54 resided within the city of Omaha. Of the 38 patients at the VAH, 27 lived within Omaha. The nine veterans and one private patient living outside Omaha resided in the adjoining areas of Nebraska or Iowa. FIGURES 1 and 2 show the localization of cases in the general area involved and in the city of Omaha. In Omaha, there was a rough correlation of geographical location of cases with lower socio-economic status, high rate of alcoholism, and number of retail liquor outlets.

Since approximately 50% of the patients in the VAH reside in Omaha, some predilection for the Omaha area is demonstrated by the fact that the Omaha population makes up 76% of the VAH myocardopathy patients. Nevertheless, the geographical localization of the patients is not sharp.

Seasonal Incidence. The initial cases were noted during December, 1964, in SJH and the VAH; a sharp increase during May and June of 1965 and of 1966 was noted. As shown in FIGURE 3, no further cases have been seen since early

TABLE 1

RACE AND SEX OF MYOCARDIOPATHY PATIENTS IN THREE HOSPITALS

Hospital	Patients Discharged per year	Caucasian Patients	Myocardiopathy Patients	
			Male	Female
Saint Joseph's	12,528	94%	14	8
Veterans Administration	5,389	93%	38	0
Douglas County				
Medical-Surgical	2,534	78%	3	1
Psychiatric	1,820	78%		

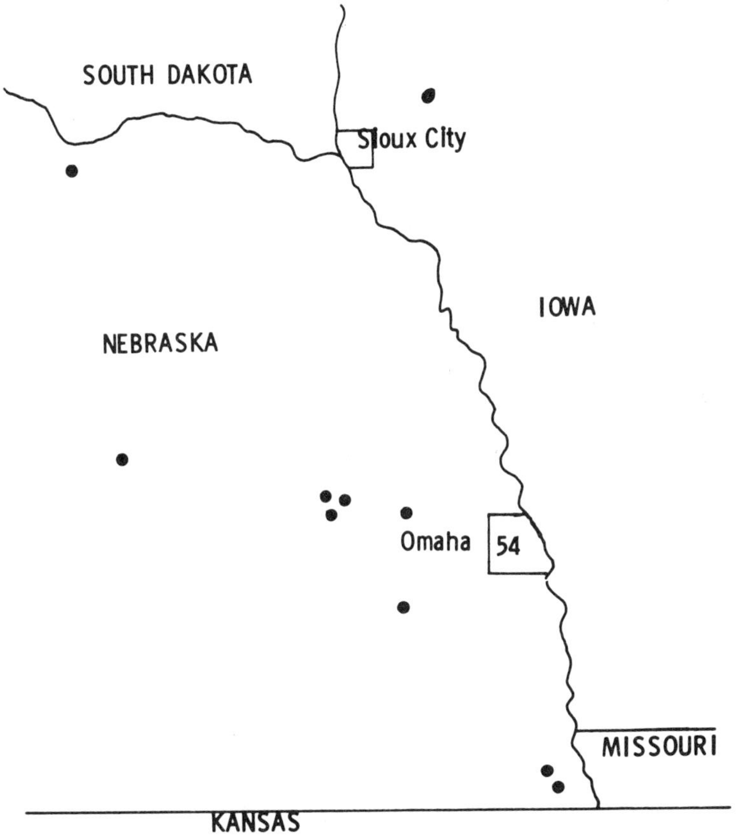

FIGURE 1. Location of cases in three-state area.

in July, 1966. The peculiar seasonal incidence is as yet unexplained. The recognized effect of elevated temperature in precipitating the appearance of beriberi heart disease may be pertinent.[5]

Patients. The age distribution of the patients is shown in FIGURE 4. The highest incidence occurred in the fifth decade of life; 23 were between 40 and 44 years of age and 45 between the ages of 35 and 49. During the same time period, in one hospital (VAH) the diagnosis of myćardial infarction was made in 220 patients. Mycardial infarction was considered to be the cause of death in 37% of these. The comparative prevalence and mortality of the described primary mycardial entity to that of coronary artery disease in this all-male population indicate its severity.

CLINICAL FACTORS

Clinical Appearance

The typical patient presented with dyspnea, abdominal pain, and edema, all of the relatively brief duration of one to two weeks. Blood pressure and pulse pressure were low, tachycardia with regular rhythm and a protodiastolic gallop

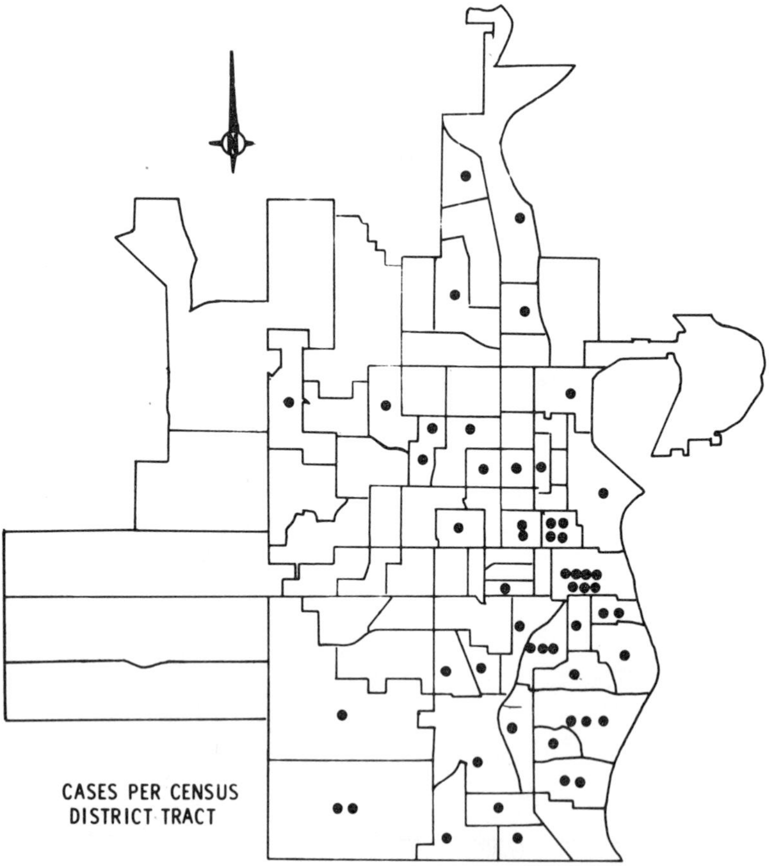

FIGURE 2. Location of cases within Omaha.

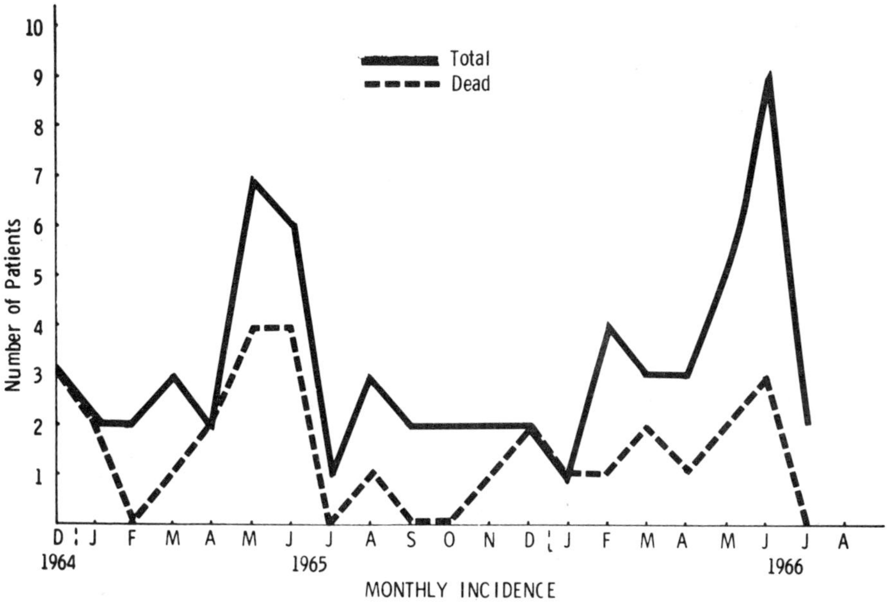

FIGURE 3. Incidence of cases per month.

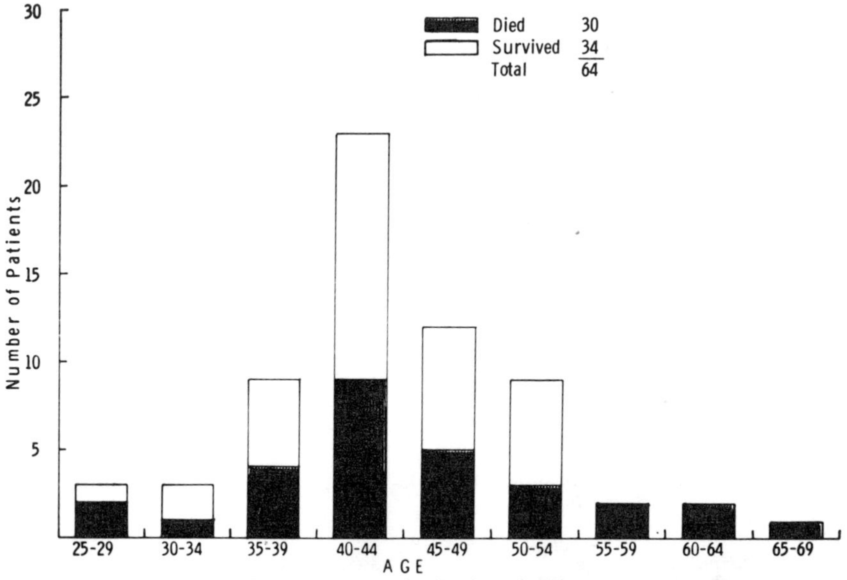

FIGURE 4. Age distribution of patients.

were present, extreme cardiomegaly with globular and configuration was common, and a peripheral cyanosis was often noted. Venous distention was marked, and hepatic enlargement with tenderness sufficient to suggest a "surgical abdomen" occurred. A detailed enumeration of symptoms and physical findings is shown in TABLES 2 and 3.

These clinical characteristics taken individually are not unusual in congestive heart failure, the absence of prior cardiac symptoms and the brief duration of illness, in addition to abdominal pain as a presenting symptom, were unusual. The predominance of signs of right-sided failure with massive cardiomegaly led to the consideration of pericardial tamponade and pulmonary embolization in the differential diagnosis. The peculiar swarthy or earthy skin color, combined with peripheral cyanosis and hepatic tenderness, was distinctive. The total constellation of symptoms and signs with the absence of other cardiac disease, rather than any one finding, led to rapid recognition of the condition after the first few cases were seen.

The findings on x-ray examination of the chest are summarized in TABLE 4. Cardiac enlargement was universally present. A globular configuration of the heart was common, suggesting pericardial effusion. Pericardial fluid was demonstrated in nine cases, in five of which it was grossly bloody. The removal of pericardial fluid consistently failed to produce a beneficial hemodynamic change. Pleural effusion was also relatively common, being present in 20 cases.

The electrocardiographic abnormalities are listed in TABLE 5. The combina-

TABLE 2

FREQUENCY OF MAJOR SYMPTOMS ON ADMISSION

Symptom	Frequency (%)*
Dyspnea	87
Weakness-fatigue	45
Abdominal pain	31
Edema	40
Nausea-vomiting	20
Chest pain	19
Cough	16
Hemoptysis	4

* Total number of patients = 64.

TABLE 3

FREQUENCY OF SIGNIFICANT ABNORMALITIES ON PHYSICAL EXAMINATION

Physical Finding	Frequency (%)*
Cardiomegaly	98
Hepatomegaly	88
Sinus tachycardia (greater than 100 beats/min)	70
Venous distention	87
Diastolic gallop	76
Edema	62
Hypotension (systolic pressure less than 90)	41
Cyanosis	25
Rales in chest	41
Paradoxical pulse	17

* Total number of patients = 64.

TABLE 4

CHARACTERISTIC FINDINGS ON CHEST X-RAYS

Findings	Frequency (%)*	
	Dead	Survivors
Cardiomegaly (generalized)	86	85
Cardiomegaly (left ventricular)	14	12
Pleural Effusion	36	12
Pulmonary vascular congestion	7	6

* A total of 62 films were reviewed: 34 from survivors and 28 from patients who died.

TABLE 5

ABNORMALITIES OF THE ELECTROCARDIOGRAMS

Abnormality	Frequency (%)*
Low voltage	59
P wave (atrial enlargement)	65
T wave, flat, cloven, inverted	49
Right axis deviation or incomplete right bundle-branch block	54
P. V. C. (frequent)	6
Supraventricular tachycardia with block	6
Left ventricular hypertrophy	3

* A total of 61 electrocardiograms were reviewed.

tion of tachycardia, low voltage, and right axis deviation or a right bundle-branch block was important in diagnosis. The comparative absence of left ventricular hypertrophy and of arrhythmias is again in contradistinction to the electrocardiograms described in other series of alcoholic myocardopathy.[6,7]

A wide variety of metabolic abnormalities were demonstrable. Among the most striking of these were the elevations of serum enzymes shown in FIGURE 5. Further study of lactic acid dehydrogenase levels indicated that the very striking elevations, those over 1,000 units, were usually of hepatic origin. In general, there was a more grave prognosis with the most extreme elevations. A second striking abnormality, that of pH and lactate accumulation, is demonstrated in FIGURE 6; the prognostic significance is clearly evident. The acidosis, lactic acid accumulation, and enzyme elevation tended to occur in the same patient and to show a correlation in degree of severity. FIGURE 7 shows the overall serum electrolyte pattern found in the patients in conjunction with blood urea nitrogen levels and the pH. The relative roles of azotemia and lactic acid accumulation in the acidosis are of particular interest.

A significant degree of hepatic dysfunction, most clearly evidenced by bilirubin retention, was encountered. This was accompanied by a definite increase in the hematocrit. These values, together with that of the serum albumin, are shown in FIGURE 8. Measurements of red cell volume and plasma volume indicated that the hematrocrit values represented a true erythrocytosis.

Additional laboratory examinations were, for the most part, less revealing. Serum iron determinations were at the lower limit of normal, (70–85 μg/100 ml), which is somewhat surprising in view of the elevated hematocrit and hepatic necrosis. Protein-bound iodine was within normal limits, and uric acid was elevated in only one patient. In one patient, an elevated serum amylase (640 Somogyi units) was noted, but pancreatitis was not present at autopsy. In 50%

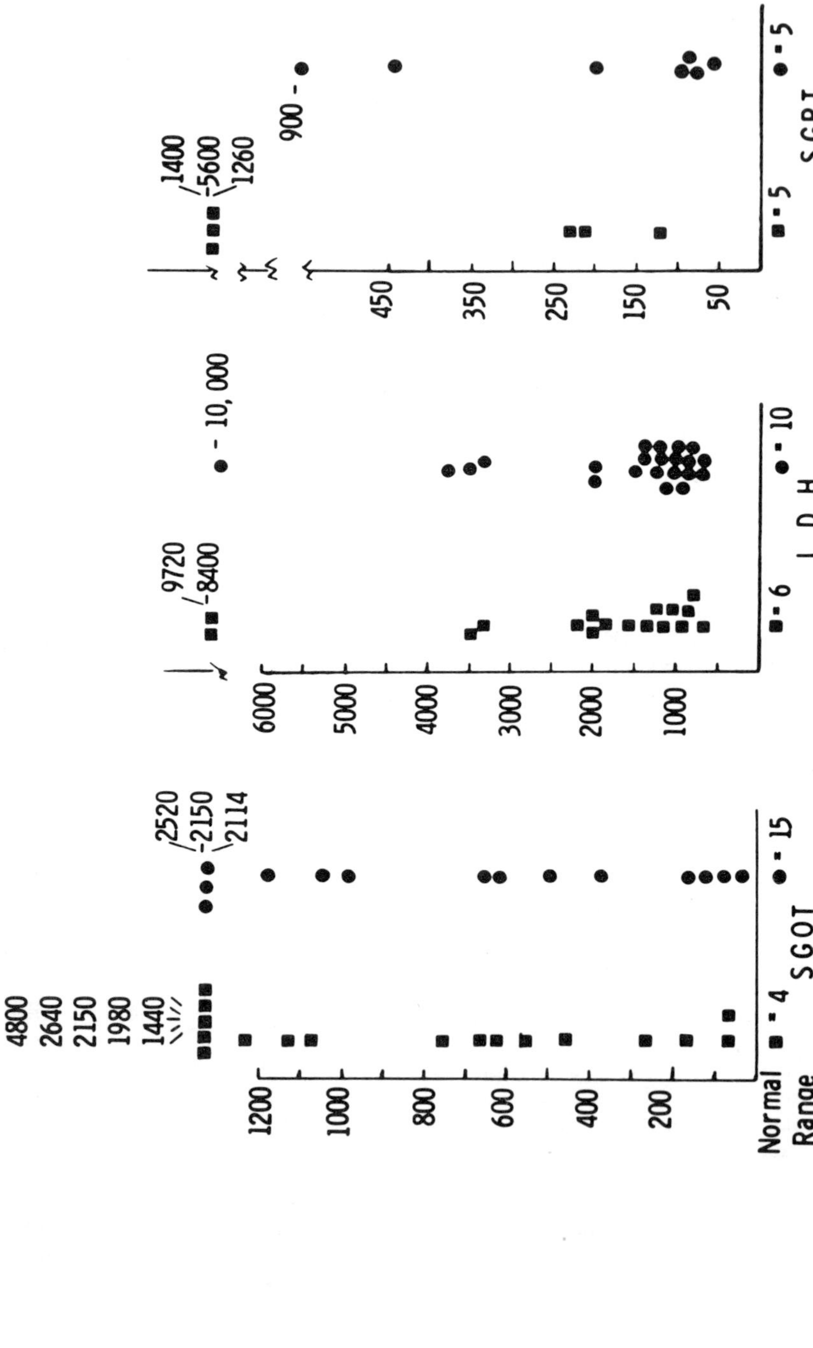

FIGURE 5. Serum enzyme values in patients. SGOT = serum glutamic oxalactetic transaminase; SGPT = serum glutamic pyruvic transaminase; LDH = lactic acid dehydrogenase. ■ = dead; ● = survivors.

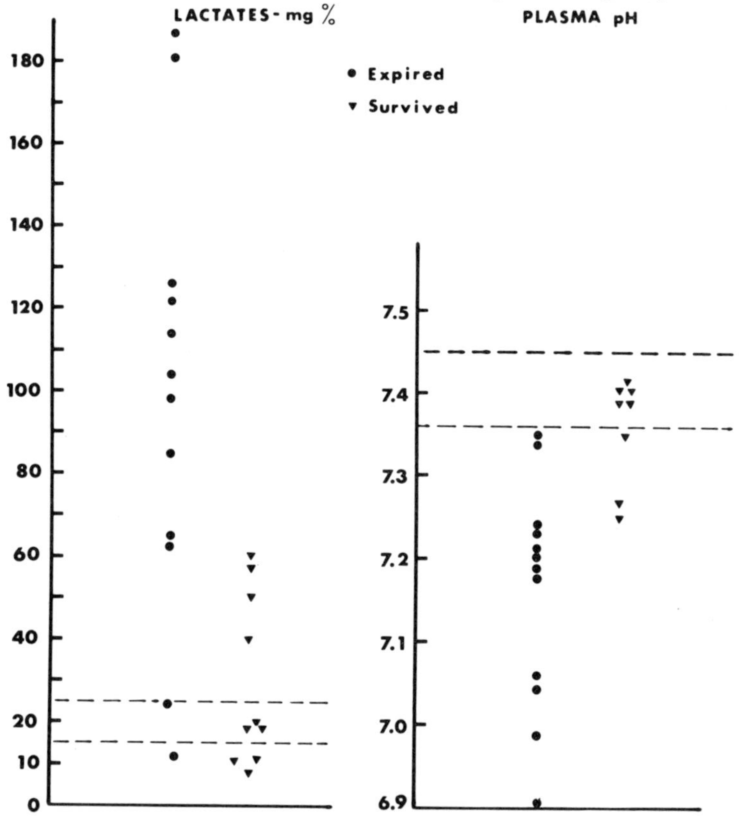

FIGURE 6. Plasma lactate and pH in patients.

of the patients, the prothrombin time was prolonged to greater than five seconds over the normal value. All alkaline phosphatase determinations were normal or slightly elevated. Serum cholesterol values were within normal limits, but seemed lower than might be expected in a predominantly male population in the stated age range.

Mild elevation of the fasting blood sugar was found in four of the patients. The only significant finding on urinalysis was proteinuria, found on admission in 50% of the patients. However, oliguria was frequent, and, when progressive, usually mirrored a failure in response to therapy, with eventual demise. There was a close correlation between diminished urine output and elevated blood urea nitrogen.

A serum triglyceride level greater than 120 mg/100 ml was found in only one subject; however, free fatty acid concentrations greater than 700 μEq occurred in six of the nine patients studied. In these nine patients, the last patients studied, other measurements were made which, although few in number will be mentioned. Serum cortisol was elevated in two of the eight tested, aldosterone excretion was normal in two, and catecholamine excretion was elevated in one of three. In six subjects, the 17-ketosteroid excretion was low (3–9 mg/24 hours), whereas the 17-ketogenic steroid excretion was within normal limits. Creatine phosphokinase was determined in only four patients and was normal in each. Serum calcium and phosphorous values were not remarkable.

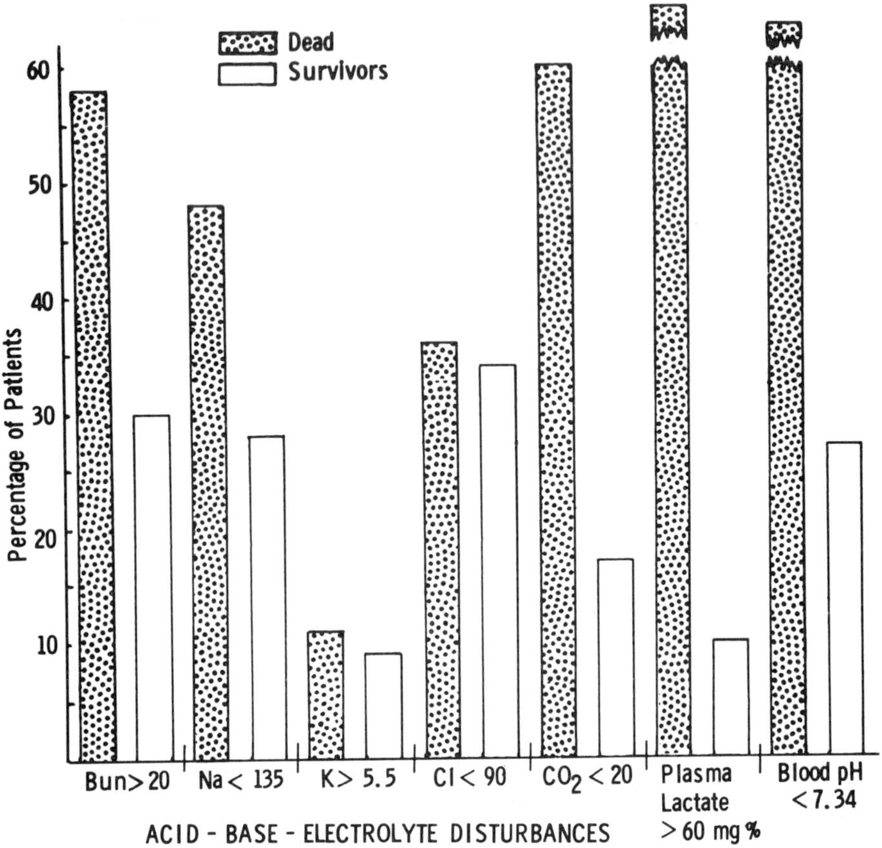

FIGURE 7. Incidence of acid-base abnormalities.

Although each of the metabolic derangements evaluated were more frequently abnormal in the group with fatal outcome, the degree of acidosis, jaundice, and impaired urea clearance had the gravest prognostic import. The rapid onset of severe cardiac failure, frequency of abdominal pain, massive cardiac enlargement, distinctive electrocardiogram without rhythm disturbance, and the unusual degree of acidosis, enzyme elevation, and hepatic dysfunction allowed decisive recognition by clinical evaluation.

Course of Disease

Of the 64 patients, 30 died. The fulminating nature of the disease is apparent from the fact that eight of the 30 died within 72 hours of admission. Vigorous therapy for congestive heart failure was carried out in each case. Acidosis, when severe, was treated by means of bicarbonate infusion, despite the presence of edema. Improvement in the respiratory distress, although transient, was noted in all patients in whom bicarbonate infusion was used. Patients surviving over 24 hours received thiamine parenterally. No dramatic response was noted in any

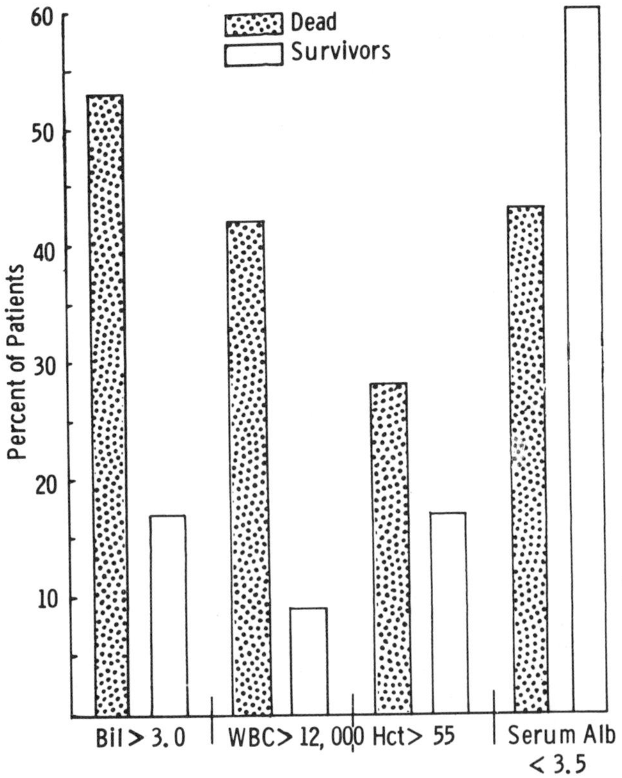

FIGURE 8. Incidence of jaundice, leukocytosis, increased hematocrit, and low serum albumin.

case. Adrenal corticosteroids were used in a few cases and also appeared to have no beneficial effect. Vasopressors were not effective in treating the hypotension, and, in fact, were suspected of causing actual clinical deterioration.

Azotemia or oliguria, or both, were frequently noted, particularly in the fatal cases. These were probably due to circulatory renal insufficiency; however, primary renal involvement has not been excluded. Most of the 36 survivors responded initially, in a satisfactory manner, to digitalis, low-salt diet, diuretics, and bed rest, in addition to thiamine. The response to phlebotomy, with the exception of one case, was generally unimpressive.

As noted previously, pulmonary embolization and pericardial tamponade were difficult diagnoses to exclude. Pericardiectomy, which was carried out in four cases because of suspected pericardial tamponade, was followed by the demise of the patient within 48 hours. One case in which a thrombus was removed by pulmonary embolectomy also died within several hour following surgery.

Although it is difficult to evaluate such things, it is our opinion that the recovering patients responded relatively slowly to therapy. Tachycardia on exercise was readily demonstrable for periods of two to three months. What pattern of cardiac function the recovered patients will eventually manifest is of great importance, particularly in establishing the relationship of this series to other cases of alcoholic myocardopathy previously described.

Pathogenesis

In the consideration of etiology and pathogenesis of the series described, it must be stressed that neither clinical nor pathological study revealed commonly recognized causes of heart failure. Coronary artery disease, hypertension, and rheumatic or congenital forms of heart disease were not found, nor were there signs of involvement of the heart in amyloidosis, collagen disease, or hemachromatosis.

Alcohol assumes a significant etiological role in descriptions of primary myocardial disease.[8-10] The diagnostic criteria for alcoholic myocardopathy vary,[11-13] and with the exception of beriberi, myocardial injury associated with alcohol is poorly understood. The frequency of alcohol ingestion, particularly beer, in the histories of our patients was impressive.

Estimated Alcohol Consumption

Estimation of alcohol consumption is notoriously invalid. In our study, we were aided by social workers who attempted to contact and correlate such information from two or three relatives or fellow workers of each patient. This estimate is shown in FIGURE 9. The average consumption of beer was about a dozen 12-ounce bottles per day for ten to 12 years. The correlation with amount or duration of drinking was not striking, although in general the highest mortality occurred in those with the greatest consumption. Approximately one-third of the patients drank other alcoholic beverages in addition to beer. This amount of alcohol is certainly immoderate; however, in our opinion, it is distinctly less than that of the cirrhotic population of the same hospitals. Seven of the 64 patients had been previously hospitalized on one occasion for the treatment of acute alcoholism.

As in the Québec series,[14] we found that one brand of beer was particularly favored by our patients. Our inability to obtain accurate historical information in some cases makes it impossible to determine exactly the predominance of this brand among our patients.

Nutritional and Deficiency Factors

In 60% of our patients, a definite history of weight loss, anorexia, and occasional vomiting and diarrhea preceded the onset of cardiac symptoms by two to six months. The weight loss ranged up to 35 lb.

Magnesium deficiency, often found in alcoholism,[15,16] was not demonstrable in our subjects. TABLE 6 gives the serum magnesium levels and urinary secretion in the last eight patients seen.

FIGURE 10 demonstrates the abnormalities of thiamine activity found. Thiamine measurements were made by the red cell transketolase method of Brin and his co-workers[17] and showed definite deficiency in eight of ten patients tested. Measurements were not performed in the others or were invalid because of prior therapy.

Abnormalities of zinc metabolism, i.e., depressed levels of zinc in the plasma and greatly increased urinary zinc excretion, previously described in alcoholic subjects, were also found. The values shown in TABLE 7 represent some of the greatest deviations from normal that we have ever encountered.

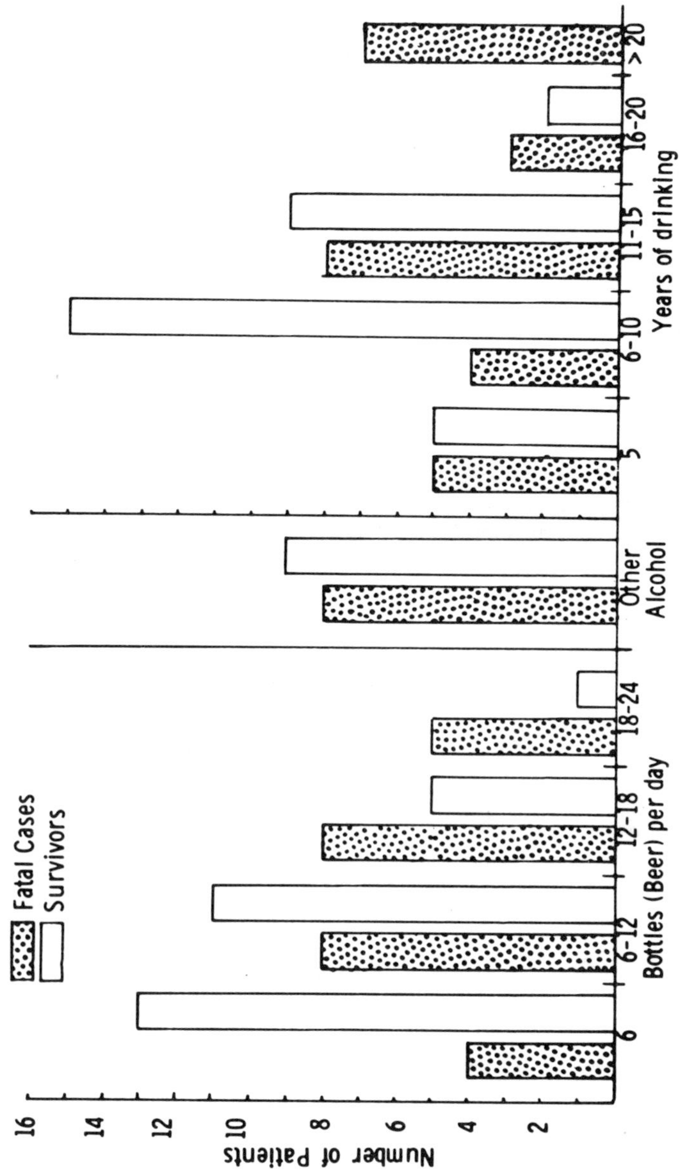

FIGURE 9. Estimated alcohol consumption in amount and duration.

TABLE 6

MAGNESIUM EXCRETION

	Serum (mg/%)*	Urine (mg/24 hr)
Normal	2.10 ± 10	60–120
L.M.	2.75	89.7
C.R.	1.93	135.4
K.R.	1.84	101.8
F.C.	1.43	125.4
A.L.	2.24	140.5
L.C.	2.19	35.5
F.H.		132.2
S.G.	2.42	35.8

* Serum values are measured in mg % or mg/100 ml.

Viral Studies

Acute and convalescent sera were examined for a rise in titer to various influenza strains in the Virology Laboratory of St. Louis University, St. Louis, Mo., through the courtesy of Dr. Goronwy O. Broun, Sr. In only one of five patients was an appreciable change in influenza antibodies noted. Injection of blood from two patients into suckling mice failed to reveal evidence of Coxsackie virus infection. We feel that these infectious agents are excluded as etiological possibilities.

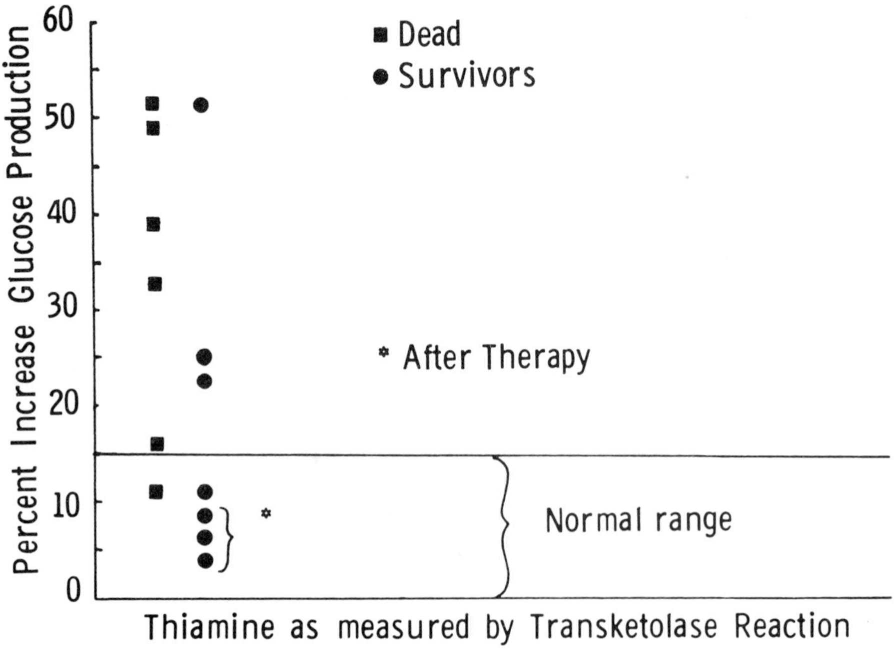

FIGURE 10. Thiamine deficiency in patients based on red cell transketolase.

TABLE 7

ZINC EXCRETION

	Serum (μg %)*	Urine (μg/24 hr)
Normal	90 ± 10	300–700
L.M.	77.0	943
C.R.	58.0	1,572
K.R.	58.6	1,332
F.C.	48.4	4,180
A.L.	79.0	1,637
L.C.	56.8	8,485
F.H.		5,313
S.G.	68.4	723
S.C.	65.4	

* Serum values are expressed in μg% or μg/100 ml.

TABLE 8

OCCUPATION OF PATIENTS ON ADMISSION

Occupation	No. of Patients
Laborer	14
Skilled trade	12
Cook-bartender	9
Unemployed	7
Housewife	6
Mechanic	6
Clerk	4
Truck driver	4
Salesman	2

Occupation

The occupation and employment of the patients at the time of admission is shown in TABLE 8. Only seven of the 64 were unemployed prior to their illness, indicating the infrequency of the deteriorated alcoholic in this series.

Beer Additives

One of the most challenging and perplexing factors common to the Québec and Omaha cases was the presence of cobalt as an additive in the beers primarily involved.[14] The chronological relation of the use of cobalt in beer to the appearance and at least temporary disappearance of the syndrome appears in FIGURE 11.

The quantitative urinary determinations of cobalt in the urine of the last few patients is shown in TABLE 9. The urinary excretion of cobalt in normal subjects is too small to be measured by atomic absorption spectrophotometry (detection to 0.004 ppm) in our laboratory. Little is known of cobalt metabolism or its urinary excretion, and the significance of the markedly abnormal cobalt excretion is uncertain at this time.

The time relationship between the addition of cobalt to beer and the appearance of the disease is slightly different in the two areas. The disease appeared in Québec shortly after initiation of its usage and disappeared abruptly with its cessation. In Omaha, a greater time-span intervened between the introduction of cobalt and the recognition of the disease. It may be of significance, in this regard, that the amount of beer consumed by the Canadian patients was much greater.[14]

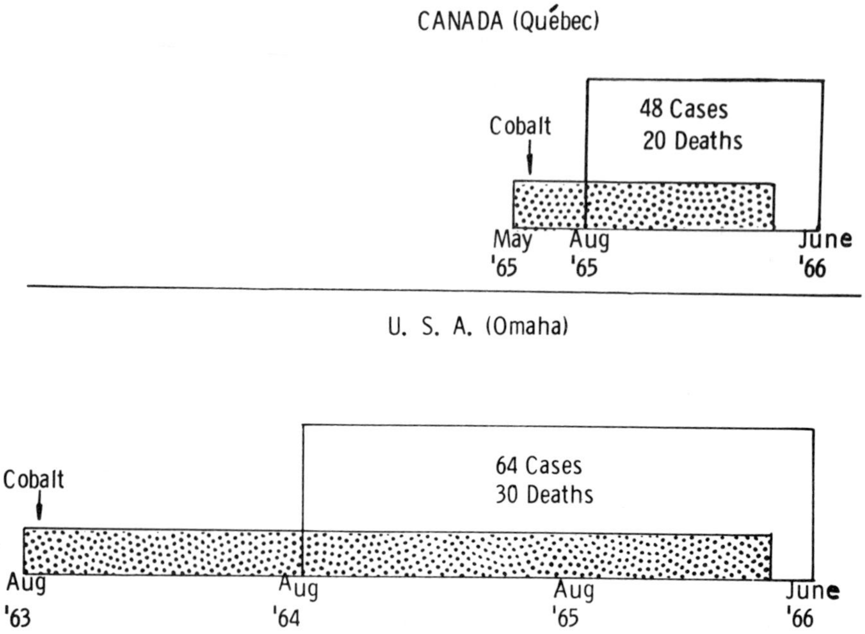

FIGURE 11. Correlation of disease with cobalt usage in the United States and Canada.

TABLE 9
URINARY COBALT EXCRETION IN MYOCARDOSIS PATIENTS

Patient	Urine Volume (ml/24 hr)	Cobalt (μg/24 hr)
L.M.	2430	143.0
C.R.	3630	72.0
K.R.	1850	48.0
F.C.	760	141.0
A.L.	4390	535.0
L.C.	1045	200.0
S.G.	840	211.0
Lue	1580	34.0

The cobalt content of the beer in Omaha was 1.1–1.2 ppm. The disease has not been seen following the removal of the cobalt from the beer. This time interval now measures six months.

DISCUSSION

The inability to define an etiological agent by clinical or laboratory examination, plus the absence of such an agent in the pathology of the myocardium, justifies a designation of idiopathic primary myocardial disease in this series. The rather striking correlation with copious alcohol ingestion and the absence of the disease entity in those not ingesting alcoholic beverages implied that these beverages might have significant pathogenetic influence.

Despite the extensive literature linking myocardial disease to alcohol ingestion, some difficulty was encountered in identifying these cases with previous description of alcoholic myocardopathy.[4-11] Among the factors that differentiated our patients were the lack of chronicity, high mortality, episodic nature, predominance of the caucasion race, beer as the primary beverage ingested, clinical aspects resembling acute right-heart failure with relative infrequency of left ventricular hypertrophy, and cardiac arrhythmias.

There are, however, striking similarities to the clinical picture in cases of beriberi heart disease described by Aalsmeer and Wenckebach,[18] as well as those of Benchimol and Schlesinger,[19] and to Shoshin beriberi.[20] Among the larger series of primary myocardial disease, that of Massumi and co-workers[21] seems to contain a significant number of cases quite similar to ours.

If the entity is considered clinically as an acute fulminating form of beriberi, several major problems are encountered. The criteria of Blankenhorn[22] for the diagnosis of beriberi heart disease, i.e., the presence of neuritis or pellagra, dependent edema, three months of inadequate diet, and response to thiamine, could not be consistently demonstrated. More disturbing to the beriberi concept is the high mortality, despite the use of parenteral thiamine, and the failure to demonstrate convincingly a brisk clinical response to thiamine, such as described by Akbarian and his associates in their meticulous study of beriberi heart disease.[23]

Only one case had definite vitamin B deficiency neuropathy (Wernicke's syndrome) in addition to myocardial failure. This seems unusual, although a relative lack of neuropathy when myocardopathy is present is well known in beriberi.[24]

Thiamine measurements by the red cell transketolase method give reasonable evidence that thiamine deficiency was present in our patients. However, similar levels of altered red cell transketolase have been described with little or no symptomatology,[25,26] and we have found similar deficiencies in alcoholic patients without neuropathy or myocardopathy.[27]

We are also impressed with the degree and frequency of acute hepatic dysfunction and the centrilobular hepatic necrosis that accompanied it. Acute beriberi heart disease has not previously been associated with such striking hepatic involvement.[28]

A major problem is the relationship of the beer additive, cobalt, to the disease entity. The most suggestive evidence of a cause-effect relationship between the two is chronological: the appearance of the disease immediately after cobalt usage and, more strikingly, the apparent abrupt cessation of the disease following the discontinuation of cobalt usage. The peculiar geographical distribution of the disease, the variation in the amount of beer ingested, the absence of the disease among brewery workers, and its apparent absence in countries where much more beer per capita is consumed, including beer containing cobalt, are not in keeping with a direct etiological influence. Cobaltous chloride is known to stimulate red cell production and to protect against the anemia that develops after experimental abscess formation.[29] In patients with anemia and chronic infections, a reticulocytosis followed by increased hematocrit and increased red cell mass resulted when cobalt therapy was given in a dosage of 100 mg per day. A dusky discoloration of the skin was noted as a side effect.[29] Cobalt is thought to stimuate erythropoiesis as a side effect of the interference with oxygen transport in erythroid cells owing to its ability to form complexes with certain amino acids, cysteine and histidine, which bind oxygen.[30]

There is little evidence of toxicity of cobalt at the dosage levels capable of inducing erythropoiesis. Absorption of orally administered salts is followed by urinary loss.[31] Intravenously administered cobalt salts are excreted in both bile and urine, but up to 5% can be found in body tissues ten days later.[32] The most common side effect of the orally administered drug has been gastrointestinal irritation.[30] Experimental doses of 200–300 mg/kg causes vomiting, diarrhea, and occasionally acute nephritis in dogs. Death from cardiac paralysis, preceded by a decrease in blood pressure and labored respirations, has also been produced experimentally.[33] The toxic effect of cobalt appears to resemble that of iron in both man and animals.[34]

It is interesting, in view of the known effect of cobalt on erythropoiesis, that an increase in the red cell mass was demonstrable in our patients. This is also seen in congestive heart failure, regardless of cause, but the degree of polycythemia described in congestive heart failure without venous shunts is usually less marked than that found in this study.

Theoretically, the severe acidosis, due at least in part to lactic acid, may arise from three contributing factors: tissue hypoxia, hepatic necrosis, and thiamine deficiency. In addition, the known activity of cobalt in inhibiting oxidative reactions may play a role.[30]

Although consideration of the myocardial failure dominated the therapeutic regimen, the enzyme elevation and incidence and degree of jaundice with right upper-quadrant abdominal tenderness and hepatomegaly were most impressive. Although perhaps explicable on the basis of acute congestion, when accompanied pathologically by a profound centrilobular necrosis without fat accumulation, a primary hepatic involvement warrants serious consideration. Descriptions of hepatic pathology in fatal cases of primary myocardial disease of any etiology indicate that this degree of hepatic necrosis is unusual. The elevation of enzymes and the degree of bilirubinemia is beyond that encountered in chronic or even acute right-heart failure.[35,36] This also suggests some as yet unexplained hepatic involvement.

A hypothesis which assumes that a particular population was conditioned to the development of acute beriberi by a variety of circumstances, including beer ingestion and thiamine deficiency, seems most plausible. However, even if minute amounts of cobalt did act as a precipitating agent, it remains to be established how and under what conditions this adverse reaction may occur. Antithiamine activity, divalent cation displacement, or inhibition of oxidative enzymes are avenues for investigation of the presumed noxious effect.

References

1. Medical News Section. 1966. Quebec's Medical Mystery. J.A.M.A. **196:** 25 & **197:** 27.
2. Dye, C. L., D. Rosenbaum, J. C. Lowe, R. H. Behnke & P. D. Genovese. 1963. Primary myocardial disease. Ann. Intern. Med. **58:** 426.
3. Sanders, V. 1963. Idiopathic disease of myocardium. Arch. Intern. Med. (Chicago) **112:** 75.
4. Burch, G. E. & J. J. Walsh. 1960. Cardiac insufficiency in chronic alcoholism. Amer. J. Cardiol. **6:** 864.
5. Wolf, P. L. & M. B. Levin. 1960. Shoshin Beriberi. New Eng. J. Med. **262:** 1302.
6. Evans, W. 1964. Alcoholic myocardiopathy. Progr. Cardiov. Dis. **7:** 151.
7. Brigden, W. & J. Robinson. 1964. Alcoholic heart disease. Brit. Med. J. **2:** 1283.
8. Fowler, N. O. & M. Gueron. 1965. Primary myocardial disease. Circulation **32:** 830.
9. Eliaser, Jr., M. & F. J. Giansiracusa. 1956. The heart and alcohol. Calif. Med. **84:** 234.
10. Alexander, C. S. 1966. Idiopathic heart disease. Amer. J. Med. **41:** 213.
11. Ferrans, V. J. 1966. Alcoholic cardiomyopathy. Amer. J. Med. Sci. **252:** 123.
12. Pintar, K., B. M. Wolanskyj & E. R. Gubbay. 1965. Alcoholic cardiomyopathy. Canad. Med. Ass. J. **93:** 103.
13. Brigden, W. 1957. Uncommon myocardial diseases. Lancet **ii:** 7006.

14. MORIN, Y. & P. DANIEL. 1967. Québec Beer-Drinkers' Cardiomyopathy: Etiological Considerations. Canad. Med. Ass. J. **97:** 926.
15. FLINK, E. B., F. L. STUTZMAN, A. R. ANDERSON, T. KONIG & R. FRASER. 1954. Magnesium deficiency after prolonged parenteral fluid administration and after chronic alcoholism complicated by delerium tremens. J. Lab. Clin Med. **43:** 169.
16. KALBFLEISCH, J. M., R. D. LINDEMAN & W. D. SMITH. 1961. Effect of ethyl alcohol administration on urinary excretion of magnesium and other electrolytes in alcoholics and normal subjects. J. Lab. Clin. Med. **58:** 833.
17. BRIN, M., M. TAI, A. S. OSTASHEVER & H. KALINSKY. 1960. The effect of thiamine deficiency on the activity of erythrocyte transketolase. J. Nutr. **71:** 273.
18. AALSMEER, W. C. & K. F. WENCKEBACH. 1929. Herz und Kreislauf bei der Beri-Beri-Krankheit. Wein Z. Inn. Med. Grenzg. **16:** 193.
19. BENCHIMOL, A. B. & P. SCHLESINGER. 1953. Beriberi heart disease. Amer. Heart J. **48:** 245.
20. WEISS, S. & R. W. WILKINS. 1937. The nature of the cardiovascular disturbances in nutritional deficiency states (beriberi). Ann. Intern. Med. **2:** 104.
21. MASSUMI, R. A., J. C. RIOS, A. S. GOOCH & D. W. DATLOW. 1965. Primary myocardial disease. Circulation **31:** 19.
22. BLANKENHORN, M. A. 1945. The diagnosis of beriberi heart disease. Ann. Intern. Med. **23:** 398.
23. AKBARIAN, M., N. A. YANKOPOULOS & W. H. ABELMANN. 1966. Hemodynamic studies in beriberi heart disease. Amer. J. Med. **41:** 197.
24. KEEFER, C. S. 1930. The beriberi heart. Arch. Intern. Med. (Chicago) **45:** 1.
25. BRIN, M. 1964. Erythrocyte as a biopsy tissue for functional evaluation of thiamine adequacy. J.A.M.A. **187:** 762.
26. DREYFUS, P. M. 1962. Clinical application of blood transketolase determination. New Eng. J. Med. **267:** 596.
27. DELANEY, R. L., H. G. LANKFORD & J. F. SULLIVAN. Thiamine, magnesium and plasma lactate abnormalities in alcoholic patients. Prco. Soc. Exp. Biol. Med. In press.
28. BLANKENHORN, M. A., C. F. VILTER, I. M. SCHEINKER & R. S. AUSTIN. 1946. Occidental beriberi heart disease. J.A.M.A. **131:** 717.
29. ROBINSON, J. C., G. W. JAMES, III & R. M. KARK. 1949. The effect of oral therapy with cobaltous chloride on the blood of patients suffering with chronic suppurative infection. New Eng. J. Med. **240:** 749.
30. BERK, L., J. H. BURCHENAL & W. B. CASTLE. 1949. Erythropoietic effect of cobalt in patients with or without anemia. New Eng. J. Med. **240:** 754.
31. COMAR, C. L. & G. K. DAVIS. 1947. Cobalt metabolism studies. IV. Tissue distribution of radioactive cobalt administered to rabbits, swine, and young calves. J. Biol. Chem. **170:** 379.
32. COMAR, C. L., G. K. DAVIS & R. F. TAYLOR. 1946. Cobalt metabolism studies. I. Radioactive cobalt procedures with rats and cattle. Arch. Biochem. **9:** 149.
33. FERRERO, S. 1939. Azione patologica e proprieta farmacologiche del cobalto; rivista pintetica. Folia Med. (Napoli) **25:** 482.
34. Goff, J. M. 1929. Cobalt as vaso-dilator. J. Pharm. Exp. Ther. **38:** 1.
35. RICHMAN, S. M., A. J. DELMAN & D. GROB. 1961. Alterations in indices of liver function in congestive heart failure with particular reverence to serum enzymes. Amer. J. Med. **30:** 211.
36. WEST, M., D. GELB, C. G. PILZ & H. J. ZIMMERMAN. 1961. Serum enzymes in disease VII. Significance of abnormal serum enzyme levels in cardiac failure. Amer. J. Med. Sci. **241:** 350.

A DISTINCTIVE MYOCARDIOPATHY OCCURRING IN OMAHA, NEBRASKA: PATHOLOGICAL ASPECTS

Henry T. Grinvalsky and Donald M. Fitch

Pathology Service of Creighton Memorial St. Joseph's Hospital
Department of Pathology of Creighton University School of Medicine
and Pathology Service of the Veterans Administration Hospital
Omaha, Neb.

Introduction

On December 21, 1964, a 51-year-old female was admitted to Creighton Memorial Saint Joseph's Hospital because of the sudden onset of rapidly progressing cardiac congestive failure; she died within 58 hours. Postmortem examination revealed the absence of significant coronary or valvular alterations and a heart unlike any other seen in the postmortem service of that institution during the previous five years. Two additional cases were seen within the next 25 days. During the 20-month period following the recording of the first case, a total of 14 cases of a distinctive cardiac lesion were recognized; in the same period of time, 12 similar cases were recorded on the postmortem services of the Veterans Administration Hospital of Omaha and the Douglas County Hospital. Our purpose in presenting the gross and light microscopical characteristics of these cases, related in time, place, clinical circumstances, personal social history, and basic morphology, is to stress their distinctiveness, in the hope that they will not be lost in the ever-expanding spectrum of so-called "alcoholic myocardiopathy."[1–7]

Material and Methods

Postmortem studies were performed on 26 of the 30 fatal cases, representing 14 from the autopsy services of the Creighton Memorial Saint Joseph's Hospital (CMSJH), 11 from the Veterans Administration Hospital (VAH) of Omaha, and one from the Douglas County Hospital (DCH). This constituted 86.6% of the fatal cases that came under clinical observation. Protocols and original histological materials were available for initial screening, but, because of the wide variation in technical qualities, recuts of the original paraffin blocks were supplemented by additional heart blocks selected from formalin-fixed wet tissue stock. Paraffin sections were cut at 5 μ, and the following standard staining procedures were utilized: hematoxylin and eosin, Masson trichrome, Snook reticulum, Weigert's resorcinfuchsin elastica, periodic acid-Schiff, alcian blue, Brown-Brenn bacterial, Goodpasture microorganism, and oil-red-O propylene glycol for fat. In addition, ten formalin-fixed preserved gross hearts were available for reevaluation from the CMSJH cases.

General Observations

Age, Race, and Sex. Age range for the entire group was from 22 to 71 years, with a mean of 46 years. The mean age of the VAH group was 41 years, compared with 48 years for the CMSJH group. All patients were caucasian, except for the youngest patient, who was an American Indian. The oldest patient was from the DCH service. Three of the fatal cases (11%) were females, reflecting the ratio of females (14%) in the entire clinical group.

Time of Survival after Hospital Admission. The time of survival can be analyzed conveniently on an hour basis. Survival span ranged from 20 minutes to

426 hours, with a median of 76 hours. The one patient surviving beyond ten days lived for 426 hours (approximately 18 days).

Seasonal variation. Major peaks of incidence in both the clinical and autopsy groups occurred between the last two weeks of April and the first week in July in two consecutive years. These peaks accounted for 42.2% of the fatal autopsied cases and 48.4% of the entire clinical group. These peaks correlated with climatological data (FIGURE 1) for the corresponding period. In late April, comfortable spring temperature and humidity give way to hot humid days. Sharp inclines in average monthly temperatures resulted from sustained temperatures of 85–90° F occurring in periods of five to seven days. Humidity discomfort resulted from a concomitant increase in precipitation, which changed from 2.6 inches in March to 6.9 and 5.5 inches in May and June of 1965 and from 0.88 inches in March to 3.6 and 5.9 inches in May and June of 1966. Secondary peaks occurred in the December–January periods in two consecutive winter seasons.

Incidence. The combined autopsy incidence for the two institutions for the 20-month period was approximately 3%. No classical cases had been observed prior to December, 1964, nor were any seen after July 10, 1966. The secondary peaks, the winter peaks, had not occurred in 1966, as might have been anticipated by the two previous December–January increases. A letter communication survey of the autopsy services of the remaining ten hospitals in the Omaha metropolitan area disclosed nine additional cases, which are not included in this study. Two institutions recorded three cases each, one institution two cases, and one institution one case. The remaining six institutions had no cases on record.

Morphological Observations

Pericardium

Eight cases (30.4%) showed normal pericardial sacs containing no abnormal fluid and having a smooth and glistening surface membrane. In 11 cases (41.9%), the sacs were lined by smooth and glistening membranes but were abnormal due to the amount of clear fluid they contained. The amounts varied between 50 cc (in three cases) and 1,000 cc, with only five cases (19%) having amounts in excess of 200 cc. In the two cases with fluid of "massive" or 1,000-cc amounts, the fluid was under tension.

In an additional seven patients, pericardiocentesis was attempted as a diagnostic or therapeutic measure; these cases deserve further comment. At postmortem, three different states were found: (1) pericarditis alone in one case; (2) pericarditis with hemopericardium in four cases; and (3) hemopericardium alone in three cases with amounts of 100, 320, and 720 cc. In these three cases, there was evidence of epicardial disruption or myocardial penetration, which was considered the cause for the accumulation of blood in the pericardial sac. Two were due to transmural penetration with intraventricular tap; in the third case (720-cc hemopericardium), only partial penetration of the wall had occurred, but prominent ecchymosis surrounded the needle tract, and a branch of the anterior coronary vein had been penetrated and oozed blood freely when the intact heart was manipulated *in situ*. In this case, the patient's clinical condition dramatically worsened after pericardiocentesis, which yielded only 200 cc of "bloody" fluid. In the one remaining case with an abnormal pericardial sac, a definite fibrinous pericarditis was unassociated with a specific inciting cause.

Histological study in the "normal " group revealed that the pericardium and epicardium was lined by serosal cells, with only slight swelling at most. A greater

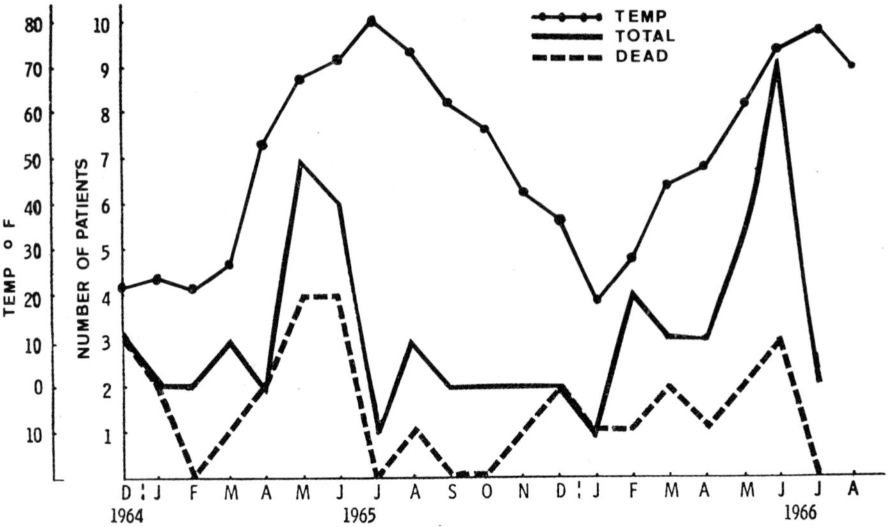

FIGURE 1. Monthly incidence of cases in relation to average monthly temperature. Total cases include all cases observed clinically, including fatal ones. Two sharp peaks in April through June of consecutive years account for 42% of the fatal cases and 48% of the total cases.

degree of serosal cell swelling occurred in the hydropericardium group. Definite serosal cell proliferation occurred in the cases in which pericardiocentesis had been attempted, and when pericarditis was present, it was of the typical and well-established fibrinous type, with associated mild or moderate inflammatory cell infiltration of the mononuclear type with an admixture of polymorphonuclear leukocytes. In the one case in which the pericarditis seemed to be an unrelated finding, the histological evidence would qualify it as an "early" or mild fibrinous variety, with a minimal inflammatory cell infiltration.

The accumulation of fluid in the pericardial sac seems to parallel the tendency for accumulation of abnormal amounts of fluid in the pleural cavities and abdomen. Otherwise, inordinate amounts of thoracic fluid were associated either with pulmonary embolism and infarction or pneumonia. An inordinate amount of ascitic fluid occurred in three cases (500, 750, and 1,000 cc), but these were found in association with hepatic cirrhosis in each instance. One other case with an unusual amount of ascitic fluid (2,000 cc) was a patient (the only one in the autopsy group who had been a readmission) who survived for ten days, and there was no cirrhohis, abnormal pleural fluid accumulation, or notable peripheral edema.

Peripheral edema was not a notable finding in the postmortem study. Case records mention this abnormal state in only six cases: two with 4+ pitting edema, two with 2+, and two with 1+. There was no mention of pedal, sacral, scrotal, or posterior dependent edema in the remaining 21 cases (79.9%).

Comment. It is apparent that patients on whom pericardiocentesis was performed did not benefit from the procedure to the degree anticipated. The patients did not seem to tolerate the procedure well, and misleading clinical findings resulted. In two cases, intraventricular aspirations of blood occurred in substantial amounts (700–800 cc), and the patients experienced no relief from the apparently successful pericardial tap. Morphologically, hemopericardium and/or pericarditis followed in a degree not commonly anticipated in pericardial tap under other conditions. Evidently, the flabbiness of the myocardium removes the usually telltale pulsating and resistent landmark sought for during the performance of pericardial tap, and lack of myocardial tone and venous vascular distention of subepicardial and intramural vessels seen in this entity encourage intrapericardial bleeding after penetration. In addition, pericardial and epicardial serosal and supporting elements appeared to be unusually hyperreactive.

Nevertheless, a clinical problem is presented when physical examination and x-ray studies disclose a prominent heart shadow with possible pericardial fluid increase. It appears that some method of relief other than violation of the integrity of the pericardial sac is advisable.[8]

Heart

Gross Examination

The appearance of the epicardium conformed to the changes described under the pericardium section. The hearts were characteristic and rather uniform in appearance. There was enlargement due to a combination of dilatation and hypertrophy (FIGURES 2 and 3), but it was the appearance of the myocardium that was distinctive. Loss of tone resulted in flabbiness to the degree that the heart generally reflected the contour of the cupped hand, and flattening was instantaneous when it was placed on the examining table. The subepicardial coronary venous vascular pattern was accentuated, with exaggeration of the hair-like tributaries, but unusual contours or conformations were not otherwise noted. Coronary ostia and arteries were generally devoid of significant atheroma formation. The myocardium of the smaller hearts was pale muddy-brown. In the larger hearts, it was pale gray-tan or pale gray-yellow, but the tigroid appearance of myocardium seen in severe and chronic anemia was absent; the gray-tan or yellow cast was rather uniform in distribution. Furthermore, the myocardium appeared to be soggy to the touch, as if it were waterlogged. Except where mural thrombi were detected (to be described in a subsequent section), the valvular and mural endocardium was delicate and translucent. Where dilatation was more striking, the trabeculae carnae were more markedly stretched, and the intervening fenestrations were rendered quite prominent.

The distribution of heart weights is presented in (FIGURE 4). Heart weights ranged between 425 and 800 g, with a mean of 600 g. A comparison of the ranges and means from the individual hospitals is worthy of mention. The range for the VAH group was 425–700 g, with a mean of 550 g; the range for the CMSJH group was 475–800 g, with a mean of 675 g. The one case from DCH had a heart weight of 725 g. The right ventricle ranged in thickness between 0.4 and 1.2 cm, with a mean of 0.6 cm; the left ventricle ranged in thickness between 0.8 and 2.5 cm, with a mean of 1.8 cm. The heart with the thinnest right ventricular wall (0.4 cm) had a left ventricular wall of 1.3 cm and weighed 600 g. The heart with the thickest right ventricular wall (1.2 cm) had a left ventricular wall of 2.5 cm and weighed 800 g. The heart with the thinnest left ventricular wall (0.8 cm) had a right ventricular wall of 0.5 cm and weighed 475 g. The heart with the thickest left ventricular wall also had the thickest right ventricular wall, as noted above. It was not possible to gain insight into the character of the heart from the thicknesses of the respective ventricular walls, although increasing thickness of the structures seemed to parallel increasing heart weight.

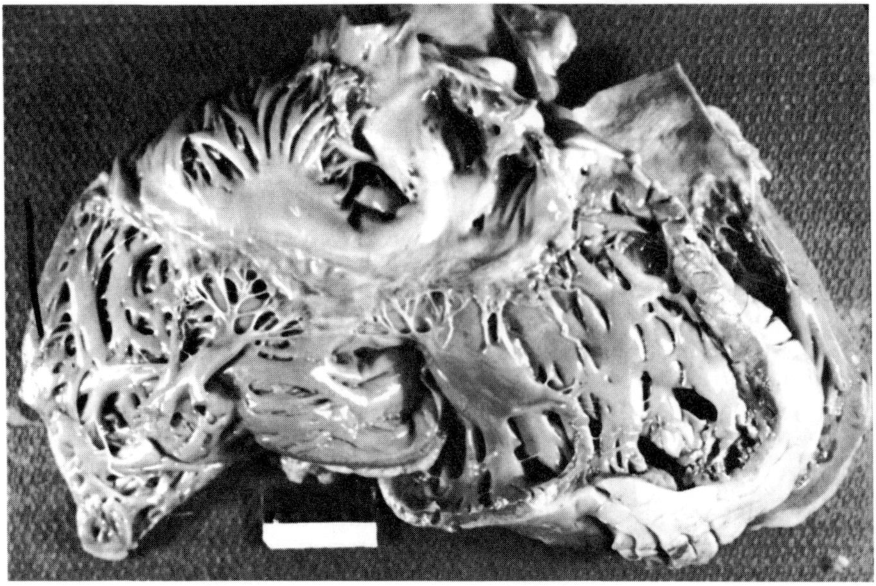

FIGURE 2. Gross specimen of right heart, showing marked chamber dilatation principally involving the ventricular component. Some index of flabbiness can be appreciated in the marked flattening of contours, especially in the intraventricular septum region.

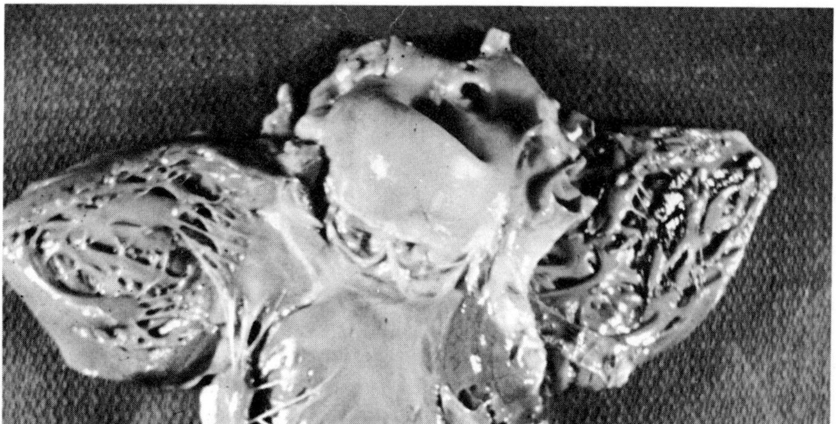

FIGURE 3. Gross specimen of left ventricle, showing dilatation and stretching of the trabeculae carnae. The intervening fenestrations are widened, and the aortic valve cusps and aorta are free of sclerotic changes. Marked flabbiness is reflected by flattening of contours.

Cardiac enlargement was generally a function of a combination of cardiac hypertrophy and chamber dilatation. TABLE 1 gives the pattern of chamber dilatation compared with heart weight. There was no single pattern noted. Only in two cases was there a right-sided dilatation dominance without a significant degree of left-heart dilatation. In most cases (six) there was a combination of both right and left ventricular dilatation, with a left ventricular dilatation dominance in four. In four cases, only a biventricular dilatation was noted in the protocols; in three cases, all chambers were recorded as dilated. It appears evident from a study of TABLE 1 that the heavier the heart the greater the degree of dilatation. This would also correlate roughly with age, since heart weight correlated with increasing age of the patients except in rare instances.

Microscopical Study

The epicardium in most instances showed some degree of swelling of the serosal lining cells, and seemingly passive, isolated subepicardial aggregates of round cells suggested foci of ectopic erythropoiesis. There also was a mild degree of serous atrophy of fat in several instances. When epicarditis occurred, as in the pericardiocentesis group, it was the typical fibrinous variety, with a relatively mild inflammatory cell infiltrate.

The general appearance of the myocardium in hematoxylin and eosin preparations indicated a tendency for hypertrophy of myocardial cells and exaggeration

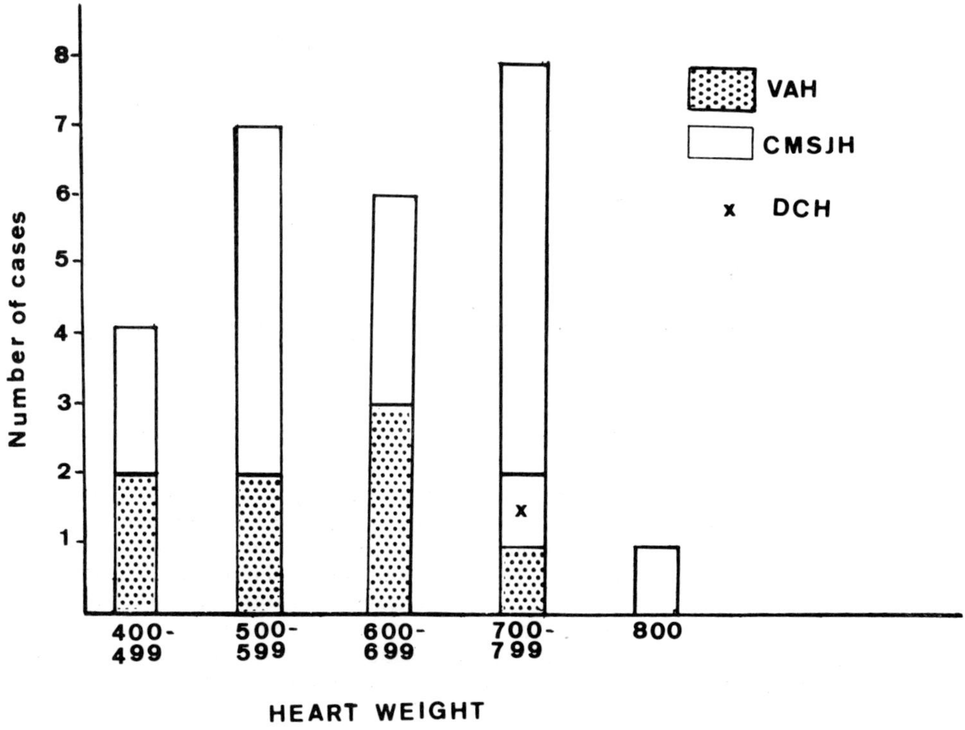

FIGURE 4. Heart weights charted against number of cases per institution.

TABLE 1

DEGREE OF CHAMBER DILATION ACCORDING TO HEART WEIGHT

Heart Wt. in Gm	RA	RV	LA	LV	BV	AC
800	X	XXXX	X	XXX		
770						XXXX
725	XXXX	XXXX		XX		
725	XXXX	XXXX		XX		
710	XX	XXXX	XX	XXXX		
700	XXXX	XXXX	X	XXXX		
650						XXXX
600		XX		XXX		
600	X				XXX	
600	XXXX	XXXX		XXX		
570	XX	XXX				
550					XX	
540	XX	XX		XXXX		
520					XXX	
500	X	XX		XXX		
500		X		X		
480		X		XX		
475						XX
475					XX	

KEY: RA= Right Atrium; RV=Right Ventricle; LA=Left Atrium; LV=Left Ventricle; BV=Biventricular; AC=All Chambers; X = Minimal; XX =Mild; XXX =Moderate; XXXX=Marked

of intercellular spaces, presumably by edema even in the milder cases. In sections from the larger hearts, the myocardial cell enlargement was more striking, especially when comparison was made with sections of "average" postmortem heart muscle processed concurrently. Nuclei showed zonal enlargement, hyperchromatism, and distortion in shape, often with delicate infoldings adjacent to foci where degenerative changes (to be described subsequently) were more prominent. Other enlarged nuclei, with undulated nuclear membranes, had central clear zones and chromatin concentrated peripherally. Binucleate forms with nucleoli in each nuclear mass were occasionally seen. There appeared to be an increase in paranuclear lipochrome pigment. In the more mildly involved cases, cytoplasm of cells tended toward pallor imparted to it by delicate vacuolization, which might be interpreted as a postmortem change at first glance. This vacuolization, however, was present even when the interval between death and postmortem fixation was short and there had been no prolonged agonal period (see results of oil-red-O fat stain in the section on Special Staining Techniques). The separation of myocardial fibers by "edema" was of varying degrees and seemed to parallel the extent of degenerative changes seen in myocardial cells. In some of the more severely involved hearts, myocardial cells were separated from their endomysial envelopes, and a prominent clear zone intervened between sarcoplasm and endomysium (FIGURE 5).

More distinctive (but not pathognomic) degenerative changes involved myocardial cells in diffuse but focal patterns varying from case to case only in the degree of involvement. Two generalizations can be made: (1) The changes to be described were commonly of such intensity, even in the mildest cases, that once recognized, they were not difficult to locate or relocate (FIGURE 6). (2) The larger the heart, the more striking the frequency, sizes, and intermixture of cellular and interstitial changes (FIGURE 7). The myocardial cell degenerative changes can be classified as vacuolar, granular, or sarcolysis. Each has its own characteristics, but in each the final result is the same: dissolution of the myofibrils and ultimate destruction of the cell involved. The basic degenerative process may affect only parts of a cell, whereas in immediately adjacent sarcoplasm, myofibrils may be accentuated and cross-striations regular and distinct. It is surprising to see

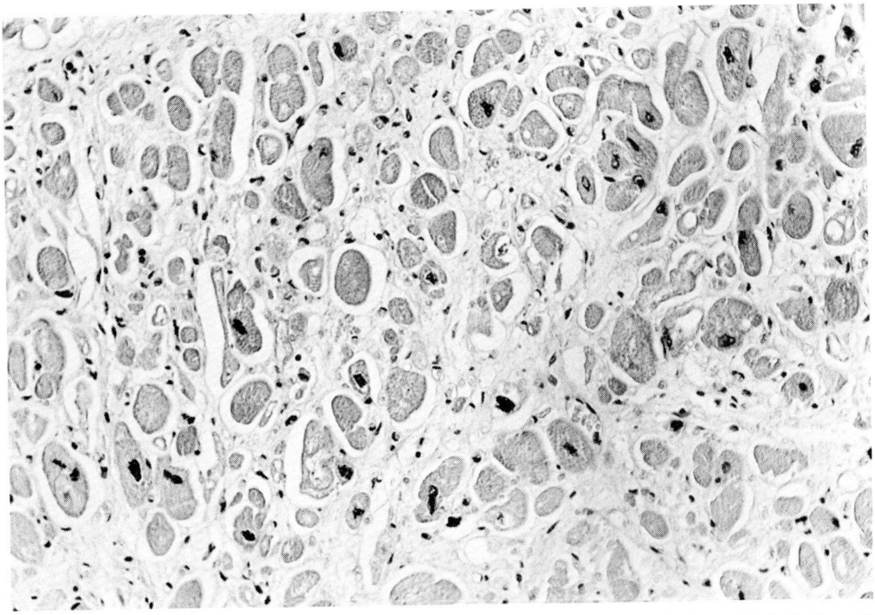

FIGURE 5. Marked separation of myocardial fibers, associated with interstitial "edema." Note reduction in bulk of many myocardial cells and prominent clear zones between endomysium and sarcoplasm. Stain: hematoxylin and eosin. × 225 (orig. mag. × 320).

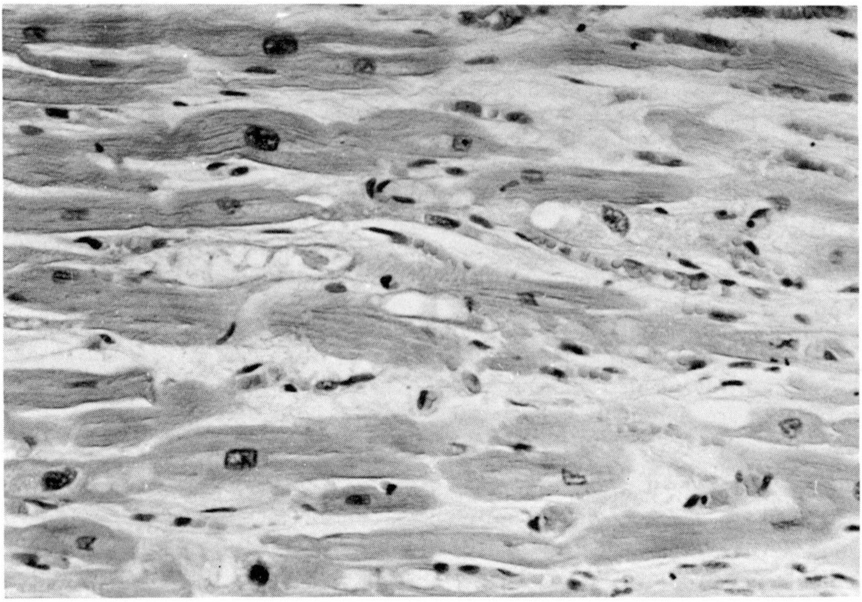

FIGURE 6. Myocardial cells reflecting hypertrophy, interspersed with cells showing vacuolar or granular degeneration. Some interstitial edema is also evident. Stain: hematoxylin and eosin. × 315 (orig. mag. × 450).

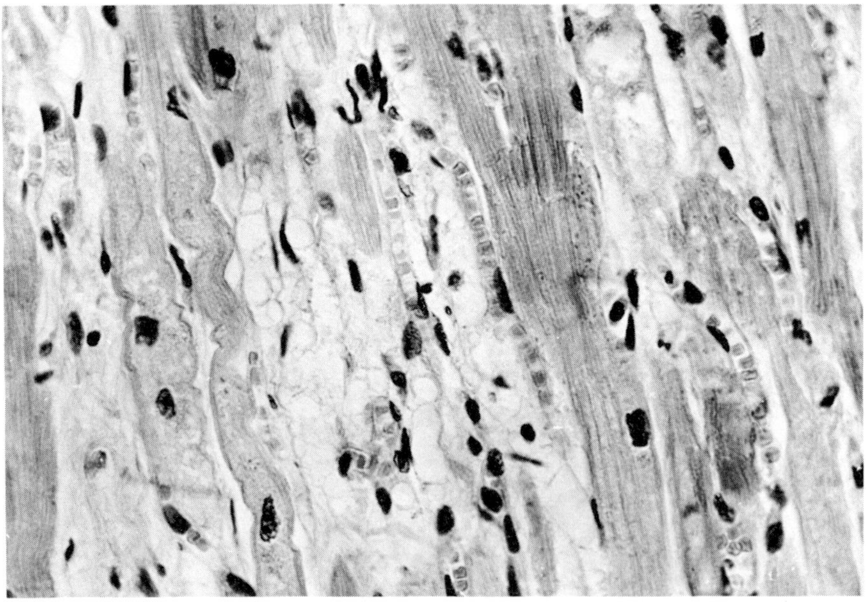

FIGURE 7. Larger clusters of myocardial cells, showing vacuolar or granular degeneration. Some nuclear enlargement and hyperchromatism is also evident. Stain: hematoxylin and eosin. × 315 (orig. mag. × 450).

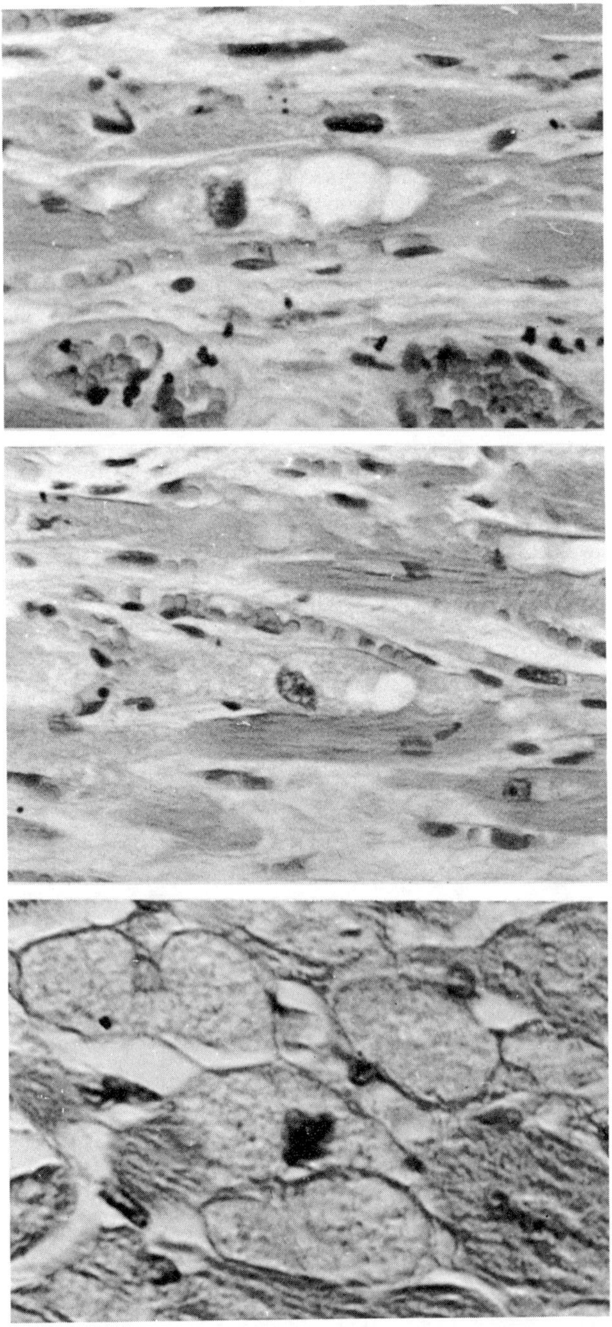

FIGURE 8. (*Top*) Adjacent or confluent vacuoles in a cell showing marked vacuolar degeneration. Stain: hematoxylin and eosin. × 520. (*Middle*) Cell showing granular degeneration, with a solitary vacuole at one angle. Stain: hematoxylin and eosin. × 520. (*Bottom*) Swollen Purkinje-like cells, characteristic of sarcolysis. Stain: hematoxylin and eosin. × 720.

the degree to which degeneration of myofibrils and sarcoplasm may occur without comparable degree of disturbance or dissolution of the nucleus of the cell. The point at which these changes become irreversible is not known.

Vacuolar Degeneration. The sarcoplasm develops vacuoles of varying sizes and concentration (FIGURE 8, top). In longitudinal section, there is no uniform pattern of localization, although the process may begin in the juxtanuclear zone. Often, a vacuole larger than the nucleus is found on either side of the nucleus, compressing and distorting it. In other instances, multiple smaller vacuoles dispersed throughout the sarcoplasm give it an eroded or moth-eaten appearance. In transverse sections, cells with vacuolar degeneration may look like "doughnuts," with a substantial "empty" hole surrounded by a rim of myofibril-poor sarcoplasm of varying width (FIGURE 9).

Granular Degeneration. The cytoplasm of cells revealing granular degeneration shows progressive conversion of myofibrils and sarcoplasm into coarsely granular acidophilic debris. Occasionally, such cells may also contain one or two small vacuoles (FIGURE 8, middle).

Sarcolysis. This change has also been referred to as myocytolysis,[9] and it involves the myocardial cell in more uniform fashion than is seen in either vacuolar or granular degeneration (FIGURE 8, bottom). Myofibrils disappear throughout the cell in diffuse fashion, and the remaining sarcoplasm has a fine dust-like evenly dispersed granularity. The nucleus may eventually appear centrally located in a relatively empty space marginated only by a narrow rim of condensed sarcoplasm hugging the endomysial envelope. This change is less likely to involve single or small clusters of cells but occurs principally in fascicular aggregates, not uncom-

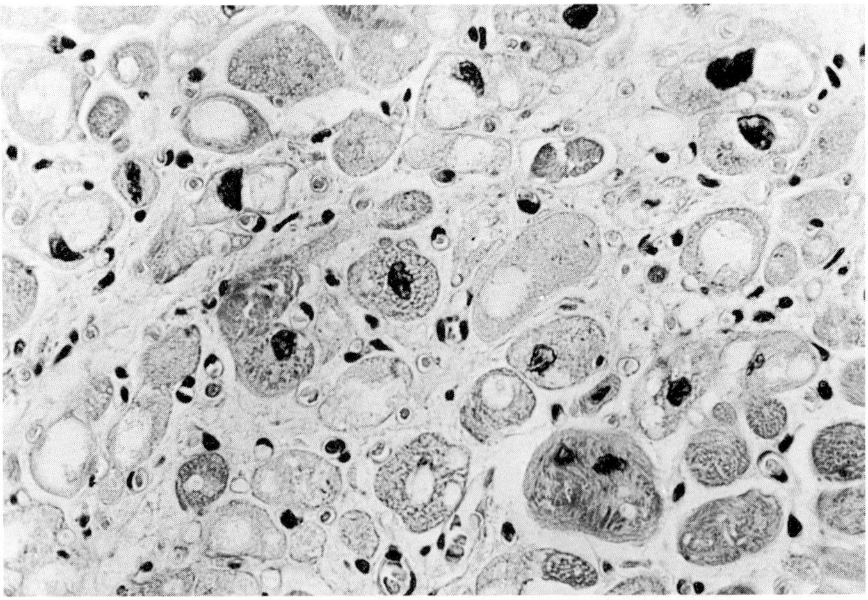

FIGURE 9. Cross-section patterns of groups of cells displaying marked vacuolar degeneration. Note "doughnut-like" appearance of some cells. Other cells show nuclear shape distortion; hyperchromatism, and enlargement. Stain: hematoxylin and eosin. × 315 (orig. mag. × 450).

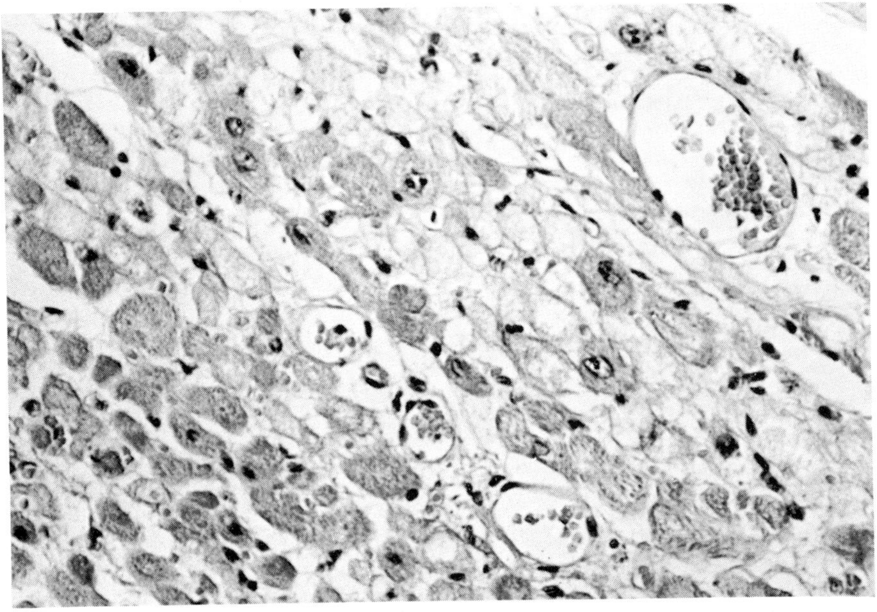

FIGURE 10. Fascicle of cells undergoing sarcolysis, adjacent to an ectatic blood vessel. The blood vessels are without notable change except for dilatation of lumens. Stain: hematoxylin and eosin. × 315 (orig. mag. × 450).

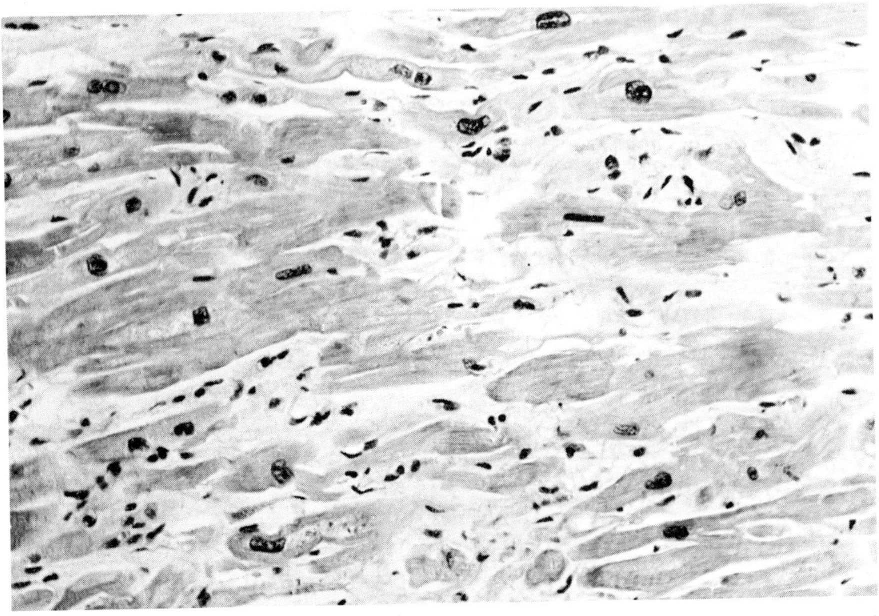

FIGURE 11. Longitudinal section of myocardium, showing small gaps in architecture caused by myocardial cell dropout. Stain: hematoxylin and eosin. × 315 (orig. mag. × 450).

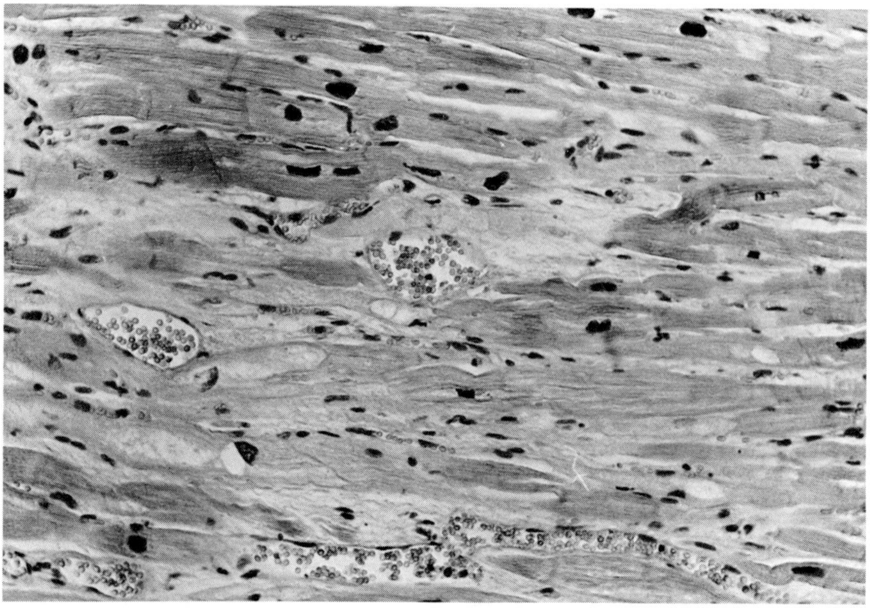

FIGURE 12. Area of pallor around ectatic blood vessel, due to loss of refractility in myocardial cells undergoing sarcolysis. Such pallor could be misinterpreted as "fibrosis." Stain: hematoxylin and eosin. × 315 (orig. mag. × 450).

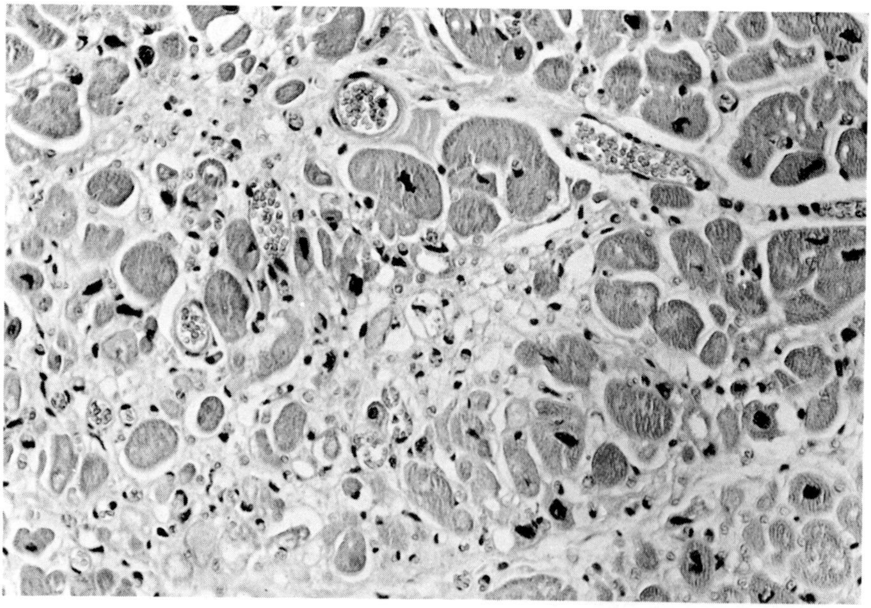

FIGURE 13. Marked variation in bulk of myocardial cells. Some cells are reduced to mere myoplastic remnants blending in with the stroma, which has become conspicuous due to disappearance of large numbers of myocardial cells. Stain: hematoxylin and eosin. × 225 (orig. mag. × 320).

monly in association with dilated perimysial venous blood vessels (FIGURE 10). The transformation of the cell causes it to look like a swollen Purkinje cell.

It is common to find that the degenerative changes described above cause cellular dropout involving only isolated cells or small clusters, producing a looseness and lack of cohesiveness in myocardial patterns. In longitudinal sections, small gaps punctuate and interrupt the myocardial synctium (FIGURE 11). In other instances, when larger groupings or even fascicles are involved, cross-section study reveals marked variation in myocardial cell bulk, and many fibers are reduced to minute islands of sarcoplasm blending in with the stroma, which becomes conspicuous (FIGURES 12 and 13). Lipochrome pigment could be found freely dispersed among the stromal elements. The progressive dissolution of myocardial cells produces an apparent increase in connective tissue, which may be erroneously interpreted as "scarring" or fibrosis. Actually, such areas represent condensation of the stroma due to widespread dissolution of myocardial cells. The collagen structure in such zones is delicate, fibrillar with distinct orientation, and often punctuated by dilated capillaries. When these areas are in contact with perimysial trabeculae, there is also striking dilatation of perimysial venous channels. Fibrosis as a reactive process with scar formation was not a distinctive feature in this group of cases, although progression of the process to a point of collagenous repair might be anticipated if the patients had survived.

The stromal pattern of edema and condensation had little associated inflammatory cell infiltration (FIGURE 14). In the rare case, few polymorphonuclear leukocytes were scattered in sparse fashion. In no case was it a predominant or eye-catching feature. Stromal (sarcolemmal) nuclei and interstitial stromal nuclei at times seemed enlarged and increased in numbers, but this change may also repre-

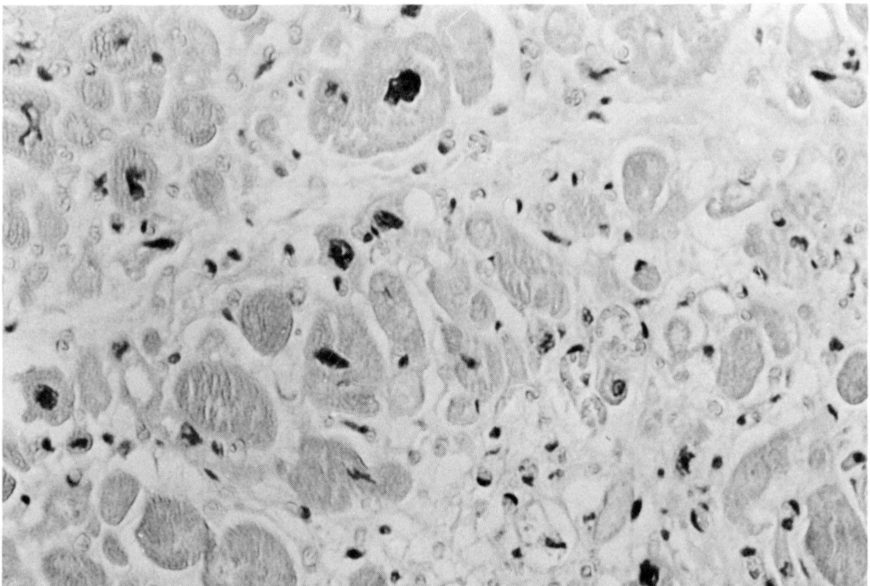

FIGURE 14. Stromal pattern of edema and condensation, but no inflammatory cell reaction associated with it. Nuclear enlargement with infolded contour and hyperchromatism is present in some myocardial cells. Stain: hematoxylin and eosin. × 315 (orig. mag. × 450).

sent condensation concentration of stromal elements due to myocardial cell dropout. In view of the notable absence of inflammatory reactive processes, it may not be proper to refer to the progressive myocardial cell changes as cellular necrosis but rather as necrobiosis when degeneration has led to cell death. In only one case was a small area of infarct-like necrosis identified. In two other cases, dystrophic calcification in individual degenerating myocardial cells was noted.

Except for vascular ectasia and mild swelling of endothelial cells, intramyocardial blood vessels were unaltered and generally disposed in somewhat edematous perimysial trabeculae. In most zones, the endocardium and underlying supporting stroma were without notable change except for looseness of architecture. When mural thrombi occupied Thebesian spaces, mild inflammation and some fibroblastic proliferation was conspicuous by contrast in the stromal lamellae.

Results of Special Staining Techniques. The most revealing findings were produced by the oil-red-O stains for fat. It must be stressed that the changes were focal in distribution but at times were surprising in degree when compared to the original hematoxylin and eosin sections. These stains revealed that the vacuolar changes in the cytoplasm of myocardial cells were principally due to the production of fat droplets (FIGURE 15). In the more delicately dispersed areas, one might consider only fat phanerosis; at the other extreme, substantial portions of myoplasm were displaced by coarser or large fat vacuoles (FIGURE 16, top). When examined by polarization microscopy, these stained frozen-section preparations revealed the presence of doubly refractile fatty acid crystals in the larger fat-filled vacuoles. In isolated fields, refractile aster-like radiations imparted to the neutral fat gave a telltale pattern indicating the presence of crystalline elements (FIGURE 16, bottom) even without the use of polarizing filters. Some small-size intracellular vacuoles did not give a positive fat reaction, indicating that they

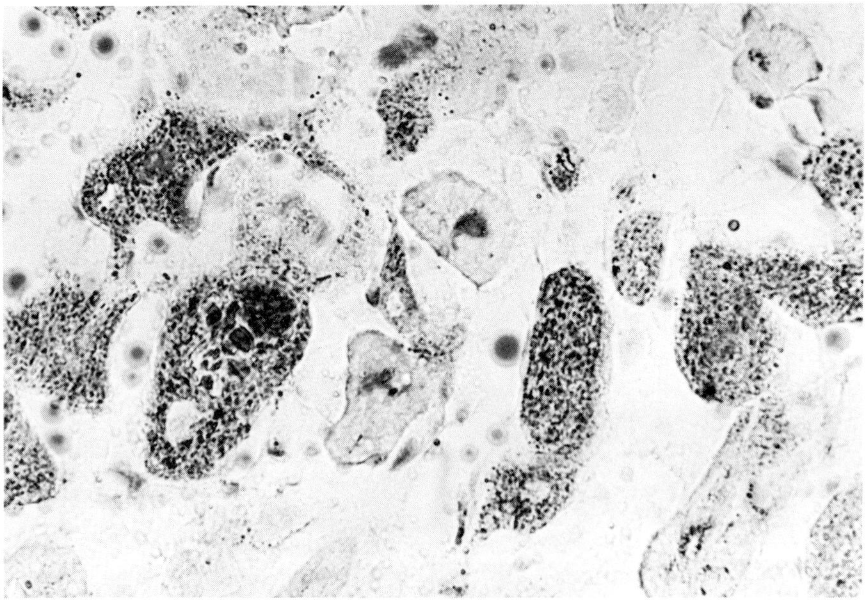

FIGURE 15. Fine and coarse globules of neutral fat (black in photo) in adjacent and scattered cells. Stain: oil-red-O. × 365 (orig. mag. × 520).

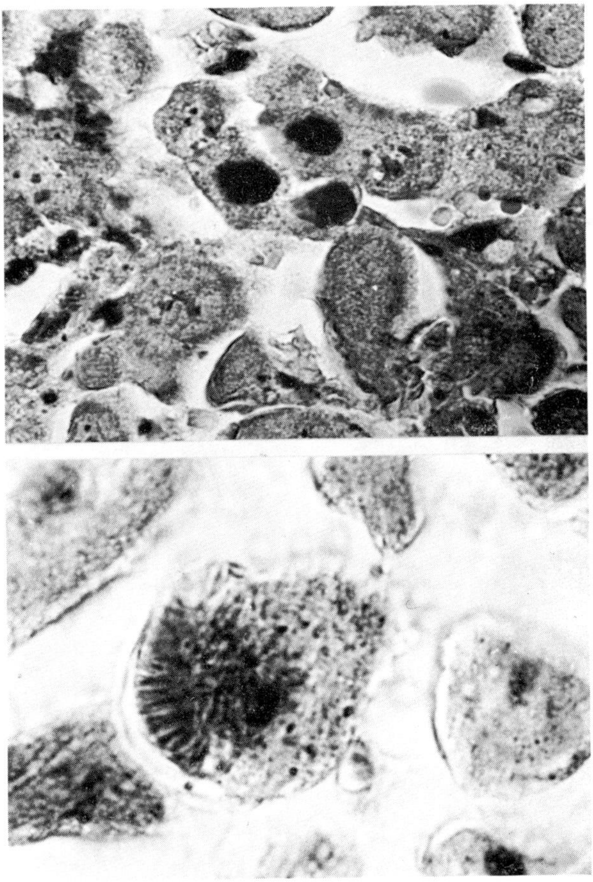

FIGURE 16. (*Top*) Single, very large globules of neutral fat (black in photo) in adjacent cells. Smaller vacuoles are evident in other cells. Stain: oil-red-O. × 520. (*Bottom*) Aster-like radiation imparted to the neutral fat by crystals that were doubly refractile under polarized light. Crystals had features compatible with triglycerides. Stain: oil-red-O. × 720.

were of a nonlipid nature. The presence of interstitial neutral fat could not be determined without reservation because of the tendency for the large amounts of intracellular fat to become partially disloged during technical preparation of the sections. Trichrome stains failed to disclose the presence of a substantial fibrosing process and supported the interpretation that a condensation of stromal elements occurred in the myocardial cell-poor areas. Stromal fibers stained here with a uniform pallor, remained distinct and delicate, and were permeated by delicate and dilated capillary channels (FIGURES 17 and 18). The connective tissue in the perivascular zones within the perimysial trabeculae was loose but stained with a normal intensity of blueness.

Reticulum stains were quite dramatic in the areas of more intense myocardial degeneration. There was almost total nonstainability of reticular fibers, and remaining myocardial cells or myoplasmic remnants were devoid of the character-

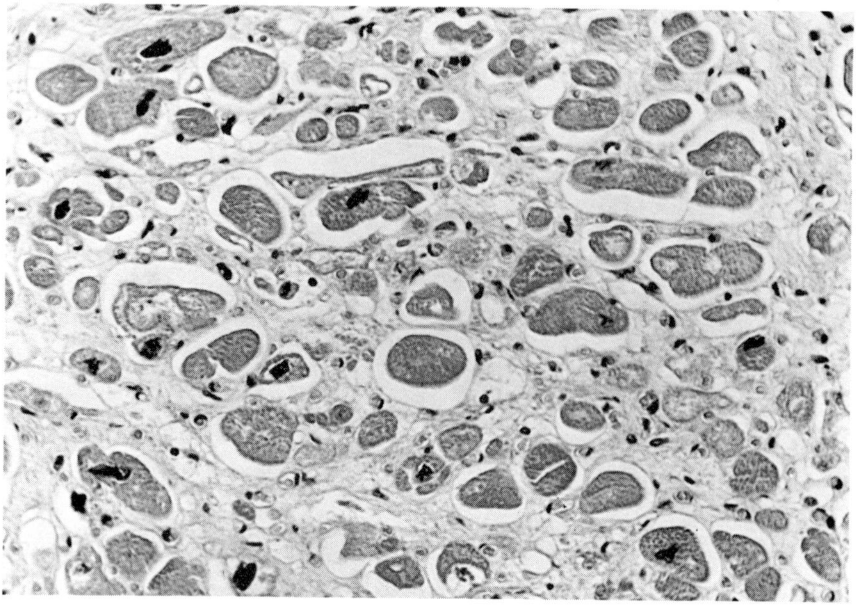

FIGURE 17. Unmasking of endomysial and epimysial connective tissue, with some "condensation." Fibers remain oriented and permeated by ectatic capillaries. Note conspicuous absence of inflammatory cell reaction. Compare with degree of unmasking in FIGURE 18. Stain: trichrome. × 225 (orig. mag. × 320).

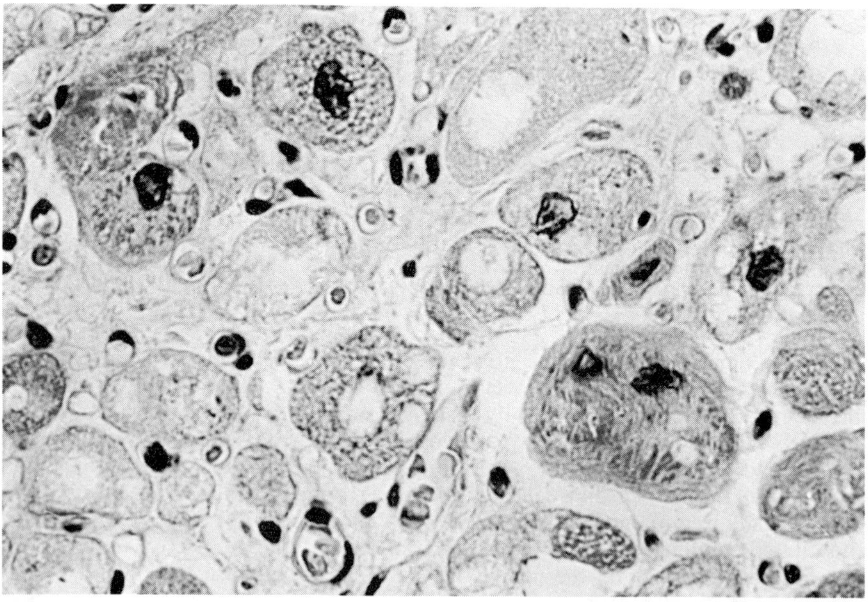

FIGURE 18. Unmasking of endomysial and epimysial connective tissue, with some "condensation." Fibers remain oriented and permeated by ectatic capillaries. Note conspicuous absence of inflammatory cell reaction. Compare with a lesser degree of unmasking in FIGURE 17. Stain: trichrome. × 315 (orig. mag. × 450).

istic endomysial reticular envelopes. In the larger trabeculae and in areas where degenerative myocardial cell changes were not conspicuous and in the subendocardial zones, reticulum fibers were not notably altered.

Periodic acid-Schiff, alcian blue, and mucicarmine preparations failed to show intracellular or interstitial concentrations of polysaccharides or mucin. Elastica, microbial Goodpasture, and Brown-Brenn preparations added nothing positive to the interpretation of the morphological findings.

Other Associated Vascular Lesions

Lesions of blood vessels other than the intrinsic mural myocardial alterations were confined to mural thrombosis or thromboembolism, which occurred in eight cases (30.1%). The distribution of the phlebothrombi or mural thrombi is shown in TABLE 2. Seven cases were seen with phlebothrombosis of the prostatic venous plexus, and five had pulmonary embolism and infarction. One case had pulmonary embolism with only patchy hyperemia, and the remaining one had no trace of embolization upon gross examination of the lungs. In two instances, concurrent right atrial mural thrombosis could have been the source for the pulmonary embolism, but the emboli were contained only in small- or medium-caliber pulmonary radicles and conformed in dimension and contours with those contained in the periprostatic venous plexus. Moran,[10] and Grabstald and Morningstar[11] stress the importance of the periprostatic venous plexus as a source of pulmonary emboli in nonsurgical patients, citing a 29.9% incidence in one study (Moran). The incidence in our study is 27%. In one remaining case, pulmonary embolism was found in association with right atrial appendage mural thrombosis, but no mention of the status of the periprostatic venous plexus was entered in the protocol. There was no evidence of peripheral embolization in the three cases that had mural thrombi in the left ventricle.

TABLE 2

DISTRIBUTION OF PHLEBOTHROMBI OR MURAL THROMBI

Site	No. of Cases
Periprostatic venous plexus alone	4
Periprostatic venous plexus and right atrial appendage	1
Periprostatic venous plexus, right atrial appendage, and left ventricle	1
Periprostatic venous plexus and left ventricle	1
Right atrial appendage and left ventricle	1

DISCUSSION

The presentation of cardiac failure associated with long-standing high alcoholic intake with beer preference is the common clinical denominator in the group of cases under discussion. Similar relationships (high alcoholic intake) and adverse cardiac manifestations are common in studies pertaining to occidental beriberi, and this adverse development is attributed to thiamine deficiency.[12-17] The recurrent appeal for support of a mechanism of direct alcoholic toxicity finds its adherents, but a lessening support for the nutritional and thiamine deficiency basis is not as yet notable. It cannot be denied that a direct alcoholic toxicity under some circumstances may cause morphological alterations in another dimension, but not in the magnitude disclosed in this study. Weiss,[13,14] Olson,[18] Follis,[19] and Jones[20] present some of the arguments favoring the thiamine factor mechanism as part of the multiprinciple nutritional deficiency of beriberi. In a certain percentage of cases, generally cited as 5%,[21] clinical presentation is characterized by rapidly progressing cardiac failure in individuals previously not known to have organic heart disease; often, these cases are seen as acute medical emergencies, with death supervening within a short period of clinical observation. This form of beriberi heart disease is referred to as the acute fulminating (shöshin) type. Platt[21] reasserted the seasonal relationship with climatological factors and the development of a new crop of acute fulminating cases in the Orient. He attributes this susceptibility to a lack of adaptation to early summer weather, when both temperature and humidity contribute to personal discomfort and interfere with sleep so that metabolic recuperation does not occur. It should be recalled that 42% of the autopsied cases and 48% of the total clinical cases in the present study occurred as distinct peaks in late spring and early summer (see FIGURE 1) in two consecutive years and correlated with mounting and sustained temperature and humidity indices. Other factors that may precipitate the acute fulminating form of beriberi are any cause for sudden increase in thiamine requirement, such as sustained strenuous exercise, fever, infectious disease, especially pneumonia; administration of epinephrine; and increase in carbohydrate intake without concommitant increase in thiamine in the subclinically deficient individual.[20–22] It is noteworthy that secondary peaks of incidence occurred in the December–January season, when upper respiratory infections and "flu" are common. In some cases, when reasonably reliable clinical histories were available, one could obtain information that the onset of symptoms occurred with or shortly after an attack of "flu." (In the winter season of 1964–1965, when the first cases emerged, an epidemic of adenovirus occurred in newborns in this area, and these patients had exhibited a degree of cardiac failure).

Cases of acute fulminating beriberi are included in clinical studies,[12–17,23,24] of the disease, and two cases were recently reported by Wolf and Levin.[22] The morphological findings presented in our study include the spectrum of changes seen in beriberi and duplicate the features of the shöshin type, in which pathological changes appear to be more intensified.[12–16,22,24,25] No previous reference to the occurrence of periprostatic phlebothrombosis as a source of embolism has been found (except for the work of Moran,[10] who refers to nonsurgical cases in general). The mechanism may be related to peripheral vascular dilatation, considered by Akbarian and co-workers[26] as an intrinsic component of beriberi rather than a consequence of cardiac failure. The features of hypertrophy, the character of cardiac enlargement and dilatation, and the presence of mural cardiac thrombosis have been confirmed.[15,20,25]

The lack of response to thiamine therapy may be raised as an argument against the designation of the cases in this study as beriberi. This is especially true since Blankenhorn[27] cited favorable response to thiamine therapy in the diagnostic criteria for occidental beriberi. It is appreciated that no distinct cardiac lesions may be seen in patients dying of the disease. Insofar as this is true, it has been postulated by Follis,[28] Dan and Darby,[29] Wintrobe,[30] and Jolliffe[31] that the disease is a biochemical one for an indeterminate period of time. In other words, the disease has two basic phases. For a variable period of time, only a biochemical lesion exists, without morphological counterpart visible on light microscopy. Yet, the changes recently recognized by electron microscopy[32,33] and histochemistry[34] in studies of myocardium in so-called "alcoholic myocardiopathy" may represent the early morphological counterpart during the stage when myocardial cell responsiveness is still possible with dramatic recovery. The second phase begins when the biochemical lesion gives way to morphological alteration of a degenerative type. When it occurs to the extent we have described, it seems unlikely that the myocardium would have a capacity for dramatic response to therapy. It is noteworthy that, in the simple nutritional deficiency type of beriberi occurring in the Orient, responsiveness to thiamine therapy was noted in only 75 to 80% of the patients treated, and some who did respond did so slowly.[21,35] It may be that thiamine responsiveness is a valid index to prognosis rather than being a prerequisite to the diagnosis of beriberi heart disease. It should be recalled that the second part of the number 8 criterion proposed by Blankenhorn[27] states: ". . . or autopsy findings consistent with beriberi." The anatomical changes we have discussed conform to those initially described by Wenckebach,[36,37] subsequently expanded and confirmed and finally summarized by Scotti[38] and Gould.[9]

In Omaha, almost epidemic incidence of adverse cardiac reaction occurred only during the time when cobaltous chloride was used as a beer foam stabilizer, and no additional cases have occurred since July, 1966, approximately two months after the use of cobalt was discontinued. A similar experience occurred in Québec, Canada, with a parallel relationship to the use of cobalt. The clinical courses and morphological alterations in the two separate "epidemics" appear to be identical.[39] In some of the patients in the Omaha group, urinary excretion studies for cobalt revealed substantially elevated levels. Although the role of cobalt in the pathogenesis of the cardiac lesion remains largely circumstantial, it cannot be ignored. By what mechanism could cobalt be implicated? If past clinical and experimental evidence is valid, it appears that a direct and unilateral toxicity effect is unlikely. The use of cobaltous chloride as a therapeutic agent in the various forms of refractory anemia, with administration of amounts in excess of 100 mg per day for prolonged periods, was unattended by untoward cardiac reactions of the type manifested by our patients.[40–42] (The daily intake of the more avid beer drinkers in our study did not involve more than 10–15 mg of cobalt.) In children,[42] administration of cobaltous chloride to the point of goitrogenic effect, with dosages resulting in serum concentrations of up to 195 μg%, did not produce cardiac manifestations. Hopps and co-workers,[44] utilizing dosages up to ten times the recommended adult therapeutic dose for prolonged periods, failed to produce lesions indicating toxicity effect in animals. Experimentally, it has been shown by Levy and his colleagues[45] that cobalt in animals exerts a significant inhibitory effect on enzymatic activity commonly involved in myocardial cell metabolism, especially succinoxidase, choline oxidase, cytochrome oxidase, catalase, and, under anaerobic conditions, choline and succinic dehydrogenase. It may be possible that, by a mechanism of enzyme interference, disturbances occurs in oxidative processes required for thiamine utilization, reducing the capabilities of cells to metabolize thiamine efficiently in the deficiency state.

Direct block of thiamine utilization by cobalt ion may be an alternate mechanism for its adverse action. The importance of magnesium ion in the synthesis of thiamine pyrophosphate is now recognized.[46–50] Most of the cocarboxylases are considered to be thiamine pyrophosphate-magnesium-protein compounds,[57] and the pyrophosphate in the form of cocarboxylase cannot be replaced by thiamine in pure preparations.[52] Perhaps when thiamine levels are critically low or when a competitive bivalent metallic ion such as cobalt is above critical concentrations in a state of relative thiamine deficiency, competitive cobalt ion substitution for magnesium ion occurs, with a nonfunctional thiamine complex resulting.[53] This state may develop in sudden stressful situations demanding increased cocarboxylase activity and may persist as long as the competitive ion remains above critical levels. The operation of such a blocking mechanism may partly explain the failure of response to thiamine administration in contrast to the favorable response elicited when simple thiamine dietary deprivation exists. A competitive blocking phenomenon may remain as long as the substituted ion remains above critical concentration, with return of response to therapy only after excretion or neutralization has occurred. It is possible that metallic ion interference with enzyme synthesis similar to cocarboxylase may be one mechanism by which heavy metal toxicity is generally manifested. In 1905, Dreschfeld,[54] in a discussion of frequently fatal cardiac disease in beer drinkers, made reference to the frequency with which it was observed in the Manchester, England, area and the curious disappearance of "alcoholic" heart cases coincident with a termination of a concurrent epidemic of arsenical neuritis. More recently,[55] the mechanism of arsphenamine intoxication was suggested as being mediated by a block in thiamine utilization.

Whether alcoholic intake is a necessary concomitant for an interference or blocking action by cobalt remains to be determined by experimental methods. Any form of malnutrition with thiamine deprivation may be the only prerequisite for cobalt to act in the proposed fashions. Also to be determined is whether any other elements or nutritional factors are significantly involved in the overall production of this distinctive myocardiopathy. (See section on hyperreactivity of epicardial lining and disturbance of endomysial reticulum. Could this be ascorbic acid related?)

A schema for the pathogenesis of this acute fulminating (shöshin) form of beriberi admittedly is speculative and awaits experimental confirmation, but is presented as follows: (1) high alcoholic intake (beer preference) as a predisposing or conditioning factor leading to thiamine deficiency; (2) cobalt, a contributory factor, exaggerating thiamine deficiency to the point of adverse cardiac reaction either by direct block of thiamine utilization or indirectly by interference with intracellular enzymatic functions necessary for thiamine utilization; and (3) a precipitating factor, either as infection, such as "flu;" inflammation, as in pulmonary infarction; or sudden climatic change with increased and sustained environmental temperature and humidity. This schema is in accord with that proposed by Dan and Darby[29] and Follis[28] to enable a better understanding of the interaction of factors involved in the production of beriberi.

Acknowledgments

The authors wish to express their appreciation to Sgt. George M. Alexander and Sgt. William L. Swartz, United States Air Force Hospital, Offutt Air Force Base, Omaha, Neb., for assistance in the technical preparation of the histological materials.

References

1. Brigden, W. & J. Robinson. 1964. Brit. Med. J. **2:** 1283.
2. Burch, G. & J. Walsh. 1960. Amer. J. Cardiol. **6:** 864.
3. Evans, W. 1961. Amer. Heart J. **61:** 556.
4. Ferrans, V., G. Burch, J. Walsh & R. Hibbs. 1965. Bull. Tulane Univ. Med. Fac. **24:** 119.
5. Alexander, C. 1966. Amer. J. Med. **41:** 213.
6. Gubbay, E. 1966. Canad. Med. Ass. J. **95:** 21.
7. Ferrans, V. 1966. Amer. J. Med. Sci. **252:** 89.
8. Burch, G. & J. Phillips. 1962. Amer. Heart J. **64:** 266.

9. GOULD, S. 1960. Pathology of the Heart. 2nd edit. : 500. Charles C Thomas, Publ. Springfield, Ill.
10. MORAN, T. 1947. Amer. J. Clin. Path. **17**: 205.
11. GRABSTALD, H. & W. MORNINGSTAR. 1955. Surg. Gynec. Obstet. **100**: 419.
12. SCOTT, L. & G. HERMANN. 1928. J.A.M.A. **90**: 2083.
13. WEISS, S. & R. WILKINS. 1937. Ann. Intern. Med. **11**: 104.
14. WEISS, S. 1940. J.A.M.A. **115**: 832.
15. DOCK, W. 1940. Trans. Ass. Amer. Physicians **45**: 61.
16. BLANKENHORN, M., C. VILTER, I. SCHEINKER & R. AUSTIN. 1946. J.A.M.A. **131**: 717.
17. BENCHIMOL, A. & P. SCHLESINGER. 1958. Amer. Heart J. **46**: 245.
18. OLSON, R. 1958. Fed. Proc. **17**: 3.
19. FOLLIS, R. 1956. Amer. J. Clin. Nutr. **4**: 107.
20. JONES, R. 1959. Circulation **19**: 275.
21. PLATT, B. S. 1958. Fed. Proc. **17**: 3.
22. WOLF, P. & M. LEVIN. 1960. New Eng. J. Med. **262**: 1302.
23. KEEFER, C. 1930. Arch. Intern. Med. (Chicago) **45**: 1.
24. AALSMEER, W. & K. F. WENCKENBACH. 1929. The Heart and Circulatory System in Beriberi. Urban & Schwarzenberg. Vienna, Austria.
25. LEVY, R. & W. VON GLAHN. 1937. Trans. Ass. Amer. Physicians **52**: 259.
26. AKBARIAN, M., N. YANKOPOULOS & W. ABELMANN. 1966. Amer. J. Med. **41**: 197.
27. BLANKENHORN, M. 1945. Ann. Intern. Med. **23**: 298.
28. FOLLIS, R. 1958. Fed. Proc. **17**: 3.
29. DAN, W. & W. DARBY. 1945. Physiol. Rev. **25**: 326.
30. WINTROBE, M. 1945. Arch. Intern. Med. (Chicago) **76**: 341.
31. JOLLIFFE, N. 1962. Clinical Nutrition. 2nd edit. : 2–8. Hoeber. New York, N. Y.
32. HIBBS, R., V. FERRANS, W. BLACK, D. WEILBAECHER, J. WALSH & G. BURCH. 1965. Amer. Heart J. **69**: 766.
33. ALEXANDER, C. 1966. Amer. J. Med. **41**: 229.
34. FERRANS, V., R. HIBBS, D. WEILBAECHER, W. BLACK, J. WALSH & G. BURCH. 1965. Amer. Heart J. **69**: 748.
35. HAWES, R. & C. SMITH. 1937. Brit. Med. Ass. **1**: 87.
36. WENKEBACH, K. F. 1928. Lancet **ii**: 266.
37. WENKEBACH, K. F. 1934. Das Beriberi-Herz. Pathologie und Klinik in Einzeldarstellungen. **6**: 106. Springer. Berlin, Germany.
38. SCOTTI, T. 1966. *In* Anderson's Pathology. 5th edit. **1**: 459. C. V. Mosby. St. Louis, Mo.
39. BONENFANT, J. 1966. Bull. Path. (ASCP) **7**: 297.
40. FOUNTAIN, J. & M. DALES. 1955. Lancet **i**: 541.
41. ROBINSON, J., G. JAMES & R. KARK. 1949. New Eng. J. Med. **240**: 749.
42. BERK, L., J. BURCHENAL & W. CASTLE. 1949. New Eng. J. Med. **240**: 754.
43. GROSS, R., J. KRISS & T. SPAET. 1955. Pediatrics **15**: 284.
44. HOPPS, H., A. STANLEY & A. SHIDELER. 1954. Amer. J. Clin. Path. **24**: 1376.
45. LEVY, H., V. LEVISON & A. SHADE. 1950. Arch. Biochem. **27**: 34.
46. ROGERS, E. 1962. Ann. N. Y. Acad. Sci. **98**: 412.
47. HOLZER, H., F. DA FONESCA-WOLLHEIM, G. KOHLHAW & C. W. WOENCKHAUS. 1962. Ann. N. Y. Acad. Sci. **98**: 453.
48. BROWN, G. 1962. Ann. N. Y. Acad. Sci. **98**: 479.
49. LEDER, I. 1962. Ann. N. Y. Acad. Sci. **98**: 486.
50. DEREUCK, A. & M. O'CONNOR. 1961. The Mechanism of Action of Water-Soluble Vitamins. Ciba Found. Study Group. No. 11. Little, Brown & Co., Boston. p. 78.
51. OCHOA, S. 1939. Biochem. J. **33**: 1262.
52. WOHL, M. & R. GOODHART. 1964. Modern Nutrition In Health and Disease. 3rd edit. : 383. Lea & Febiger. Philadelphia, Pa.
53. WEBB, J. 1963. Enzyme and Metabolic Inhibitors. 1st edit. **1**: 54–56, 440, & 484. Academic Press, Inc. New York, N. Y.
54. DRESCHFELD, I. 1905. Brit. Med. J. **2**: 1023.
55. RINEHART, J., L. GREENBERG & M. FRIEDMAN. 1947. Amer. J. Path. **23**: 879 (abstr.).

QUÉBEC BEER-DRINKERS' CARDIOMYOPATHY: CLINICAL AND HEMODYNAMIC ASPECTS*

Yves Morin, André Têtu, and Gaston Mercier
Department of Medicine, Laval University, Québec, Canada

On August 24, 1965, a 39-year-old stevedore was admitted to the Department of Surgery of the Hôtel-Dieu de Québec. The clinical picture was unusual. The patient complained of severe epigastric pain, with tenderness localized to the upper part of the abdomen. He was deeply cyanotic, this grayish hue was found especially in the face, neck, and abdomen. He was short of breath but lay flat in bed; above all, he was very anxious and agitated but did not present any evidence of incoherence or gross tremor. The patient admitted to drinking regularly an average of 25 pints of beer (Brand XXX) daily. His dietary habits were poor and irregular; he rarely ate on weekends (or whenever he was off from work) and ate sandwiches at other times. On physical examination of the cardiovascular system, his heart rate was regular at 115 beats per minute, and blood pressure was 80/60. Arterial pulses were symetrical but of small volume. The jugular veins were distented, and a prominent *a* wave (FIGURE 1) could easily be detected. Palpation of the precordium was negative. No murmurs could be heard on auscultation of the heart, but loud third and fourth heart sounds were obvious.

In spite of the low blood pressure and the quiet heart, a diagnosis of beriberi was made. The patient was catheterized after he had been fully digitalized and received diuretics. Instead of the high cardiac output that was expected, the cardiac index was 1.8 liters per minute and did not rise after a 25-second exercise period. The end-diastolic ventricular pressures were elevated in both ventricles. It was felt that this patient presented an unusual form of alcoholic myocardiopathy; he was treated in the usual fashion, given thiamine in large dosage, made a slow recovery, and went back to work and to beer.

However, in the next three weeks, two identical cases were seen in the same hospital and three in other centers of the city. Seven cases were admitted in October, six in November, seven in January, eight in February, six in March, and finally four in the first days of April. All cases were found in the Québec City area, and none were reported in other parts of the country.

There were 48 men and two women as patients. Most of them were middle aged. Some men were unemployed; however, most were employed as truck drivers, waiters, dock workers, and construction workers. Although this was not a constant finding, many performed heavy physical labor.

All of these patients were unusually heavy beer drinkers, and 36 had been drinking heavily for at least 20 years. The average alcoholic intake was 24 pints daily, but one patient, a truck driver, drank an average of 20 quarts of beer daily. Most patients drank beer exclusively, but six occasionally consumed other types of alcoholic beverages. Although the average patient preferred draught beer sold exclusively in taverns, bottled beer was also consumed, since taverns are closed on Sunday in Québec City.

By November, it became obvious, and this was confirmed by a governmental epidemiological survey, that all of the surviving patients who could

* Supported by a special grant from the Department of Health of the Province of Québec and by Medical Research Council grant no. 100-4M-220.

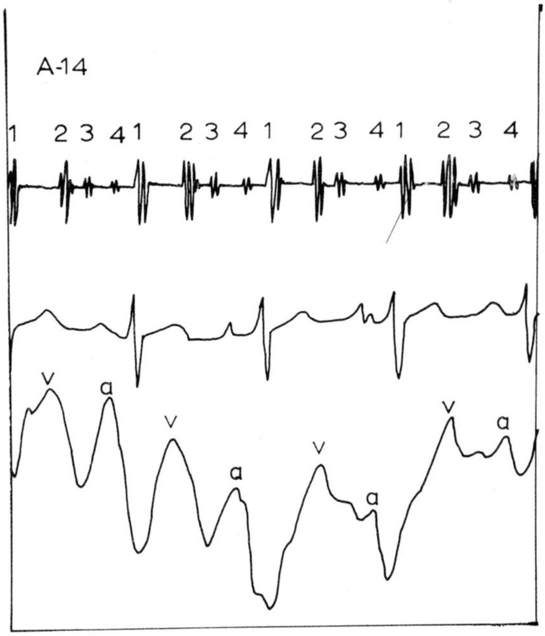

FIGURE 1. Phonocardiogram and phlebogram in the initial patient.

be questioned drank preferably (but not exclusively) Brand XXX. The XXX Brewery is in an unusual position in Québec City. It was established on the site of the oldest brewery in North America, built by Jean Talon in 1668 to help combat alcoholism among French settlers. Its excellent tasting brew was (and still is) very popular in Québec and accounts for approximately 80% of the local market. A beer of the same name is manufactured in Montreal; as far as could be ascertained, the only difference between the two products at that time was that the Québec Brand XXX beer contained approximately ten times more cobalt sulfate. This chemical has been added to some Canadian beers since July, 1965, to improve the stability of the foam. For this reason, it has been added in larger breweries only to draught beer. However, in smaller breweries, such as in Québec City, separate batches were not brewed for bottle and for draught beer; therefore, the cobalt sulfate was added to all the beer processed in the XXX Brewery. Thus, the intake of this food additive was increased to much higher levels than in Montreal.

Most patients were in good health from three months up to two weeks prior to admission. The first symptoms to appear were gastrointestinal. Every patient questioned admitted to a severe anorexia that prevented food intake and frequently limited beer consumption. Nausea and vomiting were frequent, and hematemesis was seen on seven occasions. Diarrhea was often encountered, and there were four instances of melena. Progressively, signs of heart failure appeared: shortness of breath, dry and persistent cough, thoracic and right upper quadrant abdominal pain, often very severe, and ankle edema.

On physical examination, most remarkable signs were related to the cardiovascular system: a peculiar cyanosis, limited to the face and trunk, was typical enough to permit a spot diagnosis of the condition. The fact that melanin pigment was found to be increased on skin biopsy of these patients may in part explain this unusual coloration. The heart rate was always rapid but regular; this is in contrast with other types of primary myocardiopathy, in which arrhythmias, such as auricular fibrillation, are commonly encountered. The blood pressure was low, and arterial pulses were of small volume. Arterial thrombi (or emboli) were clinically encountered in five cases and were the cases of death in two of these. Hepatomegaly, ankle edema, and jugular vein distension were seen in approximately half of the cases. Frequently, a giant *a* wave was recorded on the jugular phlebogram (FIGURE 1). The precordium was quiet.

On auscultation of the heart, murmurs of mitral and tricuspid insufficiency, often heard in more common forms of primary myocardiopathy, were rare in this disease. Third and fourth heart sounds were frequently heard, however, and, after they had disappeared with clinical improvement, could often be heard for several weeks following vigorous exercise. Pulmonary rales were heard in 27 out of 50 cases, and nine cases were admitted in frank pulmonary edema.

Of the 50 cases, 20 died. In these cases, evolution was rapid, and the clinical descriptions fit the picture of Shöshin beriberi,[1] with the exception that signs of hyperkinetic circulation such as "the powerfully undulating pulsations in the heart region, the epigastrium and the neck" and the "full arterial pulse" were not seen. However, the severe dyspnea, the anxiety and restlessness, the epigastric and precordial pain, the obvious cyanosis, and the auscultatory findings were similar. The patients died quickly, usually within 24 hours, generally in shock that did not respond to vasoactive amines, steroids, digitalis, or thiamine.

Hematological studies performed in these patients showed a hemoglobin or red blood cell count in the high normal range, and nine patients were frankly polycythemic. Four patients tested had increased blood volume. Sedimentation rate was normal in all cases. Generally, serum iron levels were low in the face of high hemoglobin. Serum electrolytes—sodium, potassium, chloride, calcium, phosphorus, and magnesium—were generally within normal limits when studied; 14 cases out of 23 tested showed lactic acidosis, with a low pH generally indicating a poor prognosis.

Liver function tests were done in the majority of cases, serum bilirubin was elevated in 23 out of 33 cases. Prothrombin time was prolonged in all patients tested, over twice control values in 16 out of 34 cases. This is somewhat surprising if one considers the frequent thrombotic complications encountered in this disease. Flocculation tests (thymol flocculation, thymol turbidity, and cephalin-cholesterol flocculation) were generally normal. Electrophoresis of serum proteins showed little disturbance; there was slight hypoalbuminemia and an important elevation of serum globulins.

The serum enzyme levels showed striking elevations and, when performed during the acute stage of the illness, confirmed the suspected diagnosis: seven patients in shock in whom serum glutamic oxalacetic transaminase was measured had levels above 2000 units. Other serum enzymes were also found to be elevated (glutamic pyruvic transaminase, lactic dehydrogenase, ornithine carbamyl transferase, isocitric dehydrogenase, aldolase). The elevation of these serum enzyme levels correlated well with the central hepatic necrosis found in the severe form of the disease and, especially in view of the high lactic dehydrogenase: bicarbonate dehydrogenase ratio and of the disproportionately elevated levels of serum ornithine carbamyl transaminase, it was felt that these unusually high serum enzyme levels were hepatic and not myocardial in origin.

Attempts to measure thiamine in the blood were not successful. Thiamine deficiency was demonstrated in 13 patients tested by one of two methods: either by comparison of the expected with the actual levels of serum pyruvic acid in relation to serum lactic acid levels or by the pyruvic acid tolerance test using a loading dose of glucose. One must interpret these results with caution, however, since thiamine deficiency, as detected by the erythrocyte transketolase determination, can be found in fasting subjects within four days.[2] Virological and immunological studies were negative. Search for toxic substances such as arsenic or lead was negative.

Electrocardiograms were performed, at least once, in 48 out of 50 patients. Electrocardiographic tracings were remarkably similar in all cases (FIGURES 2 and 3), in the acute stage as well as during the later stages of the disease. Tachycardia was the rule; arrythmias, all of them supraventricular, were seen in only three cases and then were transitory. This is, of course, in contrast to findings in other types of cardiomyopathy. Low voltage of the QRS segment in the limb leads was a constant finding, these waves not exceeding 5 millivolts, even in cases in which pericardial effusion was shown not to be present by cardiac catheterization. These minicomplexes progressively disappeared and within a month were generally replaced by evidence of left ventricular hypertrophy.

Abnormalities in the P wave were bizarre and frequent and led to heated arguments as to whether right or left atriomegaly was present. Although all types of anomalies were seen, the most frequent finding was a broad peaked P wave with right axis deviation in the limb leads with a diphasic (plus and

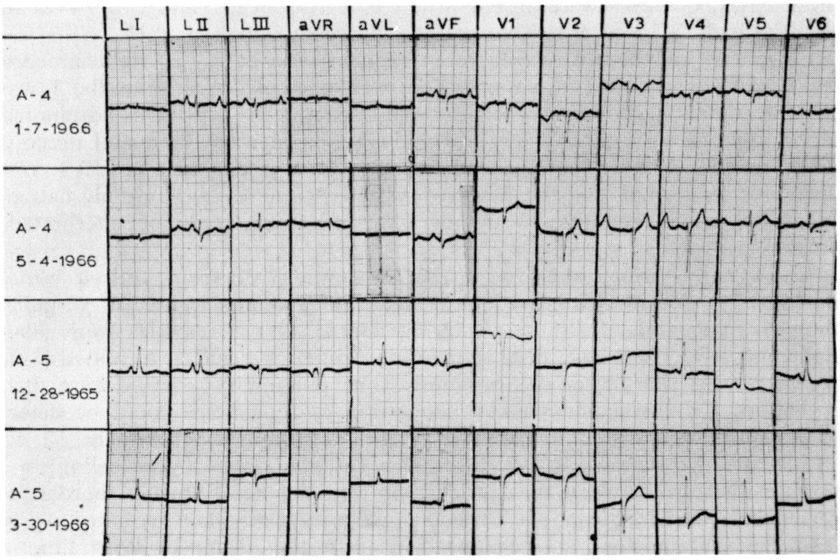

FIGURE 2. Electrocardiograms from acute and late stages of the cardiomyopathy in two patients.

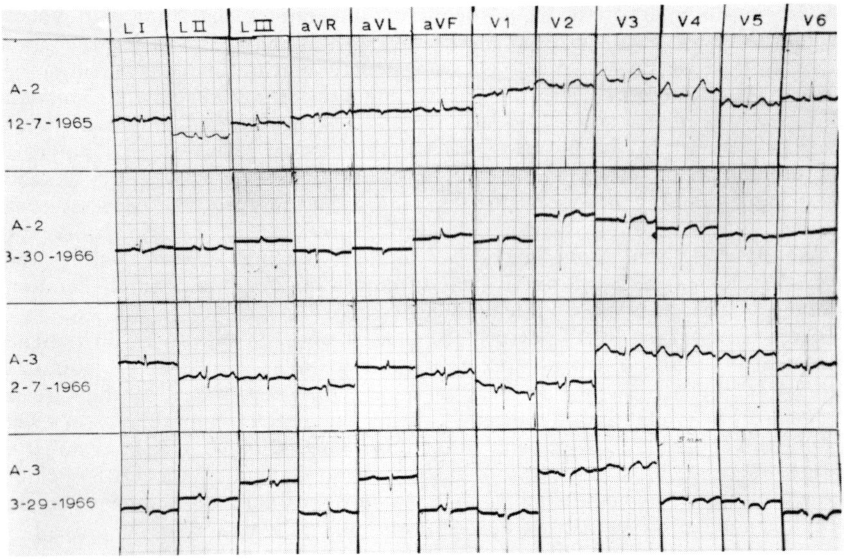

FIGURE 3. **Electrocardiograms from acute and late stages of the cardiomyopathy in two patients.**

minus) P wave in leads V1 and V2. These abnormalities also disappeared within a month.

Intraventricular conduction defects were rarely seen; there were three cases of bundle branch block. However, septal depolarization was felt to be abnormal in 22 cases; Q waves were absent in left epicardial leads, and Q-S waves were seen in leads V1 and V2. This pattern cleared up in two weeks.

Elevations of the ST wave were frequently seen in the right precordial leads, and nonspecific T wave anomalies were the rule. With time, the T waves became frankly negative, symmetrical, and "ischemic" in type. This last anomaly, in conjunction with high voltage of the QRS segment in limb and precordial leads, remained stable for two to three months. At that time, the QRS voltage decreased to normal, and the T waves in leads V4 to V6 were simply flattened. After six to nine months, 17 out of 22 cardiograms could be interpreted as normal.

Chest x-rays were taken in 46 patients, many of them with a portable machine. No specific pattern could be detected (FIGURES 4 and 5). All patients showed an enlarged heart to a varying degree, and all cavities were dilated, right and left. There was distention of the superior vena cava, and the more severe it was, the graver the prognosis. The pulmonary arteries were dilated in half of the cases, and passive congestion of lung fields could be detected in the same proportion of patients. Pleural effusion was found in 12 cases and in the two patients in whom cardiac catheterization, by revealing an abnormal distance between the catheter tip and the heart shadow border, suggested pericardial effusion; a cardiac angiogram was taken by injecting contrast material in the right atrium to confirm the diagnosis. With time, the pulmonary congestion disappeared, the heart size decreased, and, six to nine months after the onset of the illness, heart size had returned to normal.

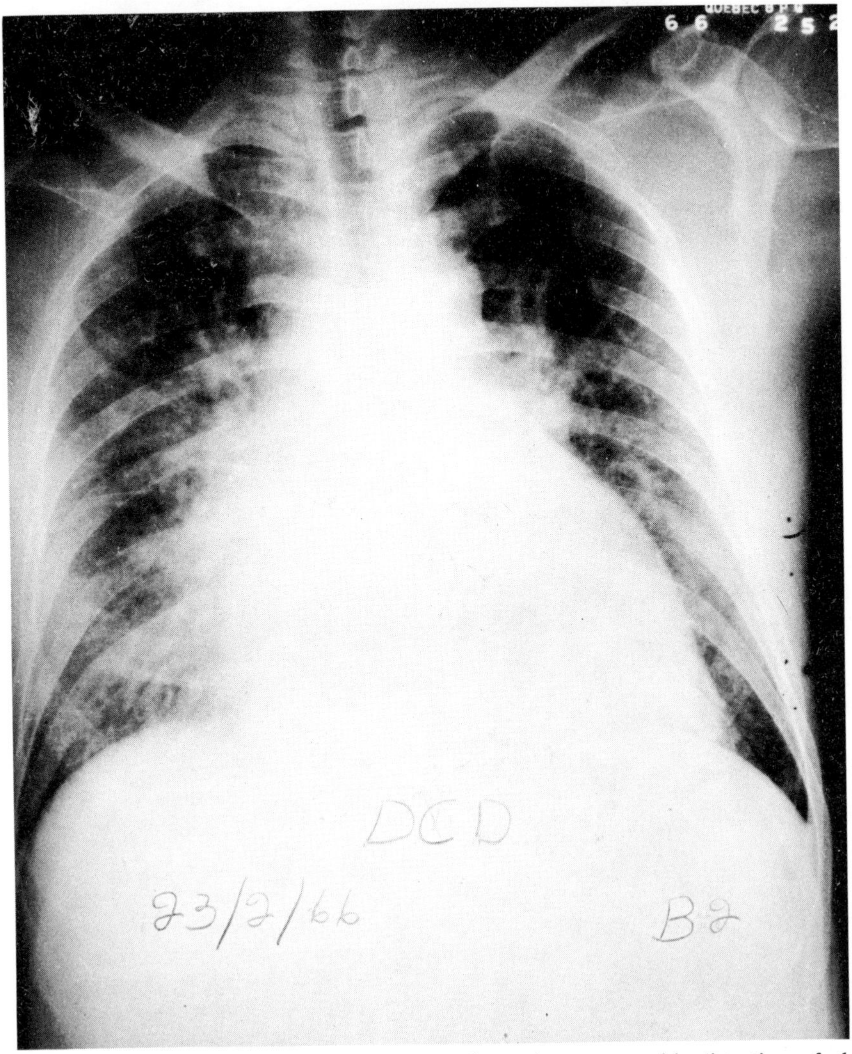

FIGURE 4. Chest x-ray, showing extreme cardiac enlargement, with distention of the great vessels and pulmonary congestion.

Hemodynamic studies were performed in 13 patients within 48 hours of admission. At the time of examination, most patients had received digitalis and diuretics but not thiamine. Cardiac outputs (FIGURE 6 and TABLE 1) were normal or low and did not increase with exercise or administration of isoproterenol (Isuprel®).† These figures are not significantly different from the cardiac index values of 136 cases of primary myocardial disease reported in the literature.[3-14] However, these results are significantly different ($p < 0.05$) from the cardiac index values of 12 cases of beriberi heart disease reported by Wagner.[15] As expected, pressures in the right ventricle (FIGURE 7) showed an

† Distributed by Winthrop Laboratories, Inc., New York, N. Y.

elevated systolic pressure, indicating increased pulmonary resistance developing as a consequence of an increased left end-diastolic pressure. The right ventricular pressure curves also indicated a decrease in ventricular compliance as the ratio of end-diastolic pressure to systolic pressure was higher than 1:3. Left ventricular pressure curves (FIGURE 8) show a low systolic pressure that was constant in the acute stage of the illness and indicated the low cardiac output in the face of normal systemic arterial resistance. However, as indicated previously, end-diastolic pressure was elevated, which is the morphology of the curve, often exhibiting the "atrial kick," that follows the giant *a* wave in the atria.

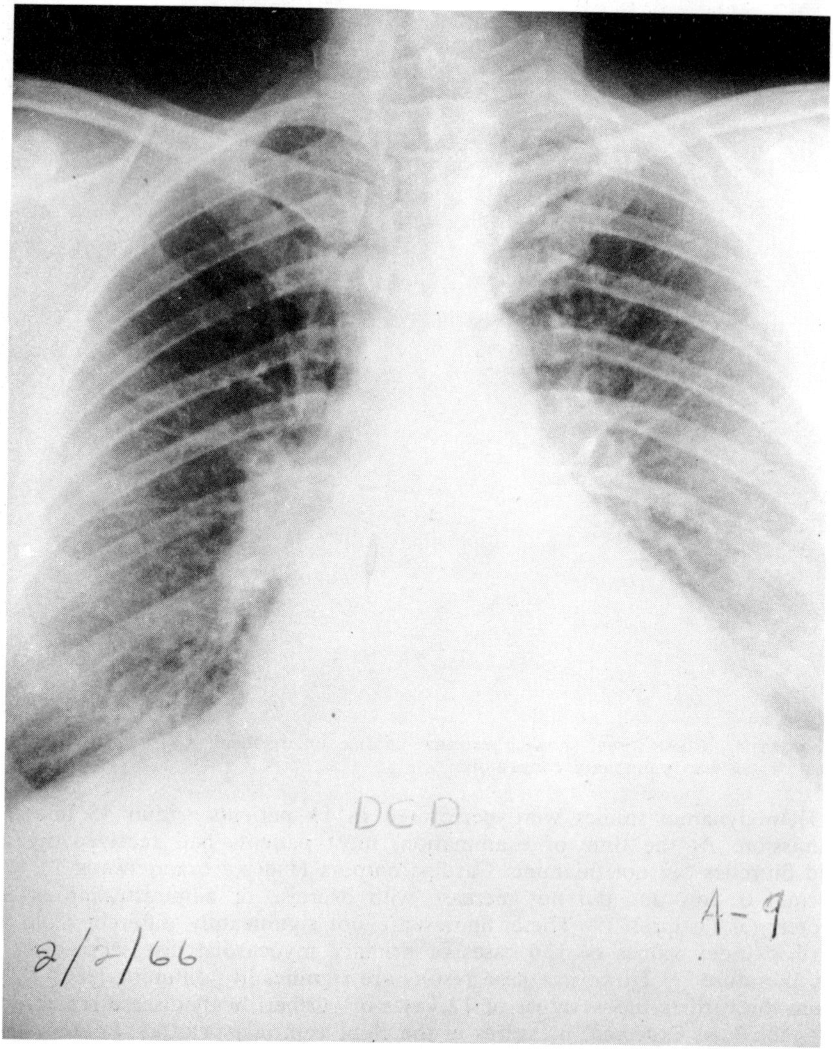

FIGURE 5. Chest x-ray, showing cardiac enlargement.

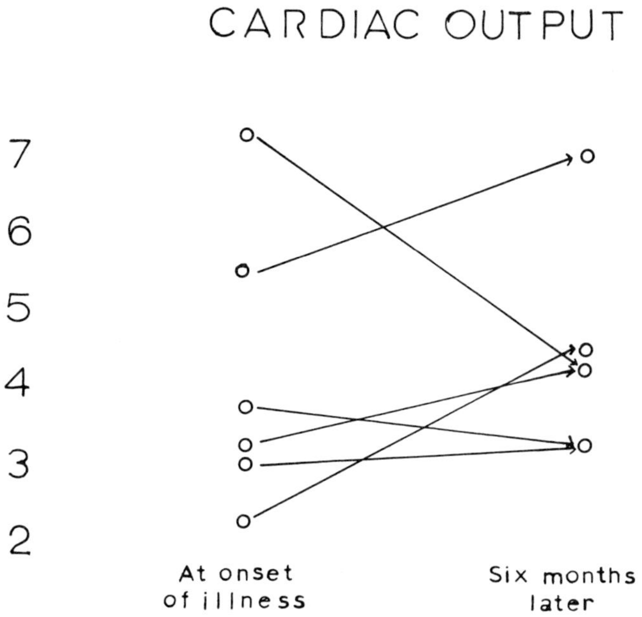

FIGURE 6. Cardiac output in six patients at onset of illness and six months later.

TABLE 1

CARDIAC INDEX VALUES*

A-5	A-14	A-7	A-8	A-1	A-6	A-3	
1.6	1.7	1.8	2.1	3.0	3.6	5.6	(Mean, 2.7)
B-6	E-10	E-9					
1.3	1.3	2.2	(Mean, 1.6)				
C-1							
4.4							

* Top line = patient number; bottom line = cardiac index, in liters per minute.

In summary, these hemodynamic studies show a normal or low cardiac output, diminished myocardial compliance, absence of myocardial response to exercise or catecholamine, and a normal peripheral resistance. The evolution of these cases was variable, and it is doubtful whether therapy had much influence on the eventual outcome. Most patients were treated with digitalis, diuretics, and thiamine. Recovery was slow and progressive.

After discharge from hospitals, patients were seen fairly regularly, although eight were lost to follow-up. The remaining subjects failed to follow diet or to take their medication regularly; most important of all, 16 out of 22 returned to their drinking habits, consuming as much beer and of the same brand as they did before. Their food habits were identical. Many of them were inebriated when seen on follow-up studies. In spite of this, none had symptoms or physical signs referable to the cardiovascular system. Electrocardiograms

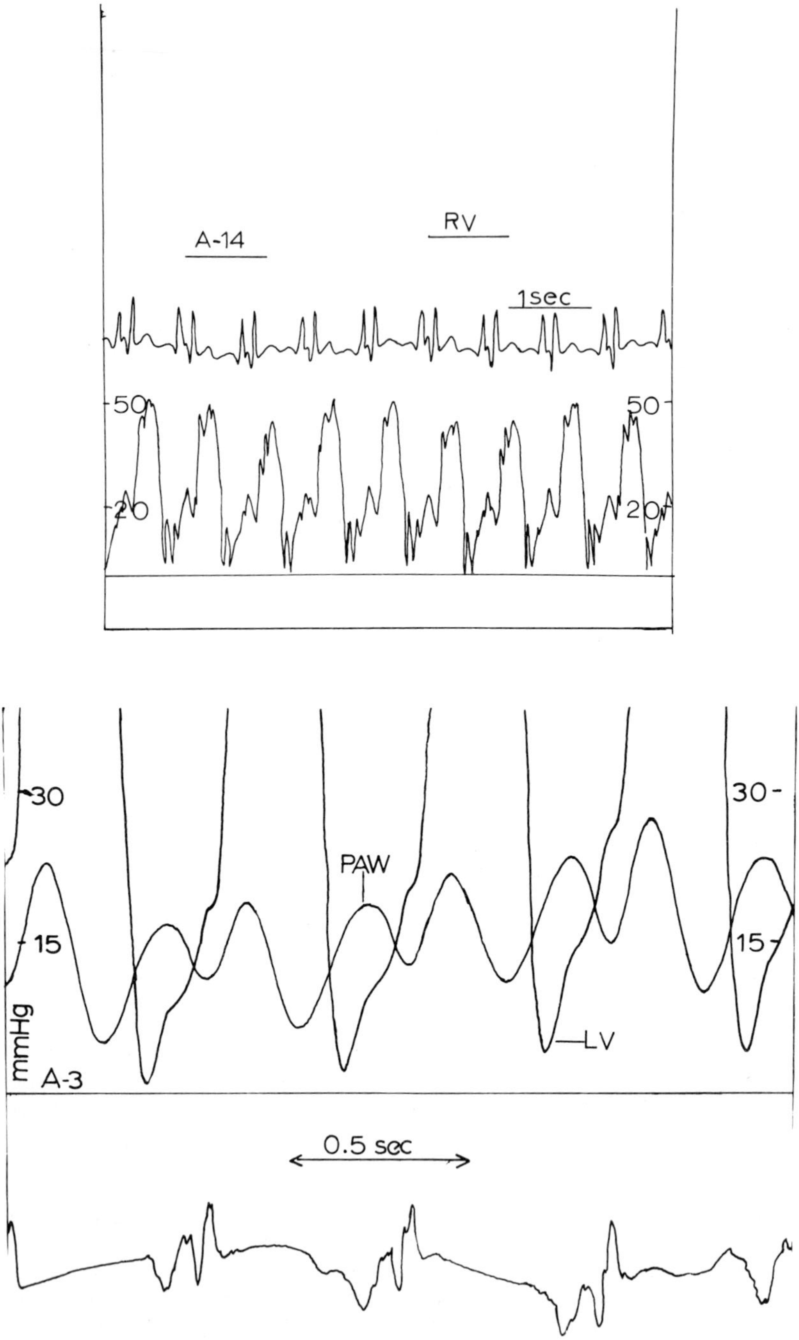

FIGURE 8. Left ventricular and pulmonary arteriolar pressure curves.

were either normal or, in five cases out of the 22, showed minor and non-specific T wave changes. Chest x-rays were all within normal limits.

Thus, between August, 1965, and April, 1966, in the Québec City area, a syndrome with definite clinical and hemodynamic features appeared. Similar cases were not seen in other parts of the country. However, one of the authors had the opportunity to examine cases in Omaha, Neb., and in Minneapolis, Minn. Other series probably exist elsewhere.

Clinically, the patients presented as cases of severe heart failure with shock, liver involvement, gastrointestinal ulcerations, and thrombotic phenomena. There is a certain similarity between this disease and beriberi heart disease. In the latter however, an abnormally high cardiac output with very low systemic resistances is a constant finding; this phenomenon would appear to be only one aspect of the disease, and myocardial involvement of the type observed in the Québec myocardosis also has been found in beriberi.[16]

The etiology of this syndrome will not be definitely established until the disease is experimently reproduced in animals. However, we feel that the epidemiological, clinical, and pathological evidence is presently strong enough to incriminate cobalt as one of the essential causative factors of this syndrome. The toxicity of cobalt has been well studied at a clinical[17] and at a cellular level,[18] but a similar syndrome has not, to our knowledge, been reported previously. The fact that cobalt, as an antianemia agent, has in the past been used extensively at much higher dosage (24 pints of Brand XXX beer would officially contain 8 mg of cobalt sulfate, while 4 tablets daily of Roncovite®‡ would represent an intake of 60 mg of cobalt chloride) without producing such a dramatic picture would tend to indicate that other factors are at play to increase the susceptibility of these patients to cobalt. The nature of these other factors is the object of our investigation at the present.

References

1. PLATT, B. S. 1958. Clinical features of endemic beriberi. Fed. Proc. **17:** 8.
2. HARO, E. N., M. BRIN & W. W. FALOON. 1966. Fasting in obesity. Thiamine depletion as measured by erythrocyte transketolase changes. Arch. Intern. Med. (Chicago) **117:** 175.
3. MASSUMI, R. A., J. C. RIOS, A. S. GOOCH, D. D. NUTTER, T. VINCENT & D. W. DATLOW. 1965. Primary myocardial disease. Report of fifty cases and review of the subject. Circulation **31:** 19.
4. GOODWIN, J. F., H. GORDON, A. HOLLMAN & M. B. BISHOP. 1961. Clinical aspects of cardiomyopathy. Brit. Med. J. **5219:** 69.
5. FOWLER, N. O., M. GUERON & D. T. ROWLANDS, JR. 1961. Myocardial Disease. Circulation **23:** 498.
6. SACKNER, M. A., D. H. LEWIS, M. J. ROBINSON & S. BELLET. 1961. Idiopathic myocardial hypertrophy. Amer. J. Cardiol. **7:** 714.
7. STORSTEIN, O. 1964. Primary myocardial disease. Acta Med. Scand. **176:** 731.
8. YU, P. N., J. COHEN, B. F. SCHREINER, JR. & G. W. MURPHY. 1964. Hemodynamic alterations in primary myocardial disease. Progr. Cardiov. Dis. **7:** 125.
9. DYE, C. L., P. D. GENOVESE, W. J. DALY & R. H. BEHNKE. 1963. Primary myocardial disease. Hemodynamic alterations. Ann. Int. Med. **58:** 442.
10. BOYD, D. L., M. E. MISHKIN, H. FEIGENBAUM & P. D. GENOVESE. 1965. Three families with familial cardiomyopathy. Ann. Intern. Med. **63:** 386.
11. GOODWIN, J. F. 1964. Cardiac function in primary myocardial disorders. Brit. Med. J. **5397:** 1527.
12. PIETRAS, T. J., W. R. MEADOWS, M. FORT & J. T. SHARP. 1965. Hemodynamic alterations in idiopathic myocardiopathy including cineangiography from the left heart chambers. Amer. J. Cardiol. **16:** 672.

‡ Distributed by Hoechst Pharmaceuticals, Montreal, Canada.

13. Wendt, V. C., T. B. Stock, R. O. Hayden, T. A. Bruce, S. Gudbjarnason & R. J. Bing. 1962. The hemodynamics and cardiac metabolism in cardiomyopathies. Med. Clin. N. Amer. **46:** 1445.
14. Bourdarias, J. P., P. Ourbak, P. Penther, L. Scebat & J. Lenegre. 1966. Étude hemodynamique des myocardiopathies non obstructives d'origine indéterminée. Acta Cardiol. (Brux.) **21:** 285.
15. Wagner, P. I. 1965. Beriberi heart disease. Physiologic data and difficulties in diagnosis. Amer. Heart J. **69:** 200.
16. Akbarian, M., N. A. Yankopoulos & W. H. Abelmann. 1966. Hemodynamic studies in beriberi heart disease. Amer. J. Med. **41:** 197.
17. Caujolle, F. & D. Meunier. 1959. Sur la toxicité du cobalt. Rev. Path. Gen. **59:** 254.
18. Dingle, J. T., J. C. Heath, M. Welb & M. Daniel. 1962. The biological action of cobalt and other metals. The mechanism of the respiratory inhibition produced by cobalt in mammalian tissues. Biochem. Biophys. Acta. **65:** 34.

QUÉBEC BEER-DRINKERS' MYOCARDOSIS: PATHOLOGICAL ASPECTS

Jean-Louis Bonenfant, Carlton Auger, Georges Miller, Jacques Chenard, and Paul-Emile Roy

Department of Pathology, Laval University, Québec, Canada

Last winter, a peculiar epidemic of myocardosis occurred in the Lower Town of Québec City, and we had the opportunity to study the pathology of some of these cases.[1-3] A total of 20 deaths occurred, and the autopsy findings in all cases revealed the same degenerative changes in the myocardium. In addition, biopsy material from heart, liver, and skeletal muscle of patients who survived was available for study. In this paper, we are limiting ourselves to a description of the cardiac and thyroid lesions. The complete data of the autopsy findings will be published elsewhere.[4]

Cardiac Findings

In all cases, the heart was uniformly increased in size and on cut section was pale and slightly brownish. In many, mural thrombi were present in one chamber or another. The coronary arteries showed a very minor degree of arteriosclerosis.

Histologically, the myocardial changes were intense and diffuse (FIGURE 1). The size and staining properties of the muscle fibers were variable; at higher magnifications, the main lesion appeared to be caused by the diminution or even the loss of the myofibrillar elements (FIGURE 2). Numerous vacuoles were present in most fibers and consisted of ill-defined central or scattered globular clearings (FIGURE 3). The major portion of the smaller vacuoles corresponded to sudanophilic inclusions (FIGURE 4). This hydropic or lipoid vacuolization was the only invariable feature present and was certainly responsible for the pale-brownish aspect of the myocardium on cut section. In addition, an interstitial edema and discrete focal fibrosis were present. One case showed rare foci of chronic inflammatory cells, polymorphonuclear eosinophils, histiocytes, and mast cells.

The periodic acid-Schiff reaction for glycogen was negative in the autopsy cases but strongly positive in the surgical material. The absence of glycogen in the autopsy material is presumably due to postmortem autolysis. The interstitial edema was less marked in the surgical specimens than in the autopsies, but this was also probably a postmortem change.

In the single case examined under the electron microscope,[5] the lesions seemed to involve chiefly the myofibrils, the sarcoplasmic reticulum, and the mitochondria. The sarcolemnal membranes, the nuclei, and the Golgi apparatus showed relatively little damage.

The myocardial changes were widespread. Many myofibrils had totally disappeared (FIGURE 5), and most of the remaining ones were fragmented. The myofibrillar substance was replaced by a rich and evenly dispersed deposit of fine particulate material, probably representing glycogen.

The mitochondria, relatively normal in number, were found scattered or in disoriented clusters, and were often bizarre in shape (FIGURE 6). Many of them were small and dense with a shrunken appearance. The smooth-surfaced sarcoplasmic reticulum of the myocardial fibers showed severe damage. The

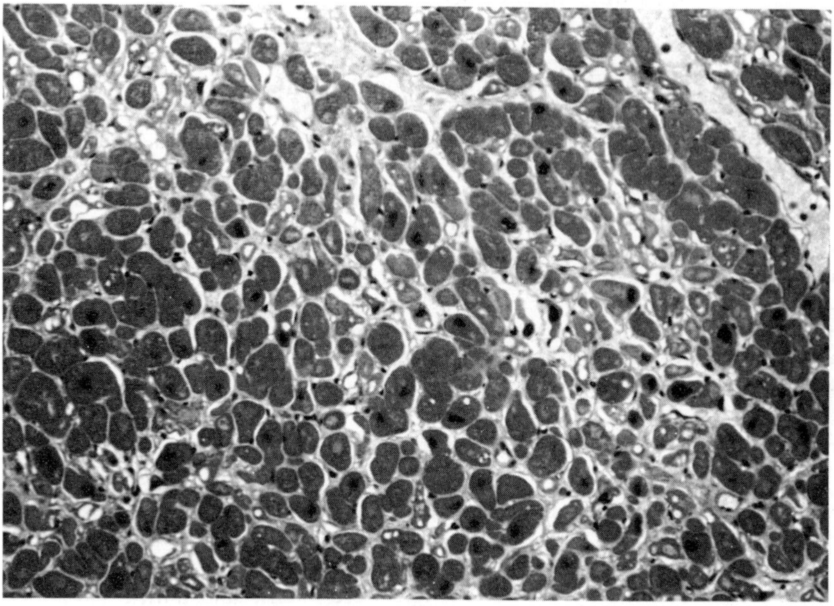

FIGURE 1. Diffuse myocardial changes and interstitial edema. Stain: hematoxylin and eosin. × 160 (orig. mag. × 200).

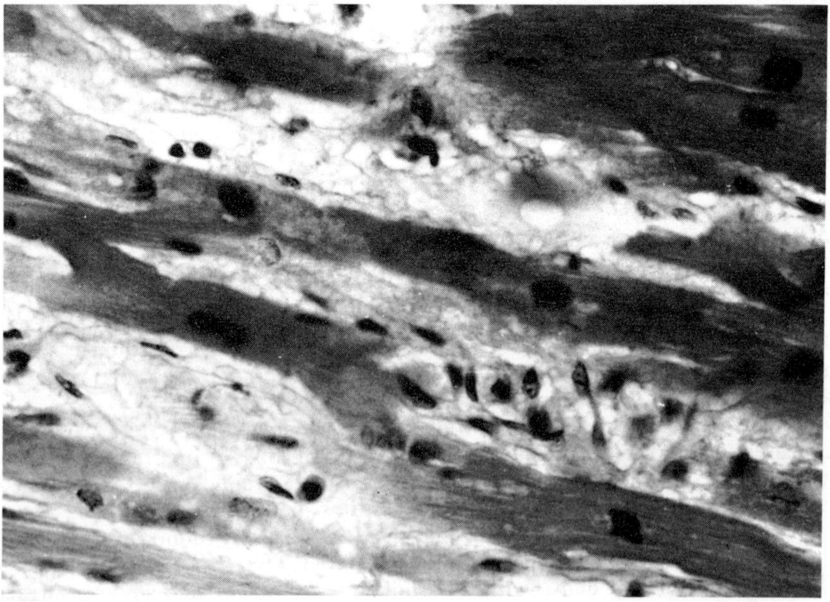

FIGURE 2. Diminution and loss of myofibrils. Stain: hematoxylin and eosin. × 320 (orig. mag. × 400).

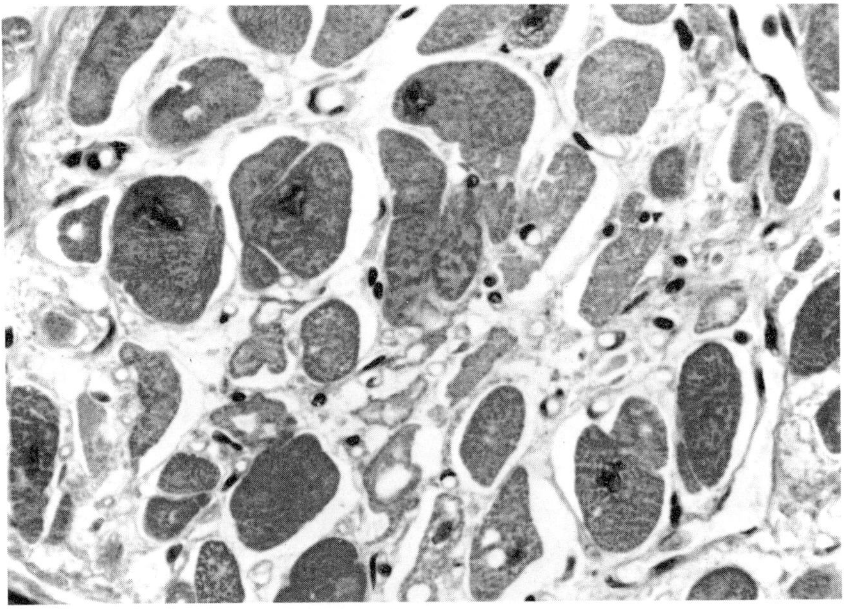

FIGURE 3. Hydropic vacuolization of the muscle fibers. Stain: hematoxylin and eosin. × 320 (orig. mag. × 400).

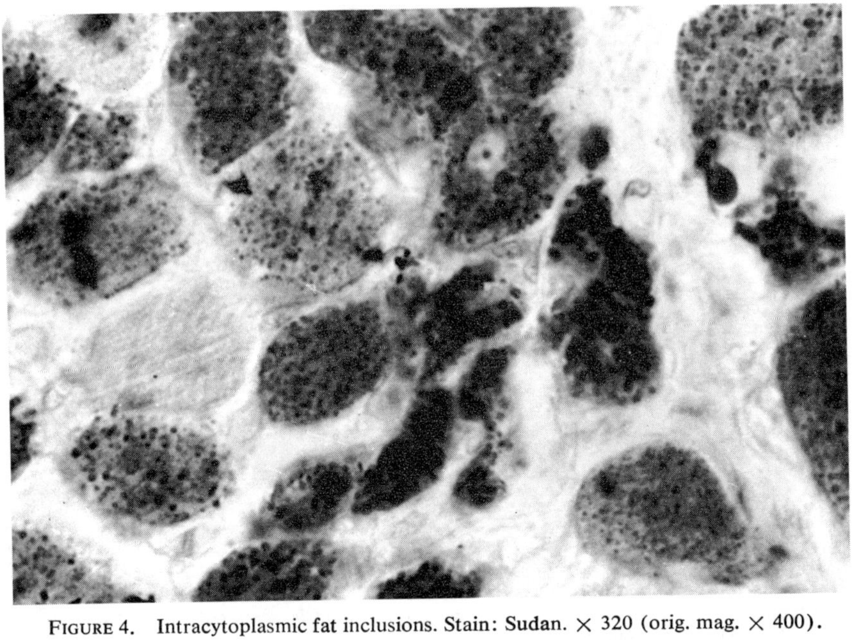

FIGURE 4. Intracytoplasmic fat inclusions. Stain: Sudan. × 320 (orig. mag. × 400).

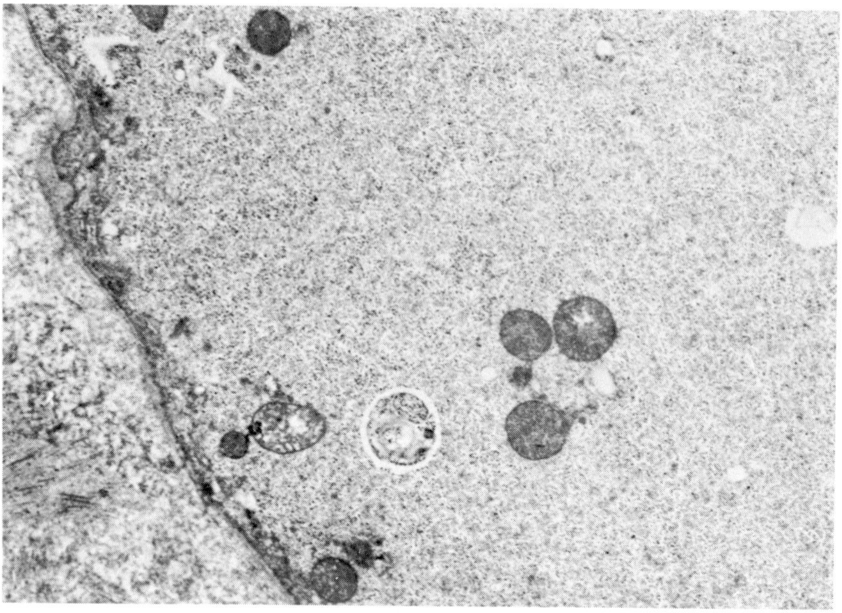

FIGURE 5. Electron micrograph, showing total disappearance of myofibrils. × 19,850 (orig. mag. × 24,800).

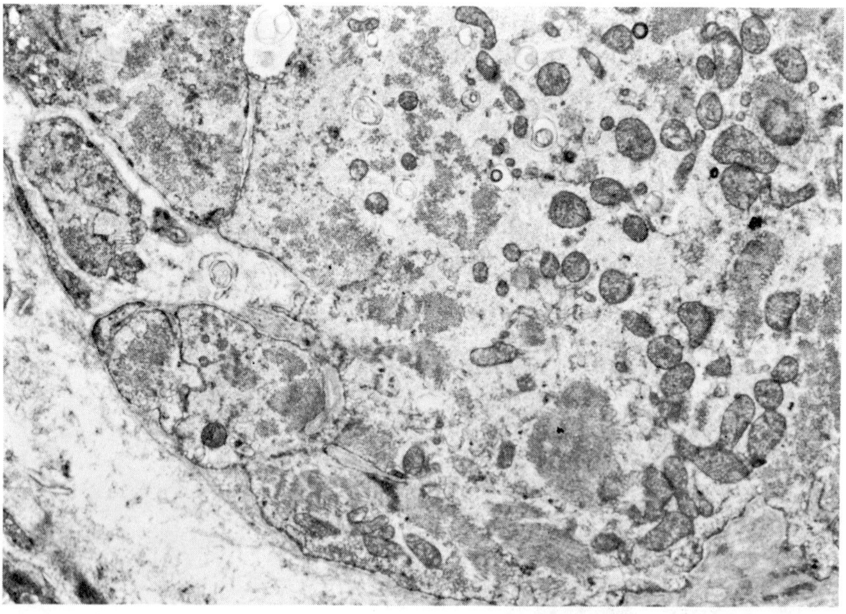

FIGURE 6. Electron micrograph, showing mitochondria scattered or in disoriented clusters. × 8,640 (orig. mag. × 10,800).

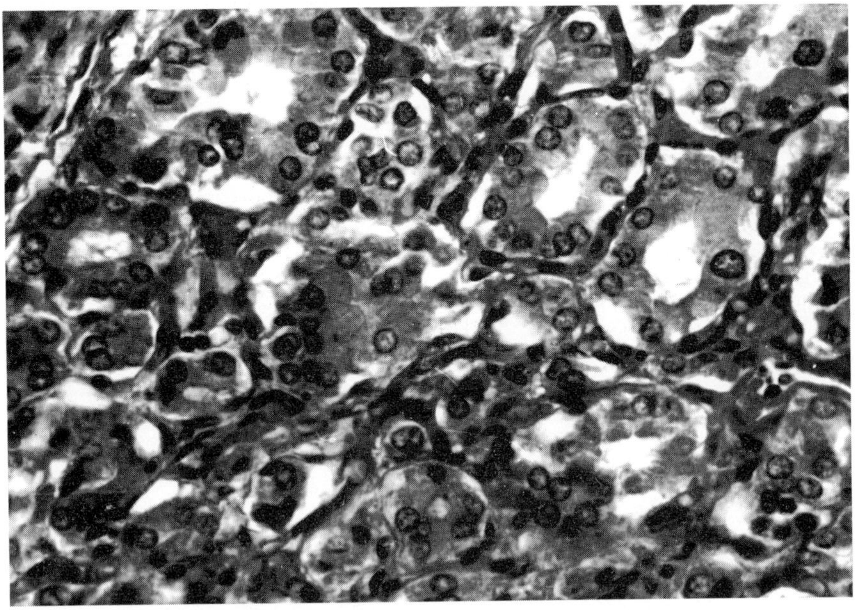

FIGURE 7. Cubic or columnar aspect of the epithelial cells of the thyroid vesicles. Absence of colloid. Stain: hematoxylin and eosin. × 320 (orig. mag. × 400).

persisting elements were swollen and formed frequently large vesicles. Occasionally, a few cells contained large electron-dense bodies suggestive of lipid.

Thyroid Findings

On gross examination, the size and color of the thyroids were unremarkable, and the changes were essentially microscopical. Colloid was often absent or scanty, granular, and vacuolated. The epithelial cells were cubic or columnar (FIGURE 7), with a clear cytoplasm containing a delicate dark granulation. The stroma was congested without any significant inflammatory infiltration. The general picture is quite similar to the changes reported in the thyroid after cobalt medication in children.[6,7]

Conclusion

These patients were ingesting from 5 to 10 mg of cobalt per day in their beer, and this chemical element must be considered in the etiology of the myocardiopathy. Incidental findings included a high frequency of inflammatory gastrointestinal lesions and central hemorrhagic necrosis of the liver.

Summary

The principal pathological features of the myocardial lesions encountered in Québec's beer drinkers were a diffuse vacuolar degeneration and myofibrilysis. In the cases where thyroid tissue was available for study, changes comparable to those found in children receiving cobalt medication were encountered. It is suggested that cobalt intoxication must be considered in the etiology of these cases of myocardosis.

References

1. Quebec's Medical Mystery. 1966. J.A.M.A. **196:** 11.
2. Quebec's Medical Mystery Spreads. 1966. J.A.M.A. **197:** 4.
3. Bonenfant, J.-L. 1966. Beer-drinker's myocardosis. Bull. Path. **7:** 297.
4. Bonenfant, J.-L., G. Miller & P. E. Roy. 1967. Québec Beer-Drinkers' Cardiomyopathy: Pathological Studies. Canad. Med. Ass. J. **97:** 910.
5. Auger, C. & J. Chenard. 1967. Québec Beer-Drinkers' Cardiomyopathy: Ultrastructural Changes in One Case. Canad. Med. Ass. J. **97:** 916.
6. Holly, R. G. 1955. Studies on iron and cobalt metabolism. J.A.M.A. **158:** 1349–1392.
7. Klinck, G. H. 1955. Thyroid hyperplasia in young children. J.A.M.A. **158:** 1347–1348.

MOLECULAR CHANGES IN MYOCARDIAL INFARCTION IN HEART MUSCLE*

Richard J. Bing, Sigmundur Gudbjarnason, Hans Tschopp, and Wolfgang Braasch
Department of Medicine, Wayne State University School of Medicine Detroit, Mich.

In the past, studies on the biochemical effect of coronary occlusion have dealt primarily with the release of enzymes by the heart muscle or with changes in substrate extraction by anaerobic cardiac tissue. Many questions, however, remain unanswered. These are concerned mainly with the possible biochemical changes occurring in infarcted muscle as a result of the reparative processes, together with the factors that govern the rates of healing and collagen formation in cardiac scar tissue in the infarcted area. In addition, there are problems concerned with the early biochemical changes in heart muscle occurring soon after infarction and with the reestablishment of circulation in the affected areas after coronary occlusion, as influenced by revascularizing procedures.

Studies on Infarcted Heart Muscle

One of the purposes of this particular study was to examine activities involved in energy metabolism and the production of metabolites for biosynthesis of subcellular constituents. Myocardial infarction was produced in dogs by ligation of several branches of the anterior and posterior descending coronary arteries, as reported elsewhere.[1] The response of heart muscle to an alteration in the biochemical environment accompanying coronary occlusion was examined by determining the activities of enzymes in the uninjured normal part of the left ventricle and in the periphery and center of the infarct. Enzymes of the glycolytic and tricarboxylic acid cycle studied were: fructose-1,6-diphosphate aldolase, glyceraldehyde-phosphate dehydrogenase, lactate dehydrogenase, malate dehydrogenase, DPN- and TPN-specific isocitrate dehydrogenase, and glutamate oxalacetate transaminase. Of these enzymes only DPN-specific isocitrate dehydrogenase is a specific mitochondrial enzyme. The activities of α-glycerophosphate dehydrogenase and of creatine phosphokinase were also determined; the hexose monophosphate shunt was represented by glucose-6-phosphate dehydrogenase and by 6-phosphogluconate dehydrogenase. The details are published elsewhere.[2,3]

During the first 120 minutes following ligation of the branches of some of the coronary arteries, the significant changes consisted of a rise followed by a decline in the ratio of phosphorylase a to total phosphorylase and in a fall in creatine phosphokinase. 6-Phosphogluconate dehydrogenase rose markedly in the infarcted zone, and the activity of glucose-6-phosphate dehydrogenase also increased (TABLE 1). An early rise in the ratio of phosphorylase a to total phosphorylase immediately after infarction has been reported in Wollenberger;[4] Cori and Cori noticed an initial rise followed by a decline in skeletal muscle during tetanic stimulation,[5] and Klarwein and his associates from this laboratory reported similar results in fibrillating cardiac muscle.[6] It is likely that the decline in this ratio, observed 30 minutes after infarction, is the result of increased lactic

* This work was supported by United States Public Health Service grant no. HE-05043 and The Michigan Heart Association.

TABLE 1

ENZYME CHANGES AT THE PERIPHERY AND CENTER OF INFARCTED AREAS AFTER LIGATION OF LEFT CORONARY ARTERY BRANCHES COMPARED WITH NORMAL TISSUE*

Time (minutes after ligation)	Glucose-6-Phosphate Dehydrogenase		6-Phosphogluconate Dehydrogenase		Creatine Phosphokinase		Ratio of Phosphorylase a to Total Phosphorylase	
	Periphery	Center	Periphery	Center	Periphery	Center	Periphery	Center
30 min	133.6	130.7	110.8	103.9	89.8	83.8	77.6	110.1
n	7	7	7	7	5	5	4	4
60 min	107.5	117.5	107.9	126.7	102.2	132.7	89	65.4
n	5	5	5	5	5	5	6	6
120 min	125.7	115.7	125.0	169.0	89.8	42.0	50.6	33.9
n	7	7	7	7	7	7	4	4

* All values are means, expressed as a percentage of the normal values. N = number of experiments in each case.

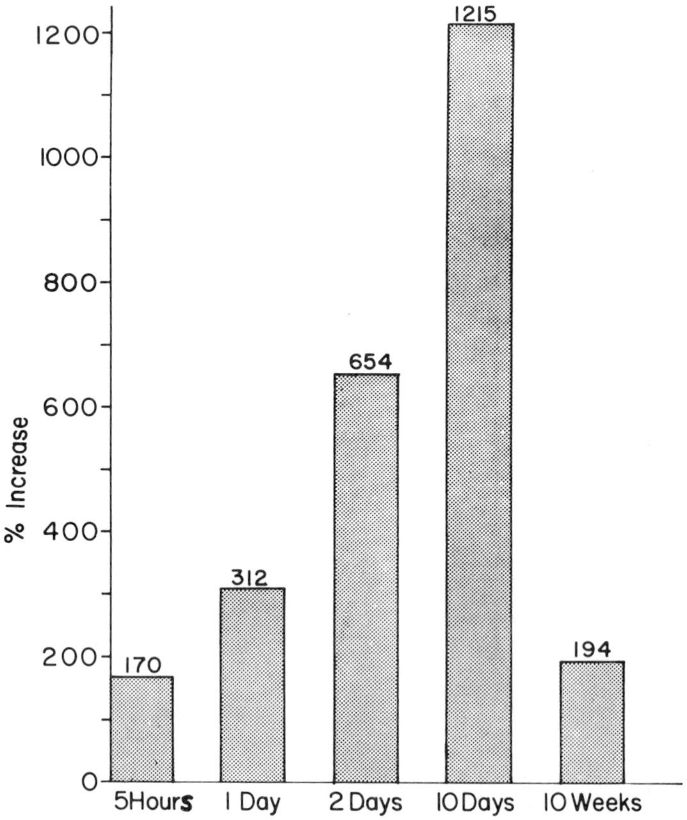

FIGURE 1. Increase in activity of glucose-6-phosphate dehydrogenase in infarcted heart muscle.

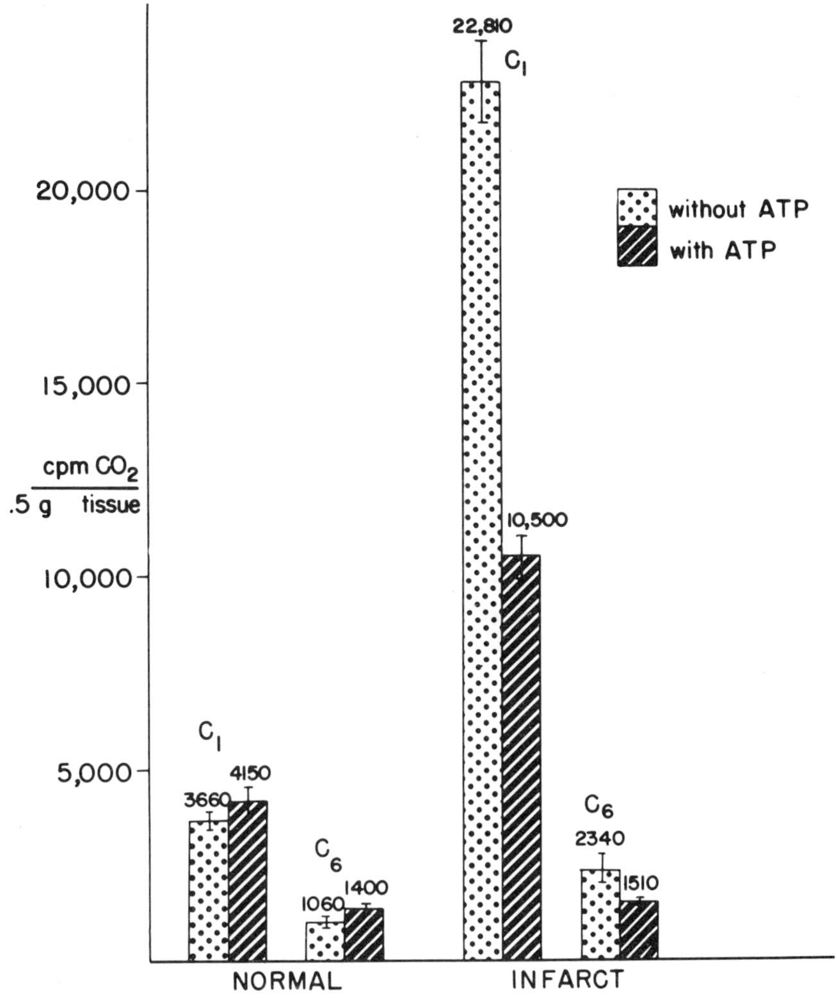

FIGURE 2. Oxidation of glucose-1-^{14}C and glucose-6-^{14}C to $^{14}CO_2$ by normal tissue and infarcted heart muscle. 2.5 ml of homogenate, representing 500 mg of tissue in 0.25 M sucrose, was incubated for 30 minutes at 37° C with 10 μc of labeled glucose. The incubations were carried out in the presence and absence of exogenous adenosine triphosphate [ATP (15 mM)].

acid in heart muscle which inactivates the enzyme system responsible for the conversion of inactive to active phosphorylase.

The early rise in 6-phosphogluconate dehydrogenase and glucose-6-phosphate dehydrogenase indicates activation of the pentose monophosphate shunt (TABLE 1); the activity of this enzyme rose to more than 1,000% of control values (FIGURE 1) in the center of the infarct ten days after infarction. In line with this observation was the finding that there was enhanced formation of $^{14}CO_2$ from glucose-1-^{14}C in the infarcted tissue (FIGURE 2). This also reflects the increased activity of the pentose monophosphate shunt. At the same time, there was some inactivation of the glycolytic and mitochondrial enzymes, as indicated by diminished activites of lactate dehydrogenase, aldolase, isocitrate dehydrogenase, and malate dehydrogenase. It appears to us that this rise in glucose-6-phosphate dehydrogenase and 6-phosphogluconate dehydrogenase occurs at a time (five hours after infarction) when infiltration of new cells cannot be observed histologically. At five hours after infarction, there was already a moderate increase in glucose-6-phosphate dehydrogenase activity in the infarcted myocardial cells (FIGURE 1). There are many difficulties in evaluating enzymes of necrotic tissue, such as changes in protein content, edema and necrosis, changes in membrane permeability, infiltration of cells, and hydrolysis and degradation; but the changes observed here are greater than those that would result from alterations in protein content alone.

The importance of this shift to the hexose monophosphate shunt lies in its numerous interconnections with other metabolic pathways. The shunt is essential for nucleic acid synthesis and for TPNH-dependent synthesis. The shunt also plays an important role in developmental processes, as demonstrated by Krahl[7] and by Burt and Wenger.[8] The significance of the hexose monophosphate shunt during the development of the pig heart was demonstrated by Jolley and his associates.[9] It is also possible that dedifferentiation and degeneration of heart muscle may play a role in initiating increased hexose monophosphate shunt activity, as observed by Fujimoto and Harary in tissue cultures.[10]

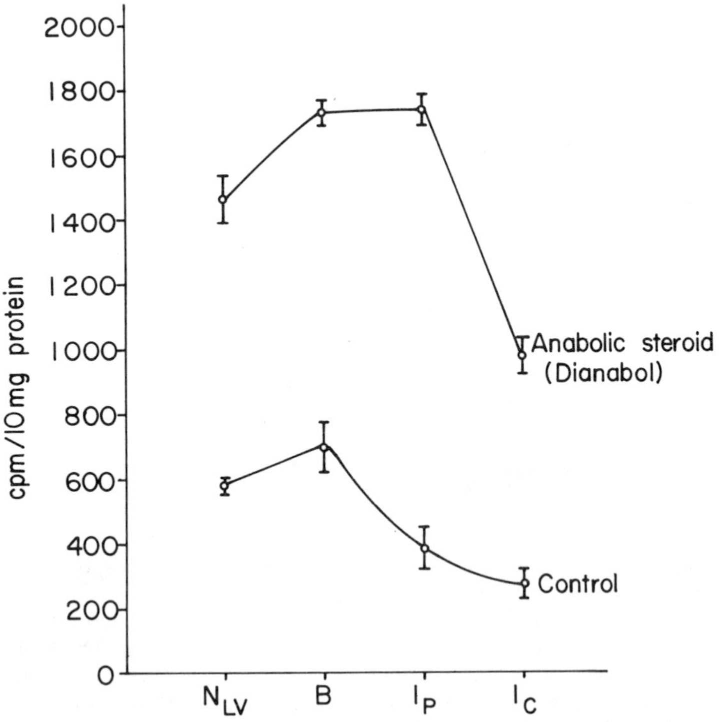

FIGURE 3. Effect of an anabolic hormone (Dianabol®) on the rate of protein synthesis in normal and infarcted heart muscle 24 hours after infarction, as reflected by glycine-2-^{14}C incorporation into the protein of infarcted muscle. N_{LV} = normal; B = borderline; I_p = periphery of infarct; I_c = center of infarct.

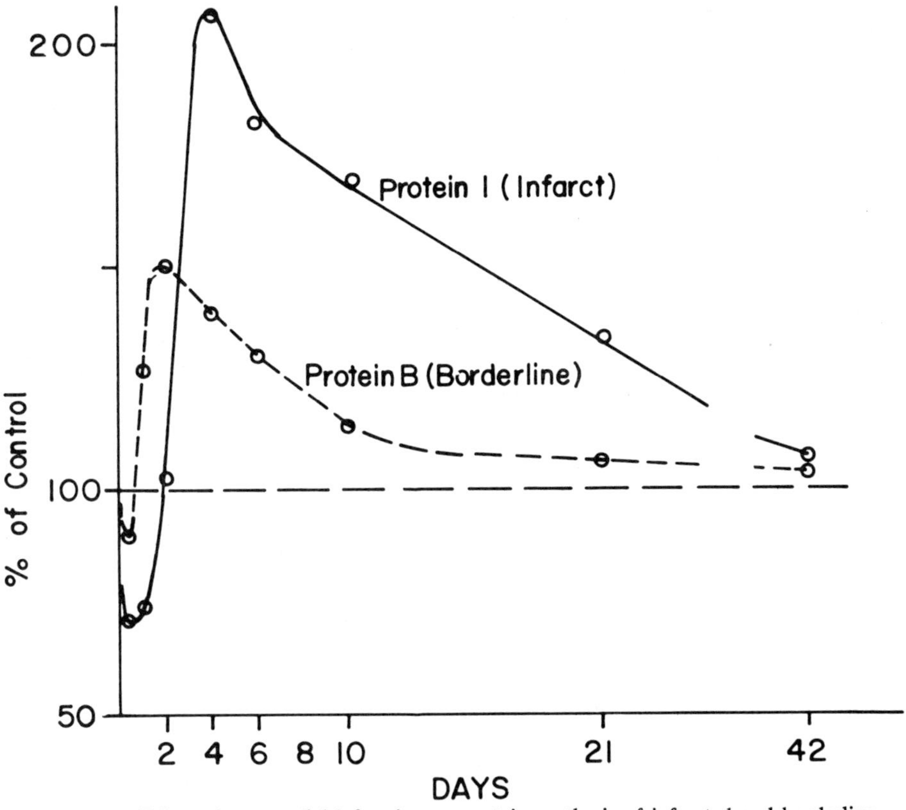

FIGURE 4. Effect of myocardial infarction on protein synthesis of infarcted and borderline tissue. Each point represents the mean value of three experiments.

Since increased activity of the pentose monophosphate shunt probably occurs in the presence of cellular processes demanding increased formation of nucleic acid, it is not surprising that administration of anabolic hormones such as methandrostenolone (Dianabol®)† to animals following ligation of branches of the coronary arteries results in an increased activity of this shunt. There is also a marked increase in the incorporation of glycine-2-^{14}C into proteins of the infarcted area following administration of this anabolic steroid (FIGURE 3). Dianabol® increased incorporation of the labeled amino acid by 233% compared with normal tissue.[11] Treatment with this compound also appeared to increase the thickness of the scar tissue and prevented the formation of aneurysms. Experiments carried out *in vitro* on infarcted and normal cardiac muscle from treated and untreated animals also showed an increased rate of protein synthesis.

In addition to the "anabolic" steroids, treatment with ascorbic acid or small amounts of insulin (10 units) with potassium chloride or glucose (the Sodi-Pallares polarizing solution) had similar effects.[11,12] The use of ascorbic acid or the Sodi-Pallares solution may be beneficial in promoting healing of the infarcted region, although at the moment there are no truly quantitative methods to

† Distributed by Ciba Pharmaceutical Co., Summit, N. J.

assess the effect of these compounds in man. The development of such methods is costly, but represents a true challenge to the clinical investigator, although at present there is little inclination for full support of these ventures.

The effect of myocardial infarction upon the overall synthesis of proteins and nucleic acid in infarcted tissue was also studied by means of observing the incorporation of glycine-2-^{14}C into protein and nucleic acids of the heart muscle of dogs.[1] FIGURE 4 illustrates the effect of myocardial infarction upon the incorporation of glycine-2-^{14}C into proteins of infarcted tissue. The incorporation into control tissue is considered 100%, and the specific activity of protein obtained from infarcted and borderline zones is related to this control sample. Immediately after coronary occlusion, the incorporation of glycine-2-^{14}C into protein decreased, but soon afterward rose again above normal. Incorporation into cardiac proteins reached a maximum of 207% of the control on the fourth day.[1] Borderline tissue showed an early increase in protein synthesis. The concentration of deoxyribonucleic acid (DNA) increased on the second day after infarction and reached a maximum of 90% above normal eight days later (FIGURE 5).

Using cell fractionation by means of differential centrifugation, four nuclear

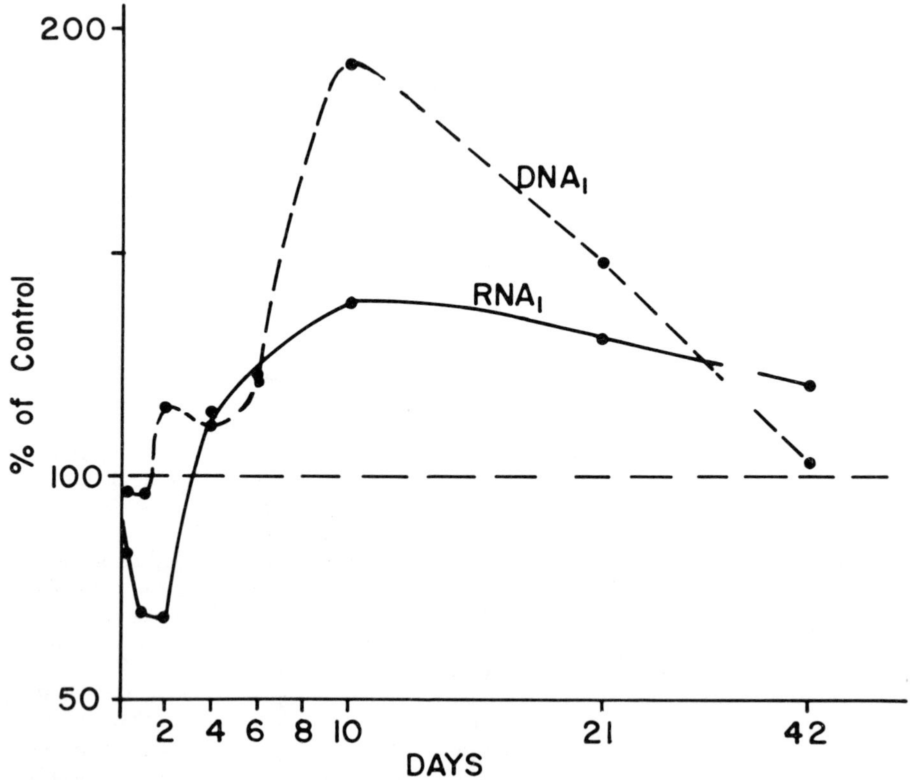

FIGURE 5. Effect of myocardial infarction on the RNA and DNA concentrations in infarcted tissue.

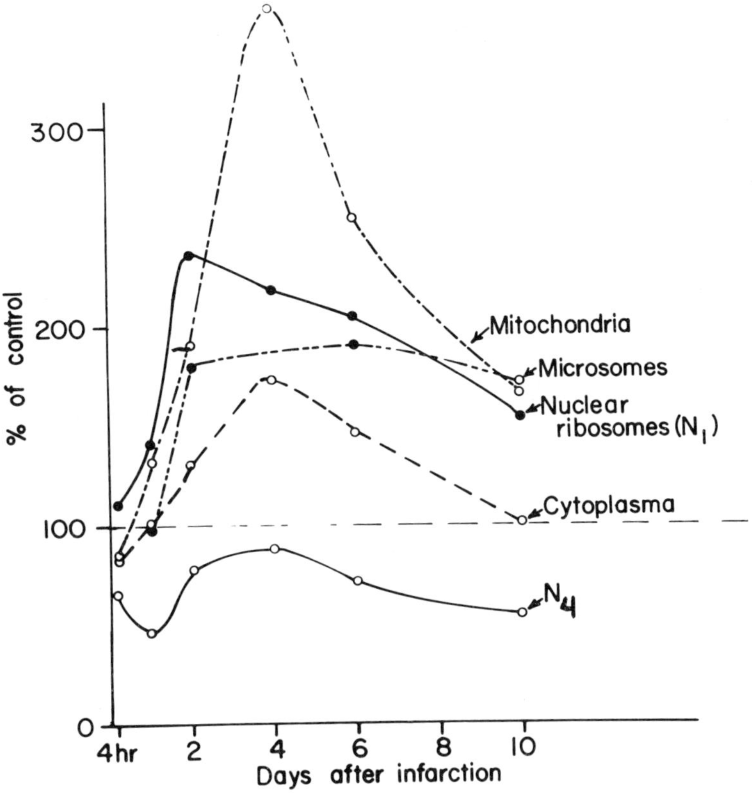

FIGURE 6. Effect of myocardial infarction on incorporation of glycine-2-^{14}C into subcellular protein fractions of infarcted tissue compared with normal left ventricular muscle of the same heart. N_4 = fraction containing the contractile protein.

fractions were obtained.[1] The first (N_1) contained mainly nuclear ribosomes; the second (N_2) contained DNA, ribonucleic acid (RNA), and nuclear proteins; the third (N_3), employing phenol extraction, resulted in an aqueous-phase RNA (p-RNA) and an interphase fraction with high activity (m-RNA); finally, the fourth portion (N_4) was obtained containing the contractile proteins.[1]

FIGURE 6 shows that incorporation into the nuclear ribosomal fraction precedes all other fractions; this is followed by incorporation into mitochondria and cytoplasmic microsomes. The N_4 fraction, containing the bulk of the contractile proteins, shows an early fall in the incorporation, which remains subnormal. FIGURE 7 demonstrates the incorporation of glycine-^{14}C into nucleic acids of infarcted tissue. The earliest increase in incorporation was observed in "nucleolar" p-RNA, followed by nuclear ribosomal RNA. The activity of the DNA fractions increased 48 hours after infarction.[1] These results indicate that the reparative process starts in the cell nuclei as early as 24 hours after infarction. An early increase in activity was seen in the nuclear ribosomal fraction and in the nucleolar p-RNA, followed by nuclear ribosomal RNA. The sequence of labeling of the protein fraction indicates a possible nuclear origin of cytoplasmic particles.[1]

The first step in the reparative process seems to be concerned with the synthesis of nuclear material, followed by reconstruction of mitochondria and microsomes.[1]

Results Obtained in Experimentally Induced Chronic Cardiac Insufficiency

The preceding results were obtained on hearts with complete and instantaneously produced coronary occlusion. In man, however, coronary artery disease is usually a slowly progressive chronic illness, with complete occlusion occurring as an end stage of a chronic pathological process. Experiments were therefore performed to study vascular capacity and capillary blood flow, together with changes in enzyme patterns, in the hearts of dogs with experimentally produced coronary artery insufficiency. Coronary insufficiency was produced by gradual constriction of the right coronary artery and of both branches of the left coronary artery by means of luminal expansion of casein plastic sleeves (ameroids), according to the method of Litvak and his associates.[13] Since the anterior septal artery originates above the constriction, the ventricular septum can be used as control. Capillary blood flow was determined by the method of Sapirstein, using rubidium-86 chloride;[14] vascular capacity was estimated with the method of Myers and Honig.[15] Revascularization was produced by implantation of an internal mammary artery, omental graft, epicardiectomy, and seropericardiec-

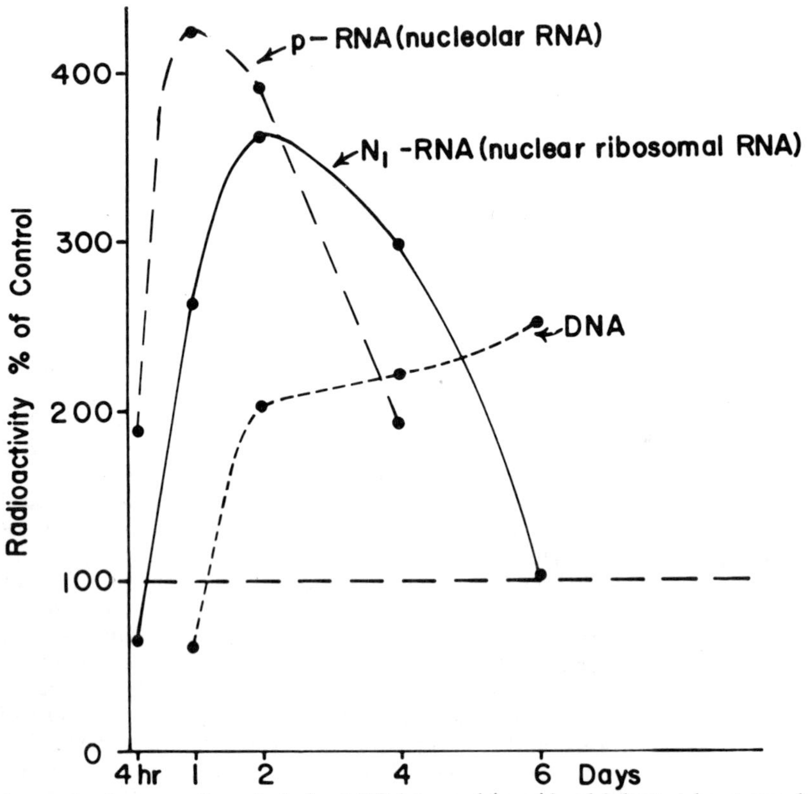

FIGURE 7. Incorporation of glycine-2-^{14}C into nucleic acids of infarcted heart muscle.

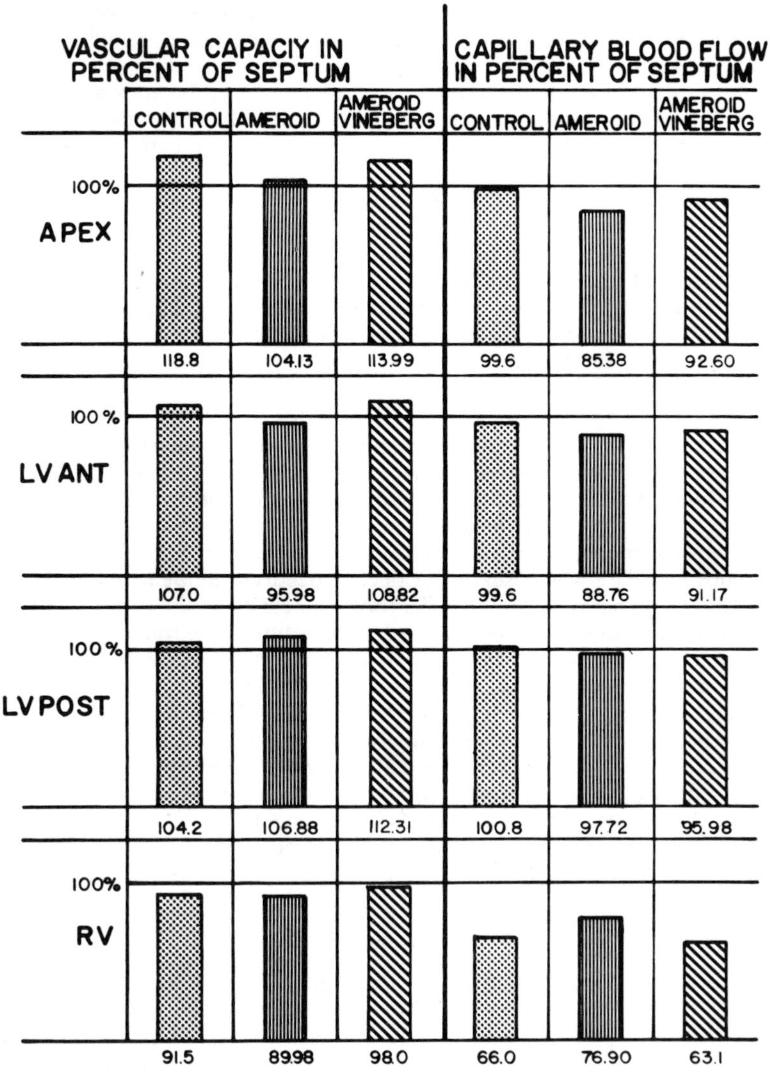

FIGURE 8. Changes in vascular capacity and capillary blood flow in coronary insufficiency produced by ameroid rings and in animals with ameroid rings and an implanted mammary artery (Vineberg operation).

tomy according to Vineberg and his colleagues.[16] In our experiments, the internal mammary artery was tunneled into the anterior aspects of the left ventricle at the same time as the ameroid sleeves were placed around the coronary arteries.

The results on relative (with respect to the septum) capillary blood flow and vascular capacity are shown in FIGURE 8. It can be seen that, with the exception of the posterior aspects of the left ventricle and of the right ventricle, ameroid constriction leads to a diminution of the capillary blood flow. Implantation of the internal mammary artery resulted in an increase in capillary blood flow above values recorded in hearts with ameroid constriction alone. Similar changes occurred in relative vascular capacity. Ameroid constriction of the coronary arteries resulted in a diminution in vascular capacity in the apex and the anterior wall of the left ventricle; this effect was either partially or completely reversed by implantation of the internal mammary artery according to the procedure of Vineberg and his associates.[16]

Although the results on enzyme activities in the hearts of these animals are thus far only preliminary, they are of some interest, since they demonstrate that, in contrast to infarcted heart muscle resulting from ligation of the coronary arteries, heart muscle of animals with ameroid constriction fails to show any significant changes in enzyme activities. This indicates that there may be marked differences between the heart muscle of animals with coronary insufficiency and those with frank myocardial infarction.

Summary

Some biochemical and vascular changes in infarcted heart muscle after rapid ligation of the coronary arteries were studied; changes were also observed in the myocardium exposed to gradual narrowing of the coronary artery, simulating coronary insufficiency. In infarcted heart muscle, a rapid increase in activity of the pentose monophosphate shunt and in the ratio of active phosphorylase to total phosphorylase was observed. A decline occurred in the activities of enzymes of the glycolytic pathway and the tricarboxylic acid cycle.

Reparative processes in the infarcted myocardium were found to be accelerated by certain anabolic substances, such as anabolic steroids, small doses of insulin, and by ascorbic acid. It was also found that reparative processes commence in the cell nucleus. The first step was the synthesis of nuclear material.

In heart muscle exposed to slowly progressive coronary occlusion, both capillary blood flow and vascular volume were diminished. The activities of enzymes of the glycolytic pathway and the tricarboxylic acid cycle, as well as those of the pentose monophosphate shunt, remained unchanged. Revascularization of the heart by implantation of an internal mammary artery led to a relative increase in capillary flow and vascular volume in some portions of the myocardium.

References

1. Gudbjarnason, S., C. De Schryver, C. Chiba, J. Yamanaka & R. J. Bing. 1964. Protein and nucleic acid synthesis during the reparative processes following myocardial infarction. Circ. Res. **15:** 320.
2. Gudbjarnason, S., C. De Schryver, G. Hunn & R. J. Bing. 1964. Changes in myocardial enzyme pattern in human heart disease. J. Lab. Clin. Med. **64:** 796.
3. Delbrück, A., E. Zebe & T. Bücher. 1959. Über Verteilungsmuster von Enzymen des energieliefernden Stoffwechsels im Flugmuskel, Sprungmuskel und Feitkörper von Locusta migratoria und ihre cytologische Zuordnung. Biochem. Z. **331:** 273.
4. Wollenberger, A. Endogenous catecholamine mobilization and the shift to anaerobic energy production in the acutely ischemic myocardium. *In* Proceedings of the International Symposium on the Coronary Circulation and Energetics of the Myocardium, October, 1966, Milan, Italy. S. Karger. Basel, Switzerland. In press.
5. Cori, G. T. & C. F. Cori. 1933. Changes in hexose phosphate, glycogen and lactic acid during contraction and recovery of mammalian muscle. J. Biol. Chem. **99:** 493.
6. Klarwein, M., K. Kako, A. Chrysohou & R. J. Bing. 1961. Effect of atrial and ventricular fibrillation and ventricular tachycardia on carbohydrate metabolism of the heart. Circ. Res. **9:** 819.
7. Krahl, M. E. 1956. Oxidative pathways for glucose in eggs of the sea urchin. Biochim. Biophys. Acta **20:** 27.

8. BURT, A. M. & B. S. WENGER. 1961. Glucose-6-phosphate dehydrogenase activity in the brain of the developing chick. Develop. Biol. **3:** 84.
9. JOLLEY, R. L., V. H. CHELDELIN & R. W. NEWBURGH. 1958. Glucose catabolism in fetal and adult heart. J. Biol. Chem. **233:** 1289.
10. FUJIMOTO, A. & J. HARARY. 1965. The effect of lipids on enzyme levels in beating rat heart cell. Biochem. Biophys. Res. Commun. **20:** 456.
11. GUDBJARNASON, S., J. C. FENTON, P. L. WOLF & R. J. BING. 1966. Stimulation of reparative processes following experimental myocardial infarction. Arch. Intern. Med. (Chicago) **118:** 33.
12. SODI-PALLARES, D., A. BISTENI, G. A. MEDRANO, M. R. TESTELLI & A. DE MICHELLI. 1963. The polarizing treatment of acute myocardial infarction. Dis. Chest. **43:** 424.
13. LITVAK, J., L. E. SIDERIS & A. M. VINEBERG. 1957. The experimental production of coronary artery insufficiency and occlusion. Amer. Heart J. **53:** 505.
14. SAPIRSTEIN, L. A. 1958. Regional blood flow by fractional distribution of indicators. Amer. J. Physiol. **5:** 193.
15. MYERS, W. W. & C. R. HONIG. 1964. Number and distribution of capillaries as determinants of myocardial oxygen tension. Amer. J. Physiol. **207:** 653.
16. VINEBERG, A. M., K. YUTAKA & W. J. PIROZYNSKI. 1966. Experimental revascularization of the entire heart. Amer. Heart J. **72:** 79.

ETIOLOGY OF CONGESTIVE HEART FAILURE IN CLINICAL MEDICINE

Raymond T. Benack
Georgetown University Medical School, Washington, D. C.

The clinical syndrome of congestive heart failure is an ill-defined collection of signs and symptoms which, when placed together, present the classical picture of congestive heart failure. Rarely in the private practice of medicine does one easily diagnose incipient or mild congestive heart failure, whereas acute pulmonary edema rarely presents a challange in diagnosis, except possibly when it occurs in conjunction with asthma. Before entering any discussion of the etiologies of congestive heart failure seen in private practice, I would like to approach the problem of the diagnosis of congestive heart failure in private practice.

A few years ago, I attempted to set up a scale on which to grade the most commonly noted signs, symptoms, and characteristics of congestive heart failure. Nearly all congestive heart failure patients had some characteristics in common. The frequency with which some characteristics occurred gave an indication of the relative importance of that particular sign or symptom. For example, congestive heart failure was never found in the absence of some underlying heart disease. Rarely, except in a few cases of primary myocardial disease, did the condition not improve with digitalis. A diastolic gallop rhythm has almost universally been accepted as being diagnostic of congestive heart failure, but the difficulty in clinically detecting this sign reduces the value one can place on it.

However, if we assign a unit value to each symptom or sign, we can develop a scale such as that shown in TABLE 1. A total of 15 points or more can be considered diagnostic of congestive heart failure. No condition other than congestive heart failure was found in which the total value of the signs and symptoms was more than 15. If each person suspected of having congestive heart failure was checked for each of the 22 signs or symptoms listed, no case of congestive heart failure would be missed.

Various other conditions that clinically resemble congestive heart failure are evaluated in TABLE 2. None of these conditions totaled 15 points or more. I have not tried to separate the criteria into major or minor ones, but I suspect that it could be done.

With this brief introduction, we can now approach the problem of congestive heart failure as seen in the clinical practice of medicine. First, it should be mentioned that an interest in congestive heart failure makes one more keenly aware of the possibility of congestive heart failure as the origin of a patient's complaints, which leads one to make a diagnosis at an earlier stage than the average physician. Second, a physician practicing internal medicine rarely encounters congestive heart failure due to congenital heart disease, except when called into consultation on children. These factors might affect a study if one wanted to know the true percentage of cases of congestive heart failure within a given population.

My presentation is not directed toward the etiologies of congestive heart failure seen in a cardiac clinic or a university medical center, where one might see the more unusual or more complicated forms of heart disease. The 112 patients discussed in this presentation represent consecutive congestive failure patients seen

TABLE 1

SCALE FOR DIAGNOSIS OF CONGESTIVE HEART FAILURE*

No.	Sign or Symptom	Points
1.	Underlying heart disease (acute or chronic)	5
2.	Clinical improvement with digitalis	5
3.	Diastolic gallop rhythm	4
4.	Pulsus alternans	2
5.	Positive hepatojugular reflex	2
6.	Orthopnea	2
7.	Paroxysmal nocturnal dyspnea	2
8.	Pulmonary rales in the absence of infection	2
9.	Dyspnea on exertion	1
10.	Elevated venous pressure	1
11.	Prolonged circulation time	1
12.	Decreased vital capacity	1
13.	Hilar congestion on chest x-ray	1
14.	Cardiomegaly	1
15.	Peripheral edema	1
16.	Pleural effusion	1
17.	Ascites	1
18.	Fatigue	1
19.	Decreased urinary output	1
20.	Anorexia, nausea, and/or vomiting	0.5
21.	Tachycardia (palpitation)	0.5
22.	Unexplained weight gain	0.5

* A total of 15 points or more is regarded as being diagnostic of congestive heart failure.

TABLE 2

CONDITIONS CLINICALLY SIMILAR TO CONGESTIVE HEART FAILURE

Conditions	Total Points*
Heart disease without congestive heart failure	8
Emphysema	5
Asthma	4
Emphysema and heart disease	9
Asthma and heart disease	10
Bronchiectasis	4

* Points according to the scale shown in TABLE 1.

during two six-month periods in private practice (TABLE 3). These periods included the winter and spring of 1965 and 1966.

The etiologies of the congestive heart failure seen during 1966 were affected by a blizzard that completely entrapped the suburbs of Washington, and by a mild but above average influenza epidemic. These two factors probably prematurely precipitated many cases of congestive heart failure due to atherosclerotic heart disease and viral myocarditis. This is apparent from a comparison with a similar period in 1965, during which there were fewer cases of viral myocarditis and atherosclerotic heart disease, although the ratio remained the same (TABLE 3).

How does one approach the problem of determining the etiology of congestive heart failure in the clinical practice of medicine? TABLE 4 lists the most common causes of congestive heart failure. Under the heading of Collagen Diseases I have placed lupus erythematosis and polyarteritis nodosa, since I find that, although these conditions may be present more frequently, other causes, such as hypertension or pulmonary disease, are more likely to be responsible for the heart failure than the diseased myocardium.

TABLE 5 gives some of the characteristics of the congestive failure patient. As can be seen, the age of onset may be useful in determining the etiology. Atherosclerotic heart disease occurs primarily in the 50-to-60-year-old patients, but is seen in those under the age of 50 with a predisposition to diabetes. Patients with evidence of myocardial infarction seem to develop congestive heart failure earlier than those with recurrent angina.

Sustained hypertension appears to precipitate congestive heart failure at an earlier age and the more severe the hypertension the sooner the onset of the heart failure. Rheumatic heart disease also precipitates congestive heart failure at an earlier age, and primary myocardial disease affects the youngest age group. Viral myocarditis may affect any age, but its predominance in the older age group appears to be related to the tendency of the older individual to develop the disease.

A careful history, a complete physical examination, electrocardiograms, chest x-rays, laboratory studies, and a good deal of intuition are all important in the determination of the exact etiology of congestive heart failure. It is also important to understand when congestive heart failure will occur.

Congestive heart failure occurs when the myocardium has sustained sufficient injury so that there is an alteration in the basic physiological processes, causing

TABLE 3

ETIOLOGY OF CONGESTIVE HEART FAILURE SEEN IN PRIVATE PRACTICE

Etiology	1966	1965
Atherosclerotic heart disease		
Myocardial infarction	15	11
Recurrent angina	14	10
Hypertensive cardiovascular disease		
Essential	5	4
Renal	1	—
Rheumatic heart disease		
Acute myocarditis	—	1
Mitral stenosis with auricular fibrillation	1	1
Mitral insufficiency	1	1
Aortic insufficiency	2	—
Mitral stenosis and mitral insufficiency with auricular fibrillation	1	2
Congenital		
Subendocardial fibroelastosis	—	1
Primary myocardial disease	3	1
Cor pulmonale		
Chronic asthma	4	2
Emphysema	4	4
Far-advanced pulmonary tuberculosis	2	1
Massive pulmonary infarction	1	—
Viral myocarditis	8	4
Rheumatoid heart disease	1	1
Subacute Endocarditis	1	—
Thyrotoxicosis	1	1
Hemachromatosis	—	1
Lupus Erythematosis	1	—
Total	66	46

TABLE 4

CAUSES OF CONGESTIVE HEART FAILURE

Atherosclerotic
  Myocardial infarction
  Recurrent angina
	Primary Myocardial Disease

Hypertensive
  Essential
  Renal
  Coarctation of aorta
  Primary hyperaldosteronism
	Cor Pulmonale
	  Chronic asthma
	  Emphysema
	  Far-advanced pulmonary tuberculosis
	  Primary pulmonary hypertension
	  Pulmonary valvular stenosis
	  Massive pulmonary infarctions
	  Tricuspid insufficiency

Rheumatic
  Mitral stenosis
  Mitral insufficiency
  Aortic stenosis
  Aortic insufficiency
	Other Cardiomyopathies
	  Myocarditia
	  Subacute endocarditis
	  Tumors of myocardium
	  Thyrotoxicosis
	  Beriberi heart disease
	  Rheumatoid heart disease
	  Hemochromatosis
	  Collagen diseases

Congenital
  Interatrial septal defect
  Interventricular septal defect
  Infundibular aortic stenosis
  Persistent atrioventricular communis
  Subendocardial fibroelastosis
  Tetralogy of Fallot
  Eisenmonger complex	

TABLE 5

CHARACTERISTICS OF PATIENTS WITH CONGESTIVE HEART FAILURE

- Atherosclerotic heart disease
  - Average age
    - Overall, 56 years
    - Diabetics, 41 years
  - Age span, 23 to 92 years
  - Duration of disease before onset of failure
    - Myocardial infarction, 3 years
    - Angina pectoris, 5 years
- Hypertensive cardiovascular disease
  - Average age, 43 years
  - Age span, 38 to 51 years
  - Duration of hypertension before onset of failure
    - Moderate hypertension (below 150/100), 8 years
    - Severe hypertension (170/110 and above), 3 years
- Rheumatic heart disease
  - Average age, 36 years
  - Age span, 46 years
  - Underlying cause
    - Acute myocarditis, 10%
    - Mitral stenosis, 30%
    - Mitral insufficiency, 20%
    - Mitral stenosis and mitral insufficiency, 10%
    - Aortic insufficiency, 10%
- Primary myocardial disease
  - Average age, 34 years
  - Age span, 19 to 43 years
- Viral Myocarditis
  - Average age, 60 years
  - Age span, 33 to 72 years

a decrease in the myocardial efficiency. This decrease in the efficiency must be greater than the normal compensatory mechanisms of the myocardium. The interval between the injury to the myocardium and the onset of heart failure is quite variable. It can vary from the simultaneous onset of heart failure with an acute myocardial infarction to an onset many years after the development of hypertension.

Atherosclerotic Heart Disease

Congestive heart failure is a frequent complication of atherosclerotic heart disease and accounts for almost 50% of the patients seen in private practice. This finding is not markedly different from previous reports that almost 50% of those dying from atherosclerotic heart disease suffer from congestive heart failure. I believe that this figure is quite accurate if every patient with documented evidence of angina pectoris is included. I realize that many cases of arrhythmias or minor T wave changes may basically have their origin in narrowing of the coronary arteries; however, I am reluctant to classify a person, particularly a young person, as having atherosclerotic heart disease without definite electrocardiogram changes compatible with an infarction, ischemia, or a positive Master's test. I also feel that there are too many other possible disease processes to consider before we classify as atherosclerotic those individuals with abnormal electrocardiograms over the age of 40. This is probably reflected in my elevated number of patients with viral myocarditis or primary myocardial disease.

Angina, in itself, is not the origin of the congestive heart failure, but recurrent angina–either frequently, within a short period of time, or moderately, over a longer period of time–often may be followed by congestive heart failure without a myocardial infarction. Particular attention must be paid to the known angina patient who begins to complain of nocturnal angina or whose angina has increased in frequency or severity without any known provocation, since this may be the first and only overt symptom of developing congestive heart failure.

I have seen atherosclerotic heart disease with congestive heart failure in individuals as young as 23 years old, with obesity and diabetes mellitus, and as old as 92 years old. The majority of cases, however, have occurred in the 50-60-year-old age group.

Hypertensive Cardiovascular Disease

Hypertension is one condition, but hypertensive cardiovascular disease is another and more important condition. It includes not only sustained elevation of the blood pressure above 140 mm Hg systolic and 90 mm Hg diastolic, but there must also be fundoscopic changes and evidence of cardiac enlargement, preferably suspected on x-ray and confirmed by electrocardiogram. This does not rule out demonstration of enlargement of the heart on clinical examination.

Although the literature abounds with discussions concerning cases of renal hypertension and primarily hyperaldosteronism, in the clinical practice of medicine the most commonly diagnosed hypertensive cardiovascular disease is essential hypertension. This diagnosis is usually arrived at after complete and sometimes extensive workup.

The average evaluation of a hypertensive patient includes routine complete blood count, blood sugar, blood urea nitrogen, urinalysis, urine concentration test, serum electrolytes, Amytal®* test, intravenous pyelogram, Regitine®† test,

* Amobarbital sodium; distributed by Eli Lilly & Co., Indianapolis, Ind.
† Phentolamine; distributed by Ciba Pharmaceutical Co., Summit, N. J.

and urinary catecholomines. In most instances, these tests can be completed on an ambulatory basis, but, when practical, a carefully planned program of evaluation can be completed within a few days of hospitalization.

If coarctation of the aorta or renal artery stenosis is suspected, a retrograde aortogram should be performed. My own personal experience is that differential catheterization studies of the kidneys have not been particularly useful in the diagnosis of hypertension of renal origin. If these studies fail to reveal any origin of the hypertension, the tentative diagnosis of essential hypertension may be given to the patient. At suitable intervals thereafter, some or all of the studies should be repeated to determine any changes which might suggest an etiology of hypertension.

Rarely does congestive heart failure follow closely the onset of hypertension, except possibly in acute toxemia of pregnancy or in malignant hypertension. More commonly, heart failure follows years after hypertension becomes well established. Since many cases of hypertension have their onset in the middle-aged individuals, care should be taken to determine whether the congestive heart failure is due to the hypertension rather than atherosclerotic heart disease. When patients were classified for this study, diagnoses of congestive heart failure due to atherosclerotic heart disease were based on the criteria mentioned previously.

In hypertension, congestive heart failure does not result as a direct injury to the myocardium, as might occur in a myocardial infarction or myocarditis. The myocardium can hypertrophy until it is several times larger and heavier than its original size. It is difficult to point out the exact point at which heart failure ensues, but, at some point, the myocardium becomes deprived of its nourishment through the strangulation of the myocardial blood vessels by the hypertrophied muscle mass or through the enlargement of the muscle mass beyond the capabilities of its vascular tissue. Once the myocardium suffers from inadequate nourishment, its cells lose their efficiency and heart failure follows.

Most commonly, the heart failure involves the left ventricle, and the symptoms are usually caused by left ventricular failure. Rarely do the symptoms occur suddenly. More characteristically, the symptoms develop gradually and over a period of time. Symptoms may, in fact, be so subtle that evidence of right ventricular failure is discovered before the physician becomes aware of the presence of left ventricular failure.

Although essential hypertension may be the most common form of hypertension, we cannot overlook the surgically correctable forms of hypertension, such as coarctation of the aorta or renal artery, pheochromocytoma, or an aldosterone-secreting tumor. If any of these are suspected, the patient is entitled to adequate angiography and laboratory evaluation. The significance of early diagnosis of these forms of hypertension is the prevention of irreversible changes in the heart and blood vessels due to prolonged hypertension.

Rheumatic Heart Disease

In this modern era of penicillin, there has been a significant decrease in the prevalence of rheumatic fever and rheumatic heart disease. However, even with the effectiveness of penicillin, we cannot overcome the laxity of the public in following instructions. Too frequently I find patients who have not taken the penicillin for the prescribed length of time. In one family alone, two children came down with rheumatic fever because the parents, despite instructions, believed that they needed the penicillin only until the children were well. The second child developed rheumatic fever even after the parents were reminded of the importance of giving the child the penicillin for the full ten days. Unfortunately, three weeks later the child was seen at home with migratory arthritis, cardiac arrhythmia, and bilateral basilar rales. Discouraging as it may be, this is an example of congestive heart failure occurring during an episode of acute rheumatic fever due to myocarditis.

Although right ventricular failure is usually seen with pure mitral stenosis, left ventricular failure may develop as a result of chronic auricular fibrillation or the development of mitral insufficiency. However, left ventricular failure is the predominant type of failure seen with aortic insufficiency or aortic stenosis. Combined right and left ventricular failure may develop as a late manifestation of the condition.

The sudden onset of congestive heart failure in a patient with previously stable rheumatic heart disease should make one suspicious of reactivation of rheumatic fever or the development of subacute bacterial endocarditis. After the age of 40, the possibility of rheumatic heart disease as the etiology of congestive heart failure is reduced, and the probability of atherosclerotic heart disease increases. Consequently, even if a patient over the age of 40 is known to have rheumatic heart disease, there is a good possibility that atherosclerotic heart disease is the cause of failure.

Primary Myocardial Disease

The patients with congestive heart failure which are a challenge in diagnosis are those with primary myocardial disease. This classification of patients seems to be enlarging as we become more aware of the condition. In my experience, failure attributable to primary myocardial disease always occurs below the age of 45 in both males and females without any prodromal symptoms. Thus, primary myocardial disease must be suspected in any individual who suddenly develops the signs and symptoms of congestive heart failure without a previous history of heart disease. However, occasionally failure may occur in a patient with a possible underlying cause. One patient with a documented history of rheumatic fever as a child but who revealed no evidence of rheumatic heart disease suddenly developed pulmonary edema, a chaotic rhythm, and an enlarged heart. All studies for rheumatic fever were negative. Similarly, there was a very poor history to suggest any viral etiology. Finally, it was found that the myocardium was unusually sensitive to digitalis. Ultimately, it was necessary to titrate the digitalis. Bed rest was the most effective treatment, and any attempt to increase his activity without adequate digitalization was followed by an exacerbation of the heart failure.

This patient was evaluated independently at three different medical centers, and each called his condition primary myocardial disease. I believe that he demonstrates the usual criteria for primary myocardial disease: cardiac enlargement, the signs and symptoms of congestive heart failure, arrhythmia, nonspecific T and ST wave changes on the electrocardiogram, absence of any underlying heart disease, unusual sensitivity to digitalis, and improvement with bed rest.

Other Myocardiopathies

Thus far, I have discussed the more common origins of congestive heart failure. Viral myocarditis was briefly mentioned. This condition seems to have its greater frequency during the winter months and an even greater rise during influenza epidemics. The possibility of viral myocarditis should be considered in older patients, who are more susceptible to the virus. One should not assume atherosclerosis or stress in the older patient who develops congestive heart failure while suffering from influenza. There is a good chance that a virus may be the underlying cause.

Other causes of congestive heart failure include lupus erythematosis, although this diagnosis is difficult to make except after reviewing the patient's course over a long period of time. One patient had evidence of some myocardopathy which had existed for at least five years before the development of hypertension.

The diagnosis of rheumatoid heart disease was made in two patients with advanced rheumatoid arthritis who developed congestive heart failure without evidence of any other forms of heart disease. In one, the diagnosis was confirmed at autopsy by the presence of granulomatosis lesions in the myocardium. Other etiologies of congestive heart failure include thyrotoxicosis and hemachromatosis.

I have not entered into any extensive discussion of cor pulmonale, but it should be pointed out that the higher than average number of cases seen was due to my dual interest in asthma and pulmonary diseases. Let my simply say that all that wheezes is not asthma, nor are all cases of respiratory difficulty in the asthmatic due to asthma. Too frequently, the asthmatic is treated for asthma when in reality he should be treated for congestive heart failure.

Summary

Congestive heart failure occurs when the myocardium has sustained sufficient injury so that there is an alteration in the basic physiological processes, causing a decrease in the myocardial efficiency. This decrease in the efficiency must be greater than the normal compensatory mechanisms of the myocardium. The interval between the injury to the myocardium and the onset of heart failure is quite variable. It can vary from the simultaneous onset of heart failure with an acute myocardial infarction or myocarditis to an onset many years after the development of hypertension.

In the clinical practice of medicine, congestive heart failure is an ill-defined collection of signs and symptoms which, when placed together, present the classical picture of congestive heart failure. This author has found it useful to assign a unit value of from 0.5 to 5 for each of the 22 most common signs, symptoms, and characteristics of congestive heart failure. The frequency with which a sign or symptom occurred gave an indication of its relative importance. If each patient suspected of having heart failure were checked for each of the 22 most common signs and symptoms, few, if any, cases of congestive heart failure would be overlooked. Similarly, many cases resembling early or incipient heart failure would be found to have not heart failure but some other noncardiac disease.

Every patient with congestive heart failure must have some underlying myocardial pathology to precipitate the condition. In most instances, a careful history, a complete physical examination, electrocardiograms, chest x-rays, laboratory studies, and a good deal of intuition are all important in determining the exact etiology.

In two six-month periods, the author saw 112 patients with congestive heart failure. Atherosclerotic heart disease accounted for 50 (44.6%) of the patients. It was present in patients between the ages of 23 to 92 years, with an average age of 56 years, although in diabetics the average age was 41 years. Congestive heart failure occurred an average of three years after a myocardial infarction and five years after the onset of recurrent angina.

Hypertensive cardiovascular disease was the underlying cause of heart failure in ten patients. Nine of the patients suffered essential hypertension, and one had renal hypertension. The average age of the hypertensive patient with congestive heart failure was 43 years (age span, 38 to 51 years). In those with moderate hypertension (below 150/100), the onset of failure was eight years after the development of hypertension; in those with severe hypertension (170/110 and above), the onset was three years after the initial diagnosis.

Rheumatic heart disease accounted for ten cases of congestive heart failure. The average age of the rheumatic heart disease patient was 36 years, but congestive heart failure occurred as early as 12 years of age, in conjunction with rheumatic myocarditis, and as late as 46 years of age, in association with pure aortic insufficiency. It has been seen in conjunction with either aortic or mitral valve involvement but seems to be more common with auricular fibrillation in conjunction with mitral valve disease.

Viral myocarditis caused congestive heart failure in 12 patients. These patients were primarily in the older age group, and the prevalence increased during a mild but definite influenza epidemic.

Primary myocardial disease seemed to affect the younger age group. The increased awareness of this condition seems to be responsible for the increased frequency with which the condition is diagnosed.

Other causes of left ventricular failure included subendocardial fibroelastosis, rheumatoid heart disease, subacute bacterial endocarditis, thyrotoxicosis, hemachromatosis, and lupus erythematosis.

A particular interest in asthma and pulmonary diseases was evident in the number of cases of cor pulmonale (18). Actually, the increased prevalence of chronic pulmonary diseases probably accounts in part for the increased prevalence of cor pulmonale.

THE IMPORTANCE OF ELECTROLYTE THERAPY IN HEART DISEASE

Demetrio Sodi-Pallares
Instituto Nacional de Cardiología de México
Mexico City, Mexico

Since 1960, my colleagues and I[1] have substantially modified the medical treatment of the cardiopathies in our cardiac patients. Digitalis compounds and diuretic drugs in heart failure, the vasodilator agents in angina and coronary insufficiency, and the hypotensive drugs and diuretics in essential hypertension have yielded their place of honor to polarizing treatment.

This treatment[2] has, in brief, the following purposes: (1) to repolarize myocardial fibers during diastole when there is diastolic depolarization; (2) to correct the deficit of intracellular potassium and excess of intracellular sodium and water; (3) to improve the intracellular metabolism, particularly the Krebs cycle, altered by hypoxia; (4) to improve muscular contraction; (5) to decrease the injury of muscle fibers, as demonstrated by the electrocardiogram (ECG); (6) to correct arrhythmias, when present; (7) to increase diuresis; (8) to correct hyponatremia and hypokalemia; (9) to correct intra- and extracellular acidosis; and (10) to improve the general condition of the patient.

Therapeutic Approach

It is convenient, at this point, to specify what is meant by polarizing treatment, since many cardiologists presently believe that the treatment depends solely on polarizing solutions. In reality, the methods are diverse, but there is no doubt that the most important aspect is the polarizing diet. In the following sections we shall examine some of the factors that constitute this therapeutic approach:

1. A low sodium-high potassium diet with adequate hydration. We suggest that two of our previous publications[2,3] concerning this diet be consulted. Fats are not reduced in this regimen.

2. Medications with an initial entropic effect[4] are to be withheld. For example, therapeutic doses of quinidine favor the retention of intracellular sodium from the first day of administration and inhibit adenosinetriphosphatase (ATPase) and phosphoglycerokinase. The word entropy in its cardiological application has been defined in another publication.[4]

3. Medications with a late entropic effect that exceeds its antientropic effect are to be avoided. The antientropic effect of digitalis[4] is indirect, but its direct entropic effect can exceed that of the antientropic effect, and the drug can be injurious. At this time, the favorable effects of the drug are not recognized, not even by the bradycardia, notwithstanding the presence of accentuated negative RST displacement in the left precordial leads.

4. Depolarizing drugs are also to be avoided, e.g. excess of diuretics. It is important not to confuse the words entropic, depolarizing, and toxic, even though the three are intimately related. The word entropic[4] fundamentally refers to an increase in the ratio Na_i/Na_e. The word depolarizing[2] refers to a diminution of the resting potential, and a decrease of the ratio K_i/K_e. Both entropic and depolarizing effects can be present at well-known therapeutic doses with drugs such as quinidine, digitalis, and diuretics. The word toxic has been defined in many books on therapeutics, but it is important to emphasize that, when the toxic effect

of a drug is present, the cellular depolarization and entropy are, generally, well advanced.

5. Recognition of extracardiac diseases that contribute to myocardial depolarization. In our experience, the principal ones are: diabetes mellitus, thyroid disorders, gallbladder diseases, liver diseases (with and without failure), renal failure, aldosteronism and adrenal failure, disturbances in acid-base equilibrium, electrolyte disorders, hypoxia at the tissue level (due to different factors), infectious processes, entropic effects of various drugs (steroids, saluretics, hypotensives, etc.), acute and chronic pyelonephritis, hiatus hernia, bone fractures (especially of the femur), anemias and other hematological disorders (leukemia, hemorrhages, etc.), collagen diseases, cerebrovascular accidents, respiratory insufficiency, vomiting and diarrhea, acute pancreatitis, "dumping" syndrome, chronic alcoholism and other intoxications (aspirin), and neoplasias.

6. Extracardiac treatments should be avoided, if possible, when they contribute to myocardial depolarization: the corticoids in rheumatic diseases, emetine as an amebacidal treatment, diets rich in sodium (such as those prescribed in diabetes), saline solutions used to correct acidosis, cathecolamines used in the treatment of shock, etc.

7. Serum potassium levels should be maintained at 4.5–5.5 mEq/l, while serum sodium values should be maintained in the low-normal or subnormal range, 135–137 mEq/l. Values of sodium higher than 140 mEq/l are evidence that the patient has not been following the diet, or that salt has not been sufficiently restricted.

8. Some polarizing mechanisms are: adequate exercise; sufficient sleep; avoidance of alcohol, cigarettes, indigestion, and constipation; i.e., a life healthy in all aspects should be maintained. Stimulation of low metabolism with thyroid preparations favors myocardial polarization.

9. Polarizing solutions are indicated in the following cardiac conditions: advanced cardiac insufficiency, recent myocardial infarction, severe cases of angina pectoris which have been unresponsive to previous polarizing treatments, dilutional hyponatremia in heart failure, renal insufficiency enhanced by cardiac conditions, unmanageable arrhythmias (particularly paroxysmal ventricular tachycardia), and shock in recent myocardial infarction.

The strength of the polarizing solutions, i.e., the concentration of glucose, quantity of insulin, and the number of milliequivalents of potassium chloride, along with instructions as to the number of days or weeks necessary for infusion, have been reported in an earlier publication.[3]

Reports in the Literature

Every year, with increasing frequency, the medical literature contains articles about "polarizing solutions." However, it seems to me that the concept of polarizing treatment has not been sufficiently understood. To reiterate, "polarizing solutions" and "polarizing treatment" are not the same thing. If given without consideration of diverse depolarizing factors, the infusion of a polarizing solution can depolarize the patient. Some of the results obtained by other authors with polarizing solutions should be mentioned.

Shimert and co-workers[5] have demonstrated reversibility of lesions in the sarcoplasm of human papillary muscle biopsies obtained during mitral valve replacement in patients treated with polarizing solutions. Sibilia and Marino,[6] using polarizing solutions with potassium aspartate, glucose, and insulin have reported marked improvement in the clinical condition and ECG of four cases of acute myocarditis, as well as improvement in patients with acute hepatitis and secondary myocardial changes.

Day[7] reported good recovery of 33 patients with myocardial infarction treated with polarizing solution. Mitra[8] studied 170 patients with a confirmed diagnosis of myocardial infarction treated with oral potassium, glucose, and subcutaneous insulin. After 14 days, the mortality in the control group was 28.2%, compared with 11.7% in the treated group.

Fabris[9] reported good clinical evolution and disappearance of precordial pain, dyspnea, and tachycardia in 13 patients with myocardial infarction, 16 with coronary disease, and two with mitral insufficiency, all treated with a polarizing solution in which potassium aspartate was present. Fritz[10] also reported good results in 50 patients with recent myocardial infarction treated with polarizing solutions.

Bobák and co-workers[11] reported preliminary experience with 16 cases of acute myocardial infarction in which polarizing solution produced rapid disappearance of precordial pain, regression of arrhythmias, and faster restitution of ECG changes. The same authors also reported good results of polarizing treatment in paralytic ileus (personal communication).

Chella[12] reported good results in the ischemic injury pattern of recent myocardial infarctions treated with polarizing solution. Germer[13] gave polarizing solution to 50 patients with recent myocardial infarction and observed an increase in systolic blood pressure and decrease in diastolic pressure, increase in systolic volume and in minute-volume, and decrease of peripheral resistance, arrhythmias, and pain. Good results were also observed in shock and in heart failure. The author believes this is due to an increase of intracellular glucose and glycogen, as well as an increase in the formation of adenosine triphosphate (ATP).

Barbiere and Parravicini[14] reported good results in different parameters of 20 patients with recent myocardial infarction treated with polarizing solutions. Similar good results were reported by Girola and co-workers[15] in 23 cases of recent myocardial infarction, and by Ratti and Sanna.[16]

Köhler[17] speaks about his own experience with the therapy of "repolarization," using either glucose, insulin, and potassium chloride or potassium-magnesium-aspartate, with or without glucose-insulin. The results, according to the author, are clinically surprising: treatment was not only biochemically and electrophysiologically successful in patients with myocardial infarction, but also especially successful in instances of "digitalis hypersensitivity," decompensated valve defects, in the postoperative phase, and in refractory cardiac insufficiency.

Nieper and Blumberger[18] polarized the heart with potassium and magnesium aspartates (1–1.5 g) in 84 patients with angina pectoris. The therapeutic results were most satisfactory in 80% of the cases, far superior to previous experience of the same authors with conventional long-term therapy. The authors also report good results obtained in cases of recent myocardial infarction, heart failure, and arrhythmias with infusions of potassium and magnesium aspartates.

Losse and his colleagues[19] demonstrated that there is an increase in sodium, potassium, and water in the erythrocytes in essential hypertension compared with healthy normotensive controls; in plasma, however, sodium and potassium levels remain normal. Serial examinations throughout the disease prove that the fall in blood pressure under appropriate low salt diet and therapeutic measures (diuretics) is paralleled by a decrease in the intracellular sodium and water; on the other hand, the potassium content tends to increase under therapy, while the chloride concentration does not differ significantly from normal, either before or after therapy. The authors insist that, salt intake has to be restricted early and consistently in the therapy of essential hypertension.

Friedman and co-workers[20] were able to show that the sodium gradient between the extracellular space and the smooth muscle cell is decisive for the tone of the cell; an increasing gradient led to a decrease in tonus, and a decreased gradient to an increase in tonus. An intracellular sodium concentration rising above normal signified a lowering of the sodium gradient, causing a rise in tone and, consequently, an increase in blood pressure.

Laborit[21] insists that any factor capable of stimulating the functioning of the Embden-Meyerhof and Krebs pathways will be favorable to sodium extrusion. This is the case for epinephrine. Unfortunately, epinephrine exhausts the fiber of potassium and glycogen and inhibits the synthesis of glycogen. These two phenomena are also caused by anoxia. On the other hand, the combination of insulin with hypertonic glucose and potassium, originally recommended by the author, stimulates both pathways and reintegrates potassium into the cellular space.

Máté and co-workers[22] discussed the utility of the regular administration of potassium to descompensated heart patients. Potassium promotes a considerable diuresis, so that if one also maintains a diet reduced in salt, there is no need for any restriction of liquid consumption.

Larcan[23] proposed a new polarizing solution containing glucose, insulin, heparin, dibasic potassium phosphate, potassium and magnesium aspartates, cocarboxylase, cytochrome c, and, possibly, dipyridamole. The author used this solution in 40 patients with recent myocardial infarction and compared the results with those obtained in 30 patients treated by bed rest and anticoagulants and, if necessary, opiates. Greater and faster improvement was obtained in the group treated with the polarizing solution.

Day and Averill[24] stated that the polarizing solution recommended by us has a definite antiarrhythmic effect, particularly in preventing ventricular fibrillation in the acute coronary patient, and in abolishing ventricular bigeminy and frequent premature ventricular beats. They have treated 141 patients with polarizing-solution therapy. Ventricular fibrillation developed in 3.5% of this group; in contrast, 134 patients not receiving potassium drip therapy showed a 16.4% incidence of ventricular fibrillation.

Kanther[25] studied the effect of potassium-magnesium-aspartate in 22 individuals submitted to hypoxic respiration in two comparable test series taken before and after three days of treatment with 2 dragées of potassium-magnesium-aspartate four times daily (289.28 mg of organically bound potassium). In five persons with healthy hearts (17–39 years old), a distinct decrease of the hypoxic T wave and QRS changes was shown after the administration of potassium-magnesium-aspartate. In 12 clinically confirmed heart patients (hypertension, coronary atherosclerosis, and coronary insufficiency) between 40 and 65 years old, there was a more than 100% reduction in the hypoxic loss of the T wave amplitude under the therapeutic regimen.

Pillen[26] emphasizes that potassium-magnesium-aspartate has proved to be an excellent basic treatment for all kinds of myogenic cardiac insufficiency, especially for combating any form of hypoxic or anoxic myocardial damage. Kenter and Falkenhahn[27] treated 97 patients with fresh myocardial infarction using potassium-magnesium-aspartate. Comparison with a control group showed that mortality was reduced by 50% and pain, shock syndrome, and dysrhythmia regressed more rapidly with the polarizing therapy.

Bronzini and Scotti[28] treated 40 patients with recent myocardial infarction using the polarizing solution with glucose, potassium, and insulin. The alterations in rhythm were of low incidence and rapidly disappeared. The mortality diminished from 45 to 32.5%, and ECG stability was obtained in 25 days, on the average. Curcio and Bonaventura[29] reported four cases of gigantic negative T waves, which rapidly improved or disappeared with polarizing solution.

One of the most interesting current articles on the effect of polarizing treatment in recent experimental myocardial infarction was written by Gudbjarnason and his associates.[30] The authors studied the incorporation of glycine-2-^{14}C into the protein of cardiac muscle as a measure of the rate of protein synthesis. Myocardial infarction was produced in dogs by ligation of branches of the anterior and posterior descending coronary arteries. Samples were obtained from infarcted tissue, borderline tissue, and normal left and right ventricular muscle. Treatment with insulin increased the incorporation of glycine-2-^{14}C into the protein of infarcted tissue by 94%, 24 hours after infarction. Treatment with bovine growth hormone raised the incorporation by 168%, and treatment with a combination of growth hormone and insulin raised the incorporation by 251%. Treatment with an intravenous infusion of glucose, insulin, potassium chloride, coenzymes, and vitamins increased protein synthesis in infarcted muscle seven hours after infarction by 173%. Repeated infusion led to a further rise in incorporation 24 hours after infarction (188%). Treatment with ascorbic acid increased protein synthesis in the center of the infarct by 122%, 24 hours after infarction, and treatment with the anabolic steroid methandrostenolone augmented incorporation into the center of the infarct by 249%.

In a few publications,[31–33] the results with polarizing solutions are not as favorable as those previously mentioned. In most of these communications, nothing is said in relation to the diet; in addition, the methodology used for the administration of the solutions is not the one recommended by our group after years of clinical and experimental work. It may be that those authors have not fully appreciated the concepts of polarization and entropy in relation to the cell, and they easily confuse polarizing therapy with the administration of inadequate polarizing solutions.

Clinical Results

The last part of this communication will deal with some of our results obtained in private practice as well as in hospitals.

Patients with Essential Hypertension

All patients (50 cases) were submitted to a low sodium (350 mg per day) and high potassium diet, generally with a substantial daily ingestion of water (around 2 l). At the same time, potassium chloride (1.5–3 g) was given orally. If the patient was reluctant to be on such a strict diet, we allowed him 1 g of sodium chloride per day, but, in order to counterbalance this indulgence, 0.5 g of clorothiazide was given before breakfast. The depolarizing effect of such a low dose this diuretic is minimal in comparison with the polarizing effect of the whole regime of treatment, including other antientropic measures (adequate physical exercise, regular resting hours, anabolic compounds, vitamins, etc.). Our results are summarized in FIGURE 1. The excellent results obtained with this second degree of polarizing therapy can easily be appreciated.

In ten out of 50 cases, the diastolic blood pressure rose again when the patients went off the diet. A good response was reobtained when this group returned to the polarizing regime. The incidence of symptoms before and after treatment is shown in TABLE 1. Only three of the patients had no complaints prior to the diet regimen. Following treatment, 35 patients became asymptomatic.

Patients with Angina Pectoris

This group of 24 patients was placed under the same therapeutic regimen as the patients with essential hypertension. In 18 patients, the pain entirely disappeared during the first week. In four patients, the pain was markedly reduced, appearing

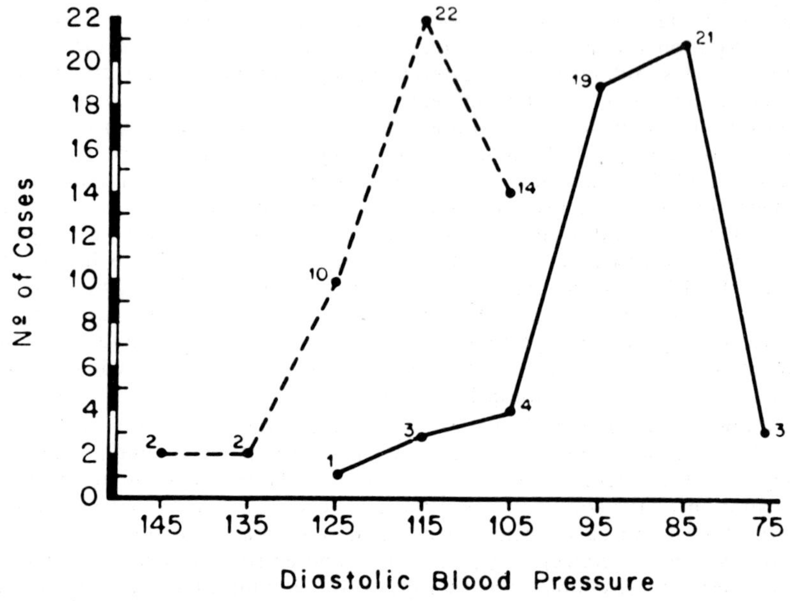

FIGURE 1. Results obtained before (dashed line) and after (solid line) polarizing treatment in 50 patients with essential hypertension. There were 28 men and 22 women among the patients. The age range was 42–74 years, with an average of 56 years.

TABLE 1

FREQUENCY OF SYMPTOMS IN 50 PATIENTS WITH ESSENTIAL HYPERTENSION*

Symptom	Before Treatment	After Treatment
Headache	19	3
Palpitations	15	1
Dizziness	13	2
Dyspnea	10	—
Angina	10	4
Premature beats	9	1
Tinnitus	8	5
Muscular cramps	5	—
Asthenia	4	—
Paresthesias	3	—
Unconsciousness	1	—
Aphasia	1	1
Myodesopsias	1	—
Epistaxis	1	—
No symptoms	3	35

* Numbers add up to more than 50 since most patients had more than one symptom.

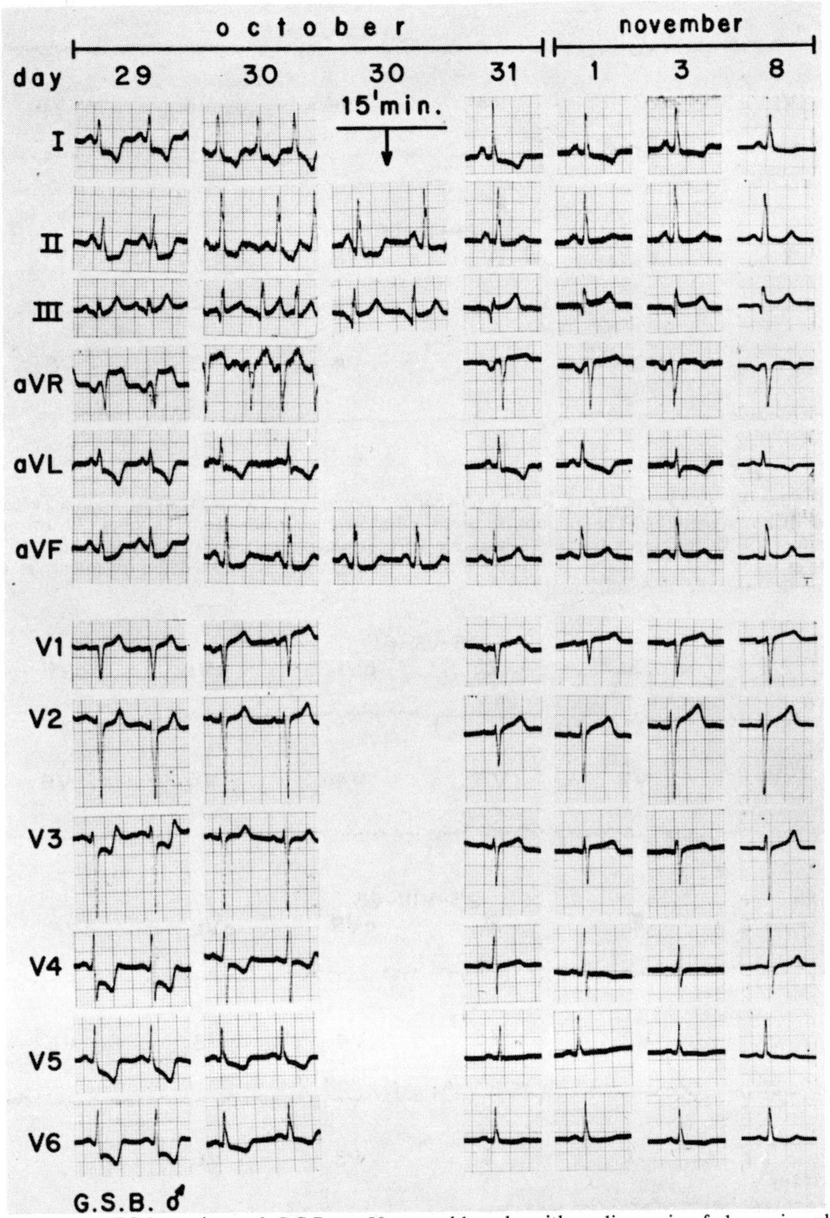

FIGURE 2. ECG tracings of G.S.B., a 50-year-old male with a diagnosis of dynamic subaortic stenosis with subintrant angina. The patient received polarizing solution from October 29 through November 8, in addition to the polarizing diet. Note the disappearance of the subendocardial injury of the left ventricle by the presence of negative RST displacement in leads I, II, aVL, aVF, and V3 through V6 on October 29, and absence of it on November 8. The angina pectoris also disappeared.

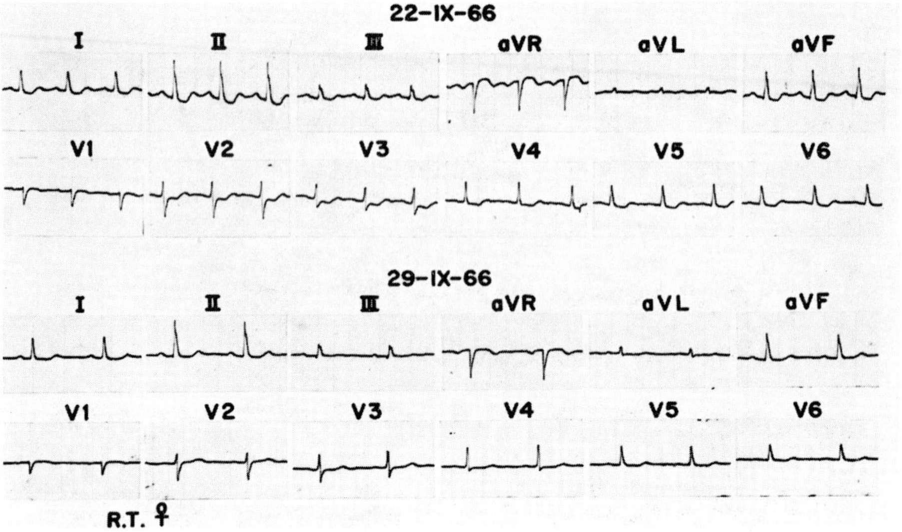

FIGURE 3. ECG tracings of R.T., a 60-year-old female with a diagnosis of angina pectoris and diabetes mellitus. The patient received polarizing solution from October 22 through October 29. In the upper tracing, a negative RST displacement seen in leads V2 through V6 and in leads I, II, II, and aVF. In the second tracing, there is marked improvement, at the same time the angina disappeared.

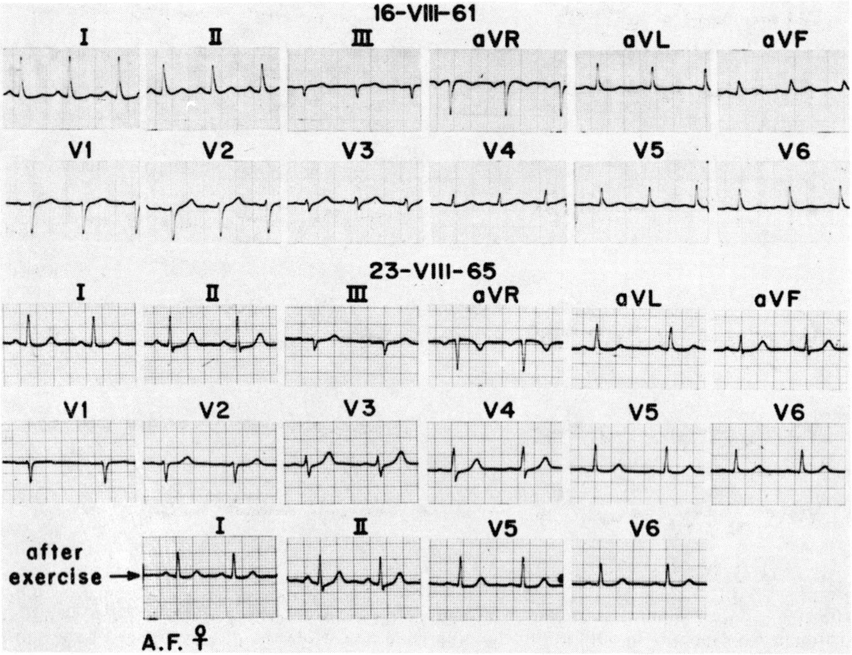

FIGURE 4. ECG tracings of A.F., a 30-year-old female with a diagnosis of rheumatic aortic insufficiency and angina pectoris. The polarizing diet eliminated the attacks of angina in one week. Note the marked improvement in the last tracing.

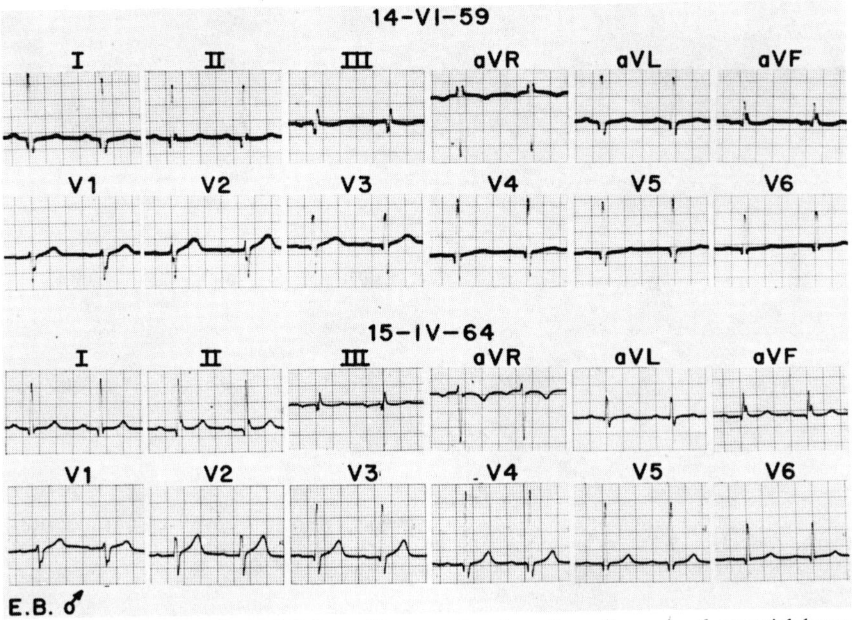

FIGURE 5. ECG tracings of E.B., a 48-year-old male with a diagnosis of essential hypertension (210/140 mm Hg). The main complaints were precordial pain, headache, and palpitations. After two months of polarizing therapy, the blood pressure dropped to 165/115 mm Hg, and there were no more symptoms. Note the marked improvement of the tracing after five years of therapy.

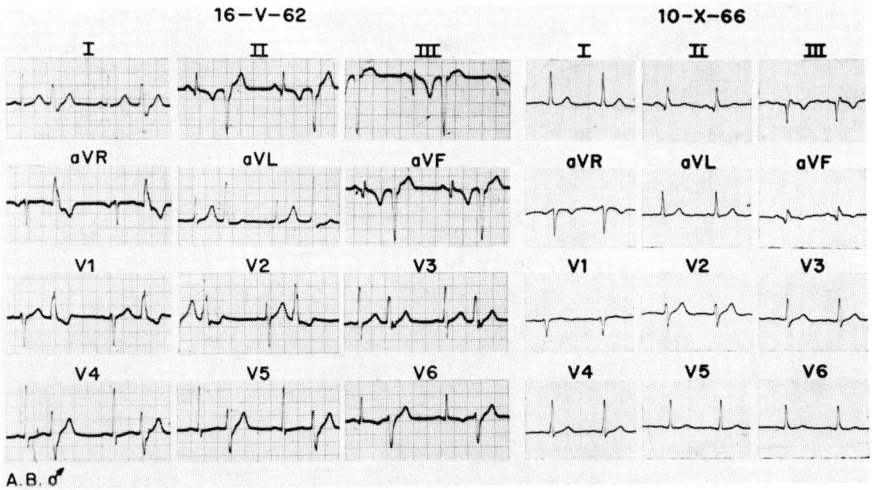

FIGURE 6. ECG tracings of A.B., a 45-year-old male with a diagnosis of posterior-inferior myocardial infarction with residual angina. The patient was kept on a polarizing diet for years. Note the disappearance of the bigeminism and of the lateral subepicardial ischemia.

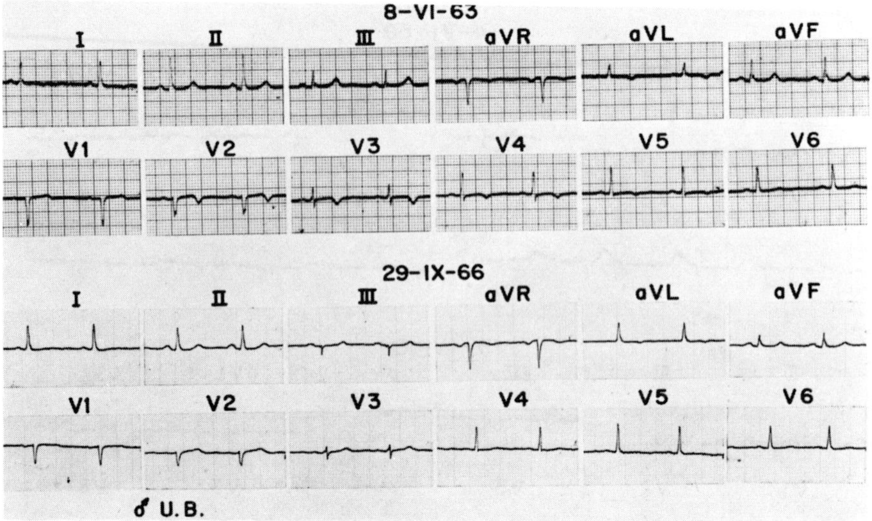

FIGURE 7. ECG tracings of U.B., a 53-year-old male. The patient complained of precordial pain for two years. With the polarizing treatment, the angina disappeared in less than two months. Note the marked improvement of the tracing after three years of therapy.

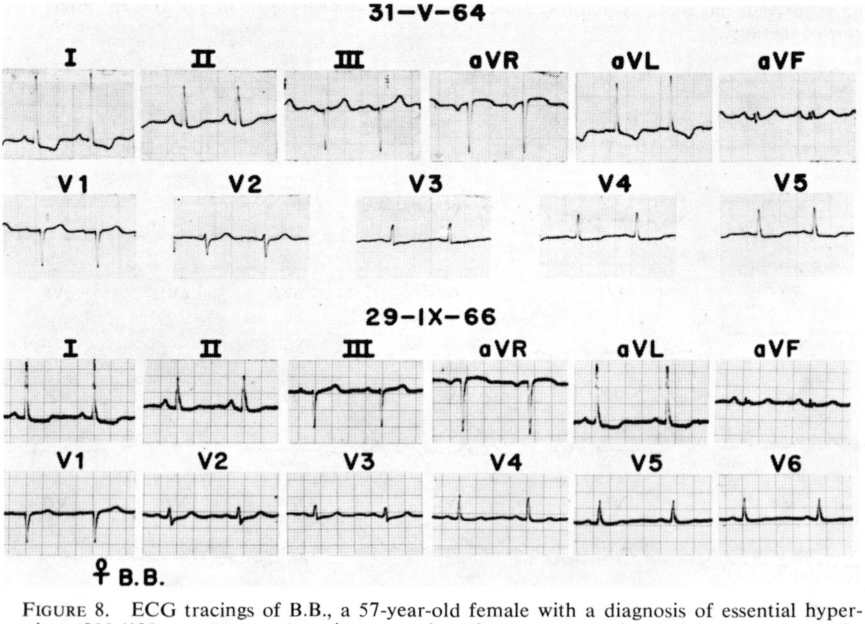

FIGURE 8. ECG tracings of B.B., a 57-year-old female with a diagnosis of essential hypertension (230/120 mm Hg) and angina pectoris. After one year of polarizing treatment, the blood pressure dropped to 160/70 mm Hg, and the angina disappeared. Note the marked improvement of the tracing after two years of treatment.

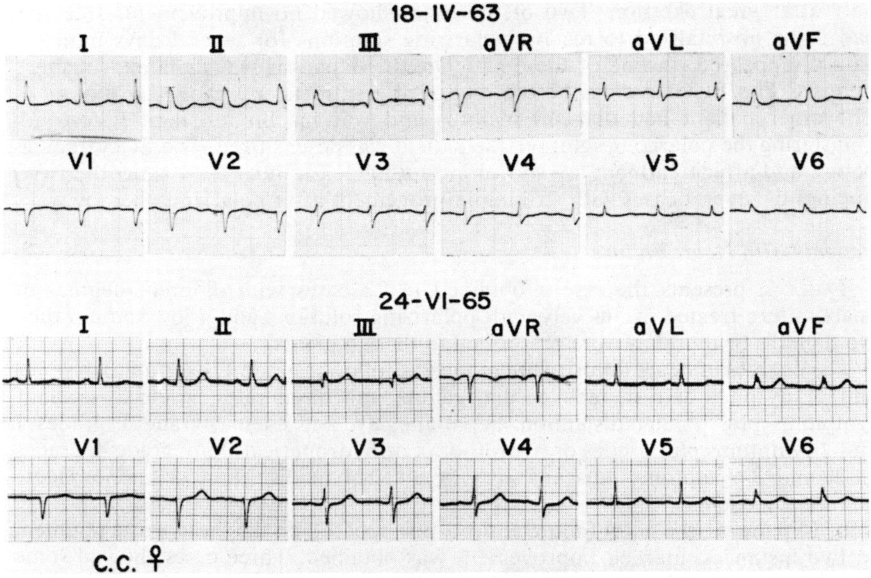

FIGURE 9. ECG tracings of C.C., a 56-year-old female with a diagnosis of essential hypertension (200/110 mm Hg). The main complaints were precordial pain and repeated epitaxsis. After one month of treatment, all the complaints disappeared, and the blood pressure dropped to 170/90 mm Hg. Note the marked improvement of the tracing after two years of therapy.

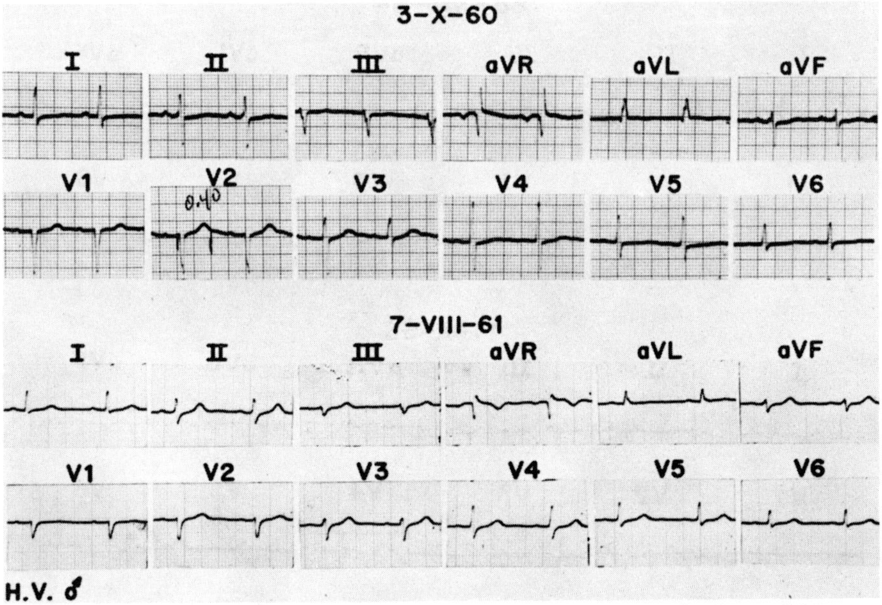

FIGURE 10. ECG tracings of H.V., a 42-year-old male with a diagnosis of essential hypertension (200/120 mm Hg). The main complaints were headache and palpitations. After few months of polarizing treatment, the blood pressure dropped to 130/80 mm Hg, the complaints disappeared and the tracing markedly improved.

only after great exertion. Two of the cases showed no improvement, and they had to be hospitalized to receive polarizing solutions for several days until the pain disappeared. In one of these patients, the diagnosis was dynamic subaortic stenosis. The ECG tracings before and after treatment are shown in FIGURE 2. The other patient had diabetes mellitus and was insulin resistant. Before administering the polarizing solution, the patient was desensitized. The ECG tracings before and after treatment are shown in FIGURE 3. FIGURES 4–14 show the ECG tracings of several cases with striking improvement after polarizing therapy.

Patients with Heart Failure

TABLE 2 presents the results obtained in 22 cases with different degrees of heart failure treated exclusively with polarizing solutions and a low sodium diet. No digitalis or diuretics were prescribed to these patients.

The degrees of heart failure were graded as follows: grade 1, exertional dyspnea and/or dyspnea at rest, tachycardia, gallop, and basal rales; grade 2, grade 1 symptoms plus jugular distention, hepatomegaly, and edema; grade 3, grades 1 and 2 symptoms plus ascites or hydrothorax or hydropericardium; grade 4, grades 1, 2, and 3 symptoms plus anasarca or electrolyte disturbances and/or acute pulmonary edema.

In 14 patients, the heart failure entirely disappeared on the therapeutic regimen. In two instances, marked improvement was obtained. Three cases showed some improvement (grade 1 of heart failure). In one case, the results were negative with the polarizing treatment, and two of the patients died.

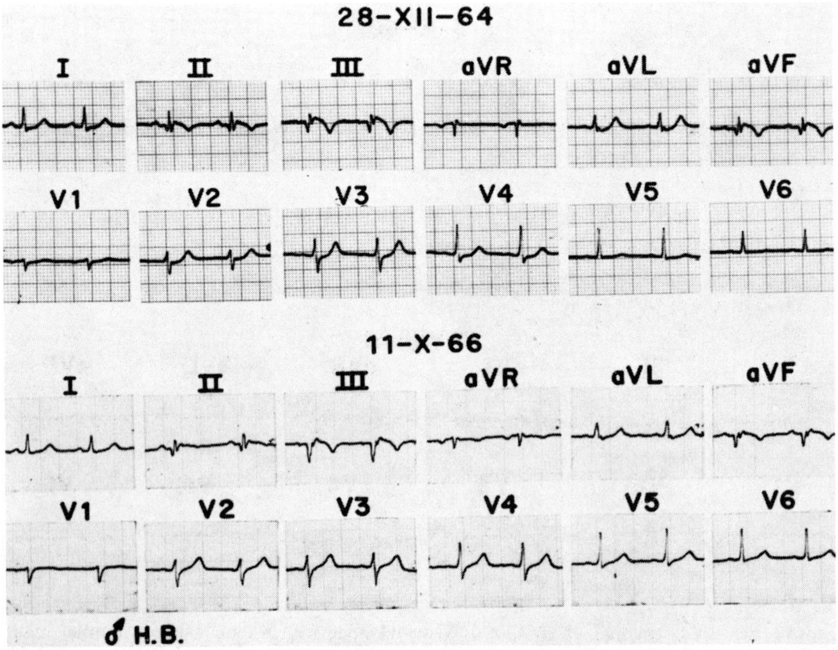

FIGURE 11. ECG tracings of H.B., a 64-year-old male with a diagnosis of posterior-inferior infarction with residual angina pectoris. With polarizing treatment, the pain disappeared, as did the anterolateral ischemia.

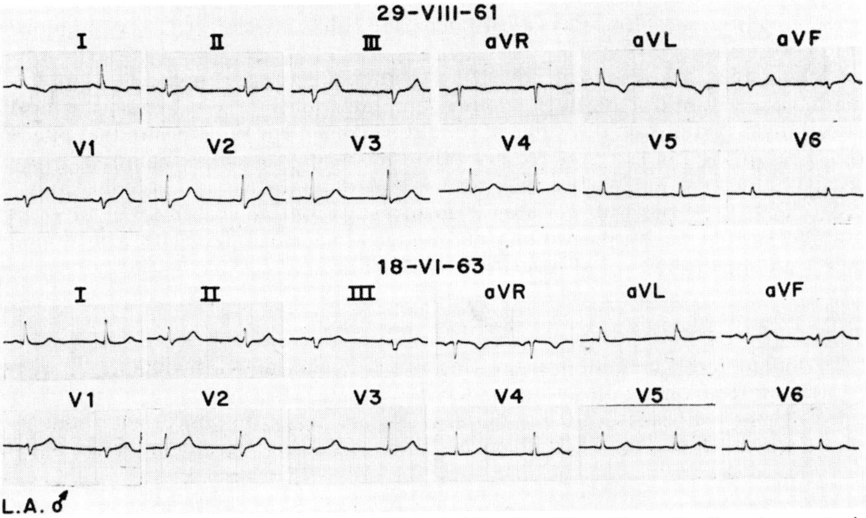

FIGURE 12. ECG tracings of L.A., a 56-year-old male with a diagnosis of angina pectoris for two years. After polarizing treatment, the pain disappeared in two weeks. Note that the negative T waves in leads I and aVI that were present in the first tracing disappeared in the last record.

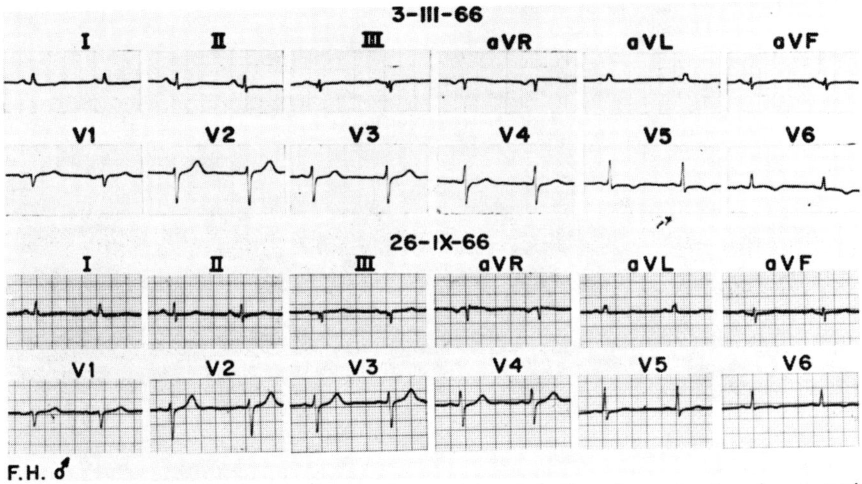

FIGURE 13. ECG tracings of F.H., a 59-year-old male with a diagnosis of angina pectoris for one year. The pain disappeared in two weeks with polarizing therapy. After six months, marked reduction of the anterolateral ischemia was obtained.

Cases 21 and 22 deserve special mention. Case 21 showed a marked electrolyte disturbance (Na, 109 mEq, and K, 6.3 mEq in the serum). The polarizing solution given without potassium was ineffective for four days; during the fifth day, however, diuresis increased to 10 l, with 5 l on the sixth day (marked negative water balance). The high diuresis corrected the electrolyte disturbance and the heart failure. Case 22 showed repeated attacks of pulmonary edema, and the patient improved only after digitalis and diuretics were withdrawn and the polarizing treatment alone (four days with polarizing solutions and diet) was administered.

In this paper, the results of polarizing treatment on recent myocardial infarction have not been discussed. Previous communications,[2,7,8,22,30] to date the most serious investigations on this subject, should be consulted. We are sure that polarizing therapy is far superior to any other medical procedure in most cardiovascular ailments, but we are well aware that it is not easy to convince other researchers. We believe that a long-term investigation on a large series of cases must be carried on by the leading cardiological societies, but with a profound understanding of the basis of polarizing treatment.

Conclusions

To conclude this communication, I believe it would be worthwhile to reiterate a statement from one of our recent papers.[4]

In revising our cardiovascular therapy, we are seriously concerned about its future possibilities. This has influenced our decision to search for better path-

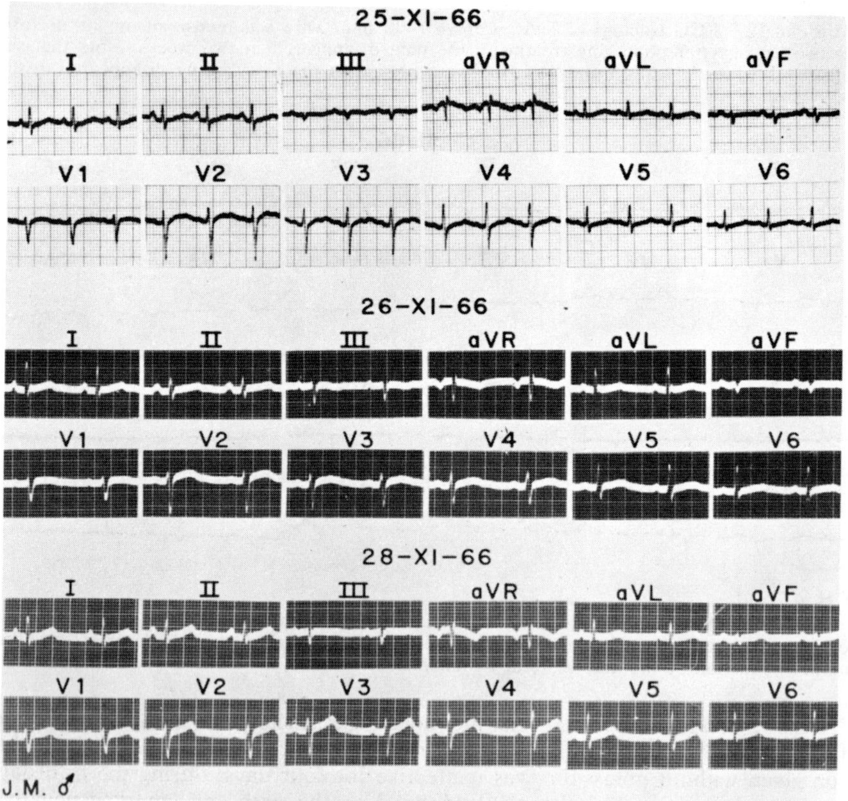

FIGURE 14. ECG tracings of J.M., a 36-year-old male with a diagnosis of angina pectoris for several months. The tracing became normal, and the pain entirely disappeared after three days of infusion of polarizing solution. (This case was not included in the groups discussed in the text.)

TABLE 2

RESULTS OBTAINED IN 22 PATIENTS WITH HEART FAILURE TREATED WITH POLARIZING SOLUTION AND LOW SODIUM DIET

Case No.	Age	Sex	Main Diagnosis	Degree of Heart Failure* Before Treatment	Degree of Heart Failure* After Treatment	Days on Polarizing Solution
1	53	M	Essential hypertension and coronary disease	2	0	15
2	31	M	Chronic cor pulmonale	2	0	9
3	65	M	Sclerotic heart disease	3	0	11
4	65	M	Syphilitic aortitis with aortic insufficiency	3	3	9 (The patient died)
5	10	F	Rheumatic heart disease	2	0	20
6	75	M	Sclerotic heart disease	3	0	8
7	44	M	Rheumatic heart disease and chronic cor pulmonale	2	0	8
8	68	M	Sclerotic heart disease	2	0	6
9	62	M	Sclerotic heart disease and chronic cor pulmonale	3	2	20
10	17	F	Rheumatic heart disease	2	2	20
11	62	F	Sclerotic heart disease and chronic cor pulmonale	3	0	16
12	51	M	Rheumatic heart disease	4	3	10
13	68	M	Chronic heart pulmonale	3	3	4 (The patient died)
14	70	F	Sclerotic heart disease and chronic cor pulmonale	3	2	9
15	51	M	Chronic cor pulmonale and essential hypertension	2	0	11
16	58	F	Rheumatic heart disease	2	0	8
17	65	M	Sclerotic heart disease	2	0	19
18	44	F	Rheumatic heart disease	3	1	20
19	83	M	Chronic cor pulmonale	3	1	10
20	55	F	Sclerotic heart disease and essential hypertension	2	0	15
21	54	F	Myocardial infarction and diabetes	4	0	8
22	75	F	Sclerotic heart disease and myocardial infarction	4	0	4

* Heart failure graded from 0 to 4.

ways with more satisfactory effects. As long as our knowledge fails to attain its ultimate goal, preventive medicine, we believe that therapy must be carried out according to three principles in addition to the classical ones:

1. Therapy must act at the cellular level. The logic of this point is based on current knowledge of electrophysiology, biochemistry, and pathology, has shown the fundamental importance of events occurring at the cellular level, i.e., the resting and action transmembrane potentials, the metabolic cycles of Embden-Meyerhof and Krebs, the ultrastructure, etc. The polarizing treatment proposed by our group takes some of these aspects into consideration.

2. Therapy must be Hippocratic, i.e., *primum non nocere,* or first do not harm. Unfortunately, most of our drugs such as the steroids, thiazides, antihypertensive agents, anticoagulants, fibrinolytics, and antiarrhythmics, have some harmful effects. On the other hand, cardiovascular therapy ought to be in accordance with natural laws, such as fixing the proper diet and imposing adequate hygienic measures. To recapitulate, we must avoid, as much as possible, cellular aggression which is often iatrogenic or derived from what we have named "the twentieth century disease," the consequence of improper living habits in our present era. We might add that the potent drugs used today in cardiology can easily produce this cellular iatrogenic effect.

3. Therapy, at least in its final result, must be antientropic.

References

1. Sodi-Pallares, D., B. L. Fishleder, F. Cisneros, M. Viscaíno, A. Bisteni, G. A. Medrano, B. Polansky & A. De Micheli. 1960. A low sodium, high water, high potassium regime in the successful management of some cardiovascular diseases. Canad. Med. Ass. J. **83:** 243.
2. Sodi-Pallares, D., A. Bisteni, G. A. Medrano, A. De Micheli, J. Ponce de León, E. Calva, B. L. Fishleder, M. R. Testelli & B. L. Miller. 1966. The polarizing treatment in cardiovascular conditions. Experimental basis and clinical applications. *In* Electrolytes and Cardiovascular Disease. E. Bajusz, Ed. **2:** 198–238. S. Karger. Basel, Switzerland.
3. Sodi-Pallares, D. & B. L. Miller. 1966. A therapeutic approach at cellular level in cardiovascular disorders. Geriatrics **21**(1): 107–116.
4. Sodi-Pallares, D., J. Ponce de León, F. Cisneros, A. Bisteni & G. A. Medrano 1966. Entropy and cardiology, Geriatrics **21**(12): 138–142.
5. Schimert, G., O. R. Hunt, M. Lillenstein & J. C. Brennan. 1966. Sodium potassium ratios in papillary muscle biopses obtained during mitral valve replacement. J. Thorac. Cardio. Surg. **52:** 126.
6. Sibilia, D. & M. Marino. 1966. La terapia polarizzante nelle miocarditi acute infantili. XXVI Congr. Soc. Ital. Cardiol. **1:** 21.
7. Day, H. W. 1965. Effectiveness of an intensive coronary care area. Amer. J. Cardiol. **15:** 51.
8. Mittra, B. 1965. Potassium, glucose and insulin in treatment of myocardial infarction. Lancet **ii:** 607.
9. Fabris, C. 1966. Contributo allo studio della terapia polarizzante nelle miocardiopatie anossiche. Cardiol. Prat. **17:** 75.
10. Fritz, E. 1965. Untersuchungen zur Behandlung des Miokardinfarktes mit Insulin-Glukose-Infusionen. Z. Kreislaufforsch. **54:** 2744.
11. Bobák, J., B. Navratil & Potysová. 1966. Lecba ischemické srdecni choroby polarizujici smesi glukozy s draslikem a inzulinem. Léceni **XII:** 156.
12. Chella, S., G. Dalli, E. Palla & P. Pucci. 1965. Modificazioni del quadro elettrocardiografico da sovraccarico ventricolare indotte dalla somministrazione di soluzione polarizzante. Therapeutikon **6:** 457.
13. Germer, W. D. 1965. Estudios sobre el tratamiento del infarto del miocardio con infusiones de glucosa-insulina. Versión Castellano Z. Kreislaufforsch. **68:** 5.
14. Barbieri, D. & M. Parravicini. 1964. Ulteriori osservazioni sul trattamento dell'infarto acuto del miocardio con infusione venosa di una soluzione polarizzante. Minerva Med. **55:** 1.
15. Girola, M., A. Vestri & M. Cerea. 1965. Tratamento dell'infarto del miocardio con le soluzioni polarizzanti di potasio, glucosio e insulina. Minerva Cardioangiol. **13:** 3.
16. Ratti, G. & G. P. Sanna. 1963. L'infarto del miocardio dal Punto di vista elettrico e ionico. Meccanismo d'azione ed effetti delle soluzioni polarizzanti. **35:** 345.
17. Köhler, J. A. 1966. The importance of recent biochemical-electrophysiological discoveries. Potassium ion and myocardium *"extra situ"* for clinical electrocardiography. *In* Electrolytes and Cardiovascular Diseases. E. Bajusz, Ed. **2:** 61–99. S. Karger, Basel, Switzerland.
18. Nieper, H. A. & K. Blumberger. 1966. Electrolyte transport therapy of cardiovascular diseases. Experimental and clinical basis. *In* Electrolytes and Cardiovascular Diseases. E. Bajusz, Ed. **2:** 141–173. S. Karger. Basel, Switzerland.

19. Losse, H., H. Wehmeyer & H. Zumkley. 1966. The behavior of the intracellular electrolytes in arterial hypertension. Investigations on erythrocytes. *In* Electrolytes and Cardiovascular Diseases. E. Bajusz, Ed. **2**: 174–197. S. Karger, Basel, Switzerland.
20. Friedman, S. M., R. H. Rosenman & S. C. Freed. 1959. Sodium gradient, smooth muscle tone and blood pressure regulation. Circ. Res. **7**: 44.
21. Laborit, H. 1966. New physiological concepts of cardiovascular functions. Therapeutic consequences. *In* Electrolytes and Cardiovascular Diseases. E. Bajusz, Ed. **2**: 239–259. S. Karger. Basel, Switzerland.
22. Máté, K., G. Birtalan, I. Horváth, V. Nemes, E. Löwey & E. Benedek. 1966. Clinical experiences in the application of electrolytes in cardiopathies. *In* Electrolytes and Cardiovascular Diseases. E. Bajusz, Ed. **2**: 260–276. S. Karger. Basel, Switzerland.
23. Larcan, A. 1966. Pathophysiological basis and practical application of a "metabolic" therapy of myocardial infarction. *In* Electrolytes and Cardiovascular Diseases. E. Bajusz, Ed. **2**: 277–301. S. Karger. Basel, Switzerland.
24. Day, H. W. & K. Averill. 1966. Recorded arrythmias in an acute coronary care area. Dis. Chest **49**: 113.
25. Kanther, R. 1966. Compensation of hypoxia in the human heart muscle by means of potassium-magnesium-aspartate. *In* Electrolytes and Cardiovascular Diseases. E. Bajusz, Ed. **2**: 324–328. S. Karger. Basel, Switzerland.
26. Pillen, D. 1966. Experiences with potassium-magnesium-aspartate therapy. *In* Electrolytes and Cardiovascular Diseases. E. Bajusz, Ed. **2**: 386–394. S. Karger. Basel, Switzerland.
27. Kenter, H. & A. Falkenhahn. 1966. Management of myocardial infarction with potassium-magnesium-aspartate. *In* Electrolytes and Cardiovascular Diseases. E. Bajusz, Ed. **2**: 420–429. S. Karger. Basel, Switzerland.
28. Bronzini, A. & G. Scotti. 1964. Effetti dell'infusione di glucosia, insulina e cloruro di potassio nell'evoluzione clinica ed elettrocardiografica dell'infarto del miocardio nel vecchio. Minerva Med. **55**: 1040.
29. Curcio, R. & S. Bonaventura. 1966. Onda T negativa gigante: Studio clinico-elettrocardiografico in quattro casi di cardiopatie ischemiche. Bol. Soc. Ital. Cardiol. **XI**: 309.
30. Gudbjarnason, S., J. C. Fenton, P. L. Wolf & R. J. Bing. 1966. Stimulation of reparative processes following experimental myocardial infarction. Arch. Intern. Med. (Chicago) **118**: 33.
31. Dixon, S., S. Hyde, R. P. Leonard & R. C. Schlant. 1965. Failure of glucose-insulin-potassium infusion to modify the consequences of acute coronary artery ligation. J. Thorac. Cardiov. Surg. **49**: 762.
32. Melloni, G. F., C. Baratta & R. Marangoni. 1964. Modificazioni elettrolotiche plasmatiche ed urinarie nell blocco atrioventricolare in corso di terapia "ripolarizzante" e cortisonica. XXV Congr. Soc. Ital. Cardiol., Roma, 1964. **1**: 97.
33. Salinas, P., F. Santucci & A. Colonna. 1965. Primi resultati della terapia dell'infarto cardiaco acuto con soluzione polarizzante glucosio-insulina-potassio. Bol. Soc. Ital. Cardiol. **10**: 230.

CONCLUDING REMARKS

Eörs Bajusz
Bio-Research Institute, Cambridge, Mass.

The contributors to this monograph have presented many new observations on fine-structural characteristics of heart muscle, on alterations that occur in the chemical workshop of cardiac cells, and even on experimentally induced and spontaneous cardiomyopathies previously nonexistent or unrecognized. Nevertheless, my concluding remarks were prepared with mixed emotions, for we are faced not only with new data and accomplishments demanding further analysis and clarification, but also with still unresolved problems from the past. Moreover, it appears to me that the increased interest in cardiomyopathies has compounded confusion in terminology, so that experimentalists, pathologists, and clinicians often find it difficult to understand one another. Therefore, it will probably prove more useful to omit a review of the specific data of the individual presentations and, rather, to outline my own views on the current status of some aspects of the study of heart-muscle disease.

Although our present knowledge, regrettably, permits no definite conclusions as to the pathogenesis of most experimentally induced cardiomyopathies, their relationship, if any, to spontaneous heart-muscle diseases in man and animals, or their interrelationships with one another, pertinent studies have produced a number of generally significant observations, on the one hand, and reemphasized our current difficulties, on the other. I believe that one of the most significant achievements of modern investigative cardiology is the demonstration that myocardial degeneration can be induced in laboratory animals, not only by direct interference with coronary circulation, but also by dietary means, administration of cardiotoxic chemicals, induction of hemodynamic alterations, exposure to emotional and physical stress, and many other techniques.

Since most of these cardiotoxic compounds and conditions, including dietary deficiencies, result in no significant morphological changes in the normal structure of coronary vessels, it is generally assumed that the necroses thus induced are the result of biochemical alterations that affect the metabolism of myocardial cells. However, if an attempt is made, on this basis, to distinguish between occlusive cardiac necrosis (i.e., myocardial infarct) and nonocclusive or metabolic cardiac necrosis (i.e., cardiomyopathy), several problems arise.

1. At the level of light microscopy, no clear pathological distinction, except for a subendocardial localization of many metabolic lesions, can be established between a primary heart-muscle degeneration and that resulting from coronary occlusion in autopsy materials.

2. Myocardial infarct, or ischemic necrosis, may develop not only as the secondary consequence of coronary artery occlusion, but through a variety of other mechanisms (e.g., increased oxygen requirement of cardiac muscle cells and other discrepancies between oxygen supply and need).

3. In the pathogenesis of a number of cardiomyopathies, several etiological factors apparently act simultaneously; they may affect either the metabolic component alone, the vascular component alone, or both, and they may act individually or in combination.

For example, it was postulated that isoproterenol-induced myocardial degeneration stems from a relative ischemia caused by the combination of a metabolic and a vascular factor, increased myocardial oxygen requirement and decreased coronary blood flow. Until the precise role and importance of these two factors have been established, objections cannot be raised, at least theoretically, when the cardiac lesion normally elicited by isoproterenol is designated as either "cardiomyopathy" or "myocardial infarct." Unfortunately, but inevitably, the terms under discussion themselves embody the uncertainties we are trying to resolve.

The lack of criteria for the morphological differentiation between a primarily degenerative and a primarily inflammatory process constitutes another great obstacle to progress. A disease that is purely degenerative at its inception may, in a matter of a few days, assume the appearance of an inflammatory disease due to the occurrence of natural reparative processes; conversely, myocarditis (true inflammation) may eventually result in muscle fiber degeneration. As we have seen, there is a characteristic morphological finding of myolysis, or myofibrillar degeneration, in a number of experimental and spontaneous cardiomyopathies. This distinct form of heart-muscle pathology is usually, although not consistently, accompanied by interstitial mononuclear cell proliferation, but by little, if any, polymorphonuclear cell invasion. Even such a primarily degenerative lesion was repeatedly designated as myocarditis in this monograph, as it is done customarily by pathologists elsewhere. It is, of course, very misleading to diagnose an inflammation secondary to myocardial degeneration as myocarditis; this term implies an infectious process to the clinician.

In spite of such difficulties, the studies using disease models revealed that most, if not all, cardiotoxic agents and conditions are potential pathogens, and their adverse effects upon the heart muscle depend on other (sensitizing or desensitizing) factors. Thus, when the mechanisms governing the resistance vs. susceptibility of heart muscle to diseases rather than the mechanisms of action of pathogens are analyzed, new avenues for possible prevention and treatment appear. However, before dealing with the cardiomyopathy problem from this novel point of view, let me explain the achievements of ultrastructural research.

Since, at the light microscopical level, the heart muscle reacts, with minor variations, in a manner essentially identical to many diverse types of injury, the illusion was cherished that the use of electron microscopy would help or even solve the causation of cardiomyopathies. This hope has not been fulfilled as yet. It seems that various metabolic and physicochemical disturbances may induce quite dissimilar fine-structural alterations in the affected myocardial cell; conversely, however, disparate pathogenic agents may damage the intracellular organelles in similar fashion, suggesting certain common pathways of cellular injury. Thus, although cellular necrosis may evolve along different pathways from an ultrastructural point of view, there is little specificity in the changes elicited by a given injurious agent. Unfortunately, therefore, even at the ultrastructural level, the morphological appearance of the heart-muscle lesion is of little value, if any, regarding differential diagnosis, mainly because it depends largely on the time of detection (i.e., duration of survival from onset of myocardial injury) and also on many other, often uncontrollable, factors.

For example, we have seen that ischemia causes at least two kinds of necrobiosis. In the center of the ischemic area, the edematous cardiac muscle cells gradually undergo cytolysis, whereas at the periphery of the affected region, the morphological changes begin with a contraction of portions of the myofibrils and terminate in coagulation necrosis. These and cognate observations indicate that the quality of structural damage depends not only on the nature of the eliciting agent, but also on the modifying influence of local and systemic factors. It has been classically shown in this monograph that the structural and chemical manifestations of cell death are greatly accelerated in states of transient ischemia, suggesting that diminished blood flow and impaired diffusion contribute to the delayed development of overt necrosis in an area of permanent ischemia.

We must search further to find a convergence upon some hidden step in myocardial metabolism, if, in fact, one exists. The divergence of ultrastructural abnormalities hitherto disclosed does not exclude the possibility that, at some as yet only imagined level of sophistication, all examples of myocardial degeneration have a common origin.

It seems important to recognize that in every situation thus far reported, except in potassium deficiency, the mitochondria were structurally severed; the sarcoplasmic reticulum was also easily damaged by numerous stimuli. In fact, an evaluation of the available data in functional terms, and within our present conceptual restraints, suggests that the most sensitive part of the cardiac-muscle cell to injury probably is the electrolyte-dependent system of the sarcoplasmic reticulum, followed by the organizer, or nucleus, and the intracellular nutrition and energy mechanism-conducting organelle, the mitochondrion, in that order. The contractile element, or myofilament, has proved to be one of the most resistant components in many types of myocardial injury. It has been suggested that, under favorable conditions, the structural alterations of the sarcoplasmic reticulum represent reversible changes, whereas there seems to be little doubt that mitochondrial failure plays an important role in causing the muscle cell to enter a stage of irreversible injury.

Unfortunately, structural components of the heart other than muscle cells and coronary vessels have received little attention as yet. Hence, I was drawn by the interesting hypothesis that certain agents and pathogenic constellations would be cardiotoxic merely because they act on the "transit-zone" between the myocardial capillary lumen and the muscle fibers, causing permeability changes and thus impeding the transport of metabolites into the muscle cells.

Ultrastructural research, especially when combined with histochemical and cytochemical techniques, may be expected to open new avenues to explore the complex problems of cardiomyopathies. Nevertheless, the mere fact that examining electron micrographs can initiate new ideas should by no means be taken as proof that these ideas are correct. Although the nonspecialist is understandably prone to accept micrographs as being sufficiently obvious and concrete – and thus proof positive of the validity of any speculation – the specialist must be more selective, and frequently pose fundamental questions: What are artifacts? What are the reliable equivalents of living matter? Do fixatives alter structural patterns in intact and injured cells in an identical manner? Are images that merely appear beautiful to us also true?

The possibility that early discernible ultrastructural changes such as enlargement and vacuolization of the sarcoplasmic reticulum and swelling and degeneration of mitochondria are already associated with significant shifts in myocardial electrolyte concentrations deserves further analysis. In any event, several additional experimental and clinical observations suggest that present-day concepts concerning the role of electrolytes in the genesis of heart-muscle disease require a basic reevaluation. The earlier belief that ion alterations such as a loss of potassium and magnesium from the myocardial cells and the uptake of extra sodium and calcium are merely secondary consequences of cellular necrosis can no longer be held. Distortions of intracellular electrolyte gradients seem to be important components of many, if not all, types of disturbance in cardiac metabolism resulting in fatal conduction defects, myocardial degeneration, or heart failure.

Proof of the essential role of potassium and magnesium ions in the maintenance of functional and structural integrity of the heart muscle can be found in experiments in which diets deficient in one or both of these minerals were fed to laboratory animals. Potassium and/or magnesium deficiency was shown to cause severe disturbances in cardiac function, degeneration of myocardial fibers, and cardiac death. Although there is now little doubt that the cardiovascular effects of potassium and magnesium deficiencies in animals are mirrored in humans, scant attention is still being paid to the large numbers of experimental studies indicating that even a transient decrease in myocardial potassium and magnesium concentration is important, because it greatly sensitizes the heart muscle to the necrotizing effect of the most diverse cardiotoxic influences; conversely, a dietary excess of potassium and/or magnesium protects the heart against the induction of functional and structural abnormalities. Although the question of how these electrolytes exert their protective action is still unsettled, recent observations are compatible with the hypothesis that either an alteration in the ion permeability of the cell membrane or an interference with the function of active transport systems for electrolytes, including the so-called sodium pump mechanism, constitutes an early (prenecrotic) phase of myocardial injury, under which conditions the electrolyte levels in the blood are of immediate importance to the severed muscle cells.

It is reasonable to suggest, on the basis of experimental findings, that the ability of one individual to successfully resist potentially cardiotoxic episodes and the susceptibility of another to develop fatal degenerative changes in the heart muscle are largely dependent on the ionic balance of the myocardium. Nevertheless, it is impossible to explain the pathogenesis of necrotizing cardiomyopathies by the oversimplified theory that various sensitizing factors predispose the heart muscle to hypokalemia and/or hypomagnesemia, and that the structural alterations precipitated by different means are merely the results of aggravated potassium and magnesium deficiencies. It is more likely that, in addition to potassium and magnesium, several other cations and anions interplay with hormonal and neuroendocrine effects in the mechanism governing the resistance vs. disease susceptibility of the heart muscle. It appears that electrolytes play a conditioning (sensitizing and desensitizing) rather than a causative role in the development of myocardial degeneration. In any event, the fact remains that, by giving large amounts of potassium and magnesium to laboratory animals, protection can be obtained against otherwise lethal cardiotoxic influences.

Although great caution must always be applied in extrapolating findings from animals to man, clinical observations are already available on the therapeutic and prophylactic effectiveness of potassium and magnesium in relation to cardiac morbidity and mortality. For my part, although I cannot yet fully accept verything that recently has been claimed concerning the metabolic and clinical effects of electrolytes, I feel that the long-range prevention of ischemic heart disease and other types of cardiomyopathies by prolonged administration of potassium and magnesium salts is a promising possibility worthy of investigation.

It should be kept in mind by clinical investigators that it may be misleading to speak in terms of daily electrolyte requirements, since we do not know what factors govern these requirements. Experimental stiudies have clearly shown, for instance, that the cardiovascular effects of both potassium deficiency and potassium excess depend, among other factors, on the amount of sodium and magnesium ingested. Furthermore, dietary intake and cellular nutrition should not be intermixed, since cellular deficiency may occur even when the dietary supply is adequate. Under the influence of potentially cardiotoxic episodes, the nutritional requirement of cardiac-muscle cells increases insofar as the need for certain cations (potassium and magnesium ions) is concerned, and the customary dietary intake may be insufficient to satisfy this increased demand.

In the field of cardiomyopathies, the terminal long-term problem is often congestive heart failure, a condition responsible for the high degree of morbidity and mortality in our population. Although we know that a number of anatomical and biochemical abnormalities may accompany cardiac failure, a distinction between aberrations that cause cardiac insufficiency and those that result from it is a constant challenge. There is little doubt that potassium depletion is already present in the majority of patients with chronic heart disease who have not been in congestive failure. During the development of myocardial insufficiency, changes do take place in the characteristics of cell membranes and also in the amount of intracellular ionic and organic constituents but there is as yet no direct evidence that these changes alone cause cell malfunction in heart failure. Much more work remains to be done, and, if further advances are to be made, they will be due to the continued cooperation among disciplines.

At this point I would like to emphasize that it seems essential to conduct our experiments under conditions kept as close to the physiological as possible, with no disrespect for the "anesthetized and isolate" methods employed so often in the past. Despite the important contributions made by analytical techniques (such as biochemical determinations requiring cell destruction, or sensitive electric measurements that demand rupture of the cell membrane), is it occasionally necessary to use investigative methods that result in no significant change in the physiological state of the cell or organ and in the response of the cardiovascular system as a unit. Modern instrumentation makes it possible to obtain electrocardiogram recordings or to measure cardiac output and arterial blood flow continuously in unanesthetized and freely moving animals. I predict that we will be impressed by the difference between the results obtained with these methods and those achieved through our former investigative techniques.

Analysis of the pathogenesis of any disease obviously necessitates the use of disease models in laboratory animals. Spontaneous diseases similar to, or identical to, human diseases would seem to be the most appropriate to study the fundamental aspects of pathological processes. For example, the existence in an inbred strain of hamsters of a genetically transmitted or conditioned cardiomyopathy that advances to congestive heart failure opens new avenues to the study of the sequence of events leading to cardiac insufficiency and the importance of extracardiac factors in the genesis of generalized venous congestion.

In the pathogenesis of cardiomyopathies, genetic factors probably influence the susceptibility to environmental agents that, in turn, accelerate or induce cardiac abnormalities. However, we are presently confused by the difficulty in separating and delineating genetic from environmental influences. We should interest more geneticists in the problems of cardiomyopathies; they will probably be concerned with the inheritance of disease susceptibility rather than with the inheritance of genetic diseases of the heart muscle, and they will enter areas in which the inheritance is apt to be very complex and lies outside the realm of simple Mendelian analysis. I believe that detailed investigations of the interactions between genetic and environmental factors should begin in the laboratory where the experimentalist has at his command mating systems, environments, adjustable dosage of pathogenic agents, and arrangements for varied host-pathogen interactions, i.e., the whole panoply of factors that are now recognized as important in the multicausal genesis of cardiopathies.

Anatomically, the heart muscle is an extremely complex structure, with an enormous range of biological problems. Nevertheless, I forsee the evolution of new concepts that will account for all the known facts on cardiomyopathies and resolve our seemingly unanswerable difficulties. Perhaps one of the contributors to this monograph will succeed in bridging the gap between the many scattered experimental observations, clinical findings, analytical data, and synthetic theories. I can wish you no less.

Printed in the United States of America